Bionanotechnology

About the Authors

Jie Chen, Ph.D., is a professor in the Faculty of Engineering at the University of Alberta in Edmonton, Alberta, Canada. He is a fellow of the Canadian Academy of Engineering, of the American Institute for Medical and Biological Engineering (AIMBE), and of the Institute of Electrical and Electronics Engineers (IEEE). He was presented with the Distinguished Alumni Award by the University of Maryland in College Park, Maryland, USA, from which he received his Ph.D. in electrical and computer engineering. His cross-disciplinary research explores new nanoscale device and circuit designs as well as nanotechnology for biomedical applications.

Yiwei Feng, B.S., is a Ph.D. student in Dr. Jie Chen's research group at the University of Alberta in Edmonton, Alberta, Canada. He holds a B.S. in engineering physics from the University of Alberta and has won many awards, including the APEGA Past Presidents' Medal and the Dean's Citation in Engineering. His research focuses on the design and development of microfluidic and lab-on-a-chip devices.

Scott MacKay, Ph.D., is a post-doctoral researcher in biological science at the University of Alberta in Edmonton, Alberta, Canada. He has a Ph.D. in electrical engineering (supervised by Dr. Jie Chen) and an undergraduate degree in engineering physics, both from the University of Alberta. His research interests include metabolomics, biosensor design, and converting laboratory methods and techniques to portable and automated systems.

Bionanotechnology

Engineering Concepts and Applications

JIE CHEN

YIWEI FENG

SCOTT MACKAY

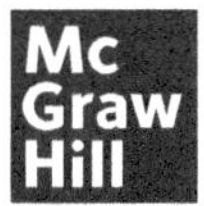

New York   Chicago   San Francisco
Athens   London   Madrid
Mexico City   Milan   New Delhi
Singapore   Sydney   Toronto

Library of Congress Cataloging-in-Publication Data

Names: Chen, Jie (Of University of Alberta), author. | Feng, Yiwei, author.
   | MacKay, Scott (Scott A.), author.
Title: Bionanotechnology : engineering concepts and applications / Jie Chen,
   Yiwei Feng, Scott MacKay.
Description: New York : McGraw Hill, 2022. | Includes bibliographical
   references and index.
Identifiers: LCCN 2021060515 | ISBN 9781260464146 (hardcover) |
   ISBN 9781260464153 (ebook)
Subjects: MESH: Nanotechnology | Bioengineering
Classification: LCC R857.N34 | NLM QT 36.5 | DDC 610.28—dc23/eng/20220106
LC record available at https://lccn.loc.gov/2021060515

McGraw Hill books are available at special quantity discounts to use as premiums and sales promotions or for use in corporate training programs. To contact a representative, please visit the Contact Us page at www.mhprofessional.com.

Bionanotechnology: Engineering Concepts and Applications

1 2 3 4 5 6 7 8 9 CCD 27 26 25 24 23 22

ISBN   978-1-260-46414-6
MHID   1-260-46414-8

This book is printed on acid-free paper.

Sponsoring Editor Robin Najar	**Copy Editor** Yashoda Rawat, MPS Limited
Editing Supervisor Stephen M. Smith	**Proofreader** Lakshmi Venky, MPS Limited
Production Supervisor Pamela A. Pelton	**Indexer** Michael Ferreira
Acquisitions Coordinator Elizabeth M. Houde	**Art Director, Cover** Jeff Weeks
Project Manager Anamika Singh, MPS Limited	**Composition** MPS Limited

Contents

Preface   ix
Acknowledgments   xi

CHAPTER 1

Introduction   1

1.1   Nanomaterials   2
1.2   Microfluidics   4
1.3   DNA and RNA Technology   5
1.4   Lab-on-a-Chip Devices   6
1.5   Outline of the Book   8
1.6   References   8

CHAPTER 2

Microfluidics I: Forces, Thermodynamics, and Fluid Flow   11

2.1   Introduction   11
2.2   Forces   13
    2.2.1   Fundamental Forces   13
    2.2.2   Gravity   14
    2.2.3   Dipole-Dipole Forces   15
    2.2.4   Capillary Forces   16
2.3   Thermodynamics   19
    2.3.1   Derivatives in Cylindrical Coordinates   20
    2.3.2   The Heat Equation   22
    2.3.3   Joule Heating in a Cylindrical Capillary   23
2.4   Mechanical Forces   24
    2.4.1   Reynolds Number   24
    2.4.2   Newton's Law of Viscosity   25
2.5   Pressure-Driven Flow (PDF)   25
2.6   Electro-Osmotic Flow (EOF)   28
    2.6.1   Debye Length   29
    2.6.2   Electro-Osmotic Flow (EOF) Equation   34
    2.6.3   Zeta Potential   36
2.7   Problems   38
2.8   References   44

CHAPTER 3

Microfluidics II: Fluid Transport and Applications   47

3.1   Diffusion   47
3.2   Electrophoretic Flow (EPF)   49
3.3   Dielectrophoretic (DEP) Force   53
    3.3.1   Theory of Dielectrophoresis (DEP)   54
    3.3.2   Electrical Properties of Microtubules   64
3.4   Comparison of Fluid Transport Methods   66
3.5   Applications   67
    3.5.1   Separation by Diffusion   67
    3.5.2   Cell Capture and Separation by Dielectrophoresis (DEP)   68
    3.5.3   Isoelectric Point (pI)   76
    3.5.4   Gel Electrophoresis   78
3.6   Problems   80
3.7   References   89

CHAPTER 4

Optical Detection and Quantum Dots   91

4.1   Introduction to Optics   91
4.2   Optical Detection and Fluorescence   94
4.3   Quantum Dots   100
    4.3.1   Theory of Quantum Dot Fluorescence   100
    4.3.2   Structure of Quantum Dots   106
    4.3.3   Properties of Quantum Dots   107
    4.3.4   Applications and Challenges of Quantum Dots   109
4.4   Problems   112
4.5   References   116

CHAPTER 5

DNA and RNA Bionanotechnology   117

5.1   Introduction to DNA and RNA   117
    5.1.1   DNA: An Overview   119
    5.1.2   RNA: An Introduction   123
    5.1.3   DNA Dissociation   124
5.2   Polymerase Chain Reaction (PCR)   127
    5.2.1   Polymerase Chain Reaction (PCR) Procedure   128
    5.2.2   Modeling the Polymerase Chain Reaction (PCR)   130
    5.2.3   Primer Selection with GenBank and BLAST   131
    5.2.4   Reverse Transcription–Polymerase Chain Reaction (RT-PCR)   135
5.3   Detection of DNA Mutations   137
    5.3.1   Heteroduplex Analysis (HA)   137
    5.3.2   Single-Strand Conformation Polymorphism (SSCP)   138
5.4   DNA Sequencing   138
    5.4.1   Sanger DNA Sequencing   138
    5.4.2   Maxam-Gilbert DNA Sequencing   142
    5.4.3   Second and Third Generation DNA Sequencing   145
5.5   RNA Sequencing and Synthesis   146

5.6   DNA Self-Assembly   148
5.7   DNA Tweezers   151
5.8   CRISPR Gene Editing   153
        5.8.1   CRISPR-Cas Systems   153
        5.8.2   CRISPR-Cas9 Procedure   154
        5.8.3   Applications and Challenges of CRISPR Gene Editing   155
5.9   Problems   156
5.10   References   160

CHAPTER 6

Lab-on-a-Chip Bionanotechnology and Micro/Nano Fabrication   163

6.1   Overview of Lab-on-a-Chip Devices   163
        6.1.1   Introduction to Lab-on-a-Chip Devices   163
        6.1.2   The Market for Lab-on-a-Chip Devices   165
6.2   Lab-on-a-Chip Biosensors   165
        6.2.1   Design of Lab-on-a-Chip Biosensors   165
        6.2.2   Lateral Flow Lab-on-a-Chip Biosensors   168
        6.2.3   Non-Faradaic Impedimetric Lab-on-a-Chip Biosensors   171
        6.2.4   Breakthroughs and Challenges of Lab-on-a-Chip Biosensors   174
6.3   Organ-on-a-Chip Devices   176
        6.3.1   Introduction to Organ-on-a-Chip Devices   176
        6.3.2   Working Principles of Organ-on-a-Chip Devices   178
        6.3.3   Applications of Organ-on-a-Chip Devices   180
        6.3.4   Breakthroughs and Challenges of Organ-on-a-Chip Technology   182
6.4   Micro/Nano Fabrication Techniques   185
        6.4.1   Substrates and Overview of Micro/Nano Fabrication   185
        6.4.2   Thin Film Deposition and Growth   187
        6.4.3   Pattern Transfer   194
        6.4.4   Surface Treatments, Modification, and Planarization   222
6.5   Micro/Nano Fabrication of Microfluidic and Lab-on-a-Chip Devices   226
        6.5.1   Fabricating Interdigitated Electrode Biosensor Microchips   226
        6.5.2   Fabricating Microfluidic Platforms   229
        6.5.3   Fabricating CMOS Lab-on-a-Chip Devices   241
6.6   References   247

CHAPTER 7

Applications of Bionanotechnology   251

7.1   Equivalent Circuit Models for Mechanical, Fluidic, and Thermal Systems   251
        7.1.1   Equivalent Parameters   251
        7.1.2   Equivalent Circuit Components   256
        7.1.3   Applying Equivalent Circuits for Modeling Microsystems   259
7.2   Polymerase Chain Reaction Microreactors   269
        7.2.1   Batch PCR Microreactors   270
        7.2.2   Continuous-Flow PCR Microreactors   283
        7.2.3   Comparison of Batch and Continuous-Flow PCR Microreactors   286
7.3   Diabetic Glucose Monitoring with Bionanotechnology   287
        7.3.1   Fluorescence-Based Minimally Invasive Glucose Monitoring   288
        7.3.2   Reverse Iontophoresis-Based Non-Invasive Glucose Monitoring   290
7.4   Bacteriophage Therapy   292
        7.4.1   Bacteriophage Therapy Procedure   292
        7.4.2   Applications of Bacteriophage Therapy   293
7.5   Biomedical Applications of Nanoparticles   295
7.6   Targeted Cancer Therapies and Drug Delivery Systems   296
        7.6.1   Nanoparticle-Mediated Thermal Cancer Therapy   297
        7.6.2   Targeted Cancer Treatment with Carbon Nanotubes   302
        7.6.3   Ultrasound-Aided Phase-Shift Nanodroplets for Cancer Drug Delivery   304
        7.6.4   Applications of DNA Nanotechnology in Targeted Cancer Treatment   306
7.7   Mitochondria-Targeted Delivery of 2,4-Dinitrophenol by Nanoparticles   307
7.8   Neural Implants and Brain–Machine Interfaces   309
7.9   Applications of Bionanotechnology in Crop Agriculture   312
7.10   References   314

CHAPTER 8

Computer Simulations with COMSOL Multiphysics® Software   319

8.1   Lab #1: 2D Simulation of Interdigitated Electrodes   319
        8.1.1   COMSOL Multiphysics® Software Tutorial #1   319
        8.1.2   Lab Assignment #1   328
8.2   Lab #2: 3D Simulation of Interdigitated Electrodes   330
        8.2.1   COMSOL Multiphysics® Software Tutorial #2   330
        8.2.2   Lab Assignment #2   334
8.3   Lab #3: Tracing Dielectrophoretic Particle Motion   336

8.3.1   COMSOL Multiphysics® Software
            Tutorial #3   336
8.3.2   Lab Assignment #3   341

APPENDIX A
Abbreviations   345

APPENDIX B
Units in SI (International System of Units)   349

APPENDIX C
Fundamental Physical Constants   351

APPENDIX D
Sign Convention for Fluid Flow   353

APPENDIX E
Coordinate Systems   355

APPENDIX F
Complex Numbers   357

Index   359

Preface

Bionanotechnology is an emerging field which utilizes the tools of nanotechnology to solve problems in biomedicine and biology. The application of bionanotechnology has enabled revolutionary improvements in a wide range of sectors ranging from healthcare to environmental science and agriculture. Examples include the development of portable medical diagnostic tools and biosensors such as microfluidic and lab-on-a-chip devices, targeted therapies and drug delivery systems for treating cancer and other diseases, high-through-put devices for rapid drug discovery and screening, miniature environmental and food monitoring systems, and nanomaterials for biomedical imaging enhancement. The range of applications of bionanotechnology is rapidly growing. Some novel applications that have emerged include cell capture and sorting, personalized cancer treatments, improved DNA and RNA sequencing, DNA amplification in microreactors, gene delivery, neural implants, and targeted nanomaterial-based fertilizers/pesticides.

Bionanotechnology is a multidisciplinary subject. In this book, we integrate a variety of disciplines that are involved in bionanotechnology and present them in a cohesive way so that senior undergraduate engineering students, graduate students, and readers who are interested in bionanotechnology can understand this multidisciplinary subject. These disciplines include materials science, micro/nano fabrication, general physics, fluid flow, electromagnetics, thermodynamics, molecular biology, immunology, biochemistry, and organic chemistry. This book contains complete discussions on microfluidics, lab-on-a-chip systems, quantum dots, DNA/RNA biotechnology, micro/nano fabrication techniques, the modeling/simulation of microsystems, and bionanotechnology-based biosensors, targeted therapies, and drug delivery systems.

Bionanotechnology: Engineering Concepts and Applications presents bionanotechnology from an engineering perspective. The purpose of this book is to correlate the theories and concepts of bionanotechnology with practical applications. Thus, fully solved examples along with problem sets, real-world case studies, and engineering design methodologies are provided throughout this book. Also, for instructors of classes using this book as a text, a solution manual for the problem sets is available at www.mhprofessional.com/ Bionanotechnology.

Jie Chen
Yiwei Feng
Scott MacKay

Acknowledgments

xi

We gratefully acknowledge the contributions of many people to the completion of this book. We thank (listed in alphabetical order by last name) Carter Behm, Ryan Brooks, Fraser Bulbuc, Xianglou Chen, Alex Deans, Nikhil Deshpande, Haley Dittmann, Ryan Fang, Pablo Gonzalez-Vasquez, Emily Gruber, Tianxiang Jiang, Jacob Johnsen, Liam McRae, Tamara Micevic, Ryan Moro, Sahil Patel, Kim Qiu, Jori Romans, Matthew Thiessen, and Songhui Zhang for their contributions to this book. Particular thanks go to Riley Stuermer for his contribution to the section about dielectrophoresis. We would also like to thank (in alphabetical order) Fraser Bulbuc, Xinyue Chen, Gareth Davies, Haley Dittmann, Ryan Fang, Shyama Gandhi, Pablo Gonzalez-Vasquez, Lukas Menze, Kaustubh Sinha, Zuyuan Tian, Meng Xiao, Xuanjie Ye, and Songhui Zhang for contributing to some of the examples and problems found throughout the book. We thank Zuyuan Tian for helping to obtain permissions for figure reprints. Finally, our sincere thanks go to Senior Acquisitions Editor Robin Najar and the production team at McGraw Hill for helping us with the publishing of this book.

Bionanotechnology

CHAPTER 1

Introduction

The combination of biology and engineering has a history spanning many centuries. In the 13th century, invisible substances were postulated by Roger Bacon to be responsible for the decay of food and the cause of diseases. The hypothesis was not confirmed until microbes were discovered by Antony van Leeuwenhoek in the 17th century following the invention of the optical microscope.[1] Microscopes are among the fundamental tools for microbiology—the study of bacteria, fungi, algae, protozoa, and viruses. In the 20th century, the combination of biology and engineering has created a number of key non-invasive medical imaging technologies such as computerized tomography (CT), positron emission tomography (PET), and magnetic resonance imaging (MRI).

In 1959, the concept of nanotechnology was first introduced by the famous theoretical quantum physicist and Nobel Prize laureate Richard Feynman.[2] Since then, nanotechnology has gained many new and important applications in a number of fields ranging from biomedicine to microelectronics. The newly developed engineering field of nanotechnology aims to create nanomaterials with features ranging from 1 nm to 100 nm in size (Figure 1-1).

The combination of biology and nanotechnology created the field of bionanotechnology, also known as nanobiotechnology. Bionanotechnology is the application of nanotechnology to solve biological and medical problems. As such, bionanotechnology is a highly interdisciplinary field lying at the intersection of nanoscale engineering, nanomaterials technology, biomedical engineering, molecular biology, and applied physics.

Some of the most common applications of bionanotechnology (Figure 1-2) include portable biosensors (e.g., microfluidic and lab-on-a-chip devices) for detecting and quantifying microorganisms or biomolecules, targeted drug delivery and targeted therapies with bionanomaterials (e.g., for curing cancer and antibiotic-resistant bacterial infections), environmental and food monitoring with nano-biosensors, enhanced cell and tissue imaging

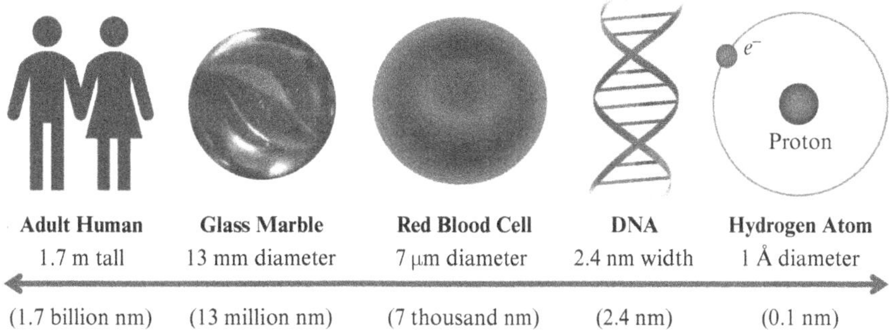

Figure 1-1   Nanotechnology aims to create nanomaterials ranging from 1 nm to 100 nm in size.

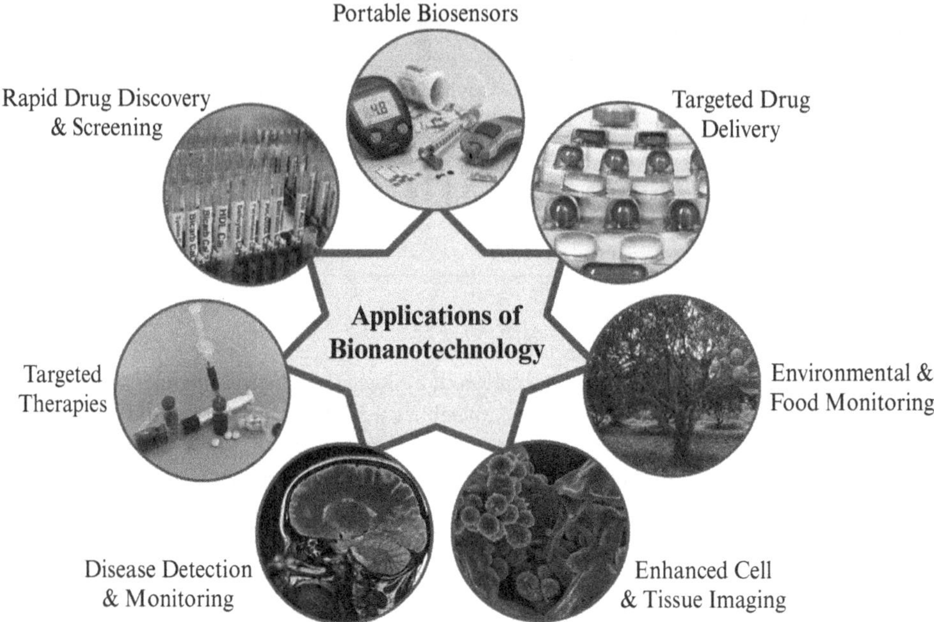

Figure 1-2   Some of the most common applications of bionanotechnology.

(e.g., quantum dots for biological labeling), disease detection and monitoring (e.g., continuous glucose monitoring for diabetes), as well as rapid drug discovery and screening (e.g., with organ-on-a-chip devices or array-type microchips).[3-10]

As an emerging technology, the research and application scope of bionanotechnology is rapidly spreading. More recent applications of bionanotechnology include—but are not limited to—cell capture and sorting, personalized cancer treatments, improved DNA and RNA sequencing, DNA amplification in microreactors, gene delivery, neural implants, and targeted nanomaterial-based pesticides.[11-16]

1.1 NANOMATERIALS

The basic building blocks of nanomaterials include graphene, carbon nanotubes, nanoparticles, semiconductor nanowires, and quantum dots. In addition, composite (i.e., hybrid) nanomaterials formed from a combination of these basic building blocks are also commonly used.

- *Graphene:* Graphene (Figure 1-3a) is a versatile two-dimensional material whose strength is about five times that of the strongest steel (the Young's modulus is $\sim 10^{12}$ Pa for graphene and $\sim 2 \times 10^{11}$ Pa for steel), even though the density of graphene (~ 2.27 g/cm^3) is significantly lower than the density of steel (~ 8.05 g/cm^3).[17,18] Graphene can conduct heat and electricity without much loss. Interesting and useful phenomena, such as the bipolar transistor effect and ballistic transport of charges, can be observed in graphene.[19]

- *Carbon Nanotubes:* Carbon nanotubes (CNTs) are cylindrical tubes of carbon formed by a catalytic growth process. A nanometer-scale drop of molten iron is a common catalyst. CNTs can behave either like a conductive metal wire or like

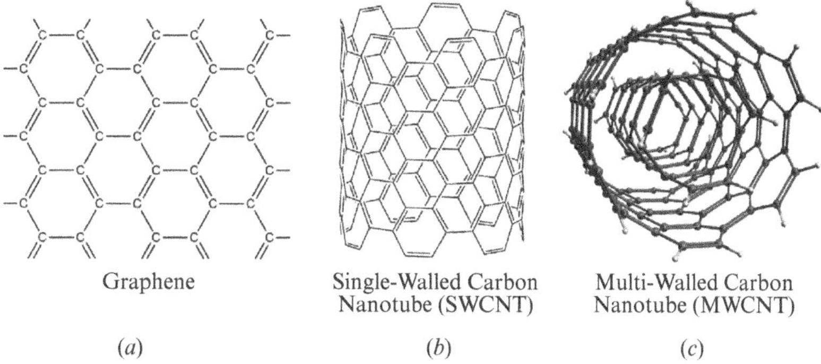

Figure 1-3   The structure of (a) graphene, (b) a single-walled carbon nanotube (SWCNT), and (c) a multi-walled carbon nanotube (MWCNT).

a semiconductor. There are two types of CNTs: single-walled carbon nanotubes (SWCNTs) and multi-walled carbon nanotubes (MWCNTs). A SWCNT is a sheet of graphene rolled up as a cylindrical tube (Figure 1-3b), while a MWCNT (Figure 1-3c) is formed by multiple layers of graphene sheets wrapped on each other in a concentric cylindrical shape. The size of SWCNTs is within the range of 0.6 to 1.8 nm in diameter and 3 to 30 μm in length. The 3D structure formed by many SWCNTs has a density of 1.33 to 1.40 g/cm^3. SWCNTs have a tensile strength of 45 billion Pa, which is over 20 times higher than that of high-strength steel alloys (~2 billion Pa). SWCNTs can be bent at large angles and re-straightened without damage. SWCNTs can carry a current density of 1 billion A/cm^2, or three orders of magnitude higher than copper wires which can carry a maximum current density of about 1 million A/cm^2. These superb mechanical and electrical properties along with high surface area enable the potential application of CNTs in biosensing, bioimaging, photothermal therapy, tissue engineering, drug/gene delivery, and lab-on-a-chip devices.[20-22]

- *Nanoparticles:* Nanoparticles are solid or hollow particles with sizes between 1 nm and 100 nm. These particles have a wide range of applications in biology and medicine (Figure 1-4a). For example, antibodies and DNA can be coated on the outside

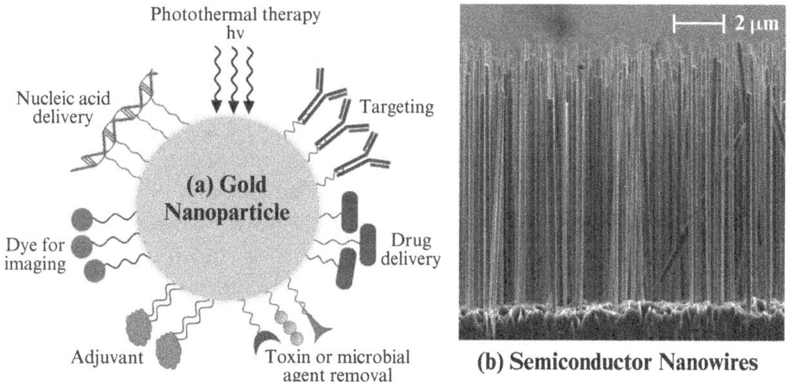

Figure 1-4   (a) The various biomedical applications of gold nanoparticles. (*The illustration is reprinted with permission from S. Bagheri et al.*[25]) (b) Colorized micrograph of gallium nitride semiconductor nanowires grown on a silicon substrate. (*The image is from L. Mansfield [NIST].*[26])

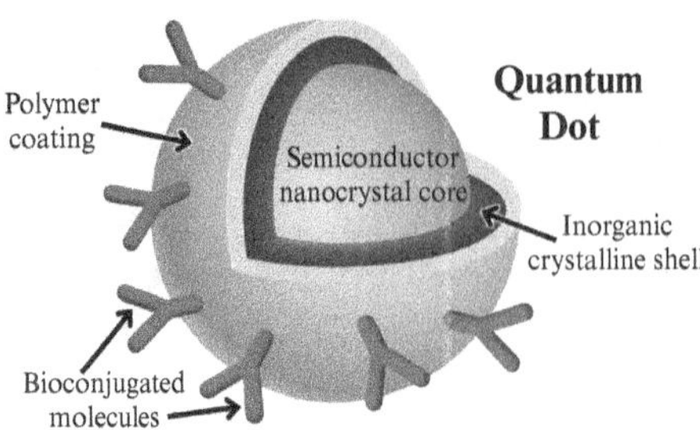

Figure 1-5   The structure of a multi-layer quantum dot (QD) designed for biomedical applications.

of solid nanoparticles for sensing or for targeted treatments. Also, hollow nanoparticles loaded with medication can be used for drug delivery.[23] In mRNA-based COVID-19 vaccines, liposomes (hollow spherical lipid nanoparticles) are used to deliver mRNA molecules into human cells.[24]

- *Semiconductor Nanowires:* Semiconductor nanowires (Figure 1-4b) are similar to carbon nanotubes (CNTs), but they are solid crystalline fibers instead of hollow tubes. They are fabricated via catalytic growth from a vapor or liquid phase. Unlike three-dimensional semiconductor materials, semiconductor nanowires have unusual quasi one-dimensional electronic properties. Promising applications include improved lithium-ion batteries and sensors.[27]

- *Quantum Dots:* Quantum dots (QDs) are artificial nanoscale crystals (Figure 1-5) with desirable optical properties. QDs exhibit fluorescence, and can be designed to re-emit light of different wavelengths after absorbing incident light. This property is beneficial for biological and medical applications.[28]

1.2 MICROFLUIDICS

Microfluidics involves the control and manipulation of tiny volumes (microliters to picoliters) of fluids in a system of channels with widths ranging from hundreds of nanometers to a few millimeters. Since its inception in the 1990s, the broad discipline of microfluidics has grown exponentially, becoming an integral part of modern biotechnology and nanotechnology. Microfluidics can be used to manipulate, transport, filter, mix, and/or separate tiny amounts of sample fluids. To carry out these tasks, a microfluidic platform utilizes pressure-driven flow, electrokinetic forces (e.g., electro-osmosis, electrophoresis, and dielectrophoresis), diffusion, centrifugal forces, capillary forces, or a combination of these forces.

Microfluidic platforms are commonly found on lab-on-a-chip devices (e.g., glucose and pregnancy test strips), organs-on-chips, and microarrays for accelerating drug discovery and screening. Additionally, microfluidic platforms are employed for improving biomedical assays, enhancing drug and gene delivery, as well as many other biotechnological and biomedical applications.[8,29] For example, microfluidic platforms can be used to sort and capture single cells, as shown in Figure 1-6. Microfluidics is a key topic in bionanotechnology, and underpins the working principles of bionanotechnological devices.

In general, shrinking down a macroscale fluidic system to create a microfluidic system will likely fail. Due to the small scales of microfluidic systems, fluid in such microsystems may behave in counter-intuitive ways. For instance, pressure-driven flow is rendered far less effective while the effect of diffusion is increased in microfluidic systems. In addition, fluid flow in microfluidic systems tends to be highly laminar, which makes fluid mixing

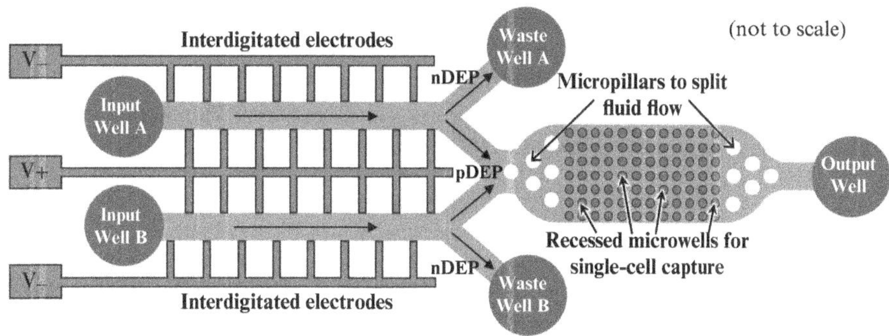

Figure 1-6   A microchip designed to selectively capture single cells using dielectrophoresis powered by interdigitated electrodes, which utilizes a microfluidic platform.

much more difficult. Thus, special design considerations are necessary when engineering microfluidic devices.

1.3   DNA AND RNA TECHNOLOGY

Deoxyribonucleic acid (DNA) and ribonucleic acid (RNA) together form one of the most important topics in biology. DNA and RNA are found in all cellular life, including humans, and contain the blueprints for synthesizing proteins which in turn form the building blocks of living organisms along with the processes needed to keep them alive. DNA consists of a sequence of nucleotides formed into a double helix structure (Figure 1-7). The exact sequence of nucleotides in DNA determines the shape, amino acid sequence, and functions of synthesized proteins in addition to how the processes in human bodies are regulated. The nucleotide sequence of a very long strand of DNA, such as the DNA sequence of a chromosome, can be grouped into genes. The combination of all of the genes of an organism forms its genome. Genomes are challenging to understand, but shedding light on genomes is important as they control the fate of all organisms, including humans.

DNA sequence determination has become a central tool in the medical and biological sciences. For instance, screening for genetic diseases (e.g., cancer, sickle cell disease, cystic fibrosis, and glaucoma) can help with preventative treatments. Sequencing the cancer genomes of cancer patients can help identify potential treatments. DNA sequencing can also be used to detect pathogens and microbes (e.g., bacteria, viruses, fungi, and parasites) in the human body, food, and the environment. In forensics, genetic sequencing helps catch criminals. In biology, it can help us understand how DNA determines cellular and protein function.

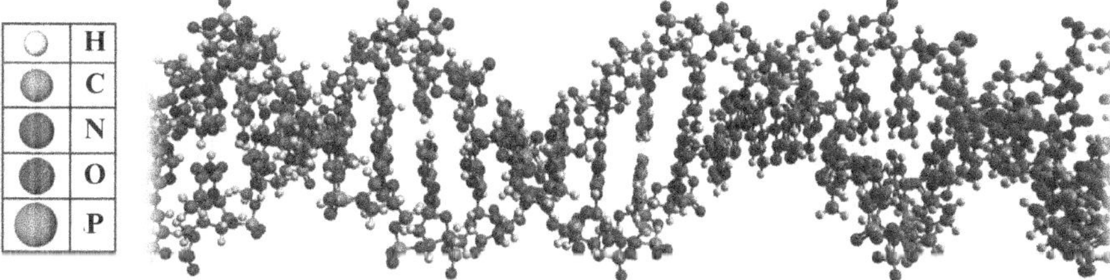

Figure 1-7   The molecular structure of double-stranded DNA.

Like DNA, RNA sequencing and quantification have also become increasingly important in biomedicine. They can be used to determine the presence, viral load, genomes, and mutations of RNA viruses (e.g., coronaviruses, influenza, rabies, HIV, and hepatitis C), study gene expressions, and screen for RNA biomarkers resulting from diseases such as cancer and diabetes.

1.4 LAB-ON-A-CHIP DEVICES

In 1945, the first-generation of computer named ENIAC was made. Consisting of 18,000 vacuum tubes and weighing about 27 tons, it occupied 167 m^2 and consumed 150 kW of electricity for operation. However, its clock speed was only 100 kHz. In September 2016, the iPhone 7 was introduced by Apple Inc. It consisted of 3.3 billion transistors, weighed only 138 g, but had a clock speed of up to 2.34 GHz. Since 1971, integrated circuits (ICs) have followed Moore's law, which states that the transistor density on integrated circuits doubles every 18 months. Because of the rapid advancement of ICs, communications and the Internet have also experienced rapid growth. However, as the silicon transistor size in ICs approaches physical limits with gate lengths below 5 nm, semiconductor nanofabrication technologies are about to hit the so-called "red brick wall." Thus, researchers are considering developing 3D ICs as well as ICs for other applications.

One of the applications is the advancement of lab-on-a-chip (LOC) devices because they share many fabrication techniques with ICs. LOC devices utilize integrated microchips that can perform standard laboratory functions to replace (or supplement) traditional wet laboratory assays. Analogous to how IC microchips can be used to create portable computers and smartphones, LOC microchips can be applied to create portable wet laboratories. Traditional biological labs require a large number of potentially expensive assays and generate a correspondingly significant amount of waste. In addition, biological experiments are time-consuming and require costly equipment and extensively trained operators. Advantages of LOCs include miniaturization, automation, and cost-effectiveness. LOCs are also easy to use and are highly portable, allowing tests to be performed anywhere. In addition, LOCs require far fewer assays and generate far less waste. Depending on the specific design, LOCs can be configured for many different purposes, such as organ mimicry or biosensing.

LOC devices can be designed for biosensing, such as the one shown in Figure 1-8. The success of LOC biosensors depends on the accurate detection of biomarkers which

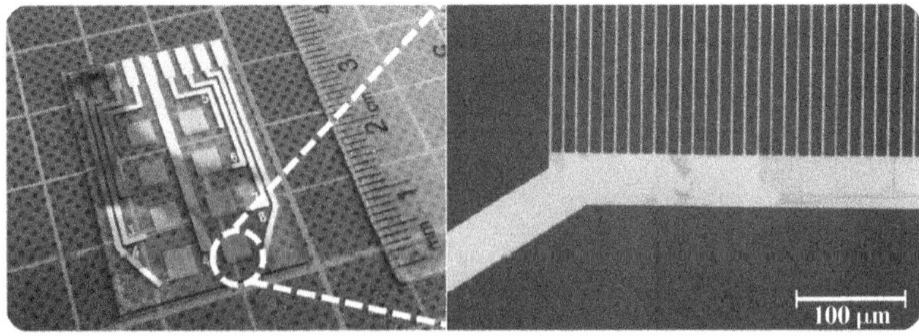

Figure 1-8   (Left) The microchip of an impedimetric lab-on-a-chip biosensor device. (Right) Optical microscope image of the gold interdigitated electrodes on the microchip responsible for biosensing. (*The photographs are provided by Prof. Jie Chen's group.*)

are biomolecules including genes, proteins, and metabolites which signal the presence or absence of medical conditions and diseases. Commonly used commercial LOC devices include glucose meters for monitoring diabetes and pregnancy test strips. Successful LOCs possess high accuracy, excellent reproducibility between users, small size, portability, and include internal power sources. LOCs aim to be easy to use and need minimal sample pre-processing. They can also be connected to wireless networks. LOCs should ideally be affordable (<$10 dollars per test) and can provide fast test results (<20 min). Each LOC may have multiple wells or inlets that allow multiple tests to be completed in parallel simultaneously. These results are then analyzed using calibrated algorithms or with machine learning methods. LOCs can be used for testing urine, saliva, blood, or serum. In addition to biomedical applications, LOCs can also be applied in food safety, smart agriculture, and environmental monitoring.

Another category of LOC devices is the organ-on-a-chip (OOC), which is designed to mimic the behavior of one or more organs *in vitro* (i.e., outside of a living organism). An OOC device is created by merging a microfluidic chip with live cells and tissues, combining micro/nano fabrication with tissue engineering. By mimicking human organs, OOC devices can be used to study the origins and progression of human diseases, the impact of gene expressions, and the role of biomolecules such as proteins or toxins. Additionally, OOC devices can be used to screen drug candidates and test medical devices *in vitro*. By eliminating the need for animal and human testing in pre-clinical and early clinical trials, OOC systems can greatly speed up drug and medical device development as well as elucidate our understanding of human physiology. An example of a sophisticated multi-organ OOC system is illustrated in Figure 1-9.

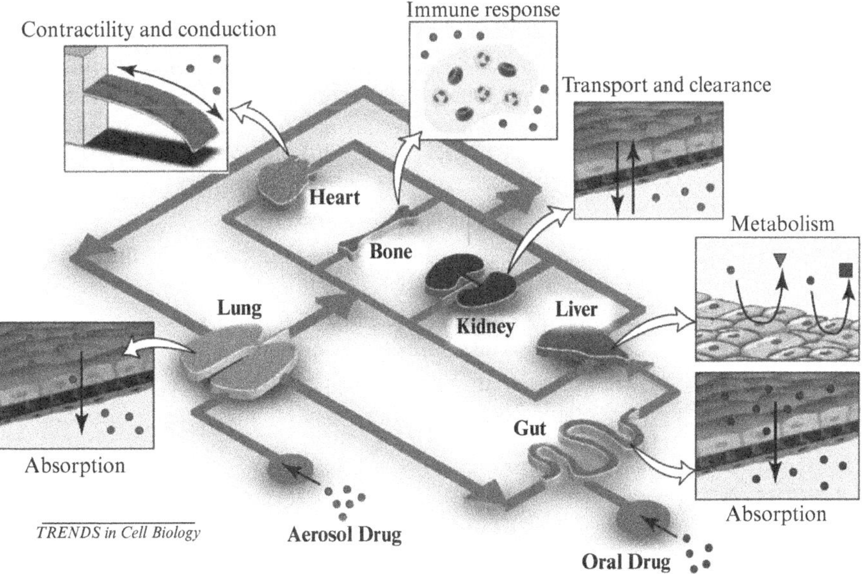

Figure 1-9 A multi-organ organ-on-a-chip (OOC) system which incorporates the functions of the human lung, heart, bone, kidney, liver, and gut. This system can be used to test the effects of aerosol drugs and oral drugs on the human body. (*The illustration is reprinted with permission from D. Huh et al.*[30])

1.5 OUTLINE OF THE BOOK

This book presents the fundamental engineering concepts and applications of bionanotechnology. The content of the book is presented in eight chapters covering fluid transport methods, microfluidics, optical detection, quantum dots, DNA and RNA bionanotechnology, the design and micro/nano fabrication of microfluidic and lab-on-a-chip devices, and the applications of bionanotechnology.

This chapter briefly introduced the background knowledge of nanomaterials, microfluidics, DNA and RNA technology, lab-on-a-chip devices, and some important applications of bionanotechnology. The details of bionanotechnology and its applications based on an engineering perspective are presented in the subsequent chapters.

Chapters 2 and 3 focus on microfluidics, which forms the basis for many lab-on-a-chip technologies and other bionanotechnological devices such as cell sorters and biomolecule separation systems. The two chapters cover fluid transport methods, the fundamentals of moving fluids in microfluidic systems, fluid thermodynamics, fluid mixing, and applications such as gel electrophoresis and cell separation.

Chapter 4 is dedicated to optical detection. The chapter covers methods of optical detection, fluorescence, and the theory and applications of quantum dots (QDs).

Chapter 5 focuses on DNA and RNA bionanotechnology. As this is an engineering book, it is assumed that readers are primarily from engineering backgrounds and only have preliminary knowledge of biotechnology. Thus, the chapter introduces DNA and RNA, followed by more advanced topics including polymerase chain reaction (PCR) techniques, DNA and RNA sequencing, the emerging field of DNA machinery, and CRISPR gene editing.

Chapter 6 is devoted to lab-on-a-chip (LOC) bionanotechnology and micro/nano fabrication. Lab-on-a-chip devices include microfluidic systems, miniaturized biosensors, micro total analysis systems (μTAS), and organ-on-a-chip (OOC) systems. The chapter covers the working principles, design, and fabrication of LOC devices. In particular, the design of LOC devices combines many of the topics discussed in the book such as microfluidics, nanomaterials, optical detection, and DNA machinery. Chapter 6 also discusses a wide range of micro/nano fabrication processes used in the semiconductor and microelectronics industries, and how they are applied in the fabrication of microfluidic and LOC devices.

Chapter 7 covers the applications of bionanotechnology. This content serves two main purposes: to present real-world case studies and applications of the theory in the previous chapters, and to tie together the topics from the previous chapters.

Chapter 8 introduces the use of computer simulation to analyze simple bionanotechnological devices consisting of interdigitated electrodes. These interdigitated electrodes can be used as biosensors (i.e., transducers) within lab-on-a-chip systems as well as platforms to separate and capture cells or particles. In particular, COMSOL Multiphysics® simulation software is introduced and is used for the simulations, which solves partial differential equations describing physical phenomena using the finite element method.

1.6 REFERENCES

[1] S. Kumar, *Essentials of Microbiology*, 1st ed. New Delhi, India: Jaypee Brothers Medical Publishers, 2016.

[2] R. P. Feynman, "There's plenty of room at the bottom," *Engineering and Science*, vol. 23, no. 5, pp. 22–36, 1960.

[3] M. Primozic, Z. Knez, and M. Leitgeb, "(Bio)Nanotechnology in Food Science-Food Packaging," *Nanomaterials*, vol. 11, no. 2, article 292, 2021.

[4] M.-X. Zhao and E.-Z. Zeng, "Application of functional quantum dot nanoparticles as fluorescence probes in cell labeling and tumor diagnostic imaging," *Nanoscale Research Letters*, vol. 10, pp. 1–9, 2015.

[5] R. Langer and N. A. Peppas, "Advances in biomaterials, drug delivery, and bionanotechnology," AIChE *Journal*, vol. 49, no. 12, pp. 2990–3006, 2003.

[6]   T. Nagamune, "Biomolecular engineering for nanobio/bionanotechnology," *Nano Convergence*, vol. 4, article 9, 2017.

[7]   C. Knoblauch, M. Griep, and C. Friedrich, "Recent advances in the field of bionanotechnology: An insight into optoelectric bacteriorhodopsin, quantum dots, and noble metal nanoclusters," *Sensors*, vol. 14, no. 10, pp. 19731–19766, 2014.

[8]   S. Damiati, U. B. Kompella, S. A. Damiati, and R. Kodzius, "Microfluidic devices for drug delivery systems and drug screening," *Genes*, vol. 9, no. 2, article 103, 2018.

[9]   D. Mark, S. Haeberle, G. Roth, F. von Stetten, and R. Zengerle, "Microfluidic lab-on-a-chip platforms: requirements, characteristics and applications," *Chemical Society Reviews*, vol. 39, no. 3, pp. 1153–1182, 2010.

[10]   M. Taguchi, A. Ptitsyn, E. S. McLamore, and J. C. Claussen, "Nanomaterial-mediated Biosensors for Monitoring Glucose," *Journal of Diabetes Science and Technology*, vol. 8, no. 2, pp. 403–411, 2014.

[11]   B. Huang, F. Chen, Y. Shen, K. Qian, Y. Wang, C. Sun, et al., "Advances in targeted pesticides with environmentally responsive controlled release by nanotechnology," *Nanomaterials*, vol. 8, no. 2, article 102, 2018.

[12]   A. Samanta and I. L. Medintz, "Nanoparticles and DNA—a powerful and growing functional combination in bionanotechnology," *Nanoscale*, vol. 8, no. 17, pp. 9037–9095, 2016.

[13]   D. R. Gossett, W. M. Weaver, A. J. Mach, S. C. Hur, H. T. K. Tse, W. Lee, et al., "Label-free cell separation and sorting in microfluidic systems," *Analytical and Bioanalytical Chemistry*, vol. 397, no. 8, pp. 3249–3267, 2010.

[14]   C. Zhang and D. Xing, "Miniaturized PCR chips for nucleic acid amplification and analysis: Latest advances and future trends," *Nucleic Acids Research*, vol. 35, no. 13, pp. 4223–4237, 2007.

[15]   D. Scaini and L. Ballerini, "Nanomaterials at the neural interface," *Current Opinion in Neurobiology*, vol. 50, pp. 50–55, 2018.

[16]   D. Branton, D. W. Deamer, A. Marziali, H. Bayley, S. A. Benner, T. Butler, et al., "The potential and challenges of nanopore sequencing," *Nature Biotechnology*, vol. 26, no. 10, pp. 1146–1153, 2008.

[17]   C. Lee, X. Wei, J. W. Kysar, and J. Hone, "Measurement of the elastic properties and intrinsic strength of monolayer graphene," *Science*, vol. 321, no. 5887, pp. 385–388, 2008.

[18]   G. Gedler, M. Antunes, T. Borca-Tasciuc, J. I. Velasco, and R. Ozisik, "Effects of graphene concentration, relative density and cellular morphology on the thermal conductivity of polycarbonate-graphene nanocomposite foams," *European Polymer Journal*, vol. 75, pp. 190–199, 2016.

[19]   F. Schwierz, "Graphene transistors," *Nature Nanotechnology*, vol. 5, no. 7, p. 487, 2010.

[20]   W. Yang, P. Thordarson, J. J. Gooding, S. P. Ringer, and F. Braet, "Carbon nanotubes for biological and biomedical applications," *Nanotechnology*, vol. 18, no. 41, article 412001, 2007.

[21]   H. Zare, S. Ahmadi, A. Ghasemi, M. Ghanbari, N. Rabiee, M. Bagherzadeh, et al., "Carbon Nanotubes: Smart Drug/Gene Delivery Carriers," *International Journal of Nanomedicine*, vol. 16, pp. 1681–1706, 2021.

[22]   P. G. Collins and P. Avouris, "Nanotubes for electronics," *Scientific American*, vol. 283, no. 6, pp. 62–69, 2000.

[23]   J. Jeevanandam, A. Barhoum, Y. S. Chan, A. Dufresne, and M. K. Danquah, "Review on nanoparticles and nanostructured materials: History, sources, toxicity and regulations," *Beilstein Journal of Nanotechnology*, vol. 9, no. 1, pp. 1050–1074, 2018.

[24]   G. Gregoriadis, "Liposomes and mRNA: Two technologies together create a COVID-19 vaccine," *Medicine in Drug Discovery*, vol. 12, article 100104, 2021.

[25]   S. Bagheri, M. Yasemi, E. Safaie-Qamsari, J. Rashidiani, M. Abkar, M. Hassani, et al., "Using gold nanoparticles in diagnosis and treatment of melanoma cancer," *Artificial Cells Nanomedicine and Biotechnology*, vol. 46, pp. S462–S471, 2018.

[26]   L. Mansfield. "Semiconductor Nanowires," U.S. NIST [Online]. Available: https://www.nist.gov/image/nanotechnologyelectronicsnanowiresthatemituvlightjpg, 2006.

[27]   J. Arbiol and Q. Xiong, Eds., *Semiconductor Nanowires: Materials, Synthesis, Characterization and Applications*. Oxford, UK: Woodhead Publishing Ltd., 2015.

[28]   A. P. Alivisatos, "Semiconductor clusters, nanocrystals, and quantum dots," *Science*, vol. 271, no. 5251, pp. 933–937, 1996.

[29]   N. Convery and N. Gadegaard, "30 years of microfluidics," *Micro and Nano Engineering*, vol. 2, pp. 76–91, 2019.

[30]   D. Huh, G. A. Hamilton, and D. E. Ingber, "From 3D cell culture to organs-on-chips," *Trends in Cell Biology*, vol. 21, no. 12, pp. 745–754, 2011.

CHAPTER 2

Microfluidics I: Forces, Thermodynamics, and Fluid Flow

2.1 INTRODUCTION

As pointed out in Section 1.2, microfluidics is the control and manipulation of fluids inhabiting a system of microchannels and microchambers. A microfluidic component is designed to carry out a fluidic unit operation, such as fluid transport, filtering, mixing, separation, or manipulation. Common examples of microfluidic components include microchannels, inlets, outlets, microchambers, micro-valves, micro-mixers, micro-dispensers, micro-filters, and micro-pumps.

A microfluidic platform is comprised of a set of microfluidic components. Figure 2-1 illustrates an example of a microfluidic platform. Microfluidic platforms are integral to the functions of many lab-on-a-chip devices such as portable biosensors for rapid and inexpensive medical diagnosis, organs-on-chips for replacing cell cultures and live animal tests, and microarrays for accelerating drug discovery and screening. Microfluidic systems are also employed to assist drug and gene delivery, increase the throughput and lower the costs of medical, biological, and biochemical assays, improve single-cell analysis, and even help synthesize microparticles and microfibers. Furthermore, microfluidic platforms are vital components of many biotechnological and biomedical devices such as cell capture and sorting microchips, electrophoresis microchips for biomolecule separation and DNA sequencing, and biochemical microreactors. Thus, knowledge of microfluidics is required to understand the working principles of bionanotechnological devices.[2-6]

The most commonly used microfluidic methods include pressure-driven microfluidics, centrifugal microfluidics, droplet microfluidics, digital microfluidics, and capillary microfluidics. In pressure-driven microfluidics, air or hydraulic pressure is applied to move fluids through microchannels. Pressure-driven microfluidics is commonly used in commercial products such as the GeneXpert® system by Cepheid—a fully automated molecular diagnostic platform. Centrifugal microfluidics uses centrifugal force to move fluids, such as the centrifugal separation of red blood cells and serum from blood shown in Figure 2-2. A digital polymerase chain reaction (PCR) system manufactured by Thermo Fisher Scientific uses droplet microfluidics. Capillary microfluidics uses capillary force to move fluids, which is utilized by Abbott Laboratories' Alere Triage® instrument.[7]

When dealing with fluids and fluid transport in most biomedical applications, special design considerations are often necessary for engineering working devices. As the volumes of fluids are small, biomedical devices must be small as well. Microfluidics is one of the

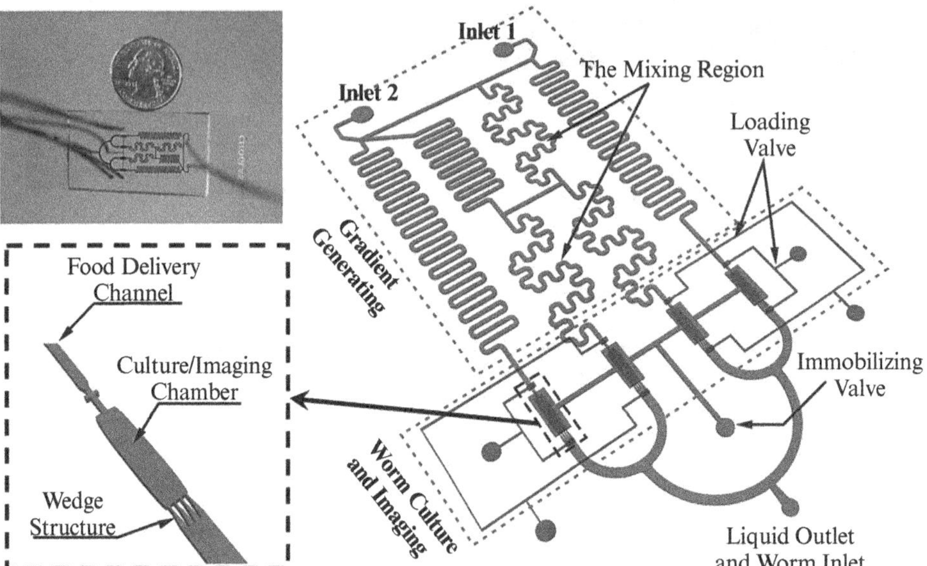

Figure 2-1   A microfluidic platform for testing the effect of dietary restriction on organism lifespan, which employs a combination of microchannels, microchambers, inlets, outlets, micro-mixers, and micro-valves. The microfluidic platform automatically feeds nematode worms (*C. elegans*) with different concentrations of bacterial food supplied through inlets 1 and 2. The worms are fluorescently labeled, and the status of the worms (i.e., whether alive or dead) is determined using optical fluorescence microscopy. As shown in the top left photograph, the size of this microfluidic chip is 50 mm (length) × 24 mm (width). (*The figure is reprinted with permission from A. Ge et al.*[1])

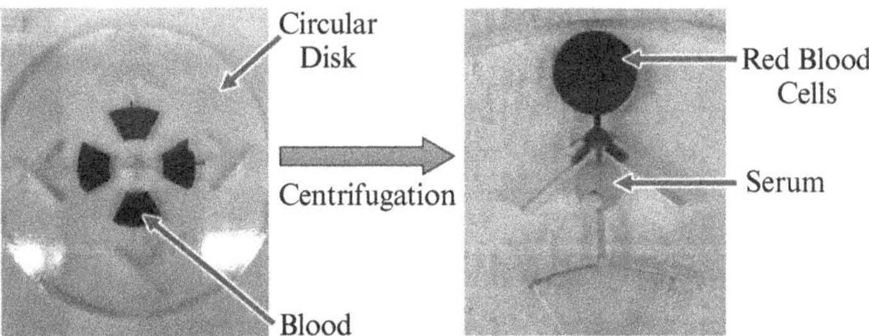

Figure 2-2   Centrifugal force for moving fluids: (left) blood is loaded into the chamber; (right) blood is separated into red blood cells and serum after centrifugation. The radius of the disk is about 3 cm for integration on a lab-on-a-chip device. (*The photographs are provided by Prof. Jie Chen's group.*)

cornerstones of biomedical technology. In their most simple form, microfluidic systems serve to transport fluids from one place to another. Fluid transport is vital in lab-on-a-chip technologies for moving biological samples from collection areas to active areas on the chip for analysis and testing.[8] Microfluidics also plays an important role in other applications, including passive valves for transporting exact volumes of fluid,[9] working in systems to separate different components present in a fluid sample,[10] or for sample purification.[11]

Creating a microfluidic system is rarely as simple as just shrinking down a regular-sized fluidic system. As the scale of the system decreases, it may act in counter-intuitive ways. For disposable microfluidic chips that are used only once, designs have to be both cheap and operate with low-power consumption, which excludes the use of traditional valves. Conventional methods for moving fluids become ineffective in microfluidic systems, and

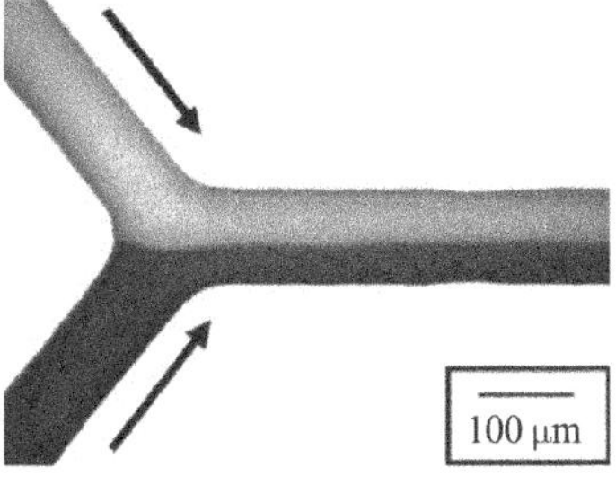

Figure 2-3 An example of laminar flow, where liquids flow without mixing. (*The image is reprinted with permission from E. R. Choban et al.*[13])

components such as hand-operated valves become impractical. One representative example illustrating the difference is the occurrence of turbulent versus laminar flow regimes. In macroscopic fluidic systems, it is taken for granted that when two different fluids are added into a system, they become mixed. However, this is not always the case for microfluidics. Under certain conditions and with the appropriate scale, fluid viscosity, and flow speed, fluid flow becomes laminar. With laminar flow, all components of the fluid move only in the direction of fluid flow, and there are no interactions between different components of the fluid. In the laminar flow regime, two different fluids can enter a single channel, and exit the channel without mixing (Figure 2-3). This can be problematic when an application requires mixing, such as processes that require a specific chemical reaction, or dilution to take place. In these cases, separate components must be specifically made to allow fluids to become mixed.[11,12] On the other hand, the lack of mixing can also be advantageous. For example, specific ingredients in a fluid can be isolated through diffusion into an adjacent buffer without mixing the original fluid and buffer (please refer to Section 3.5.1).[11]

2.2 FORCES

2.2.1 Fundamental Forces

There are four fundamental forces in the universe.

(1) The *strong nuclear force* is by far the strongest fundamental force, and has the shortest range. It holds the nuclei of atoms together against the electrical repulsion between protons. All protons and neutrons are each comprised of three quarks held together by gluons, a manifestation of the strong nuclear force. The strong nuclear force is responsible for the energy released during nuclear fission and nuclear fusion reactions.

(2) The *electromagnetic force* is the second strongest fundamental force, and has infinite range. It acts between electrically charged particles and between magnets, and can manifest as light (i.e., electromagnetic waves). Electromagnetic forces hold atoms and molecules together through the electrical attraction between electrons and atomic nuclei. Moreover, electromagnetic forces are responsible for chemical bonding, intermolecular forces, and all chemical processes.

(3) The *weak nuclear force* is the second weakest fundamental force, and has short range. It governs particle decay such as radioactive decay and neutrino interactions. The weak nuclear force is partially responsible for nuclear fission and nuclear fusion reactions.

(4) *Gravity* is by far the weakest fundamental force, and has infinite range. It acts between objects with mass. Gravity is so weak that it is only easily noticeable with respect to celestial bodies and objects such as planets, stars, galaxies, and black holes.

For bionanotechnological systems, electromagnetic forces and gravity are the most significant. Aside from pressure-driven flow caused by gravitational pressure differentials, all other fluid transport mechanisms in the context of microfluidics are caused by electromagnetic forces. Due to the sheer mass of the Earth, gravity strongly influences the behavior of nanoscale objects and liquids.

2.2.2 Gravity

Gravity is a long-range and universal force, and is the weakest force among the four fundamental forces mentioned before. Gravity acts between any two pieces of matter in the universe.

$$F = G\frac{m_1 m_2}{r^2} \tag{2.1}$$

where F is the force due to gravity between two masses (m_1 and m_2) being a distance r apart. The gravitational constant is $G = 6.674 \times 10^{-11}$ N·m²/kg².

EXAMPLE 2-1   An object falls from a height of 54 m onto the ground in 3.32 s. If there is no initial velocity, what is the acceleration of the falling object? If the radius of the Earth is 6371 km, what is the mass of the Earth?

Solution   Because there is no initial velocity, the acceleration can be calculated using

$$d = \frac{1}{2}at^2 \quad \Rightarrow \quad a = \frac{2d}{t^2} = \frac{2(54 \text{ m})}{(3.32 \text{ s})^2} = 9.80 \text{ m/s}^2$$

The object falls to the ground due to gravity. Denoting m_o as the mass of the object and m_e as the mass of the Earth, we get

$$F = G\frac{m_o m_e}{r^2} = m_o a$$

Simplifying the equations above, we obtain the mass of the Earth m_e as follows.

$$m_e = \frac{ar^2}{G} = \frac{(9.80 \text{ m/s}^2)\,(6371 \times 10^3 \text{ m})^2}{6.674 \times 10^{-11} \text{ N} \cdot \text{m}^2/\text{kg}^2} = 5.96 \times 10^{24} \text{ kg} \quad \blacktriangle$$

Gravity plays an important role in microfluidic systems. For the liquid in any column, gravity exerting on the liquid generates a vertical pressure (Figure 2-4). The pressure difference ΔP_g due to gravity between the top and bottom of a column of fluid with height Δh is given by

$$\Delta P_g = \rho_m g \Delta h \tag{2.2}$$

where ρ_m is the density of the liquid (for water $\rho_m = 10^3$ kg/m³) and the acceleration due to gravity is $g = 9.81$ m/s².

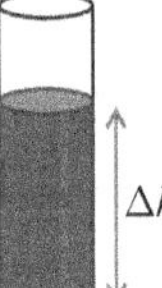

Figure 2-4   Pressure differential of a column of liquid due to gravity.

2.2.3 Dipole-Dipole Forces

Intermolecular forces, such as dipole-dipole forces, are in general very weak compared to intramolecular forces. Dipole-dipole forces are the attractive forces between the positively charged region of a polar molecule and the negatively charged region of another polar molecule. For instance, an ammonia molecule (NH_3) has both $N^{\delta-}$ (the negative region) and $H^{\delta+}$ (the positive region). Dipole forces pull them together. The same holds true for a water (H_2O) molecule. Both NH_3 and H_2O are polar molecules with slightly positive sides $\delta+$ and a slightly negative side $\delta-$ (Figure 2-5). In a water molecule, the oxygen atom has a partial negative charge and the two hydrogen atoms have partial positive charges, as oxygen has a higher electronegativity than hydrogen. The dipole-dipole force exists when the positive side of a polar molecule attracts the negative side of another polar molecule.

Dipole-dipole forces can be described by the van der Waals force, while the Lennard-Jones potential $U(r)$ determines the bond lengths in molecules:

$$U(r) = 4\epsilon\left[\left(\frac{\sigma}{r}\right)^{12} - \left(\frac{\sigma}{r}\right)^{6}\right] \tag{2.3}$$

where ϵ is the depth of the potential well, r is the distance of separation between both particles which is measured from the center of one particle to the center of the other particle (Figure 2-6), and σ is the "hard-shell" diameter of the potential (the distance at which the potential of the system is zero, i.e., the x-intercept). The bond length is the value of r at minimum potential.

Hydrogen bonding is the intermolecular attraction between hydrogen (H) atoms and a highly electronegative atom such as nitrogen (N), oxygen (O), or fluorine (F). Hydrogen bonding is an especially strong dipole-dipole force, which is essential in DNA linkages between A-T and C-G. Note that C-G bonding (triple bonding) is stronger than A-T bonding (double bonding) (Figure 2-7).

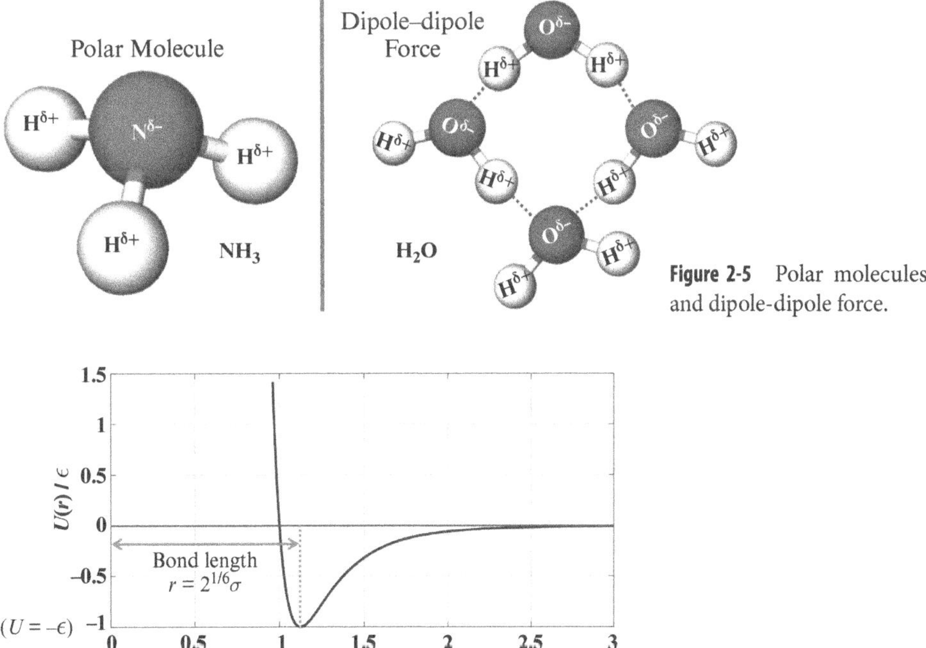

Figure 2-5 Polar molecules and dipole-dipole force.

Figure 2-6 Lennard-Jones potential diagram. The minimum energy is $U(r = 2^{1/6}\,\sigma) = -\epsilon$.

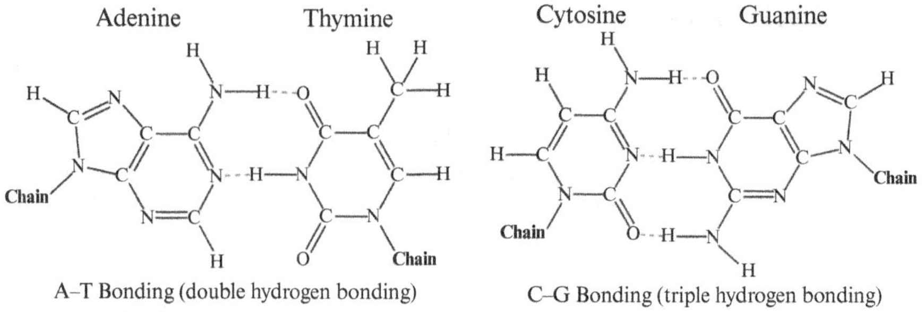

Adenine   Thymine   Cytosine   Guanine

A–T Bonding (double hydrogen bonding)   C–G Bonding (triple hydrogen bonding)

Figure 2-7   Hydrogen bonding binds adenine (A) to thymine (T), and cytosine (C) to guanine (G).

EXAMPLE 2-2   The unequal sharing of electrons between atoms in a molecule results in molecular dipoles. $\mu = Q \cdot r$ is the dipole moment of the bond, where Q is the charge, and r is the distance of separation. The potential energy between two polar atoms can be described by

$$U(r) = -\frac{2\mu_1\mu_2}{4\pi\epsilon_0 r^3} \tag{2.4}$$

where $\epsilon_0 = 8.854 \times 10^{-12}$ F/m is the permittivity of free space. Calculate the potential energy of the dipole-dipole interaction between two HF molecules being 5Å apart, given that the dipole moment of HF molecules is 1.92 debye (1 debye $= 3.3356 \times 10^{-30}$ C · m).

Solution   The dipole moment of the HF molecules is

$$\mu = (1.92)(3.3356 \times 10^{-30} \text{ C} \cdot \text{m}) = 6.404 \times 10^{-30} \text{ C} \cdot \text{m}$$

Based on the potential energy equation, we have

$$U = -\frac{2\mu_1\mu_2}{4\pi\epsilon_0 r^3} = -\frac{2 \cdot (6.404 \times 10^{-30} \text{ C} \cdot \text{m})^2}{4\pi(8.854 \times 10^{-12} \text{ F/m})(5 \times 10^{-10} \text{ m})^3} = -5.90 \times 10^{-21} \text{ J} \quad \blacktriangle$$

2.2.4 Capillary Forces

Whether taking the form of plastic or glass tubes or being built directly into lab-on-a-chip systems, capillaries such as microchannels are essential in microfluidics. These small channels can help transport fluids from one place to another, deliver samples to testing platforms, move solutions around for different chemical reactions, or clear away excess buffers. How do the fluids move through the capillaries? The easiest way is through capillary force—a force generated from surface tension or surface free energy which can draw fluids through capillaries.

Capillary forces are related to the contact angle of the material on which the capillary is formed. The contact angle is a measure of the wettability of solid surfaces. For example, a contact angle of $\theta_c = 0°$ indicates that liquid spreads over the solid surface with perfect wettability (Figure 2-8, left). Conversely, a contact angle of $\theta_c = 180°$ indicates that the solid surface repels the liquid, causing the liquid to form spherical droplets on the solid surface (Figure 2-8, right). Capillary surfaces fall between these two extremes. Figure 2-8 (middle) shows the wetting of a solid surface described by Young's equation:

$$\gamma_{LG} \cos \theta_c = \gamma_{SG} - \gamma_{SL} \tag{2.5}$$

where γ_{LG} is the liquid–gas surface tension, γ_{SG} is the solid–gas surface tension, γ_{SL} is the solid–liquid interfacial tension, and θ_c is the contact angle.

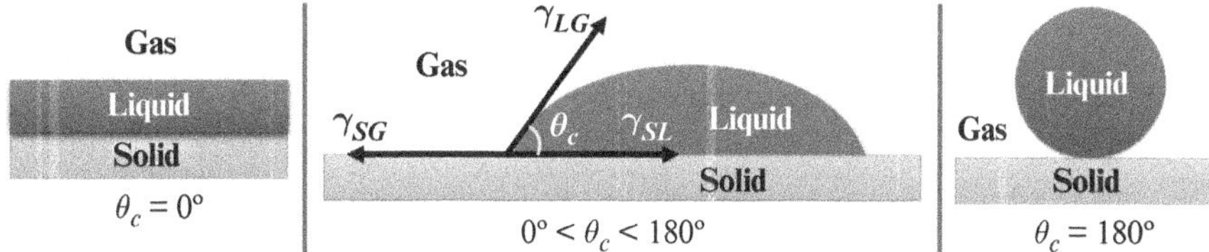

Figure 2-8 Wetting of solid surface described by Young's equation.

To illustrate surface tension, let us look at the water–air surface within a glass capillary. Water molecules at the surface interact with both bulk water molecules and air molecules. The attractive cohesive interaction forces (i.e., intermolecular forces) between water molecules is greater than the interaction force between water and air molecules. These interactions result in a net force which drags the surface water molecules toward the bulk water. Therefore, the surface water molecules undergo internal pressure and have more energy than the bulk water molecules. The surface energy per unit area, or the force per unit length is called surface tension.

In a capillary, a meniscus is formed, whose shape is dependent on the liquid in the capillary as well as the capillary material (Figure 2-9, left) through energy minimization with the surface. For liquid mercury in a glass capillary, a ∩-shaped meniscus is formed because the adhesive force between mercury and glass is weaker than the cohesive force of mercury. Conversely, a ∪-shaped meniscus is formed for water in a glass capillary because the adhesive force between water and glass is stronger than the cohesive force of water.

Let us consider a segment of fluid within a cylindrical capillary having a radius of r_0, where the liquid naturally forms a meniscus through surface energy minimization (Figure 2-9, right). To counteract the pressure difference at the liquid-gas interface, the walls of the capillary must exert a force per unit circumference (or perimeter) on the capillary, which is proportional to the amount of surface with which the edge of the liquid is in contact. The surface tension is denoted by gamma (γ) with units of N/m. Therefore, the total force exerted by this surface interaction to counterbalance the pressure difference and maintain the liquid's profile is (assuming a circular cross-section capillary)

$$F = \gamma\left(2\pi r_0\right) \tag{2.6}$$

There is another factor we have to consider as well: the contact angle of the liquid on the solid surface. Due to the contact angle, a meniscus surface is formed, which limits the interaction between the surface and the liquid. An interface with a 0° contact angle has no impedance to the surface interaction, whereas one with a 180° contact angle has no surface interaction at all. Therefore, the final total force is

$$F = 2\pi r_0 \gamma_{LG} \cos\theta_c \tag{2.7}$$

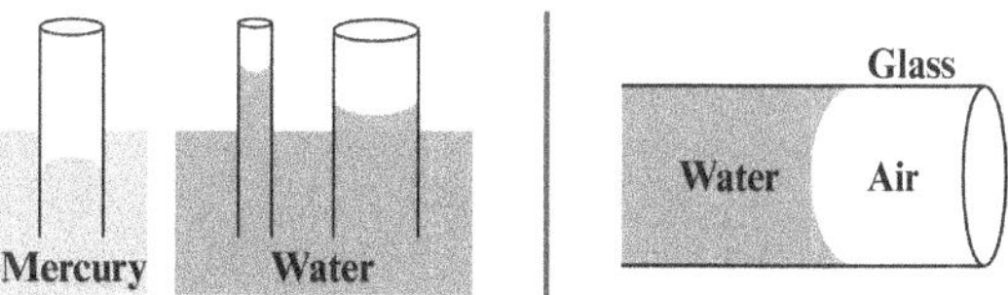

Figure 2-9 (Left) Capillary action of water compared to mercury in vertical glass capillaries. (Right) Representation of the glass–water–air interfaces in a horizontal capillary.

where γ_{LG} is the liquid–gas surface tension, and θ_c is the contact angle. For any capillary (such as a microchannel) having a constant cross-sectional perimeter $L_{channel}$ and area $A_{channel}$, the capillary pressure $P_{capillary}$ is given by

$$P_{capillary} = \frac{F}{A} = \frac{\gamma_{LG}\cos\theta_c L_{channel}}{A_{channel}} \tag{2.8}$$

For a cylindrical capillary with radius of r_0, the capillary pressure is

$$P_{capillary} = \frac{\gamma_{LG}\cos\theta_c L_{channel}}{A_{channel}} = \frac{\gamma_{LG}\cos\theta_c\left(2\pi r_0\right)}{\left(\pi r_0^2\right)} = \frac{2\gamma_{LG}\cos\theta_c}{r_0} \tag{2.9}$$

For a rectangular capillary with width w and height h, the perimeter is $L_{channel} = 2(h + w)$ and the cross-sectional area is $A_{channel} = wh$. Hence, the pressure for a rectangular capillary is

$$P_{capillary} = \frac{2(h+w)\gamma_{LG}\cos\theta_c}{wh} = 2\gamma_{LG}\cos\theta_c\left(\frac{1}{h} + \frac{1}{w}\right) \tag{2.10}$$

It can be seen from Equations (2.8) to (2.10) that when $0° \le \theta_c < 90°$, the pressure is positive. The positive pressure or force is useful for filling capillaries (e.g., microchannels) with buffer and sample solutions because no extra external mechanisms are required. Under this positive pressure condition, capillaries will automatically fill themselves. Conversely, when $90° < \theta_c \le 180°$, the pressure or force is negative. Instead of a force pulling liquid into the capillary, the liquid is pushed out, and external pressure is required to fill the capillary. This negative pressure case can be advantageous as well, as negative capillary pressures can be used to create passive valves in microfluidic systems. At $\theta_c = 90°$, there is no capillary pressure. By varying the diameter of a capillary and applying certain pressures (as shown in Figure 2-10), liquids can be pushed in and out of very specific areas of a system by applying the appropriate pressure.

Capillaries also exist in the human body. Blood vessels in the human body are classified as arteries, veins, and capillaries. Capillaries are tiny blood vessels that connect arteries and veins. Their primary function is to exchange materials (e.g., oxygen, nutrients, carbon dioxide, and waste) between the blood and body tissues.

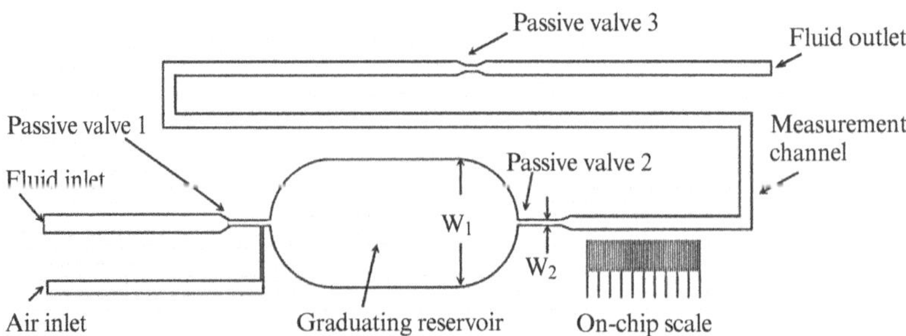

Figure 2-10 A microfluidic system that uses changes in capillary diameter to create pressure-controlled valves. (*The schematic is reprinted with permission from A. Puntambekar et al.*[9])

EXAMPLE 2-3 A square microchannel with an edge length of $w = h = 100\ \mu\text{m}$ is attached to a vertical buffer-filled supply well. The microchannel is 5 cm long. The fabrication process has led to a contact angle (with water) of 110°. If the water-air surface tension is 72 mN/m, to what height Δh does the water have to be filled in the well in order to fill the microchannel?

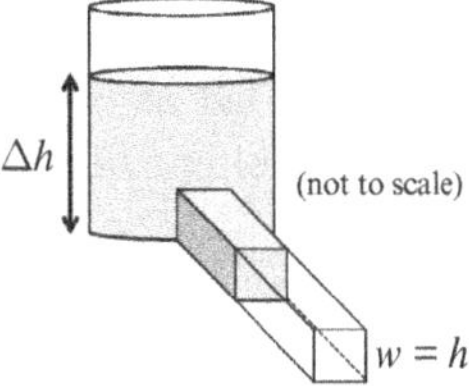

Solution   The pressure required to fill a square microchannel is calculated using Equation (2.10):

$$P = 2\gamma_{LG}\cos\theta_c\left(\frac{1}{h} + \frac{1}{w}\right) = 2(72\,\text{mN/m})\cos(110°)\left(\frac{1}{100\ \mu\text{m}} + \frac{1}{100\ \mu\text{m}}\right) = -985\ \text{Pa}$$

The negative pressure indicates that this is a required pressure (the pressure is not actually negative). This threshold pressure is caused by the gravitational force of the water in the well. Therefore, the required height Δh of water in the well is

$$\Delta P_g = \rho_m g \Delta h \;\Rightarrow\; \Delta h = \frac{\Delta P_g}{\rho_m g} = \frac{985\ \text{Pa}}{\left(10^3\,\text{kg/m}^3\right)\left(9.81\,\text{m/s}^2\right)} = 10.0\ \text{cm} \quad \blacktriangle$$

2.3 THERMODYNAMICS

The energy diagrams shown in Figure 2-11 represent the energy landscapes for a given system comprised of the *same* population of atoms. In an energy diagram, the vertical axis denotes the system's energy level while the horizontal axis represents the system's configuration. The configuration refers to a particular spatial arrangement of atoms in the system. For any given system comprised of the same population of atoms, the energy landscape of the system depends on how the population of atoms is arranged in space.

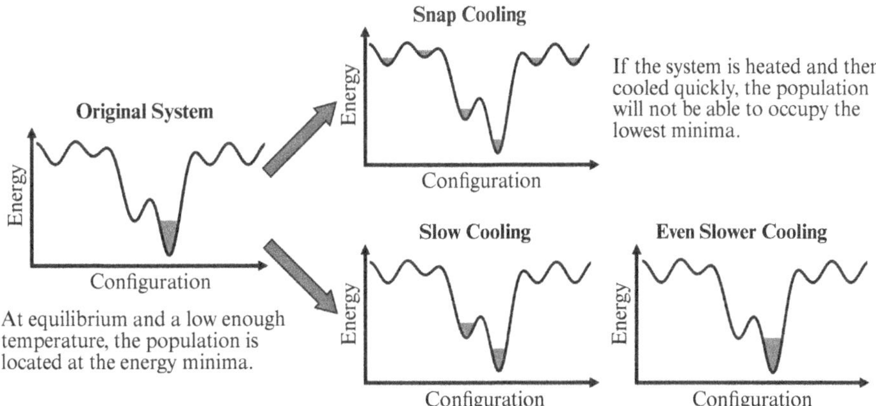

Figure 2-11   Energy diagrams for a system comprised of the same population of atoms. The vertical axis denotes energy level, while the horizontal axis represents configuration.

At equilibrium and low enough temperature, the population is located at the energy minima. The system will generally try to take the lowest energy configuration (i.e., populate the lowest energy minima), but this is not always the case. If the system is heated to a high temperature (energy is added) and is then cooled quickly, the population will not be able to exclusively occupy the lowest minima, but also settle into local minima at higher energy levels. On the other hand, if the same system is cooled slowly, the population can reach the lower minima. Let us consider a population of silica (SiO_2) particles at different temperatures. When molten silica is snap-cooled, an amorphous solid (i.e., glass) forms. However, when molten silica is cooled very slowly, a solid crystal (i.e., quartz) will form (the lowest energy state).

2.3.1 Derivatives in Cylindrical Coordinates

Before discussing the heat equation, let us review how to perform derivatives in cylindrical coordinates. Cylindrical coordinates are especially useful for modeling microfluidic systems containing cylindrical channels and capillaries. We can transform between Cartesian coordinates (x, y, z), cylindrical coordinates (ρ, φ, z), and spherical coordinates (r, θ, φ) using the identities in Appendix E. The forward and reverse coordinate transformations between Cartesian coordinates and cylindrical coordinates are as follows.

Forward transform (Cartesian to cylindrical): $\rho = \sqrt{x^2 + y^2}$, $\varphi = \arctan(y/x)$, $z = z$ (2.11)

Reverse transform (cylindrical to Cartesian): $x = \rho \cos \varphi$, $y = \rho \sin \varphi$, $z = z$ (2.12)

The mutually orthogonal unit vectors in cylindrical coordinates $\left(\hat{\rho}, \hat{\varphi}, \hat{z}\right)$ are

$$\hat{\rho} = \frac{x\hat{x} + y\hat{y}}{\rho} = \cos\varphi\hat{x} + \sin\varphi\hat{y} \qquad \hat{\varphi} = \hat{z} \times \hat{\rho} = -\sin\varphi\hat{x} + \cos\varphi\hat{y} \qquad \hat{z} = \hat{z} \quad (2.13)$$

EXAMPLE 2-4   Prove that $\hat{\varphi} = -\sin\varphi\hat{x} + \cos\varphi\hat{y}$. Also, compute $\partial\hat{\rho}/\partial\rho$ and $\partial\hat{\rho}/\partial\varphi$.

Solution   Letting $\det(M)$ represent the determinant of matrix M, we have

$$\hat{\phi} = \hat{z} \times \hat{\rho} = \overbrace{[0 \ \ 0 \ \ 1]}^{\hat{x} \ \ \hat{y} \ \ \hat{z}} \times \overbrace{[\cos\varphi \ \ \sin\varphi \ \ 0]}^{\hat{x} \ \ \hat{y} \ \ \hat{z}} = \det\left(\begin{vmatrix} \hat{x} & \hat{y} & \hat{z} \\ 0 & 0 & 1 \\ \cos\varphi & \sin\varphi & 0 \end{vmatrix}\right) = -\sin\varphi\hat{x} + \cos\varphi\hat{y}$$

The first-order derivatives $\partial\hat{\rho}/\partial\rho$ and $\partial\hat{\rho}/\partial\varphi$ are computed as follows:

$$\frac{\partial\hat{\rho}}{\partial\rho} = \frac{\partial}{\partial\rho}(\cos\varphi\hat{x} + \sin\varphi\hat{y}) = \frac{\partial}{\partial\rho}(\cos\varphi) \ \hat{x} + \frac{\partial}{\partial\rho}(\sin\varphi) \ \hat{y} = 0$$

$$\frac{\partial\hat{\rho}}{\partial\varphi} = \frac{\partial}{\partial\varphi}(\cos\varphi\hat{x} + \sin\varphi\hat{y}) = \frac{\partial}{\partial\varphi}(\cos\varphi) \ \hat{x} + \frac{\partial}{\partial\varphi}(\sin\varphi) \ \hat{y} = -\sin\varphi\hat{x} + \cos\varphi\hat{y} = \hat{\varphi} \qquad \blacktriangle$$

We can get the following first-order derivatives:

$$\frac{\partial \hat{\rho}}{\partial \rho} = 0 \qquad\qquad \frac{\partial \hat{\varphi}}{\partial \rho} = 0 \qquad\qquad \frac{\partial \hat{z}}{\partial \rho} = 0$$

$$\frac{\partial \hat{\rho}}{\partial \varphi} = -\sin\varphi\,\hat{x} + \cos\varphi\,\hat{y} = \hat{\varphi} \qquad \frac{\partial \hat{\varphi}}{\partial \varphi} = -\cos\varphi\,\hat{x} - \sin\varphi\,\hat{y} = -\hat{\rho} \qquad \frac{\partial \hat{z}}{\partial \varphi} = 0$$

$$\frac{\partial \hat{\rho}}{\partial z} = 0 \qquad\qquad \frac{\partial \hat{\varphi}}{\partial z} = 0 \qquad\qquad \frac{\partial \hat{z}}{\partial z} = 0$$

Because the position vector is $r = x\,\hat{x} + y\,\hat{y} + z\,\hat{z} = \rho\,\hat{\rho} + z\,\hat{z}$, we have

$$dr = d\left(\rho\,\hat{\rho} + z\,\hat{z}\right) = d\left(\rho\,\hat{\rho}\right) + d\left(z\,\hat{z}\right) = d\rho\,\hat{\rho} + \rho\,d\hat{\rho} + dz\,\hat{z} + z\,d\hat{z}$$

$$dr = d\rho\,\hat{\rho} + \rho\left(\frac{\partial \hat{\rho}}{\partial \rho}\cancel{d\rho} + \frac{\partial \hat{\rho}}{\partial \varphi}d\varphi + \frac{\partial \hat{\rho}}{\partial z}\cancel{dz}\right) + dz\,\hat{z} + z\left(\frac{\partial \hat{z}}{\partial \rho}\cancel{d\rho} + \frac{\partial \hat{z}}{\partial \varphi}\cancel{d\varphi} + \frac{\partial \hat{z}}{\partial z}\cancel{dz}\right)$$

$$dr = d\rho\,\hat{\rho} + \rho\,d\varphi\,\hat{\varphi} + dz\,\hat{z}$$

where we used $d\hat{\rho} = \dfrac{\partial \hat{\rho}}{\partial \rho}d\rho + \dfrac{\partial \hat{\rho}}{\partial \varphi}d\varphi + \dfrac{\partial \hat{\rho}}{\partial z}dz$ and $d\hat{z} = \dfrac{\partial \hat{z}}{\partial \rho}d\rho + \dfrac{\partial \hat{z}}{\partial \varphi}d\varphi + \dfrac{\partial \hat{z}}{\partial z}dz$

For the gradient operation on variable u, we have

$$du = \nabla u \cdot dr = \left[(\nabla u)_\rho\,\hat{\rho} + (\nabla u)_\varphi\,\hat{\varphi} + (\nabla u)_z\,\hat{z}\right] \cdot \left[d\rho\,\hat{\rho} + \rho\,d\varphi\,\hat{\varphi} + dz\,\hat{z}\right]$$

$$du = (\nabla u)_\rho\,d\rho + (\nabla u)_\varphi\,\rho\,d\varphi + (\nabla u)_z\,dz = \frac{\partial u}{\partial \rho}d\rho + \frac{\partial u}{\partial \varphi}d\varphi + \frac{\partial u}{\partial z}dz$$

Matching the two sides of the equation above, we obtain

$$(\nabla u)_\rho = \frac{\partial u}{\partial \rho} \qquad\qquad (\nabla u)_\varphi = \frac{1}{\rho}\frac{\partial u}{\partial \varphi} \qquad\qquad (\nabla u)_z = \frac{\partial u}{\partial z}$$

Therefore, the gradient operator ∇ in cylindrical coordinates is given by

$$\nabla = \nabla_\rho\,\hat{\rho} + \nabla_\varphi\,\hat{\varphi} + \nabla_z\,\hat{z} = \frac{\partial}{\partial \rho}\hat{\rho} + \frac{1}{\rho}\frac{\partial}{\partial \varphi}\hat{\varphi} + \frac{\partial}{\partial z}\hat{z} \qquad (2.14)$$

For the Laplacian operator ∇^2 in cylindrical coordinates (the proof is left as an exercise), we have

$$\nabla^2 = \nabla \cdot \nabla = \frac{1}{\rho}\frac{\partial}{\partial \rho}\left(\rho\frac{\partial}{\partial \rho}\right) + \frac{1}{\rho^2}\frac{\partial^2}{\partial \varphi^2} + \frac{\partial^2}{\partial z^2} \qquad (2.15)$$

2.3.2 The Heat Equation

In general, the heat equation in 3D is

$$c_h \rho_m \frac{\partial T}{\partial t} = \kappa \nabla^2 T + S \tag{2.16}$$

where c_h is the specific heat capacity, κ is the thermal conductivity, S is the heat generation per unit volume, T is the temperature, and ρ_m is the mass density.

As an example, let us consider a block of material that is heated on one side (Figure 2-12). The heating describes the "S" term. The solution to the differential equation will give the temperature of the material as a function of space and time.

Taking the time-independent solution $\partial T / \partial t = 0$ (or a steady state) into consideration, we can simplify Equation (2.16) to

$$0 = \kappa \nabla^2 T + S \tag{2.17}$$

To maintain the equality, the source term of the temperature distribution must be the negative of the input heat. All of the heat must be accounted for (total is zero). From Equation (2.17), we have

$$-\kappa \nabla^2 T = S \tag{2.18}$$

In this book, we primarily deal with cylindrical channels where a heating source is applied to one side of the capillary. By changing the spatial coordinates to cylindrical coordinates and still assuming that the thermal conductivity is spatially invariant in the channel, we get the heat equation

$$c_h \rho_m \frac{\partial T}{\partial t} = \kappa \left[\frac{1}{r} \frac{\partial}{\partial r}\left(r \frac{\partial T}{\partial r} \right) + \frac{1}{r^2} \frac{\partial^2 T}{\partial \varphi^2} + \frac{\partial^2 T}{\partial z^2} \right] + S \tag{2.19}$$

Here, r is the direction radially outward from the center of the channel, ϕ is the angle around the capillary, and z is the direction along the capillary. At the steady state, the left term is zero.

$$0 = \kappa \left[\frac{1}{r} \frac{\partial}{\partial r}\left(r \frac{\partial T}{\partial r} \right) + \frac{1}{r^2} \frac{\partial^2 T}{\partial \varphi^2} + \frac{\partial^2 T}{\partial z^2} \right] + S \tag{2.20}$$

Since the variation is only along the r direction (radially from the capillary center), the equation becomes

$$-\frac{1}{r} \frac{d}{dr}\left(\kappa r \frac{dT}{dr} \right) = S \tag{2.21}$$

This equation is for the steady-state temperature distribution, which by definition is time-independent and eliminates the time derivative of temperature.

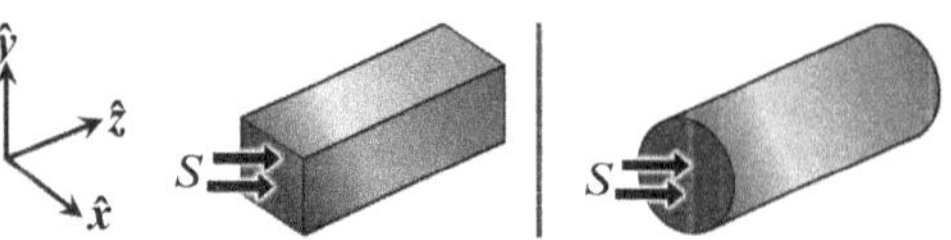

Figure 2-12 (Left) Heating a rectangular-shaped block on one side. (Right) Heating a cylindrical-shaped block on one side.

2.3.3 Joule Heating in a Cylindrical Capillary

Let us consider the source heating term (S) when there is a constant applied voltage (V) and current (I) on the capillary. We treat the capillary as a resistor, with its resistance R determined by the electrical resistivity of the fluid in the capillary, and we find the power dissipation p given the applied voltage.

$$p = IV = \frac{V^2}{R} \tag{2.22}$$

where $R = \rho_r d / A$, with ρ_r being the electrical resistivity, d the length of the capillary, and A the cross-sectional area of the capillary. Or,

$$p = \frac{V^2 A}{\rho_r d} \tag{2.23}$$

Remember that the term S is defined as the power per unit volume. Dividing the power p by the total volume of the capillary Ad and noting that the electric field within the capillary is $E = V/d$, we have

$$S = \frac{p}{Ad} = \frac{V^2}{\rho_r d^2} = \frac{E^2}{\rho_r} \tag{2.24}$$

By replacing the S term in Equation (2.21) with Equation (2.24), we get

$$-\frac{1}{r}\frac{d}{dr}\left(\kappa r \frac{dT}{dr}\right) = \frac{E^2}{\rho_r} \tag{2.25}$$

For a cylindrical capillary (e.g., microchannel) with radius r_0 having a fixed surface temperature of T_0, the temperature in the capillary is (the derivation is left as an exercise)

$$T(r) = \frac{E^2 r_0^{\,2}}{4\rho_r \kappa}\left(1 - \frac{r^2}{r_0^{\,2}}\right) + T_0 \tag{2.26}$$

EXAMPLE 2-5 What is the maximum voltage that can be applied across a 5-cm-long cylindrical microchannel with a radius of 200 μm if the microchannel is filled with a water-like liquid with a boiling point of 100°C, electrical resistivity of $\rho_r = 10^2\ \Omega\cdot\text{m}$, and thermal conductivity of 0.6 W/(K·m)? Assume that the outer wall of the microchannel is a perfect heat sink held at 25°C.

Solution Here we assume that the limiting factor in the applied voltage is Joule heating of the liquid in the capillary. For the sake of simplicity, we also assume that nothing in the system flows until the liquid reaches its boiling point. The temperature of the liquid based on Joule heating is expressed in Equation (2.26). Based on this equation, the maximum temperature is at the center of the channel ($r = 0$). Also, the electric field across the channel is calculated using $E = V/d$ with d being the length of the channel. Thus,

$$T(0) - T_0 = \frac{E^2 r_0^2}{4\rho_r \kappa} = \frac{V^2 r_0^2}{4d^2 \rho_r \kappa}$$

$$V = \sqrt{\frac{4d^2 \rho_r \kappa \left[T(0) - T_0\right]}{r_0^2}} = \sqrt{\frac{4(5\ \text{cm})^2 (10^2\ \Omega\cdot\text{m})[0.6\,\text{W}/(\text{K}\cdot\text{m})](100°\text{C} - 25°\text{C})}{(200\ \mu\text{m})^2}} = 33.5\ \text{kV}$$

Such a high voltage is not practical for driving fluid in microsystems. This heating technology might be applicable to drilling oils in the petroleum industry. ▲

2.4 MECHANICAL FORCES

2.4.1 Reynolds Number

Fluid flow can be laminar, transitional, or turbulent depending on the speed of flow (Figure 2-13). Fluid flow tends to be laminar at low speed and turbulent at high speed. The Reynolds number (Re) of a fluidic system is a dimensionless parameter that is directly related to the inertia of the system. Therefore, this parameter can be used to determine whether a system will experience turbulent flow or laminar flow. The Reynolds number is defined as

$$\mathrm{Re} = \frac{\text{inertial force}}{\text{viscous force}} = \frac{\rho_m L v}{\eta} \tag{2.27}$$

In Equation (2.27), ρ_m is the mass density of the fluid, η is the dynamic viscosity of the fluid, v is the fluid velocity, and L is the characteristic length scale of the system. For cylindrical capillaries and pipes, L is normally equal to the diameter of the circular cross-section. In systems with non-cylindrical geometries, L is not a single set value in the system, such as the radius of a capillary or length of a channel, but rather a more general term relating to the size of the overall system. For microfluidic systems, for example, L is on the order of microns (i.e., micrometers). For this reason, the Reynolds number is a general characteristic of fluidic systems and is used to determine how the system will behave.

- *Re < 2100:* A Reynolds number less than 2100 represents a system where laminar fluid flow likely dominates. Laminar fluid flow is characterized by smooth and layered fluid motion, a lack of fluid mixing, and absence of fluid instabilities such as eddies. Laminar flow occurs in small-sized systems with relatively low fluid velocity, as is the case for microfluidic systems. Given a characteristic length L on the scale of microns and average fluid velocity, microfluidic systems normally have a Reynolds number significantly less than 100, meaning that they are well within the range of laminar flow.

- *2100 ≤ Re ≤ 4000:* A Reynolds number between 2100 and 4000 indicates a system that likely experiences transitional fluid flow, where fluid behavior is in between that of laminar flow and turbulent flow.

- *Re > 4000:* A Reynolds number greater than 4000 usually denotes a system experiencing turbulent fluid flow. Turbulent fluid flow exhibits chaotic fluid instabilities such as eddies and significant fluid mixing. As seen in Equation (2.27), turbulent flow occurs in systems having high-density fluids, faster fluid flow, lower dynamic viscosity, and/or larger overall characteristic size.

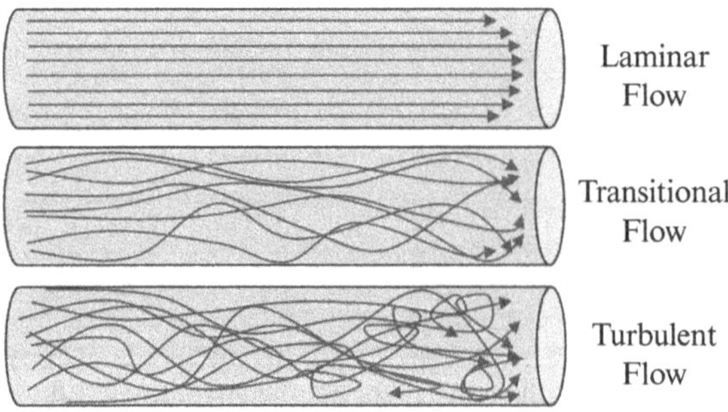

Figure 2-13   Laminar, transitional, and turbulent flows.

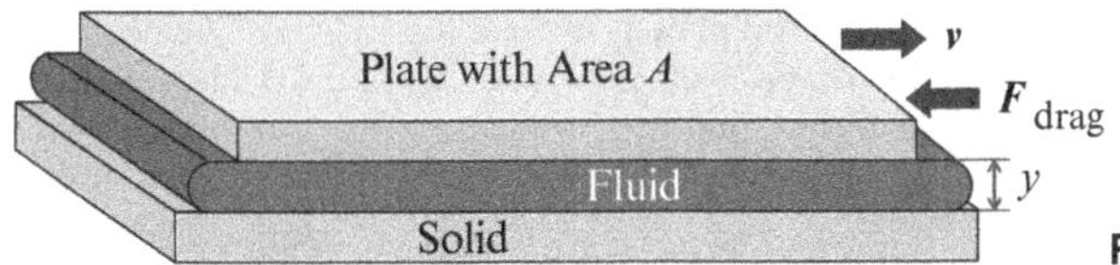

Figure 2-14   Newton's law of viscosity.

EXAMPLE 2-6   Prove that the Reynolds number is dimensionless.

Solution   The Reynolds number as defined in Equation (2.27) is

$$
\text{Re} = \frac{\text{inertial force}}{\text{viscous force}} = \frac{\rho_m L v}{\eta} \quad \Rightarrow \quad [\text{Re}] = \frac{(\text{kg/m}^3)(\text{m})(\text{m/s})}{\text{kg/(m} \cdot \text{s})} \text{ is dimensionless}
$$

where ρ_m is the fluid mass density with units of kg/m^3, L is the characteristic length scale of the system with units of m, v is the fluid velocity with units of m/s, and η is the dynamic viscosity of the fluid with units of Pa $\cdot$ s. In SI units, the pascal is Pa $=$ kg/(m $\cdot$ s^2), so that Pa$\cdot$s $=$ kg/(m$\cdot$s). $\blacktriangle$

2.4.2 Newton's Law of Viscosity

A Newtonian fluid, by definition, has a shear stress F/A proportional to the velocity gradient dv/dy. The proportionality constant is the dynamic viscosity represented by η. Namely,

$$
\eta = \left| \frac{F/A}{dv/dy} \right| \tag{2.28}
$$

where the absolute value sign is required because the dynamic viscosity η cannot be negative.

Figure 2-14 shows Newton's law of viscosity where a plate with an area A is moved with a constant velocity v on a layer of the liquid with thickness y, and a drag force F_{drag} is exerted by the liquid. The fluid in Figure 2-14 can be visualized as layers of molecules between the two plates (Figure 2-15). The top layer sticks perfectly to the top plate (no-slip condition). When the top plate is moved, it drags the top layer of molecules in the fluid with it, and the top layer drags the next layer at a different rate. The viscosity of the fluid is determined by how well each layer moves the next layer along. From Equation (2.28), it is clear that a fluid with infinite viscosity (e.g., a solid) has $dv/dy = 0$, so each layer moves the layer below it perfectly with no delay. In a fluid with zero viscosity (e.g., a gas) such that $dv/dy \to \infty$, only the top layer moves and it does not drag any other layer along with it at all.

2.5 PRESSURE-DRIVEN FLOW (PDF)

It is important to know how forces move fluids in bionanotechnological applications. In such applications, many processes involve diagnostic testing and require different microfluidic technologies. For instance, dissimilar chemical purification and chemical analysis methods need different microfluidic technologies as they involve the transport, separation, and mixing of small volumes of fluids.

Although capillary forces are sufficient for filling capillaries or for making passive valves, other techniques have to be employed to effectively get fluids moving in microfluidic systems. These techniques can be used to get sample across chips, or are used for more active chemical analysis, separation, or fluid mixing. Some of these methods for fluid

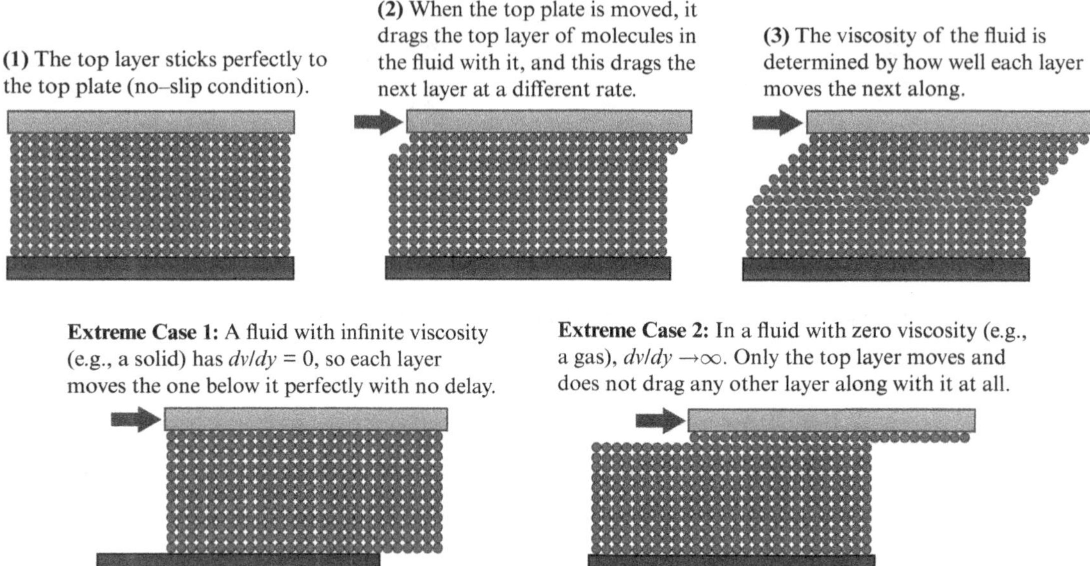

Figure 2-15   The viscosity of the fluid is determined by how well each layer moves the next layer along.

flow are similar to making liquids move through larger systems, but there are some key differences and factors that come into play when the small scales of microfluidic systems are considered. The motion of a fluid as a result of forces acting on it is described by the Navier-Stokes equation

$$\rho_m\left(\frac{\partial \boldsymbol{v}}{\partial t} + \boldsymbol{v}\cdot\boldsymbol{\nabla}\boldsymbol{v}\right) = \boldsymbol{\nabla}\cdot\boldsymbol{T} + \boldsymbol{F} - \boldsymbol{\nabla}P \tag{2.29}$$

where fluid ρ_m is the mass density, $\boldsymbol{v}$ is the fluid velocity, $\boldsymbol{T}$ is the stress tensor, $\boldsymbol{F}$ is the force per unit volume applied to the fluid (sometimes denoted as $\boldsymbol{f}$), and P is the pressure. The left- and right-hand sides of the Navier-Stokes equation (2.29) are in units of N/m^3, or equivalently kg/m^3·m/s^2. Equivalently, $\boldsymbol{F}$ could also be expressed as $\rho_m\boldsymbol{a}$, where $\boldsymbol{a}$ is the body acceleration.

Equation (2.29) can be simplified in the case of non-compressible fluids. In non-compressible fluids, the only entries in the stress tensor ($\boldsymbol{T}$) that are non-zero are shear stresses (off-axis forces) as any perpendicular forces acting on the fluid are counteracted (it does not compress, but it can flow). For these fluids, the shear force on the fluid can be related directly to its viscosity. In Equation (2.29), the stress tensor term $\boldsymbol{T}$ describes the effect of shear forces. For non-compressible fluids, we have

$$\boldsymbol{T} = \eta\boldsymbol{\nabla}\boldsymbol{v} \quad \Rightarrow \quad \boldsymbol{\nabla}\cdot\boldsymbol{T} = \boldsymbol{\nabla}\cdot(\eta\boldsymbol{\nabla}\boldsymbol{v}) = \eta\boldsymbol{\nabla}\cdot\boldsymbol{\nabla}\boldsymbol{v} = \eta\boldsymbol{\nabla}^2\boldsymbol{v}$$

$$\rho_m\left(\frac{\partial \boldsymbol{v}}{\partial t} + \boldsymbol{v}\cdot\boldsymbol{\nabla}\boldsymbol{v}\right) = \eta\boldsymbol{\nabla}^2\boldsymbol{v} + \boldsymbol{F} - \boldsymbol{\nabla}P \tag{2.30}$$

where η is the dynamic viscosity of the fluid. Although this equation is rather complex and cumbersome, it will be simplified and used in several ways as part of derivations in understanding how various applied forces can lead to fluid flow in microfluidic systems.

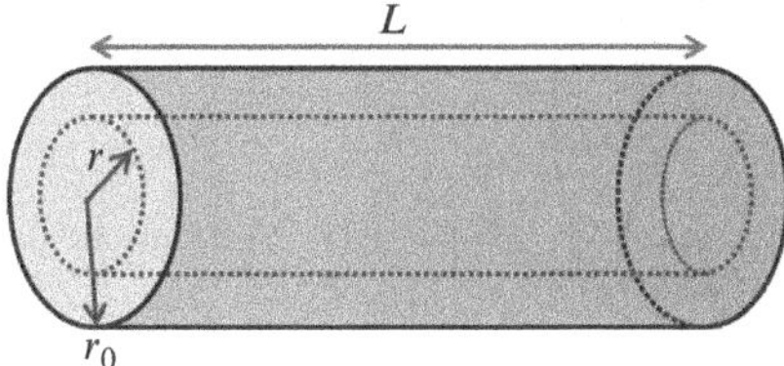

Figure 2-16 The capillary is divided into concentric cylinders for the derivation.

Equation (2.30) describes the motion of a non-compressible fluid due to a force acting on it. In reality, how can we apply the force to move the fluid? Perhaps the most obvious answer is to apply some pressure. Physically pushing fluids works perfectly well in plumbing. Using pumps to move water and letting the force of gravity do the work are other choices. So, can we do the same thing in microfluidics? The short answer is yes. However, there are some important factors we have to consider when moving to the micro-domain.

Let us focus on pressure-driven flow. Pressure-driven flow (PDF), also called Hagen-Poiseuille flow, can be derived for a non-compressible fluid in a cylindrical capillary using Newton's law of viscosity.[14] First, the entire inner area of the capillary with radius r_0 is broken into smaller cylinders with radius r (Figure 2-16). If pressure is applied to fluid in the capillary, the force pushing fluid through the cylinder is $F = A_{\text{cross}} \Delta P = \pi r^2 \Delta P$, where ΔP is the pressure drop across the length L of the cylinder. Next, we apply Newton's law of viscosity along the interface of the fluid's edge. We have

$$\eta = \left| \frac{F/A}{dv/dr} \right| = -\frac{F/A}{dv/dr} \tag{2.31}$$

where the negative sign arises from dv/dr being negative; that is, the fluid velocity v decreases as r increases toward the edge of the cylinder. The dynamic viscosity η must be non-negative.

$$\eta = -\frac{\left(\pi r^2 \Delta P\right)/\left(2\pi r L\right)}{dv/dr} \quad \Rightarrow \quad \frac{dv}{dr} = -\frac{r\Delta P}{2L\eta} \quad \Rightarrow \quad dv = -\frac{r\Delta P}{2L\eta} dr$$

The speed of pressure-driven fluid flow in the entire capillary can be found by integrating the equation above. Namely,

$$v_{\text{PDF}}(r) = \int dv = -\int \frac{r\Delta P}{2L\eta} dr = \frac{-\Delta P}{4L\eta} r^2 + C$$

The integration constant C is obtained by imposing the boundary (no-slip) condition that there is no fluid movement at the surface of the capillary: $v_{\text{PDF}}(r_0) = 0$.

$$v_{\text{PDF}}(r) = \frac{\Delta P\left(r_0^2 - r^2\right)}{4L\eta} \tag{2.32}$$

Equation (2.32) shows the pressure-driven flow (PDF) velocity of the fluid in a capillary (e.g., microchannel) under an applied pressure differential ΔP as a function of the position r along the radius of the capillary. The PDF speed $v_{\text{PDF}}(r)$ is greatest at the center of the capillary ($r = 0$) and decreases to zero at the edges ($r = r_0$). This results in a parabolic flow profile (Figure 2-17).

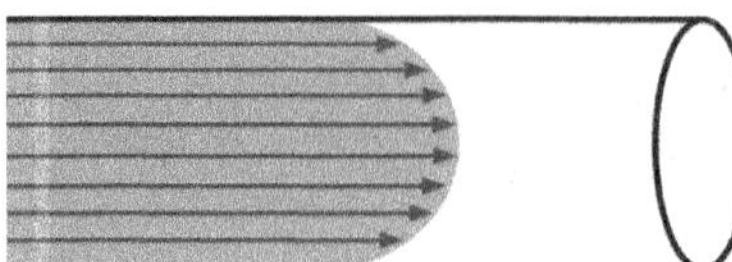

Figure 2-17   A parabolic flow profile in a capillary.

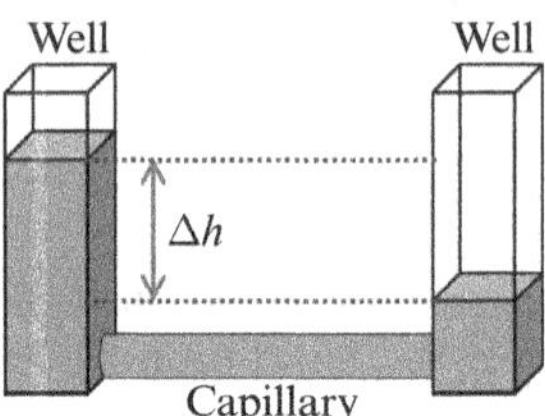

Figure 2-18   The height difference between two wells attached by a capillary generates a gravitational pressure differential, causing flow in the capillary. Without any other applied forces, the buffer level in the two wells will eventually equalize.

The total flow Q_{PDF} (volumetric flow rate) across the entire capillary due to pressure-driven flow is useful and it can be calculated by integrating the flow $v(r)$ over the entire area of the capillary. Thus,

$$Q_{PDF} = \iint_{Area} v_{PDF}(r)\, dA = \int_0^{2\pi} \int_0^{r_0} \frac{\Delta P(r_0^2 - r^2)}{4L\eta}\, r\, dr\, d\theta = \frac{2\pi\Delta P}{4L\eta}\left(r_0^2 \frac{r^2}{2} - \frac{r^4}{4}\right)\Big|_0^{r_0}$$

$$Q_{PDF} = \frac{\pi r_0^4 \Delta P}{8L\eta} \tag{2.33}$$

As seen in Equation (2.33), the total flow Q_{PDF} depends on the fourth power of the radius r_0 of the capillary, indicating that the effect of capillary size greatly exceeds that of the pressure, making pressure-driven flow not very useful in microfluidics where r_0 is tiny. An example in biology is the "fight or flight" response, where blood flow is increased in small capillaries much more effectively by the capillaries dilating rather than by raising blood pressure.

The pressure differential for pressure-driven flow is often supplied by gravity (Figure 2-18). The differences in fluid levels between columns at the inlet and outlet of capillaries result in a force that drives the flow. The pressure differential due to gravity ΔP_g is related to the column height Δh and gravitational acceleration $g = 9.81$ m/s² by

$$\Delta P_g = \rho_m g \Delta h \tag{2.34}$$

2.6 ELECTRO-OSMOTIC FLOW (EOF)

Pressure-driven flow is not always an effective means of moving fluids since it heavily depends on the capillary radius and has a parabolic flow profile, which is not ideal for some applications. So, what is an effective method for moving fluids in a microfluidic system? One method is electro-osmotic flow (EOF). This method uses an applied electric field to push a thin charge layer of ions along the capillary's inner surface, which drags along the rest of the fluid. EOF can be finely tuned and controlled, with the resulting velocity being directly proportional to the applied electric field. Also, unlike the parabolic profile of pressure-driven flow, EOF causes almost all the fluid across the radius of the capillary to travel at the same speed, making the steady transport of samples and buffers much easier. This "plug flow" can be used to inject a segment of sample-containing buffer (the sample may be a chemical, biomolecule, DNA, etc.) into a channel with the buffer on either side. EOF can

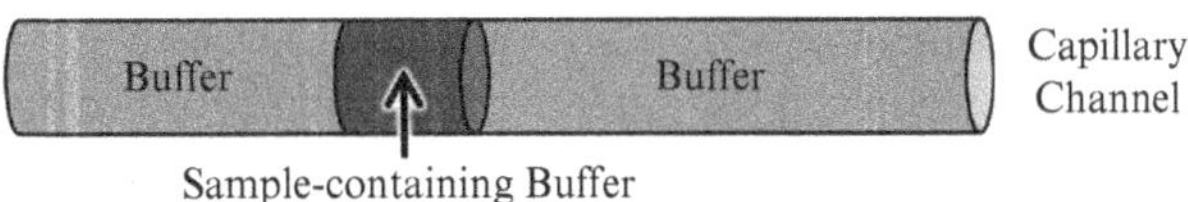

Figure 2-19   "Plug flow" of a segment of sample-containing buffer across a capillary channel.

make this plug of material stay completely intact as it travels across the capillary, which is useful for separating and mixing fluids as well as testing and imaging samples (Figure 2-19).

To understand how to establish and control the formed mobile ion layer for this EOF mechanism to work, we will take a detour through colloids first by diving into Debye screening and zeta potentials.

2.6.1 Debye Length

Debye length is a characteristic length that describes regions of electrical screening. In colloids, this region represents an area where free charges in the continuous phase gather around the charges on a droplet of the dispersed phase. The gathered charges cancel out the charges on the droplet (Figure 2-20), effectively making the droplet "electrically invisible" to charges outside the region defined by the Debye length. Debye length is an important factor in many systems, including colloids, microfluidics, and especially in plasma engineering. Any system with charged bodies interacting with a continuum of dispersed free charges experiences electrical screening and has a characteristic Debye length as a result.[15,16]

The simplest case for deriving and explaining electrical screening and Debye length is a stationary point charge (q) surrounded by a sea of positive and negative free charges, like in an ionic solution or plasma (Figure 2-20).

The stationary charge attracts and repels the free charges, establishing an electric potential defined by Poisson's equation

$$\nabla^2 \phi = \frac{-\rho_c}{\epsilon} \quad \text{with} \quad \epsilon = \epsilon_r \epsilon_0 \tag{2.35}$$

For this system, ϕ is the electric potential, ϵ is the permittivity, $\epsilon_0 = 8.854 \times 10^{-12}$ F/m is the permittivity of free space, ϵ_r is the relative permittivity (also known as the dielectric constant), and ρ_c is the volume charge density describing the charge distribution of the system. In this case, the charge density can be described by the finite negative (e.g., electrons) and positive (e.g., ions) charges which surround the stationary charge. Thus,

$$\rho_c = e\left(n_i - n_e\right) \;\Rightarrow\; \nabla^2 \phi = e\frac{n_e - n_i}{\epsilon} \tag{2.36}$$

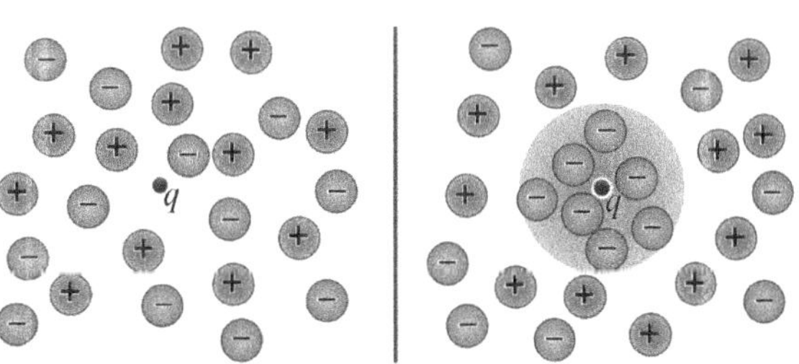

Figure 2-20   (Left) A fixed point charge q in a sea of mobile positive and negative charges. (Right) When q is positive, negative charges gather around the fixed positive charge, and mobile positive charges are repelled. The potential of the fixed charge is canceled out over the area of the large circle due to the gathered charges. The area outside the circle, therefore, is unaffected by the fixed charge and is effectively electrically neutral.

where e is the elementary charge, n_e is the number density (i.e., number per unit volume) of negative charges, and n_i is the number density of positive charges. It is assumed that all ions are singularly charged. The number of charges in a given volume n_e and n_i can be predicted using the Maxwell-Boltzmann distribution given by

$$n_e = n_{e0} \exp\left(\frac{e\phi}{k_BT}\right) \qquad n_i = n_{i0} \exp\left(-\frac{e\phi}{k_BT}\right) \tag{2.37}$$

Here, n_{e0} and n_{i0} are the initial number density distributions of negative and positive charges, respectively, k_B is the Boltzmann constant, and T is the temperature of the system. A differential equation for the potential can be derived by combining Equation (2.37) for the free charges and Poisson's equation for the system given by Equation (2.36) and making the following two assumptions:

(1)   The overall charge of the background fluid is neutral. Thus, $n_{i0} = n_{e0} = n_0$ and

$$\nabla^2\phi = e\frac{n_e - n_i}{\epsilon} = \frac{e}{\epsilon}n_0\left[\exp\left(\frac{e\phi}{k_BT}\right) - \exp\left(\frac{-e\phi}{k_BT}\right)\right] = \left(\frac{n_0e}{\epsilon}\right)2\sinh\left(\frac{e\phi}{k_BT}\right)$$

(2)   Because thermal energy dominates over the electric potential, $\dfrac{e\phi}{k_BT} \ll 1$. We get

$$\nabla^2\phi = \frac{2n_0e}{\epsilon}\sinh\left(\frac{e\phi}{k_BT}\right) \cong \frac{2n_0e}{\epsilon}\frac{e\phi}{k_BT} = \frac{2n_0e^2}{\epsilon k_BT}\phi$$

By defining the Debye screening length λ_{DB}, we obtain

$$\lambda_{DB} \equiv \sqrt{\frac{\epsilon k_BT}{2n_0e^2}} \quad (2.38) \qquad \nabla^2\phi = \frac{2n_0e^2}{\epsilon k_BT}\phi = \left(\frac{1}{\lambda_{DB}}\right)^2\phi \tag{2.39}$$

where n_0 is the univalent number density of ions. Equation (2.39) can be solved in spherical coordinates for the potential as a function of the distance from the fixed charge. In spherical coordinates, the Laplacian ∇^2 is given by (refer to Appendix E)

$$\nabla^2\phi = \frac{1}{r^2}\frac{\partial}{\partial r}\left(r^2\frac{\partial\phi}{\partial r}\right) + \frac{1}{r^2\sin\theta}\frac{\partial}{\partial\theta}\left(\sin\theta\frac{\partial\phi}{\partial\theta}\right) + \frac{1}{r^2\sin^2\theta}\frac{\partial^2\phi}{\partial\varphi^2}$$

Since there is radial symmetry for a fixed-point charge surrounded by a sea of mobile charges, we have

$$\nabla^2\phi = \frac{1}{r^2}\frac{d}{dr}\left(r^2\frac{d\phi}{dr}\right) = \left(\frac{1}{\lambda_{DB}}\right)^2\phi$$

This ordinary differential equation has the general solution

$$\phi(r) = \frac{A}{r}\exp\left(\frac{-r}{\lambda_{DB}}\right) + \frac{B}{r}\exp\left(\frac{r}{\lambda_{DB}}\right)$$

where A and B are constants. The potential should be zero as $r \to \infty$, so $B = 0$. Letting $A = \psi_0$, where ψ_0 has units of $[\text{V}\cdot\text{m}]$, the electric potential $\phi(r)$ of an electrically screened point charge as a function of distance r is

$$\phi(r) = \frac{\psi_0}{r}\exp\left(\frac{-r}{\lambda_{DB}}\right) \tag{2.40}$$

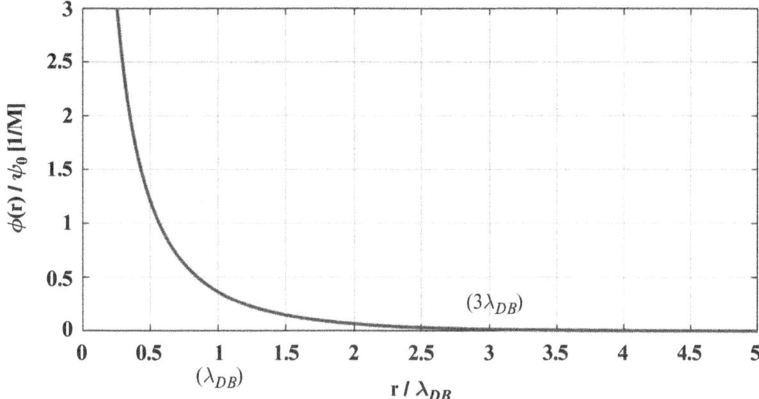

Figure 2-21   Electric potential versus distance of an electrically screened point charge. The electric potential diverges to infinity very close to the point charge (at $r = 0$), and drops off quickly with distance. The potential is not zero at the Debye length, but effectively drops to zero at around $3\lambda_{DB}$.

From Coulomb's law for a point charge, we have

$$\phi_{\text{point charge}}(r) = \frac{1}{4\pi\epsilon}\frac{Q}{r} \quad \Rightarrow \quad \phi_{\text{point charge}}(r = 0) = \pm\infty$$

Therefore, when $r = 0$, $\phi_{\text{point charge}}$ should diverge and approach infinity (the sign depending on whether the point charge Q is positive or negative). This is consistent with Equation (2.40), where the sign depends on whether ψ_0 is positive or negative (i.e., whether the point charge is positive or negative). That is,

$$\phi(r) = \frac{\psi_0}{r}\exp\left(\frac{-r}{\lambda_{DB}}\right) \quad \Rightarrow \quad \phi(r = 0) = \pm\infty$$

Close to the charge (where r is small), the potential of the point charge dominates, so that the potential looks like a regular point charge. However, as r gets closer to the Debye length, the decay term starts to dominate, and the potential quickly drops. At a distance of about $r = 3\lambda_{DB}$, the potential $\phi(r)$ drops off to nearly zero (Figure 2-21). Therefore, other charges far away from the charged particle are completely unaffected, and the particle is effectively screened.

EXAMPLE 2-7   The concept of Debye screening is also very important in understanding emulsions (such as mayonnaise) in which two usually immiscible substances are combined to form a stable matrix. In the case of mayonnaise, the emulsion is formed between oil and water and is stabilized by egg yolk. In this emulsion, small oil droplets are dispersed in the surrounding water. Under normal conditions, the hydrophobic oil droplets would coalesce to form a separate oil layer. However, due to Debye screening, the oil droplets cannot "see" each other and cannot merge to form a distinct separate layer. For the sake of simplicity, let us treat an oil droplet as a point charge (with charge q) in pure water (pH $= 7$). Assume that the water has a relative permittivity (dielectric constant) of 80 and neglect the effect of any stabilizers.

(a) What is the Debye length in this system at room temperature (298 K)?

(b) What would be the Debye length of the system if the water contains 0.1 mM of salt (NaCl), assuming that the relative permittivity remains the same?

Solution

(a) Water at pH 7 means that the concentration of both hydrogen and hydroxide ions is 10^{-7} M. Therefore, the univalent charge number density is

$$n_0 = \left[6.022 \times 10^{26}\,\text{L/(mol}\cdot\text{m}^3)\right]\left(10^{-7}\,\text{M}\right) = 6.022 \times 10^{19}\ \text{m}^{-3}$$

The Debye length can be calculated from Equation (2.38) as follows.

$$\lambda_{DB\ (\text{original})} = \sqrt{\frac{\epsilon k_B T}{2 n_0 e^2}} = \sqrt{\frac{80\left(8.854 \times 10^{-12}\,\text{F/m}\right)\left(1.38 \times 10^{-23}\,\text{J/K}\right)\left(298\text{K}\right)}{2\left(6.022 \times 10^{19}\ \text{m}^{-3}\right)\left(1.6 \times 10^{-19}\ \text{C}\right)^2}} = 972\ \text{nm}$$

(b) For salt water, we can combine the ions from salt and those initially in the water. Thus, the univalent charge number density is

$$n_0 = \left[6.022 \times 10^{26}\,\text{L/}\left(\text{mol}\cdot\text{m}^3\right)\right]\left(0.1\ \text{mM} + 10^{-7}\,\text{M}\right) = 6.028 \times 10^{22}\ \text{m}^{-3}$$

$$\lambda_{DB\ (\text{with salt})} = \sqrt{\frac{\epsilon k_B T}{2 n_0 e^2}} = \sqrt{\frac{80\left(8.854 \times 10^{-12}\,\text{F/m}\right)\left(1.38 \times 10^{-23}\,\text{J/K}\right)\left(298\text{K}\right)}{2\left(6.028 \times 10^{22}\ \text{m}^{-3}\right)\left(1.6 \times 10^{-19}\ \text{C}\right)^2}} = 30.7\ \text{nm}$$

Therefore, the addition of 0.1 mM of salt (NaCl) decreased the Debye length λ_{DB} by a factor of ~32. ▲

Emulsions and colloids are stabilized by electrostatic interactions. Reducing the Debye screening length weakens the electrostatic interactions. Therefore, the addition of salt destabilizes emulsions.[17]

Now, we move from a point charge to a charged plane. When immersed in liquid, materials such as glass gain a surface charge. This fixed charge layer forms on the inside of capillary walls. Similar to the point charge, with a buffer in the channel containing free ions, there is a mobile charge distribution around the fixed charged plane. Free ions will be drawn to or pushed away from the fixed charges, screening and canceling out the effect of the fixed charges (Figure 2-22). We will follow the same procedure as for the point charge to derive the electric potential as a function of the distance away from the charged wall.

First, the electric potential ϕ can be described using Poisson's equation (2.35). Furthermore, this charge distribution can be represented by summing the Boltzmann distributions of every free charged entity in the system (i.e., the cations and anions in the buffer within a capillary). We have

$$\nabla^2 \phi = \frac{-\rho_c}{\epsilon} = -\frac{1}{\epsilon}\sum_i n_i e z_i \exp\left(\frac{-z_i e \phi}{k_B T}\right) \tag{2.41}$$

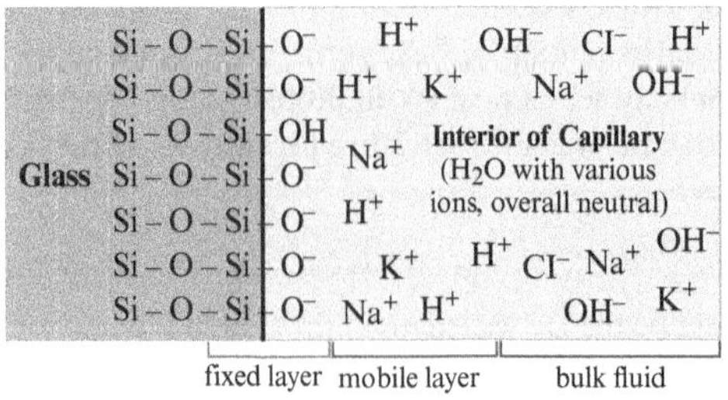

Figure 2-22 A glass surface gains a negative charge in an aqueous environment. The resulting electrically screened system has a fixed charge layer and a mobile layer of free-floating ions. Here, the fixed layer is negatively charged, the mobile layer is positively charged, and the bulk fluid is overall electrically neutral.

where ϕ is the electric potential, ϵ is the permittivity, ρ_c is the volume charge density, n_i is the initial number density distribution of the ith charged element, e is the elementary charge, z_i is the charge of the ith element (e.g., $+1$ for singly charged cations and -1 for singly charged anions), k_B is the Boltzmann constant, and T is the temperature of the system.

Equation (2.41) is a general expression, which considers any number of different free charged species in the system based on their charge and initial distribution. For the sake of simplicity, here we will only consider the case where ions are singularly charged, and the number of positive ions equals the number of negative ions, for total electrical neutrality. Thus, $z_1 = -z_2 = 1$ and $n_1 = n_2 = n_0$. We have

$$\nabla^2\phi = \frac{en_0}{\epsilon}\left[\exp\left(\frac{e\phi}{k_BT}\right) - \exp\left(\frac{-e\phi}{k_BT}\right)\right] \tag{2.42}$$

At this stage, it is the same as with the point charge, and we just need to simplify this equation using the same assumptions and approximations as before to get

$$\nabla^2\phi = \frac{2e^2n_0}{\epsilon k_BT} = \frac{1}{\lambda_{DB}^2}\phi(y) \quad \text{with} \ \lambda_{DB} = \sqrt{\frac{\epsilon k_BT}{2n_0e^2}} \tag{2.43}$$

Now, instead of solving the equation in spherical coordinates, we solve it to obtain the potential at a distance y away from the fixed charge wall, with the boundary condition that the potential at the wall is ϕ_0. The Laplacian ∇^2 simplifies to the second derivative as follows:

$$\nabla^2\phi(y) = \frac{d^2\phi(y)}{dy^2} = \frac{1}{\lambda_{DB}^2}\phi(y) \quad \text{with} \ \phi(0) = \phi_0$$

From which the following solution can be obtained:

$$\phi(y) = \phi_0\exp\left(\frac{-y}{\lambda_{DB}}\right) = \zeta\exp\left(\frac{-y}{\lambda_{DB}}\right) \tag{2.44}$$

Again, like in the case of electrical screening around a point charge, the potential of a screened surface is the same as the case without screening close to the charged surface, but it decreases exponentially with the distance away from the surface. In this case, the potential at the surface, ϕ_0, is also called the zeta potential and is denoted as ζ.

There are a few more methods other than the Poisson-Boltzmann method shown above for deriving electrical screening. Those methods are sometimes more suitable for specific systems or are more accurate, but at the expense of much more complex calculations. For instance, the Poisson-Nernst-Planck (PNP) method is most suitable for finite element analysis simulations. The software can track the motion of individual ions in a solution to find the overall potential of these ions as they are influenced by a charged body. While rigorous, it requires the use of simulation software to calculate electrical screening. Its derivation starts with Poisson's equation (2.35), the same way as the Poisson-Boltzmann method. Again, ρ_c is the volume charge density contributed by the ions in solution. ρ_c is related to the concentration of each type of ion in the solution by

$$\nabla^2\phi = \frac{-\rho_c}{\epsilon} \quad \text{with} \ \rho_c = eN_A\sum_i c_iz_i \tag{2.45}$$

Here, c_i is the molar concentration of each ion as a function of location in the system, e is the elementary charge, N_A is Avogadro's number, and $z_i = q_i/e$ is the charge number (i.e., valence). Initially, the distribution of ions is uniform. However, the ions will drift because of the applied voltage, resulting in variations of the overall concentration. The change in the molar concentration c_i of each ion over time t is described by the Nernst-Planck equation

$$\frac{\partial c_i}{\partial t} = \boldsymbol{\nabla} \cdot \left[D_i \boldsymbol{\nabla} c_i - c_i \boldsymbol{u} + \frac{D_i z_i e}{k_B T} c_i \left(\boldsymbol{\nabla} \phi + \frac{\partial \boldsymbol{A}_M}{\partial t} \right) \right] \tag{2.46}$$

where D_i is the diffusion coefficient of the ion, $\boldsymbol{u}$ is the fluid velocity, k_B is the Boltzmann constant, T is the temperature, and $\boldsymbol{A}_M$ is the magnetic vector potential. Since the fluid is stationary ($\boldsymbol{u} = \boldsymbol{0}$) and there are no significant magnetic fields ($\boldsymbol{A}_M = \boldsymbol{0}$), this equation can be simplified as

$$\frac{\partial c_i}{\partial t} = \boldsymbol{\nabla} \cdot \left[D_i \boldsymbol{\nabla} c_i + \frac{D_i z_i e}{k_B T} c_i \boldsymbol{\nabla} \phi \right] \tag{2.47}$$

Using these equations, the concentrations of ions c_i can be calculated over time based on the electric potential ϕ, and then a new potential ϕ can be calculated based on the new ion concentrations c_i. This process repeats until the potential stabilizes and electrical screening is established.

2.6.2 Electro-Osmotic Flow (EOF) Equation

Debye lengths and electrical screening are important in fluid flow because of electro-osmotic flow (EOF). EOF provides an effective way to transport fluids, which is among the many applications and consequences of electrical screening. Electrical screening in microfluidic capillaries (e.g., microchannels) combined with an applied voltage results in EOF.

In the derivation of electrical screening over a charged surface, it was pointed out that the conclusions could also be used to describe electrical screening established on the inside of a capillary filled with an ion-containing buffer. In this case, the inside of the capillary is the charged surface and an oppositely charged mobile layer of ions forms beside this surface. By applying a DC voltage along the capillary from one end to the other end, the established longitudinal electric field pushes the charged mobile layer of ions along the capillary. From the discussion of viscosity before, we know that if a layer of fluid moves, it drags other layers of the fluid along with it. In this case, the moving layer of mobile ions then drags along the rest of the fluid along with them. Figure 2-23 illustrates how EOF works.

To better control EOF for its application in microfluidic systems, we need to know the factors influencing EOF. We can start with the Navier-Stokes equation

$$\rho_m \left(\frac{\partial \boldsymbol{v}}{\partial t} + \boldsymbol{v} \cdot \boldsymbol{\nabla} \boldsymbol{v} \right) = \eta \nabla^2 \boldsymbol{v} + \boldsymbol{F} - \boldsymbol{\nabla} P \tag{2.48}$$

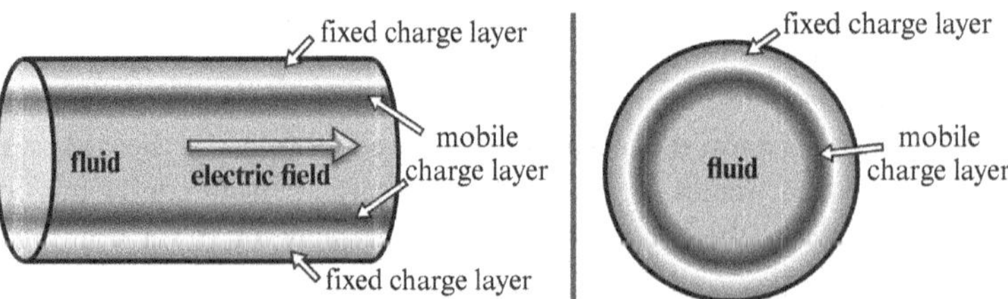

Figure 2-23   The fixed and mobile charge layers that form in a capillary. (Left) Lateral view showing the charge layers along the capillary wall and the direction of the applied electric field for EOF. The direction of the electric field together with the sign of the zeta potential of the capillary wall determines the direction of fluid flow. (Right) Cross-sectional view of the capillary showing the fixed and mobile charge layers.

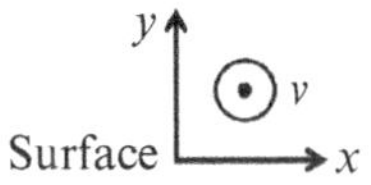

Figure 2-24   For EOF flow along a capillary, the x-axis is along the inner surface of the capillary, the y-axis points toward the center of the capillary, and the direction of fluid flow is down the capillary (out of the page).

We simplify this equation by making the following assumptions. First, the flow is in steady state, such that $\partial v / \partial t = 0$. Second, the direction of flow is down the capillary only and therefore is perpendicular to both the cross-sectional area of the capillary and the y-(radial) direction (Figure 2-24). Hence, the dot product $v \cdot \nabla v$ is zero (the proof is left as an exercise). Finally, due to the small scales involved, the effects of pressure in this case are negligible.

$$\rho_m \left(\frac{\partial \cancel{v}}{\cancel{\partial t}} + \cancel{v \cdot \nabla v} \right) = \eta \nabla^2 v + F - \cancel{\nabla P}$$

After simplification, we are left with

$$\eta \nabla^2 v = -F \tag{2.49}$$

The force acting on the fluid per unit volume (F) caused by an externally applied electric field (E) is dependent on the volume charge density of the fluid (ρ_c), which describes the charge distribution. Thus,

$$\eta \nabla^2 v = -F = -\rho_c E \tag{2.50}$$

As we have seen a few times by now, the volume charge density is related to the potential in the system described by Poisson's equation (2.35). By combining Poisson's equation and the Navier-Stokes equation with an applied electric field as shown in Equation (2.50), we get

$$\nabla^2 \phi = \frac{-\rho_c}{\epsilon} \quad \Rightarrow \quad \eta \nabla^2 v = \epsilon E \nabla^2 \phi \tag{2.51}$$

We have an expression for the potential $\phi(y)$ as a function of the distance away from the capillary wall y given by $\phi(y) = \zeta \exp\left(\frac{-y}{\lambda_{DB}} \right)$. Taking advantage of the fact that both $v = v(y) \, \hat{z}$ and $\phi(y)$ are functions of y only and thus the ∇^2 operator is just the second derivative with respect to y. Assuming that the electric field $E = E \hat{z}$ is applied longitudinally and does not depend on y, we have

$$\eta \frac{d^2 v(y)}{dy^2} = \epsilon E \frac{d^2 \phi(y)}{dy^2} \quad \text{and} \quad \frac{d^2 \phi(y)}{dy^2} = \frac{\zeta}{\lambda_{DB}^2} \exp\left(\frac{-y}{\lambda_{DB}} \right) = \frac{1}{\lambda_{DB}^2} \phi(y)$$

$$\frac{d^2 v(y)}{dy^2} = \frac{\epsilon E}{\eta} \frac{1}{\lambda_{DB}^2} \phi(y) \tag{2.52}$$

Now we find the expression for EOF by integrating Equation (2.52) twice (left as an exercise). Using the no-slip boundary condition that there is no fluid motion at the wall, or $v(0) = 0$, we obtain

$$v_{EOF}(y) = v(y) = \frac{\epsilon E}{\eta} \phi(y) + K_1 y + K_2 \quad \text{with} \quad K_1 = 0 \quad \text{and} \quad K_2 = \frac{-\epsilon E \zeta}{\eta} \tag{2.53}$$

$$v_{EOF}(y) = \frac{-\epsilon \zeta}{\eta} E \left[1 - \frac{\phi(y)}{\zeta} \right] \tag{2.54}$$

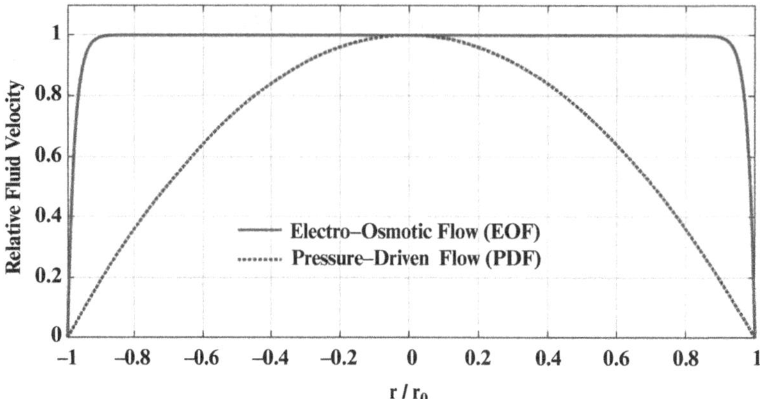

Figure 2-25   A graph comparing the velocity profiles of EOF and pressure-driven flow. Pressure-driven flow has a parabolic cross-section, with the maximum velocity at the center of the channel. EOF has a maximum constant velocity across nearly the entire channel.

At a distance greater than the Debye length ($y > \lambda_{DB}$), the potential is effectively screened out (i.e., $\phi \to 0$). Thus, the velocity is essentially a constant value for the majority of fluid in the capillary. We have

$$v_{EOF} = \frac{-\epsilon \zeta}{\eta} E = \mu_{EOF} E \quad \text{where} \quad \mu_{EOF} = \frac{-\epsilon \zeta}{\eta} \tag{2.55}$$

This is the final expression for EOF. The term $-\epsilon\zeta/\eta$, which is constant for a given system, is referred to as the EOF mobility μ_{EOF}.

Unlike the parabolic profile of pressure-driven flow in a capillary, EOF is constant when it is sufficiently far from the capillary wall. Sufficiently far from the capillary wall means more than a few Debye lengths away from the wall. In general, the Debye screening length λ_{DB} for capillary systems is on the order of nanometers to micrometers, so only a very thin layer of molecules is in the ill-defined zone close to the capillary wall. Thus, it can generally be assumed that all of the fluid is moving at the same EOF speed. Figure 2-25 shows a comparison of the velocity profiles of EOF and pressure-driven flow.

2.6.3 Zeta Potential

As stated before, the concept of zeta potential, or the electrical potential on a charged surface, is generated from the derivation of electrical screening above a charged plane. We also saw—in electrical screening over a charged plane—how a mobile charge layer of ions formed at about the Debye length away from the plane, where the potential drops to approximately zero. This concept is illustrated in Figure 2-26.

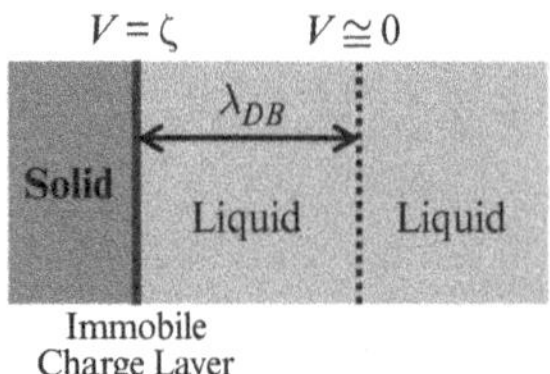

Figure 2-26   The immobile charge layer and the mobile charge layer of ions form a parallel plate capacitor, with two charged layers being separated by a dielectric.

Assuming that the immobile layer has a surface charge density of σ_c and an area of A (making its total charge $q = \sigma_c A$), the "capacitor" shown in Figure 2-26 has a voltage of

$$V = \zeta = \frac{q}{C} = \frac{\sigma_c A}{C} \tag{2.56}$$

The capacitance C and zeta potential ζ can be found using the dimensions of the system as well as the permittivity of the dielectric (in this case the liquid between the immobile and mobile charge layers). Namely,

$$C = \frac{\epsilon A}{\lambda_{DB}} \quad \Rightarrow \quad \zeta = \frac{\sigma_c \lambda_{DB}}{\epsilon} \tag{2.57}$$

Combining Equation (2.57) with the definition of electro-osmotic mobility μ_{EOF}, we get

$$\mu_{EOF} = \frac{-\epsilon \zeta}{\eta} = \frac{-\sigma_c \lambda_{DB}}{\eta} \tag{2.58}$$

All of the parameters including surface charge density σ_c, Debye screening length λ_{DB}, and dynamic viscosity η in Equation (2.58) can be controlled and engineered for a specific system. Therefore, the EOF mobility can be controlled in any application.

In addition, zeta potential is a key parameter reflecting the stability of colloids, suspensions, and emulsions—a higher zeta potential magnitude $|\zeta|$ corresponds to greater product stability. There are commercial zeta-potential analyzers which can be used to measure and calculate the zeta potential of a given material (e.g., nanoparticles). Two methods are commonly used by zeta-potential analyzers. One method measures the velocity of charged particles in an applied electrical field. The other method measures the electric charge of the moving particles by using ultrasound waves to create motion.[18]

EXAMPLE 2-8
Measuring the
Zeta Potential

A microchannel filled with a buffer solution has a voltage of V applied to the left end, with the right end grounded (Figure 2-27). The microchannel has a length of L, while the buffer has permittivity ϵ and dynamic viscosity η. At a certain time, the buffer is switched to a new buffer (with the same permittivity and viscosity) that has a different color. Assuming that EOF is the only significant source of flow and neglecting diffusion, the new buffer travels through the channel. It takes t seconds for the new color of buffer to completely fill the channel. What is the zeta potential of this system?

Solution   Assuming that only EOF is significant, the velocity of the fluid in the channel is constant and is related to the applied electric field by

$$v = v_{EOF} = \mu_{EOF} E$$

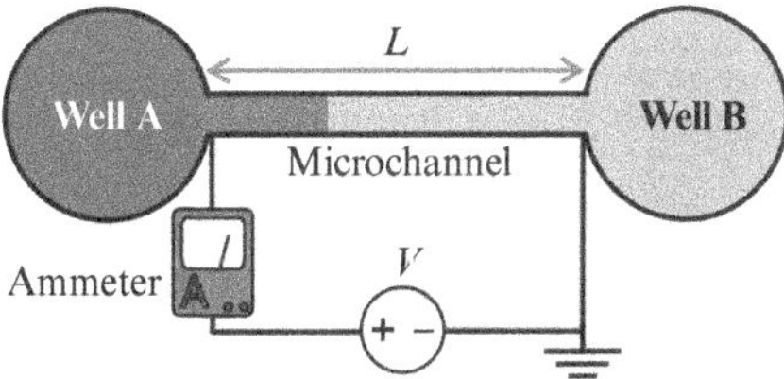

Figure 2-27   A setup for measuring the zeta potential of a microchannel system. For the sign convention, please refer to Appendix D.

In terms of the known parameters and noting the sign convention (please refer to Appendix D), we have

$$v = \mu_{EOF} E \quad \Rightarrow \quad \frac{L}{t} = \frac{-\epsilon\zeta}{\eta}\frac{V}{L} \quad \Rightarrow \quad \zeta = \frac{-\eta L^2}{V\epsilon t}$$

Note: An alternative way of measuring travel time is to let the second buffer have much higher electrical conductivity than the first buffer and to measure the change in electrical current through the channel as the new buffer is introduced. This current would steadily increase and levels off as soon as the new buffer completely fills the channel.[19] ▲

2.7 PROBLEMS

2-1 (Short-Answer). **(a)** Give an example of shear stress in liquids and solids.

(b) Would fluid in the sinusoidal pipe shown in the figure below exhibit turbulent pressure-driven flow? On what factors will that depend?

(c) Does the zeta potential (ζ) change in a wider capillary due to reduced curvature of the capillary? Why or why not?

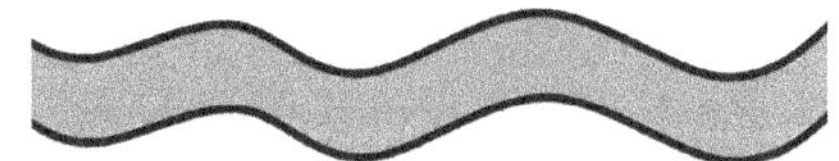

2-2. A bioMEMS device (as shown below) contains two joined microchannels that have circular cross-sections, which are capillaries with radii of 10 μm and 100 μm, respectively. The device is connected to two wells. The fabrication process has led to a contact angle (with water) of 120°. The water-air surface tension is 72 mN/m, and water has a mass density of $\rho_m = 10^3\,\mathrm{kg/m^3}$.

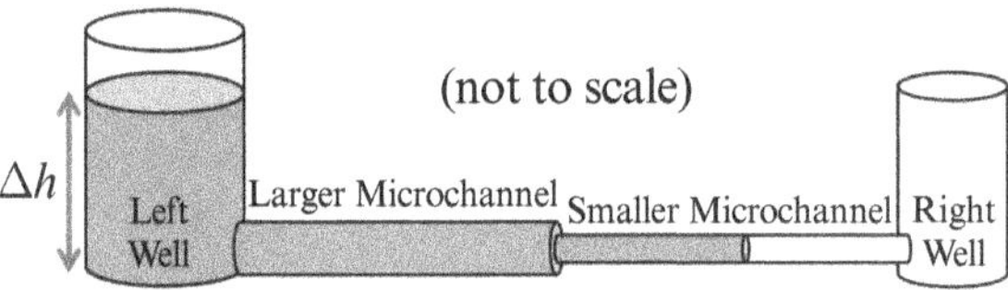

(a) How much capillary pressure is required to fill the larger microchannel with water?

(b) How much capillary pressure is required to fill the smaller microchannel with water?

(c) If a column of water (with height $h = 10$ cm) is connected to the well of the bigger channel, which channels would fill?

2-3. The microfluidic device illustrated below (reprinted with permission from A. Puntambekar et al.[9]) is designed to deliver specific volumes of fluids using pressure-driven flow and passive valves.

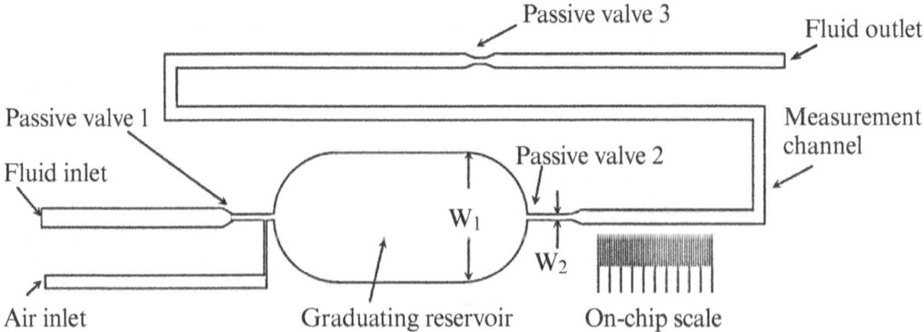

There are four main sections in the device: fluid inlet (with radius of 100 μm), graduating reservoir, measurement channel, and fluid outlet. The graduating reservoir is a large chamber for containing the designed volume of fluid. The measurement channel and fluid outlet both have a radius of 100 μm. There are three passive valves. Passive valve 1 (with radius of r_1) is in between the inlet and the reservoir. Passive valve 2 (with radius of r_2) is in between the reservoir and the measurement channel. Passive valve 3 (with radius of r_3) is in between the measurement channel and the fluid outlet. Assume that all channels are circular with direct transitions between the different channel radii, $r_3 < r_2 < r_1 < 100$ μm, the contact angle of water throughout the device is 130°, and the water-air surface tension is 72 mN/m.

(a) What pressure range is required to push fluid into the graduating reservoir (but not into the measuring channel) from the fluid input (in terms of r_1 and r_2)?

(b) After the graduating reservoir is filled, an air pressure of P is applied to move the fluid to the measurement channel. What are the minimum or maximum values of r_2 and r_3 required to ensure that the fluid stays in the measurement channel?

(c) Although it is useful in applications like this, why is pressure-driven flow not as significant (or useful) in microfluidics as in larger systems?

2-4. Millions of diabetic patients worldwide benefit from portable blood glucose meters. To test blood glucose levels, the user collects a blood sample via pinprick onto a glucometer test strip. Suppose that a hypothetical glucometer test strip design relies on a microchannel with porous walls for transporting the collected blood into the rest of the test strip. The physical properties of blood and the microchannel are $\rho_m = 1050$ kg/m³, $\gamma_{LG} = 58$ mN/m, $\theta_c = 60°$, and $L = 1.0$ cm.

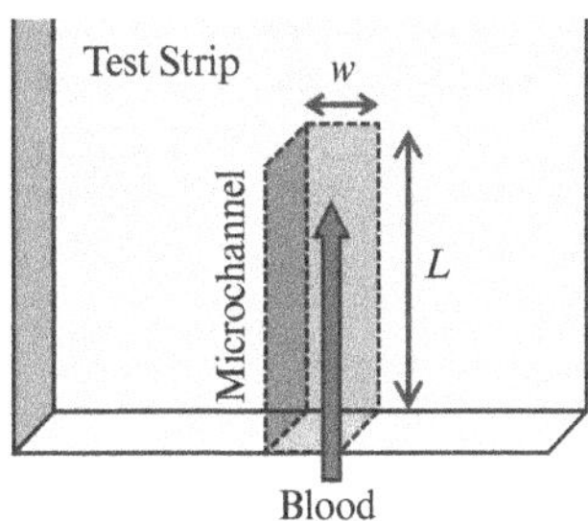

(a) List two advantages of using the microchannel with porous walls in the test strip for transporting collected blood.

(b) The microchannel has a square cross-section with side length w, and must be able to transport blood regardless of the angle the test strip is held at. To ensure that the microchannel will function as intended, how small should w be?

Hint: Consider the extreme case when the test strip is held vertically where the capillary pressure is opposed by the vertical pressure due to gravity.

2-5. Derive the Laplacian $\nabla^2 = \nabla \cdot \nabla$ in cylindrical coordinates (Appendix E) as given below.

$$\nabla^2 = \nabla \cdot \nabla = \frac{1}{\rho}\frac{\partial}{\partial \rho}\left(\rho\frac{\partial}{\partial \rho}\right) + \frac{1}{\rho^2}\frac{\partial^2}{\partial \varphi^2} + \frac{\partial^2}{\partial z^2} \quad \text{where} \quad \nabla = \left(\frac{\partial}{\partial \rho}\hat{\rho} + \frac{1}{\rho}\frac{\partial}{\partial \varphi}\hat{\varphi} + \frac{\partial}{\partial z}\hat{z}\right)$$

2-6. In spherical coordinates, prove that $\phi_{\text{wrong}}(r) = \phi_0 \exp\left(\dfrac{-r}{\lambda_{DB}}\right)$ is not the correct solution of $\nabla^2 \phi(r) = \left(\dfrac{1}{\lambda_{DB}}\right)^2 \phi(r)$, and show that the correct solution is $\phi_{\text{correct}}(r) = \dfrac{\psi_0}{r}\exp\left(\dfrac{-r}{\lambda_{DB}}\right)$.

Hint: Use the identity for ∇^2 in Appendix E. ϕ_0 and ψ_0 are constants.

2-7. A bioMEMS device is fabricated from a material having high thermal conductivity. The material behaves like a perfect heat-sink, so that the channel walls are fixed at temperature T_0. The buffer used has a resistivity of $\rho_r = 10^2$ Ω·m and a thermal conductivity (water-like) of 0.6 W/(K·m).

(a) Starting from Equation (2.25)—the time-independent heat equation in cylindrical coordinates— derive the following temperature versus radius equation in a capillary of radius r_0.

$$T(r) = \frac{E^2 r_0^2}{4\rho_r \kappa}\left(1 - \frac{r^2}{r_0^2}\right) + T_0$$

(b) If an electric field of 10^6 V/m is applied, what is the temperature at the core ($r = 0$) of the channel, assuming that the radius of the channel is $r_0 = 100$ μm?

(c) Using computer software, generate a graph of $T(r) - T_0$ versus radial position r.

2-8. Starting from the Navier-Stokes equation for a microcapillary oriented along the z-axis:

$$\rho_m\left(\frac{\partial v}{\partial t} + v \cdot \nabla v\right) = \eta \nabla^2 v + F - \nabla P \quad \text{where} \quad v = v_{\text{EOF}}(y)\,\hat{z}$$

and omitting some detailed steps, we end up with the following equation for the potential $\phi(y)$ as a function of the distance away from the capillary wall y given by

$$v_{\text{EOF}}(y) = \frac{-\epsilon\zeta}{\eta}E\left(1 - \frac{\phi(y)}{\zeta}\right) \quad \text{where} \quad \phi(y) = \zeta\exp\left(\frac{-y}{\lambda_{\text{DB}}}\right)$$

For steady-state microcapillary EOF applications with a constant applied electric field $E = E\,\hat{z}$:

(a) Why is $v \cdot (\nabla v) = 0$?

(b) Why do we assume that $\nabla P = 0$?

(c) Derive $v_{\text{EOF}}(y) = \frac{-\epsilon\zeta}{\eta}E\left(1 - \frac{\phi(y)}{\zeta}\right)$.

2-9. Consider the glass capillary section in the initial state, as shown in the figure below. Both liquids have the same physical properties, with $\epsilon = 80\,\epsilon_0$ and $\eta = 0.89 \times 10^{-3}$ Pa · s. The zeta potential of the glass surface is $\zeta = -0.15$ V. For the sign convention, please refer to Appendix D.

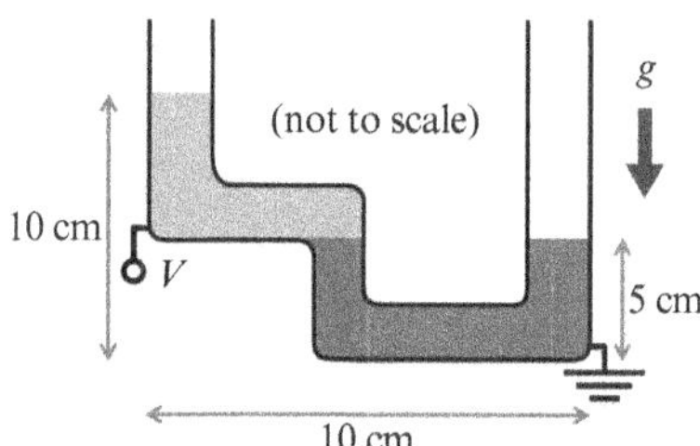

(a) If there is no applied voltage (i.e., $V = 0$), what is the position of the liquids at equilibrium?

(b) If a voltage source of $V = +3000$ V is applied across the capillary, calculate the fluid speed v_{EOF} due to EOF and draw a rough sketch of the steady state achieved.

(c) What happens if the polarity is reversed? Is there a change in profile at the intersection of the light/dark fluids right after a polarity reversal?

Note: To calculate the electric field, it is assumed that the effective length of the bottom section of the capillary tube is 10 cm + 5 cm = 15 cm. You may assume that the electric field magnitude throughout the bottom section of the capillary is constant. In reality, the electric field throughout the bottom capillary section will not be uniform due to the two bends.

2-10. Two columns are linked by a cylindrical glass capillary with length of 10 cm and radius of 100 μm. Each column is filled with 10 mm (fluid height) of a buffer, which has the same density as water. A voltage of 1000 V is applied between the columns. The zeta potential of the glass is +0.1 V. For the buffer, $\epsilon = 80\,\epsilon_0$ and $\eta = 0.89 \times 10^{-3}$ Pa · s. For the sign convention, refer to Appendix D.

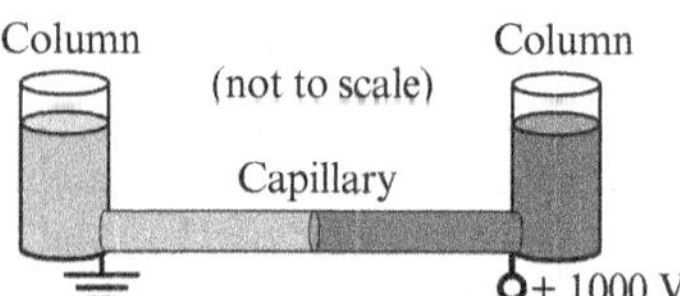

(a) How fast is the fluid flow due to EOF?

(b) Neglecting evaporation, the capillary will come to a steady state. Why?

Hint: Consider pressure-driven flow arising from the height difference of the buffer levels.

(c) At steady state, what is the height difference between the columns?

(d) Uncharged colored dyes are mixed into the columns, with light dye in the left column and dark dye in the right column. What would the capillary cross-section look like at the capillary midpoint shortly after reaching equilibrium, but before diffusion/mixing happens? Explain your answer. *Note:* Fluid in the left column (light) is at a lower height than fluid in the right column (dark).

2-11. We have a glass tube with a length of $d = 10$ mm and side dimensions of 50 μm × 50 μm (i.e., the tube cross-section is a 50 μm × 50 μm square). We want to propel liquid to elongate a red band of DNA with an initial width of 20 μm. The red DNA band sits vertically in the glass tube in pH $= 7$ pure water. Our goal is to use EOF to elongate the DNA band by varying the temperature at the top and bottom of the tube to achieve different flow rates (refer to the figures below).

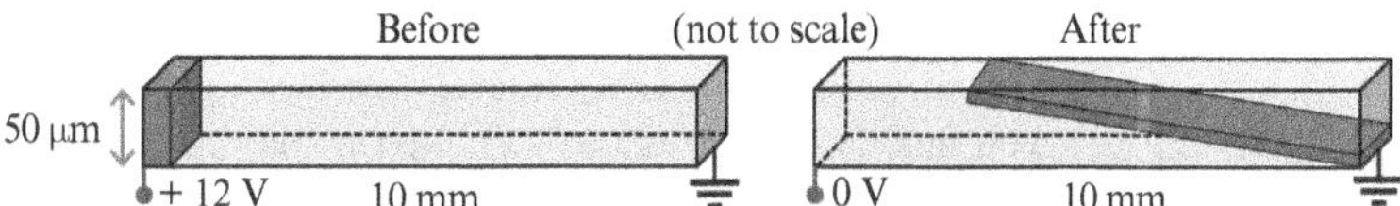

Electrical contacts on either end of the tube allow one side of the tube to be maintained at 12V DC with the other side being grounded. Large reservoirs are connected to both ends of the tube. Assume that pressure-driven flow is negligible. The double-layer capacitance formed by the charged inner glass tube surface and a mobile charge layer of ions at about one Debye length away is 150 pF. The zeta potential at the glass-liquid interface is -62 mV. A stable temperature can be provided at anywhere between 77 K using liquid nitrogen and 310 K using a hot plate. The relative permittivity of pure water is $\epsilon_r = 80$. The dynamic viscosity of pure water $\eta(T)$ is given by the following formula, where T is in kelvins [K]:

$$\eta(T) = 2.414 \cdot 10^{-5} \times 10^{\frac{247.8K}{T-140K}} \ [\mathrm{Pa \cdot s}]$$

(a) At what temperatures should we maintain the top and bottom of the glass tube to ensure maximum elongation of the DNA band? Find the dynamic viscosities at the two temperatures.

(b) Determine the velocities of the top and the bottom of the DNA band, neglecting the effects of diffusion and electrophoretic flow (EPF). For the sign convention, please refer to Appendix D.

(c) When the bottom of the DNA band reaches the right end of the glass tube, the voltage source is turned off to stop the EOF. Calculate the final elongation factor of the DNA band, namely, the final length of the DNA band divided by the original length.

2-12. Two prototype solutions X and Y (with properties given in the table below) are being tested to maximize the capillary pressure in a lab-on-a-chip device. The lab-on-a-chip device has half-cylindrical (half-circle cross-sections) microchannels with radii of $r_0 = 80$ μm and requires no external pressure or energy. The contact angle θ_c is given by the hypothetical equation:

$$\tan\theta_c = 0.5 + A\exp\left[-B\left(T + T_0\right)\right] \quad \text{where } T \text{ has units of } °C$$

(a) Calculate the contact angle θ_c for both solutions at 22°C.

(b) Calculate the liquid-gas surface tension γ_{LG} for both solutions at 22°C.

(c) Calculate the capillary pressure $P_{capillary}$ for both solutions at 22°C. Which solution should be used to maximize the capillary pressure?

Variable	Solution X	Solution Y
γ_{SL}	45×10^{-3} N/m	94×10^{-3} N/m
$\gamma_{LG} : \gamma_{SG}$	1:3	1:4
A	30	45
B	0.14/°C	0.21/°C
T_0	6°C	2°C

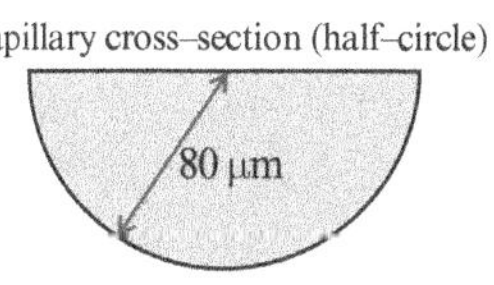
Capillary cross–section (half–circle)

2-13. You are planning an experiment at 22°C using water contained in a unique glass microchannel with the following cross-section created using isotropic etching. The boundary of the glass microchannel is marked by the top and bottom arcs. The top arc is a horizontal line and the bottom arc is defined by the following parametric equation (where all units are in [mm]).

Top Line: $y = 0$

Bottom Arc (for $y \leq 0$):

$$\left(\frac{x}{0.8}\right)^2 + \left(\frac{y-0.1}{0.5}\right)^2 = 1$$

The surface tension of the water-air interface $\gamma_{LG}(T)$ scales linearly with temperature T. From a table, you find that $\gamma_{LG}(20°C) = 72.86$ mN/m and $\gamma_{LG}(25°C) = 71.99$ mN/m. The contact angle of water on glass is $\theta_c = 35°$.

(a) Calculate the appropriate γ_{LG} value for your experiment.

(b) What is the cross-sectional area $A_{channel}$ of the microchannel?

(c) What is the capillary pressure $P_{capillary}$ in the microchannel? You can use computer software to numerically compute any difficult integrals.

2-14 (Challenging). We have a capillary oriented along the z-axis. Starting from the Navier-Stokes equation and the potential function $\phi(y)$ versus the distance away from the capillary wall y:

$$\rho_m\left(\frac{\partial \boldsymbol{v}}{\partial t} + \boldsymbol{v}\cdot\nabla\boldsymbol{v}\right) = \eta\nabla^2\boldsymbol{v} + \boldsymbol{F} - \nabla P \qquad \text{and} \qquad \phi(y) = \zeta\exp\left(\frac{-y}{\lambda_{DB}}\right)$$

with $\boldsymbol{v} = v(y)\,\hat{z}$ such that $\boldsymbol{v}\cdot(\nabla\boldsymbol{v}) = 0$. The capillary is oriented along the z-axis, and there is a constant applied electric field $\boldsymbol{E} = E\,\hat{z}$. In addition, there is a gravitational force $\boldsymbol{F}_g = mg\sin\theta\,\hat{z}$ where θ is the angle of the capillary relative to the horizontal. The pressure P is constant along the x- and y-directions, and there a constant pressure differential of $dP/dz = \Delta P/\Delta L$ along the z- (axial) direction of the capillary.

(a) Derive an expression for the steady-state fluid velocity $v(y)$, which can be split into three terms: the first corresponding to EOF, the second due to gravity, and the third due to the pressure differential.

(b) Consider a microcapillary that contains a water-based buffer solution with $\Delta P/\Delta L = 2.0$ kPa/m, $\rho_m = 1000$ kg/m³, $\eta = 8.90 \times 10^{-4}$ Pa·s, $\epsilon = 75\,\epsilon_0$, $\zeta = -50$ mV, and $\lambda_{DB} = 200$ nm. Also, the applied electric field is $E = 500$ V/m and $\theta = 10°$. Plot $v(y)$ together with each of the three terms of $v(y)$ for $0 \leq y \leq 10\,\mu$m on the same graph using software. For this scenario, how significant is each of the three terms of $v(y)$? *Note:* The dimensions of the microcapillary are larger than 20 μm.

2-15 (Challenging). A useful formula for fluid mechanics and microfluidics is the Darcy-Weisbach equation describing the loss of pressure due to fluid friction. The Darcy-Weisbach equation applies to *horizontal* channels of *uniform* diameter. While the Hagen-Poiseuille equation is only applicable to situations with laminar flow, the Darcy-Weisbach equation is applicable to both laminar and turbulent flow regimes. The Darcy-Weisbach equation for a cylindrical channel with radius r_0 is

$$\frac{\Delta P}{L} = \frac{f\rho_m\langle v\rangle^2}{r_0} \qquad \text{where} \quad f = \frac{2\tau}{\rho_m\langle v\rangle^2} \qquad \text{(Darcy-Weisbach Equation)}$$

where $\Delta P/L = (P_1 - P_2)/L$ is the pressure loss per unit length, f is the Fanning friction factor, $\langle v\rangle$ is the mean fluid velocity, ρ_m is the mass density, and τ is the shear stress due to fluid friction.

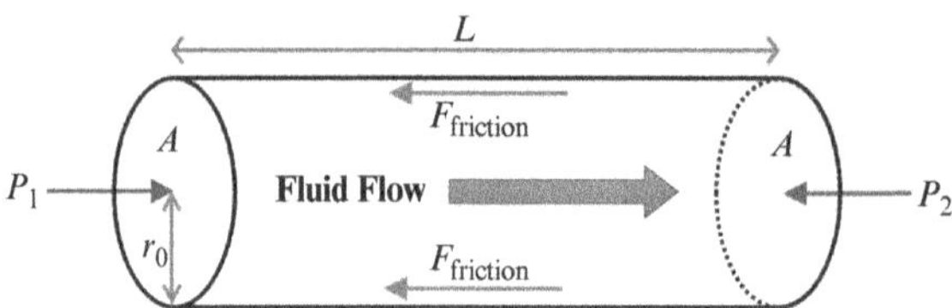

(a) Derive the Darcy-Weisbach equation using force balance and the provided expression for the Fanning friction factor f.

(b) For laminar flow in cylindrical capillaries, the Fanning friction factor is $f = 16/\text{Re}$, where Re is Reynolds number. Show that in this situation, the pressure loss due to fluid friction is equivalent to the pressure drop in pressure-driven flow (Hagen-Poiseuille flow).

2-16 (Challenging). Consider a thin rectangular channel with dimensions of $\ell \times w \times h$ where $\ell \gg h$ and $w \gg h$, as shown below. Assume that the pressure P varies only along the y-direction with a constant pressure drop of ΔP across the channel length of ℓ. Also assume that the fluid traveling through the channel is incompressible with a fluid velocity given by $\mathbf{v}_{\text{PDF}} = v(z)\,\hat{y}$. There are no external forces acting on the channel fluid.

(a) Derive the pressure-driven flow equation for $\mathbf{v}_{\text{PDF}} = v(z)\,\hat{y}$ using Newton's law of viscosity.

(b) Derive the same equation for $\mathbf{v}_{\text{PDF}} = v(z)\,\hat{y}$ using the steady-state Navier-Stokes equation.

(c) What is the total flow Q_{PDF} (volumetric flow rate) across the channel due to pressure-driven flow?

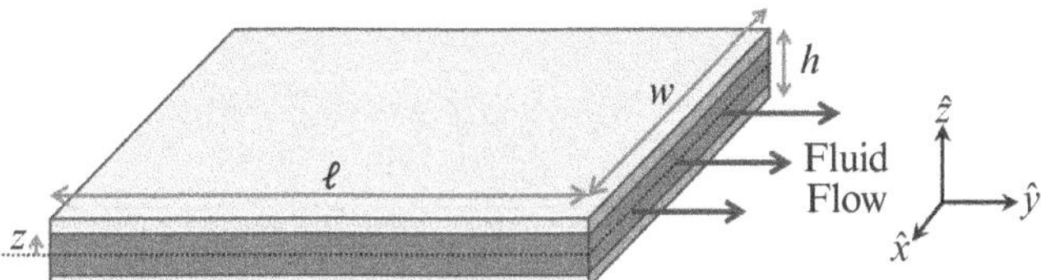

2-17 (Challenging). Another useful equation in fluid mechanics and for microfluidic systems is Bernoulli's equation for incompressible fluids, which is valid at any point along a streamline:

$$\frac{v^2}{2} + gh + \frac{P}{\rho_m} = \text{constant} \qquad \text{(Bernoulli's Equation)}$$

where (at the chosen point along the streamline) v is the fluid velocity, h is the height, g is the acceleration due to gravity, P is the fluid pressure, and ρ_m is the mass density.

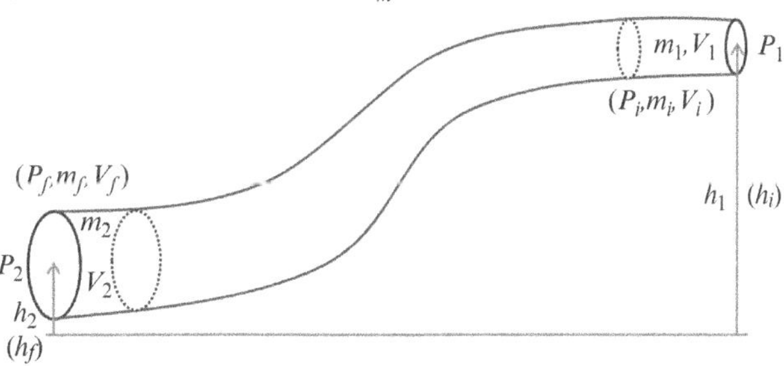

(a) Derive Bernoulli's equation using the conservation of energy and the conservation of mass.

(b) State the limitations of Bernoulli's equation.

(c) What is the maximum fluid velocity $v_{\text{PDF (max)}}$ in a cylindrical capillary due to pressure-driven flow (Hagen-Poiseuille flow)? Using Bernoulli's equation, derive another limitation for the maximum fluid velocity $v_{\text{Bernoulli (max)}}$. The fluid velocity in a cylindrical capillary cannot exceed $v_{\text{PDF (max)}}$ or $v_{\text{Bernoulli (max)}}$. Assume that the fluid starts at rest: $v_i = 0$.

(d) Derive an expression for $\Delta P^* = (P_i - P_f)^* > 0$ at which $v_{\text{PDF (max)}} = v_{\text{Bernoulli (max)}}$. Calculate ΔP^* for a water-based buffer solution with $\eta = 8.9 \times 10^{-4}$ Pa · s and $\rho_m = 1000$ kg/m³ in a cylindrical capillary with radius $r_0 = 500$ μm, length $L = 10$ cm, and height difference $\Delta h = h_i - h_f = 2.0$ cm. Using computer software, plot $v_{\text{PDF (max)}}$ and $v_{\text{Bernoulli (max)}}$ as functions of $\Delta P = P_i - P_f$.

2-18 (Challenging). Three prototype water-based buffers (A, B, and C) all with pH = 7 are tested to be used in the microchannels of a microfluidic device. The microfluidic device requires no external pressure or energy, and the contact angle θ_c between each prototype buffer and the microchannel walls is given by the theoretical equation:

$$\theta_c = \arccos\left[\frac{r_A \cos\theta_A + r_B \cos\theta_B}{r_A + r_B}\right]$$

$$\text{with} \quad r_A = \left(\frac{\sin^3(\theta_A)}{2 - 3\cos\theta_A + \cos^3(\theta_A)} \right)^{1/3} \quad \text{and} \quad r_B = \left(\frac{\sin^3(\theta_B)}{2 - 3\cos\theta_B + \cos^3(\theta_B)} \right)^{1/3}$$

where θ_A and θ_B are physical parameters that depend on the buffer and the microchannel wall material. The cross-section of the microchannels is the area bounded by the top horizonal line ($y = 0$) and the bottom arc ($y = 0.001\,x^4 - 5$) as shown below. The table below lists the physical properties of each buffer with respect to the microchannel walls.

Top Line: $y = 0$

Bottom Arc (for $y \leq 0$):

$y = 0.001\,x^4 - 5$

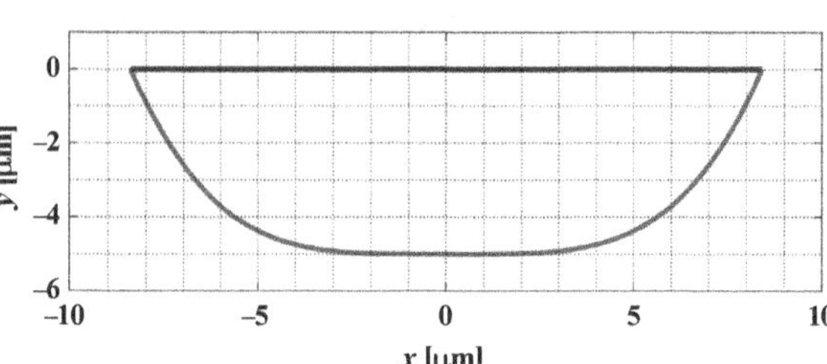

Variable	Buffer Solution A	Buffer Solution B	Buffer Solution C
γ_{LG}	70 mN/m	75 mN/m	72 mN/m
θ_A	75°	30°	65°
θ_B	120°	87°	100°
ϵ	$70\,\epsilon_0$	$70\,\epsilon_0$	$85\,\epsilon_0$
Salt concentration	2 mM of $NaCl_{(aq)}$	2 mM of $CaCl_{2(aq)}$	No salt
T	310 K	310 K	310 K
ζ	-0.17 V	-0.16 V	-0.2 V
ρ_m	1020 kg/m³	1020 kg/m³	1000 kg/m³
η	1.03×10^{-3} Pa · s	1.03×10^{-3} Pa · s	0.89×10^{-4} Pa · s

(a) Since the microfluidic device requires no external pressure, the microchannels must be able to fill themselves. Out of the three prototype buffer solutions, which solutions can automatically fill the microchannels? Justify your answer.

(b) Another requirement for the prototype buffer is that the EOF fluid velocity throughout almost the entire cross-sectional area of the microchannels must be constant. Out of three buffer solutions, which solutions satisfy this criterion?

(c) Only buffer solution B fulfills the criterion in part (a) as well as the criterion in part (b). To drive EOF for buffer solution B, assume that a DC voltage of V is applied across one microchannel with length $d = 5$ mm. What is the minimum applied DC voltage V that will cause transitional or turbulent flow? Can this voltage be practically achieved?

(d) Calculate the capillary pressure P for buffer solution B within the microchannels. Again, only buffer solution B fulfills the criterion in part (a) as well as the criterion in part (b). You may evaluate integrals numerically using computer software.

2.8 REFERENCES

[1]   A. Ge, L. Hu, X. Wang, J. Zhu, X. Feng, W. Du, et al., "Logarithmic bacterial gradient chip for analyzing the effects of dietary restriction on *C. elegans* growth," *Sensors and Actuators B: Chemical*, vol. 255, pp. 735–744, 2018.

[2]   N. Convery and N. Gadegaard, "30 years of microfluidics," *Micro and Nano Engineering*, vol. 2, pp. 76–91, 2019.

[3]   S. Damiati, U. B. Kompella, S. A. Damiati, and R. Kodzius, "Microfluidic devices for drug delivery systems and drug screening," *Genes*, vol. 9, no. 2, article 103, 2018.

[4]   Q. Smith and S. Gerecht, "Going with the flow: microfluidic platforms in vascular tissue engineering," *Current Opinion in Chemical Engineering*, vol. 3, pp. 42–50, 2014.

[5]   D. Baah and T. Floyd-Smith, "Microfluidics for particle synthesis from photocrosslinkable materials," *Microfluidics and Nanofluidics*, vol. 17, no. 3, pp. 431–455, 2014.

[6]   Y.-S. Lin, K.-S. Huang, C.-H. Yang, C.-Y. Wang, Y.-S. Yang, H.-C. Hsu, et al., "Microfluidic synthesis of microfibers for magnetic-responsive controlled drug release and cell culture," *Plos One*, vol. 7, no. 3, article 33184, 2012.

[7]   S. Sachdeva, R. W. Davis, and A. K. Saha, "Microfluidic point-of-care testing: commercial landscape and future directions," *Frontiers in Bioengineering and Biotechnology*, vol. 8, article 602659, 2021.

[8]   J. Mairhofer, K. Roppert, and P. Ertl, "Microfluidic systems for pathogen sensing: a review," *Sensors*, vol. 9, no. 6, pp. 4804–4823, 2009.

[9]   A. Puntambekar, J.-W. Choi, C. H. Ahn, S. Kim, and V. Makhijani, "Fixed-volume metering microdispenser module," *Lab on a Chip*, vol. 2, no. 4, pp. 213–218, 2002.

[10]   D. R. Gossett, W. M. Weaver, A. J. Mach, S. C. Hur, H. T. K. Tse, W. Lee, et al., "Label-free cell separation and sorting in microfluidic systems," *Analytical and Bioanalytical Chemistry*, vol. 397, no. 8, pp. 3249–3267, 2010.

[11]   H. A. Stone, A. D. Stroock, and A. Ajdari, "Engineering flows in small devices: microfluidics toward a lab-on-a-chip," *Annual Review of Fluid Mechanics*, vol. 36, pp. 381–411, 2004.

[12]   N. T. Nguyen and Z. G. Wu, "Micromixers: a review," *Journal of Micromechanics and Microengineering*, vol. 15, no. 2, pp. R1–R16, 2005.

[13]   E. R. Choban, L. J. Markoski, A. Wieckowski, and P. J. A. Kenis, "Microfluidic fuel cell based on laminar flow," *Journal of Power Sources*, vol. 128, no. 1, pp. 54–60, 2004.

[14]   A. Ostadfar, *Biofluid Mechanics: Principles and Applications*. London, UK: Elsevier Inc., 2016.

[15]   J. W. Lee, R. H. Nilson, J. A. Templeton, S. K. Griffiths, A. Kung, and B. M. Wong, "Comparison of molecular dynamics with classical density functional and Poisson–Boltzmann theories of the electric double layer in nanochannels," *Journal of Chemical Theory and Computation*, vol. 8, no. 6, pp. 2012–2022, 2012.

[16]   S. L. Carnie and G. M. Torrie, "The statistical mechanics of the electrical double layer," *Advances in Chemical Physics*, vol. 56, pp. 141–253, 1984.

[17]   G. M. Kontogeorgis and S. Kiil, *Introduction to Applied Colloid and Surface Chemistry*. Chichester, UK: John Wiley & Sons, Ltd., 2016.

[18]   "Zeta Potential Analyzers," AZoNano [Online]. Available: https://www.azonano.com/nanotechnology-equipment.aspx?cat=51, 2021.

[19]   A. Sze, D. Erickson, L. Ren, and D. Li, "Zeta-potential measurement using the Smoluchowski equation and the slope of the current–time relationship in electroosmotic flow," *Journal of Colloid and Interface Science*, vol. 261, no. 2, pp. 402–410, 2003.

CHAPTER 3

Microfluidics II: Fluid Transport and Applications

3.1 DIFFUSION

Diffusion is a commonly known process responsible for spreading and distributing molecules and particles in fluids, gases, and solids. Like capillary action and pressure-driven flow, diffusion does not have the same impact in microsystems as it does in larger systems. The effect of diffusion is dramatically increased in microsystems due to the smaller scale. The rules for diffusion are governed by Fick's laws. Fick's second law describes the diffusion of a substance with a differential equation. In 1D, Fick's second law with respect to x (x-position) and t (time) is

$$\frac{\partial N}{\partial t} = D\frac{\partial^2 N}{\partial^2 x} \;\Rightarrow\; N(x,t) = \frac{C_{\text{total}}}{2\sqrt{\pi Dt}}\exp\left(-\frac{(x-x_0)^2}{4Dt}\right) \text{ (1D)} \tag{3.1}$$

Here, $N(x, t)$ is the number density (number of particles per unit volume) distribution of the diffusing substance centered about $x = x_0$. C_{total} is a constant proportional to the total number of the diffusing particles. D is the diffusion coefficient (also known as diffusivity) of the substance with units of area per unit time, which depends on factors such as temperature and molecular weight of the diffusing substance. The solution to Fick's second law is a Gaussian function with a standard deviation of $\sigma = \sqrt{2Dt}$.

$$N(x,t) = \frac{C_{\text{total}}}{\sigma\sqrt{2\pi}}\exp\left(-\frac{(x-x_0)^2}{2\sigma^2}\right) \text{ with } \sigma = \sqrt{2Dt}\;\; (t \geq 0)\text{ (1D)} \tag{3.2}$$

This trend extends to 2D and 3D diffusions (Figure 3-1), with diffusion spreading substances outward in all directions equally. In higher dimensions, Fick's second law becomes

$$\frac{\partial N}{\partial t} = D\nabla^2 N \quad \text{and with} \quad \sigma = \sqrt{2Dt}\;\; (t \geq 0) \tag{3.3}$$

$$N(x,y,t) = \frac{C_{\text{total}}}{2\pi\sigma^2}\exp\left(-\frac{(x-x_0)^2 + (y-y_0)^2}{2\sigma^2}\right) \text{ (2D)} \tag{3.4}$$

$$N(x,y,z,t) = \frac{C_{\text{total}}}{(2\pi)^{3/2}\sigma^3}\exp\left(-\frac{(x-x_0)^2 + (y-y_0)^2 + (z-z_0)^2}{2\sigma^2}\right) \text{ (3D)} \tag{3.5}$$

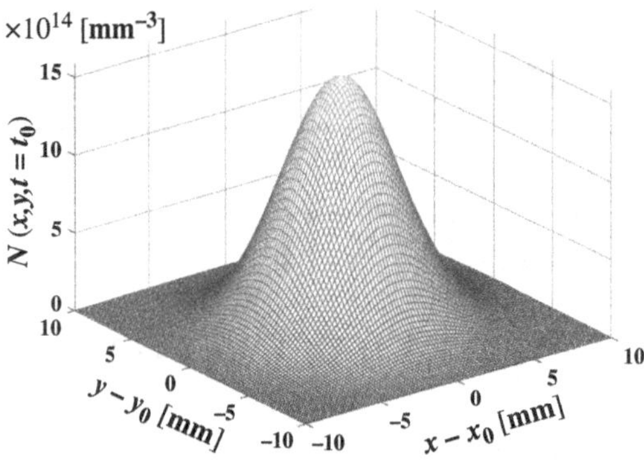

Figure 3-1   3D plot of the 2D Gaussian function describing 2D diffusion.

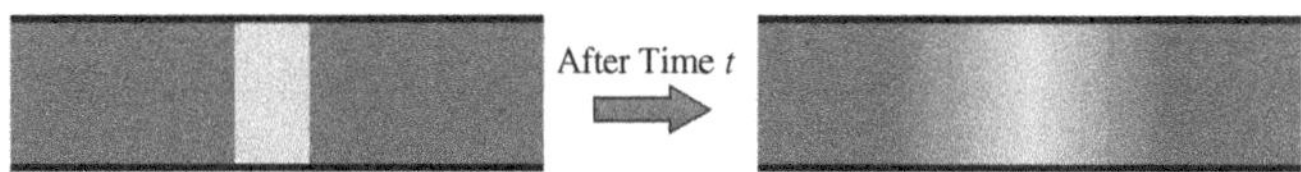

Figure 3-2   (Left) A representation of a dye band in a microchannel before diffusion. (Right) Over time, the dye diffuses equally to both sides, widening the band.

where the 2D diffusion profile $N(x, y, t)$ is centered about (x_0, y_0) and the 3D diffusion profile $N(x, y, z, t)$ is centered about (x_0, y_0, z_0). Because $\sigma = \sqrt{2Dt}$ is a statistical measure of the diffusion length, the diffusion distance $x_{\text{diffusion}}$ is defined as

$$x_{\text{diffusion}} \equiv \sqrt{2Dt} \quad (t \geq 0) \tag{3.6}$$

This equation describes how far a substance with diffusion coefficient D will travel in time t. In microfluidic applications, diffusion often takes place for "plugs," or bands of substances inside capillaries. As these bands travel down a capillary, surrounded on either side by a fluid (e.g., buffer solution), they begin to widen due to the substance diffusing into the surrounding liquid (Figure 3-2).

Under turbulent flow conditions, diffusion is highly effective at facilitating mixing. Although diffusion has much more influence in microsystems due to the smaller scale, diffusion is not a reliable way of mixing substances under laminar flow conditions. Owing to laminar flow, mixing two fluids can present a challenge within microfluidic systems. Special components sometimes have to be incorporated into a microfluidic system to facilitate mixing.[1]

EXAMPLE 3-1   Two bands of colored dye, each 50 μm wide, are initially 150 μm apart (from the center of each band) in a 500-μm-long microchannel as pictured below, where the rest of the channel is filled with a water-like buffer. One of the dye bands is red (R) with a diffusion coefficient of 10^{-10} m²/s, and the other is yellow (Y) with a diffusion coefficient of 10^{-11} m²/s. The edges of both bands have the same space (d) to the end of the microchannel.

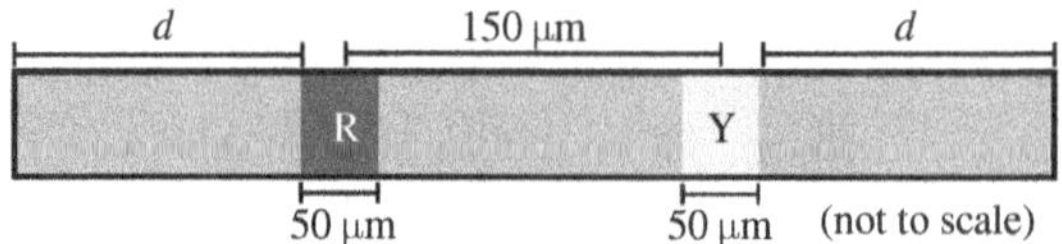

Initial conditions for the example problem.

(a) What will the channel look like after 10 s?

(b) What will the channel look like after 40 s?

(c) How long will it take for the entire channel to be orange?

Solution   We calculate the value of d first:

$$d = \frac{500\ \mu\text{m} - 150\ \mu\text{m} - 2 \times 25\ \mu\text{m}}{2} = \frac{300\ \mu\text{m}}{2} = 150\ \mu\text{m}$$

(a) For the red dye band after 10 s, the diffusion distance $x_{\text{diffusion(red)}}$ (both sides) is given by

$$x_{\text{diffusion(red)}} = \sqrt{2D_{\text{red}}t} = \sqrt{2(10^{-10}\ \text{m}^2/\text{s})(10\ \text{s})} = 44.7\ \mu\text{m}$$

Therefore, the width of the red dye band after 10 s is

$$W_{\text{red}} = 2x_{\text{diffusion(red)}} + 50\ \mu\text{m} = 2 \times 44.7\ \mu\text{m} + 50\ \mu\text{m} = 139\ \mu\text{m}$$

Similarly, the width of the yellow dye band after 10 s is

$$W_{\text{yellow}} = 2\sqrt{2D_{\text{yellow}}t} + 50\ \mu\text{m} = 2\sqrt{2(10^{-11}\ \text{m}^2/\text{s})(10\ \text{s})} + 50\ \mu\text{m} = 78.3\ \mu\text{m}$$

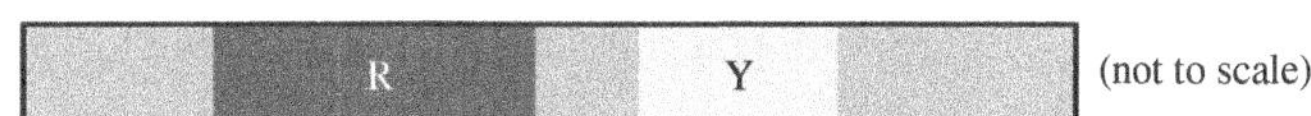

This is approximately what the channel will look like after 10 s.

(b) The width of the red dye band after 40 s is

$$W_{\text{red}} = 2\sqrt{2D_{\text{red}}t} + 50\ \mu\text{m} = 2\sqrt{2(10^{-10}\ \text{m}^2/\text{s})(40\ \text{s})} + 50\ \mu\text{m} = 229\ \mu\text{m}$$

Likewise, the width of the yellow dye band after 40 s is

$$W_{\text{yellow}} = 2\sqrt{2D_{\text{yellow}}t} + 50\ \mu\text{m} = 2\sqrt{2(10^{-11}\ \text{m}^2/\text{s})(40\ \text{s})} + 50\ \mu\text{m} = 107\ \mu\text{m}$$

There is now an orange (O) band where the two dyes mix together because

$$\frac{1}{2}W_{\text{red}} + \frac{1}{2}W_{\text{yellow}} = \frac{1}{2}(229\ \mu\text{m}) + \frac{1}{2}(107\ \mu\text{m}) = 168\ \mu\text{m} > 150\ \mu\text{m}$$

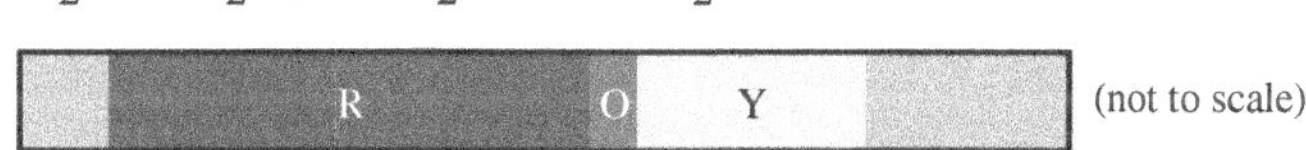

This is approximately what the channel will look like after 40 s.

(c) Since the yellow dye diffuses more slowly, the entire channel will be orange when the yellow band fills the entire channel. To travel from the edge of the band to the far side (i.e., left end), the left edge of the yellow dye will have to diffuse $d + 25\ \mu\text{m} + 150\ \mu\text{m} - 25\ \mu\text{m} = 300\ \mu\text{m}$. Therefore,

$$x_{\text{diffusion(yellow)}} = \sqrt{2D_{\text{yellow}}t} \Rightarrow t = \frac{x_{\text{diffusion(yellow)}}^2}{2D_{\text{yellow}}} = \frac{(300\ \mu\text{m})^2}{2(10^{-11}\ \text{m}^2/\text{s})} = 75.0\ \text{minutes} \quad \blacktriangle$$

3.2 ELECTROPHORETIC FLOW (EPF)

Another fluid transport technique is electrophoretic flow (EPF), which is considerably easier to understand than electro-osmotic flow (EOF). In this case, an applied electric field attracts or repels charged entities in a fluid, causing them to flow. An important distinction here is that electrophoretic flow only moves charged entities, as opposed to pressure-driven flow (PDF) or EOF, which moves virtually all of the fluid in a channel. Although electrophoretic flow alone is not effective at moving entire volumes of fluid through a channel, the ability to move specific entities in a fluid based on charge and size can be exploited in some applications (e.g., gel electrophoresis).

For a formal derivation of electrophoretic flow, we assume that a charged sphere with charge q and radius R_S is suspended in a fluid inside a channel. If an electric field $E = V/d$ is

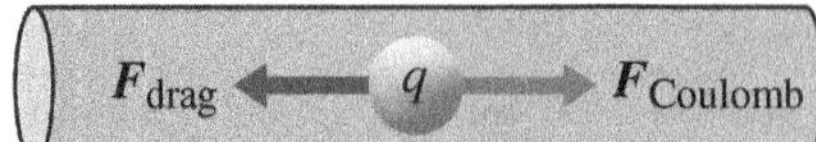

Figure 3-3   In a channel, a charged sphere suspended in fluid is pushed by a force F_{Coulomb} applied by an electric field, which is resisted by a drag force F_{drag} from the fluid in the channel.

applied along the channel by applying a voltage across the channel, a Coulomb force F_{Coulomb} will act on the charged sphere (Figure 3-3), which is

$$F_{\text{Coulomb}} = qE = \frac{qV}{d} \tag{3.7}$$

where V is the voltage applied and d is the length of the channel. The Coulomb force pushes the charged sphere through the fluid in the channel, but it is opposed by the drag force of fluid pushing against the sphere. The drag force is

$$F_{\text{drag}} = 6\pi\eta R_S v \tag{3.8}$$

This force, Stokes' drag force F_{drag}, depends on the dynamic viscosity of the fluid η, the radius of the sphere R_S, and the velocity of the sphere relative to the fluid v. Here we assume that the particles are spherical, and that fluid flow is laminar. The effective charge and radius are both affected by Debye screening effects on the molecule, which screen the charge and create a larger effective radius.

Initially, the charged sphere is at rest such that $v(t = 0) = 0$. The Coulomb force F_{Coulomb} from the applied electric field E will cause the charged sphere to accelerate until the sphere reaches a constant terminal velocity. The terminal velocity is reached when the Coulomb force F_{Coulomb} is balanced by the Stokes' drag force F_{drag}. Consider the net force F_{net} acting on the charged sphere given by

$$F_{\text{net}} = F_{\text{Coulomb}} - F_{\text{drag}} \quad \Rightarrow \quad ma = m\frac{dv}{dt} = qE - 6\pi\eta R_S v \tag{3.9}$$

$$\frac{m\,dv}{qE - 6\pi\eta R_S v} = dt \quad \Rightarrow \quad m\int \frac{dv}{qE - 6\pi\eta R_S v} = \int dt$$

$$-\frac{m}{6\pi\eta R_S}\ln|qE - 6\pi\eta R_S v| = t + C_0 \quad \Rightarrow \quad |qE - 6\pi\eta R_S v| = \exp\left[-\frac{6\pi\eta R_S}{m}(t + C_0)\right]$$

where C_0 is a constant of integration. Noting that the drag force can never be greater than the Coulomb force, we have $qE \geq 6\pi\eta R_S v$. Thus,

$$qE - 6\pi\eta R_S v = C_1 \exp\left(-\frac{6\pi\eta R_S}{m}t\right) \quad \text{where} \quad C_1 = \exp\left(-\frac{6\pi\eta R_S}{m}C_0\right)$$

$$v(t) = \frac{1}{6\pi\eta R_S}\left[qE - C_1\exp\left(-\frac{6\pi\eta R_S}{m}t\right)\right]$$

Using the initial condition $v(t = 0) = 0$, we have

$$0 = v(t = 0) = \frac{1}{6\pi\eta R_S}\left[qE - C_1\exp(0)\right] = \frac{1}{6\pi\eta R_S}(qE - C_1) \quad \Rightarrow \quad C_1 = qE$$

Putting everything together, we have

$$v(t) = \frac{qE}{6\pi\eta R_S}\left[1 - \exp\left(-\frac{6\pi\eta R_S}{m}t\right)\right] \tag{3.10}$$

Consider a typical protein molecule with net charge q in a water-based solution with the following properties: $\eta_{\text{water}} = 8.9 \times 10^{-4}$ Pa·s, $m_{\text{protein}} = 50$ kDa $= 8.3 \times 10^{-23}$ kg, and $R_{S(\text{protein})} = 2.5$ nm. A nanosecond after starting from rest (i.e., at $t = 1$ ns), we have

$$\exp\left(-\frac{6\pi\eta R_S}{m}t\right) = \exp\left[-\frac{6\pi\left(8.9\times10^{-4}\ \text{Pa}\cdot\text{s}\right)\left(2.5\ \text{nm}\right)}{8.3\times10^{-23}\ \text{kg}}(1\ \text{ns})\right] = 4.1\times10^{-220} \cong 0$$

The above result indicates that the charged protein reaches the terminal velocity almost instantly (i.e., in a timeframe shorter than a nanosecond). If the protein molecule were instead placed in a gel instead of a water-based solution, it would reach terminal velocity even more quickly because $\eta_{\text{gel}} \gg \eta_{\text{water}}$. Therefore, for the vast majority of applications, we can assume that

$$\exp\left(-\frac{6\pi\eta R_S}{m}t\right) \cong 0 \quad\Rightarrow\quad v_{\text{EPF}} = v(t) \cong \frac{qE}{6\pi\eta R_S} \tag{3.11}$$

Hence, the velocity of the charged sphere and final equation for electrophoretic flow are

$$v_{\text{EPF}} = \frac{qE}{6\pi\eta R_S} = \mu_{\text{EPF}}E \quad\text{where}\quad \mu_{\text{EPF}} = \frac{q}{6\pi\eta R_S} \tag{3.12}$$

Similar to EOF, this equation relates velocity to the applied electric field. In the same way, μ_{EPF} can be defined as the mobility, but here it is referred to as EPF mobility. This equation, of course, applies to more than just charged spheres. Charged molecules like DNA, proteins, and others also experience electrophoretic flow, with their mobilities being influenced by their charge and size. All charged particles such as ions, molecules, and nanoparticles have an effective charge q and a Stokes radius R_S. The Stokes radius R_S of a particle is the radius of an equivalent sphere with the same electrophoretic mobility and charge while moving through the same fluid. Larger particles have a larger Stokes radius, which causes larger drag force and lower EPF mobility. Therefore, different electrophoretic flow speeds are generated based on both particle charge and size. For example, the size difference of DNA molecules is essential in gel electrophoresis for DNA separation and sequencing, which will be discussed in Chapter 5.

In the presence of an electric field E, both EOF and EPF have to be considered. Summing the mobilities, we have

$$v_{\text{total}} = \mu_{\text{EOF}}E + \mu_{\text{EPF}}E = \left(\mu_{\text{EOF}} + \mu_{\text{EPF}}\right)E = \mu_{\text{total}}E \tag{3.13}$$

Again, it is important to note that EPF only affects charged bodies (e.g., charged molecules in a fluid), whereas EOF affects the entire fluid regardless of individual charges in the fluid.

EXAMPLE 3-2 A 5-cm-long cylindrical glass capillary with a radius of 100 μm links two buffer-filled wells. +5000 V is applied to the right well, and the left well is grounded. The zeta potential of the glass is 0 V. The buffer in one end of the capillary has been loaded with a sample having an initial width of 100 μm in the capillary.

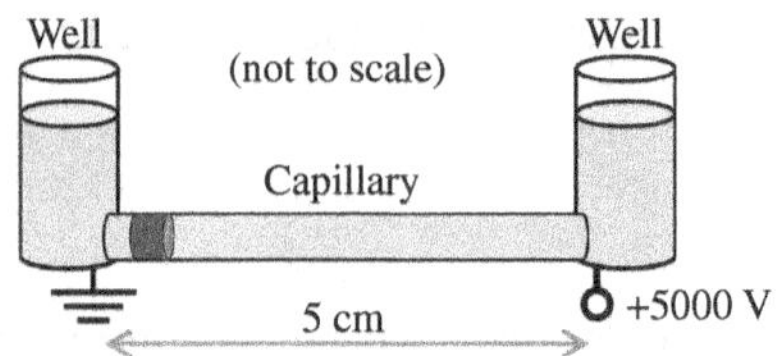

The sample contains a mixture of two different lengths of DNA, which are optically labeled and will be separated. One is 200 bps (base pairs) long and is labeled red, while the other is 202 bps long and is labeled blue. The electrophoretic mobility of the red DNA (the shorter one) is found to be -10^{-8} m²/(V·s), which scales inversely with length (i.e., where N is the length in terms of the number of base pairs). As the components arrive at the right side of the well, they are measured optically.

(a) What is the arrival time of the center of the red DNA band at the other end of the capillary? For the sign convention, please refer to Appendix D.

(b) What is the arrival time of the center of the blue DNA band at the other end of the capillary?

(c) How far apart are the centers of the bands of DNA in terms of time and distance when the center of the red DNA band reaches the other end of the capillary?

(d) If the diffusion coefficient for both DNA samples (i.e., both red-labeled and blue-labeled DNA) is 10^{-11} m²/s, approximately how wide are the bands when they reach the end of the capillary?

(e) Sketch a graph showing both red and blue intensities as a function of time as the DNA bands arrive at the end of the capillary. Emphasize the arrival time, and do not draw a long flat graph.

Solution

(a) We note that $v_{\text{EOF}} = -\dfrac{\epsilon \zeta}{\eta} E = 0$ because the zeta potential $\zeta = 0$. With the sign convention, we have

$$v_{\text{red}} = \mu_{\text{EPF(red)}} E = \left(-10^{-8}\,\frac{\text{m}^2}{\text{V}\cdot\text{s}}\right)\left(-\frac{5000\ \text{V}}{5\ \text{cm}}\right) = 0.001\ \text{m/s} \quad t_{\text{red}} = \frac{d}{v} = \frac{5\ \text{cm} - 50\ \mu\text{m}}{0.001\ \text{m/s}} = 49.95\ \text{s}$$

(b) For the blue DNA band, we have

$$v_{\text{blue}} = \mu_{\text{EPF(blue)}} E = \left(\mu_{\text{EPF(red)}} \cdot \frac{200\ \text{bps}}{202\ \text{bps}}\right) E = \frac{\mu_{\text{EPF(red)}} E}{1.01} = \frac{0.001\ \text{m/s}}{1.01}$$

$$t_{\text{blue}} = \frac{d}{v_{\text{blue}}} = \frac{5\ \text{cm} - 50\ \mu\text{m}}{(0.001\ \text{m/s}) / (1.01)} = (49.95\ \text{s})(1.01) = 50.45\ \text{s}$$

(c) $t_{\text{blue}} - t_{\text{red}} = 50.45\ \text{s} - 49.95\ \text{s} = 0.50\ \text{s}$

The distance apart is the distance from the end point that the blue band has reached to the right end of the capillary that the red band has just reached. Hence,

$$d = v_{\text{blue}}\, t_{\text{red}} = (0.001\ \text{m/s})/(1.01) \cdot (49.95\ \text{s}) = 4.9455\ \text{cm}$$

$$d_{\text{total}} = (5\ \text{cm} - 50\ \mu\text{m}) - 4.9455\ \text{cm} = 495\ \mu\text{m}$$

Alternatively, d_{total} can be found using a second method:

$$d_{\text{total}} = \left(t_{\text{blue}} - t_{\text{red}}\right) v_{\text{blue}} = (0.50\ \text{s})(0.001\ \text{m/s})/(1.01) = 495\ \mu\text{m}$$

(d) Upon reaching the end of the capillary, the widths of the DNA bands W_{red} and W_{blue} are

$$x_{\text{diffusion(red)}} = \sqrt{2Dt_{\text{red}}} = \sqrt{2(10^{-11}\,\text{m}^2/\text{s})(49.95\ \text{s})} = 31.6\ \mu\text{m}$$

$$W_{\text{red}} = 100\ \mu\text{m} + 2x_{\text{diffusion(red)}} = 100\ \mu\text{m} + 2(31.6\ \mu\text{m}) = 163.2\ \mu\text{m}$$

$$W_{\text{blue}} = 100\ \mu\text{m} + 2x_{\text{diffusion(blue)}} = 100\ \mu\text{m} + 2\sqrt{2(10^{-11}\,\text{m}^2/\text{s})(50.45\ \text{s})} = 163.5\ \mu\text{m}$$

(e) The graph below shows both the red and blue intensities as a function of time as they arrive at the end of the capillary. The Gaussian shapes of the two peaks are due to the Gaussian distributions resulting from diffusion of the red and blue DNA bands. The red and blue DNA bands will not meet because

$$\begin{cases} \dfrac{1}{2}W_{red} + \dfrac{1}{2}W_{blue} = 163.4 \ \mu m \\ d_{total} = 495 \ \mu m \end{cases} \Rightarrow \quad \dfrac{1}{2}W_{red} + \dfrac{1}{2}W_{blue} \ll d_{total}$$

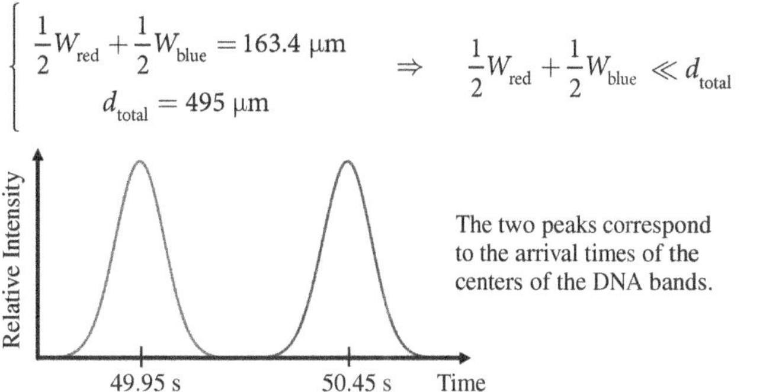

3.3 DIELECTROPHORETIC (DEP) FORCE

The basic idea behind dielectrophoresis (DEP) is to polarize particles, such as cells, in a spatially non-uniform electric field. The counterpart of DEP is magnetophoresis, in which a magnetic field instead of an electric field is applied. The major drawback of magnetophoresis is that it requires a label. In this book, we focus only on DEP. Figure 3-4 shows an example of creating a non-uniform electric field for DEP using powered microelectrodes.

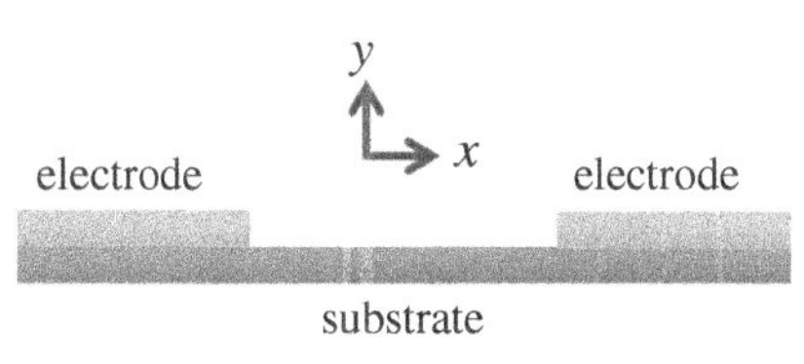

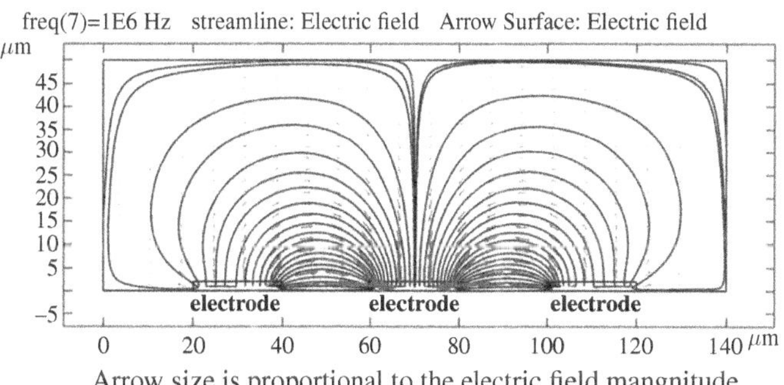

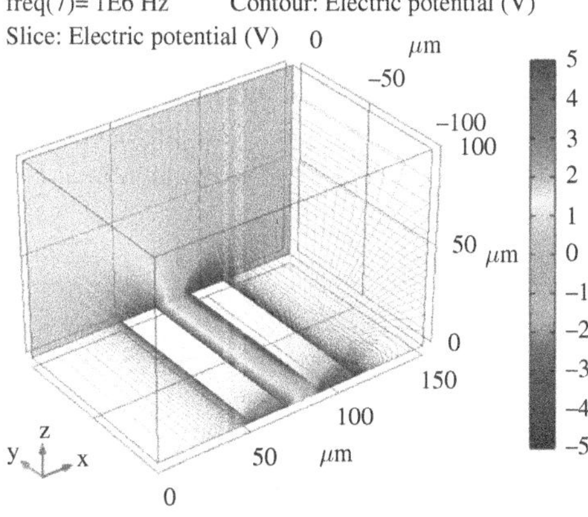

Electric potential distribution

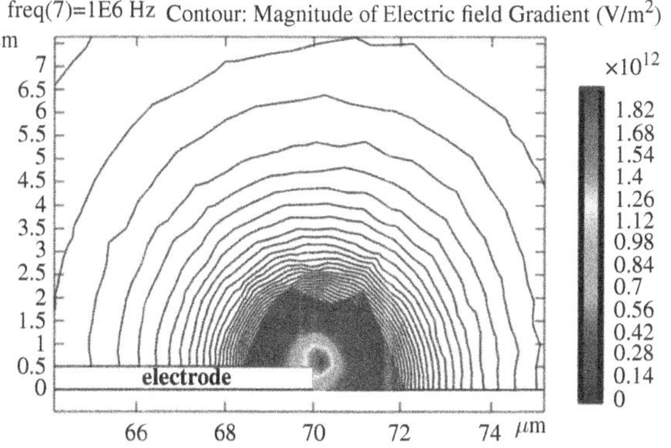

Contour plot of the electric field gradient mangnitude

Figure 3-4 Distribution of a non-uniform electric field and electric field gradient generated by two powered microelectrodes to be used for dielectrophoresis (DEP). Please refer to the lab assignments in Chapter 8 for the details. (*The plots were obtained using COMSOL Multiphysics® simulation software.*)

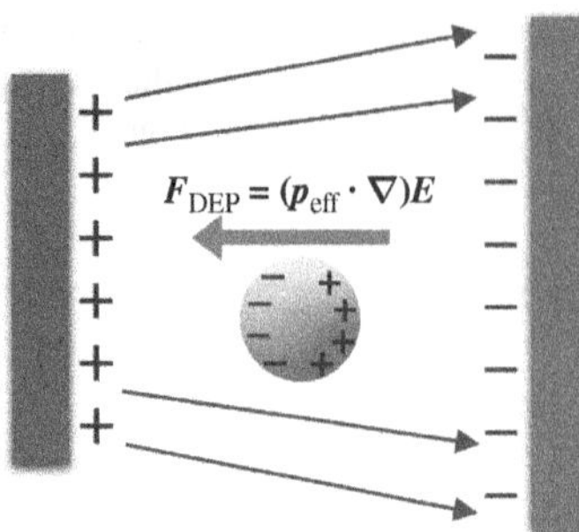

Figure 3-5   Schematic of DEP force $\boldsymbol{F}_{\mathrm{DEP}}$.

Unlike electrophoretic forces which originate from the interaction of a particle's charge with an electric field, dielectrophoresis (DEP) forces arise from the interaction of a polarized neutral particle with a non-uniform electric field. We can use DEP force (Figure 3-5) to manipulate small objects such as cells, which is fundamental to biology and biotechnology.[2] In addition to DEP force, there are other ways to manipulate cells, such as optical tweezers (the 2018 physics Nobel Prize-winning technology) and acoustic forces, which are beyond the scope of this book.

3.3.1 Theory of Dielectrophoresis (DEP)

(A) Force on an Infinitesimal Dipole

As shown in Figure 3-6, a dipole is made of a pair of equal magnitude and oppositely charged poles $+q$ and $-q$, separated by a distance given by the displacement vector $\boldsymbol{d}$ given by

$$\boldsymbol{d} = d_x\hat{\boldsymbol{x}} + d_y\hat{\boldsymbol{y}} + d_z\hat{\boldsymbol{z}} = \left(d_x, d_y, d_z\right)$$

By convention, the displacement vector $\boldsymbol{d}$ points from the negative charge to the positive charge. In the presence of a non-uniform electric field $\boldsymbol{E}$, the two charges will be generally affected by two different values of the electric field $\boldsymbol{E}(\boldsymbol{r})$ for $-q$ and $\boldsymbol{E}(\boldsymbol{r} + \boldsymbol{d})$ for $+q$, where $\boldsymbol{r} = x_0\hat{\boldsymbol{x}} + y_0\hat{\boldsymbol{y}} + z_0\hat{\boldsymbol{z}} = \left(x_0, y_0, z_0\right)$ is the position vector of $-q$.

Since the electric field is non-uniform, the force on each charge does not cancel as in the uniform field case. The net force on the dipole is given as

$$\boldsymbol{F} = q\boldsymbol{E}(\boldsymbol{r} + \boldsymbol{d}) - q\boldsymbol{E}(\boldsymbol{r}) \tag{3.14}$$

When $|\boldsymbol{d}|$ is small compared to the electric field non-uniformity, meaning that minor changes occur between the fields acting on $-q$ and $+q$, a multivariable Taylor series expansion can be used to approximate the electric field near $\boldsymbol{r}$. For a single component E_x of the electric field vector $\boldsymbol{E} = E_x\hat{\boldsymbol{x}} + E_y\hat{\boldsymbol{y}} + E_z\hat{\boldsymbol{z}} = \left(E_x, E_y, E_z\right)$, the expansion at $\boldsymbol{r} + \boldsymbol{d}$ is given by

$$E_x(\boldsymbol{r} + \boldsymbol{d}) = E_x\left(x_0 + d_x, \, y_0 + d_y, \, z_0 + d_z\right)$$

$$E_x(\boldsymbol{r} + \boldsymbol{d}) = E_x\left(x_0, y_0, z_0\right) + d_x\frac{\partial E_x\left(x_0, y_0, z_0\right)}{\partial x} + d_y\frac{\partial E_x\left(x_0, y_0, z_0\right)}{\partial y} + d_z\frac{\partial E_x\left(x_0, y_0, z_0\right)}{\partial z} + \cdots$$

$$E_x(\boldsymbol{r} + \boldsymbol{d}) = E_x(\boldsymbol{r}) + (\boldsymbol{d} \cdot \boldsymbol{\nabla})E_x(\boldsymbol{r}) + \cdots \tag{3.15}$$

Considering all three vector components E_x, E_y, and E_z of the electric field $\boldsymbol{E}$ at the position $\boldsymbol{r} + \boldsymbol{d}$, the expansion is

$$\boldsymbol{E}(\boldsymbol{r} + \boldsymbol{d}) = \boldsymbol{E}(\boldsymbol{r}) + (\boldsymbol{d} \cdot \boldsymbol{\nabla})\boldsymbol{E}(\boldsymbol{r}) + \cdots \tag{3.16}$$

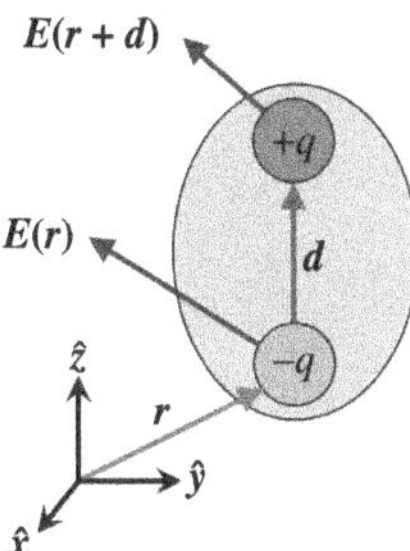

Figure 3-6   Dipole in the presence of a non-uniform electric field.

where the higher-order terms are neglected since they contain higher powers of the small quantity $|d|$. The resulting approximation for the force on the dipole from combining Equations (3.14) and (3.16) is

$$F = (q d \cdot \nabla) E(r) + \cdots \tag{3.17}$$

In the limit where $|d| \to 0$ is taken, the dipole moment $p = qd$ is small and the higher order terms of the dipole force in Equation (3.17) can be ignored (named the dielectrophoretic approximation). The force on an infinitesimal dipole is

$$F_{\text{dipole}} = (p \cdot \nabla) E(r) \tag{3.18}$$

Since this force depends on the gradient of the electric field, it is clear that uniform electric fields will not result in a net force on the dipole.

(B) Torque on an Infinitesimal Dipole
Unlike the dipole force F_{dipole}, the dipole torque T_{dipole} only depends on the electric field, not on its gradient. As such, a uniform electric field can induce a torque on an infinitesimal dipole. The torque is found from the net force acting about the center of the dipole as follows.[3]

$$T_{\text{dipole}} = \left(\frac{d}{2}\right) \times (qE) + \left(-\frac{d}{2}\right) \times (-qE) = qd \times E \tag{3.19}$$

In Equation (3.19), the dipole torque in a uniform electric field is a first-order approximation for the dipole torque in a non-uniform electric field, which is accurate when the distance between the two charges in the dipole is small.

(C) Induced Dipole Moment
Electric fields (uniform or non-uniform) can polarize a particle, even if the particle is overall electrically neutral. Such a polarized particle can be treated as a finite (non-point) dipole, and has an induced dipole moment. Using Figure 3.7 and through geometry, $r_{\pm}$ can be found in terms of (r, θ) and d.

$$r_{\pm} = \sqrt{\left(r\cos\theta \mp \frac{d}{2}\right)^2 + (r\sin\theta)^2} = \sqrt{r^2 \mp d \cdot r\cos\theta + \left(\frac{d}{2}\right)^2}$$

which, for future simplicity, can be re-expressed as

$$\frac{r}{r_{\pm}} = \left[1 \mp \frac{d}{r}\cos\theta + \left(\frac{d}{2r}\right)^2\right]^{-1/2} \tag{3.20}$$

For a finite (non-point) dipole centered at the origin with d pointing along the z-axis such that charge $\pm q$ lies on $z = \pm d/2$, the potential at a point (r, θ, φ) can be found by considering the superposition of the potentials from the positive and negative charges, as shown in Figure 3-7. The potential is independent of the azimuthal angle φ (in the x-y

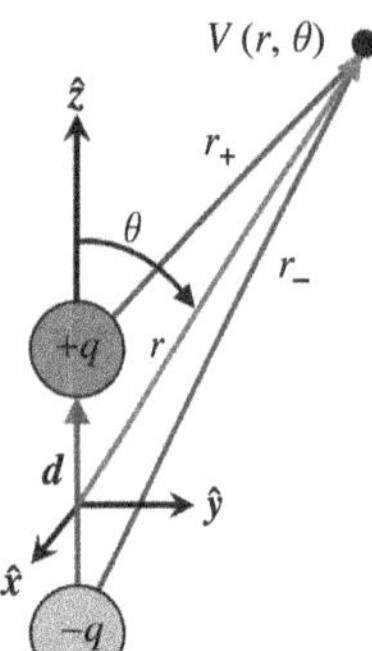

Figure 3-7 Electric potential $V(r, \theta)$ from a finite (non-point) electric dipole. Through geometry, $r_\pm$ can be found in terms of (r, θ) and d.

plane) because of the symmetry of the finite dipole. This leaves only the dependence on the radial distance r from the center of the finite dipole and the polar angle θ from the positive z-axis. Therefore, the potential $V(r, \theta)$ is

$$V(r,\theta) = \frac{q}{4\pi\epsilon_m r_+} - \frac{q}{4\pi\epsilon_m r_-} \tag{3.21}$$

where r_+ and r_- are respectively defined as the distances from the positive and negative charges to the point (r, θ, φ). ϵ_m is the electric permittivity of the medium containing the finite dipole.

Using the Taylor series expansion of $(1+x)^{-1/2}$ centered at $x = 0$:

$$(1+x)^{-1/2} = 1 - \frac{x}{2} + \frac{3x^2}{8} - \frac{5x^3}{16} + \cdots \quad \text{and with} \quad x = \left(\frac{d}{2r}\right)^2 \mp \frac{d}{r}\cos\theta, \text{ we have}$$

$$\frac{r}{r_\pm} = 1 - \frac{1}{2}\left[\left(\frac{d}{2r}\right)^2 \mp \frac{d}{r}\cos\theta\right] + \frac{3}{8}\left[\left(\frac{d}{2r}\right)^2 \mp \frac{d}{r}\cos\theta\right]^2 - \cdots = 1 \pm \left(\frac{d}{2r}\right)\cos\theta + \left(\frac{d}{2r}\right)^2\left(\frac{3\cos^2\theta - 1}{2}\right) \pm \cdots$$

$$\frac{r}{r_\pm} = P_0(\cos\theta) \pm \left(\frac{d}{2r}\right)P_1(\cos\theta) + \left(\frac{d}{2r}\right)^2 P_2(\cos\theta) \pm \cdots \tag{3.22}$$

where the coefficients are given by $P_n(\cos\theta)$, which is known as the nth Legendre polynomial. Table 3-1 lists the first few Legendre polynomials.

Combining Equations (3.21) and (3.22) and canceling common terms, the finite dipole's potential becomes

$$V(r, \theta) = \frac{qdP_1(\cos\theta)}{4\pi\epsilon_m r^2} + \frac{qd^3P_3(\cos\theta)}{16\pi\epsilon_m r^4} + \cdots = \frac{q}{2\pi\epsilon_m r}\sum_{n=1,3,5,7,\ldots}^{\infty}\left(\frac{d}{2r}\right)^n P_n(\cos\theta) \tag{3.23}$$

TABLE 3-1   The First Few Legendre Polynomials

n	$P_n(x)$	$P_n(\cos\theta)$
0	1	1
1	x	$\cos\theta$
2	$\frac{1}{2}(3x^2 - 1)$	$\frac{1}{2}(3\cos^2\theta - 1)$
3	$\frac{1}{2}(5x^3 - 3x)$	$\frac{1}{2}(5\cos^3\theta - 3\cos\theta)$

where only the odd degree terms (i.e., $n =$ odd) remain. The term corresponding to $n = 1$ is called the dipole potential V_{dipole}, which is the sole term for the potential of an infinitesimal point dipole. The next non-zero term corresponding to $n = 3$ is an octopolar correction.[3]

With the effective dipole moment given by $p_{eff} = qd$, we have

$$V_{dipole} = \frac{p_{eff}\cos\theta}{4\pi\epsilon_m r^2} \tag{3.24}$$

To represent the dipole moment induced in a particle after an electric field polarizes it, an effective dipole moment $\boldsymbol{p}_{eff}$ is chosen based on the dipole moment of a point dipole that will result in the same dipole potential V_{dipole}, if it is placed at the center of the polarized particle.

EXAMPLE 3-3 Derive the relationship between the Legendre polynomials $P_n(\cos\theta)$ and $V(r,\theta)$ using the generating function of the Legendre polynomials (below, left):

$$\left(1 - 2yz + z^2\right)^{-\frac{1}{2}} = \sum_{n=0}^{\infty} P_n(y)\, z^n \quad \text{and} \quad V(r,\theta) = \frac{q}{4\pi\epsilon_m r_+} - \frac{q}{4\pi\epsilon_m r_-}$$

Solution Using the generating function of the Legendre polynomials (above, left) and Equation (3.20):

$$\frac{r}{r_\pm} = \left[1 \mp \frac{d}{r}\cos\theta + \left(\frac{d}{2r}\right)^2\right]^{-1/2} \quad \Rightarrow \quad \begin{cases} y = \cos\theta \\ z = \pm\dfrac{d}{2r} \end{cases}$$

we obtain $\dfrac{r}{r_\pm} = \left(1 - 2yz + z^2\right)^{-1/2} = \sum_{n=0}^{\infty} P_n(y)\, z^n = \sum_{n=0}^{\infty} P_n(\cos\theta)\left(\pm\frac{d}{2r}\right)^n$

$$V(r,\theta) = \frac{q}{4\pi\epsilon_m}\frac{1}{r}\left(\frac{r}{r_+} - \frac{r}{r_-}\right) = \frac{q}{4\pi\epsilon_m}\frac{1}{r}\left[\sum_{n=0}^{\infty} P_n(\cos\theta)\left(\frac{d}{2r}\right)^n - \sum_{n=0}^{\infty} P_n(\cos\theta)\left(\frac{-d}{2r}\right)^n\right]$$

To get the difference of the two infinites sums, we cancel out all of the even terms ($n = 0, 2, 4, 6, \dots$) and double all of the odd terms ($n = 1, 3, 5, 7, \dots$). Hence,

$$V(r,\theta) = \frac{q}{4\pi\epsilon_m}\frac{1}{r}\sum_{n=1,3,5,7,\dots}^{\infty} 2P_n(\cos\theta)\left(\frac{d}{2r}\right)^n = \frac{q}{2\pi\epsilon_m r}\sum_{n=1,3,5,7,\dots}^{\infty}\left(\frac{d}{2r}\right)^n P_n(\cos\theta) \quad \blacktriangle$$

(D) Insulating Sphere in a Uniform Electric Field

An insulating dielectric spherical particle of radius R and permittivity ϵ_p is in a fluid medium of permittivity ϵ_m. An external uniform electric field $\boldsymbol{E} = E_0\,\hat{\boldsymbol{z}}$ of magnitude E_0 is directed in the z-direction which polarizes the spherical particle. The insulating sphere in uniform electric field is shown in Figure 3-8.

The electric potential outside the particle in the medium is made up of the potential $V_{external\ field}$ from the external electric field plus the dipole potential V_{dipole} from the induced dipole moment of the particle, which has the form of Equation (3.24). From these two

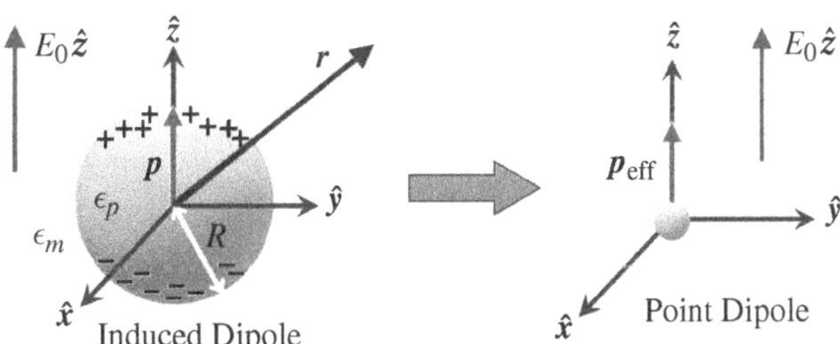

Figure 3-8 (Left) Dielectric sphere polarized with an induced dipole in a uniform electric field; (right) point dipole that satisfies the same boundary conditions.

terms, the total electric potential in the medium and outside of the particle $V_m(r, \theta)$ is postulated (using spherical coordinates) as

$$V_m\left(r, \theta\right) = V_{\text{external field}} + V_{\text{dipole}} = -E_0 r \cos\theta + \frac{A\cos\theta}{r^2} \quad \text{for} \ \ r \geq R \ \left(\text{in medium}\right) \quad (3.25)$$

where A is an unknown coefficient. Similarly, the electric potential inside the particle $V_p(r, \theta)$ is assumed to have the form

$$V_p\left(r, \theta\right) = -B\, r \cos\theta \ \text{ for } \ r \leq R \ \left(\text{in particle}\right) \tag{3.26}$$

At the boundary, the two electric potentials must be continuous. Thus,

$$V_m = V_p \ \text{ at } \ r = R \tag{3.27}$$

In integral form, Gauss's law in terms of the electric displacement vector $\boldsymbol{D}$ and the enclosed free charge $Q_{\text{free, enclosed}}$ is

$$\boldsymbol{D} = \epsilon_0 \boldsymbol{E} + \boldsymbol{P} \ \ \text{ with } \ \ \oiint \boldsymbol{D} \cdot d\boldsymbol{a} = \oiint \boldsymbol{D} \cdot \hat{\boldsymbol{n}} \, da = Q_{\text{free, enclosed}} \tag{3.28}$$

where $\boldsymbol{E}$ is the total electric field, $\boldsymbol{P}$ is the polarization density of the particle, da is an infinitesimal surface area element, and $\hat{\boldsymbol{n}}$ is the unit vector normal to the surface. From Gauss's law, we obtain a boundary condition on the radial (r) component (normal to the spherical interface) of the electric displacement vector D_r, where $\sigma_{c(\text{free})}$ represents the free surface charge density given by

$$D_{r,m} - D_{r,p} = \sigma_{c(\text{free})} \ \text{ at } \ r = R \quad \text{where} \ \ \begin{cases} D_r = D_{r,m} \ \text{ for } \ r \geq R \ \left(\text{in medium}\right) \\[2mm] D_r = D_{r,p} \ \text{ for } \ r \leq R \ \left(\text{in particle}\right) \end{cases} \tag{3.29}$$

The proof of Equation (3.29) is left as an exercise. In the case where the particle is a linear dielectric, which is assumed, the polarization density $\boldsymbol{P}$ of the particle is proportional to the total electric field $\boldsymbol{E}$ and the electric susceptibility χ_e, since $\boldsymbol{P} = \epsilon_0 \chi_e \boldsymbol{E}$. Hence, the electric displacement vector $\boldsymbol{D}$ is proportional to the electric field $\boldsymbol{E}$, with the proportionality constant being the material permittivity ϵ as shown below.

$$\boldsymbol{D} = \epsilon_0 \boldsymbol{E} + \boldsymbol{P} = \epsilon_0 \boldsymbol{E} + \epsilon_0 \chi_e \boldsymbol{E} = \epsilon_0 \left(1 + \chi_e\right) \boldsymbol{E} = \epsilon \boldsymbol{E} \ \ \ \text{ with } \ \ \epsilon = \epsilon_r \epsilon_0 = \epsilon_0 \left(1 + \chi_e\right) \tag{3.30}$$

Since the sphere is an insulator, there is no free surface charge such that $\sigma_{c(\text{free})} = 0$. Using Equations (3.29) and (3.30), we obtain the condition for the radial (r) component of the electric field E_r:

$$\sigma_{c(\text{free})} = 0 \quad \Rightarrow \quad D_{r,m} = D_{r,p}$$

$$\epsilon_m E_{r,m} = \epsilon_p E_{r,p} \ \text{ at } \ r = R \quad \text{where} \ \ \begin{cases} E_r = E_{r,m} \ \text{ for } \ r \geq R \ \left(\text{in medium}\right) \\[2mm] E_r = E_{r,p} \ \text{ for } \ r \leq R \ \left(\text{in particle}\right) \end{cases} \tag{3.31}$$

The electric field E_r in the radial direction can be found with the partial derivative of the potentials V as follows:

$$E_{r,m} = -\frac{\partial V_m}{\partial r} = E_0 \cos\theta + \frac{2A\cos\theta}{r^3} \quad \text{for} \ \ r \geq R \ \left(\text{in medium}\right) \tag{3.32}$$

$$E_{r,p} = -\frac{\partial V_p}{\partial r} = B\cos\theta \ \ \text{ for } \ r \leq R \ \left(\text{in particle}\right) \tag{3.33}$$

From Equations (3.25) to (3.33), the unknown A and B are found as (the proof is left as an exercise)

$$A = \frac{\epsilon_p - \epsilon_m}{\epsilon_p + 2\epsilon_m} R^3 E_0 \quad \text{and} \quad B = \frac{3\epsilon_m}{\epsilon_p + 2\epsilon_m} E_0 \tag{3.34}$$

Matching Equation (3.24) with the dipole term of Equation (3.25), we get the effective dipole moment $\boldsymbol{p}_{\mathrm{eff}}$ of the insulating spherical particle polarized in an external uniform electric field $\boldsymbol{E} = E_0\,\hat{\boldsymbol{z}}$:

$$V_{\mathrm{dipole}} = \frac{p_{\mathrm{eff}}\cos\theta}{4\pi\epsilon_m r^2} = \frac{A\cos\theta}{r^2} \quad \Rightarrow \quad p_{\mathrm{eff}} = 4\pi\epsilon_m A = 4\pi\epsilon_m \frac{\epsilon_p - \epsilon_m}{\epsilon_p + 2\epsilon_m} R^3 E_0$$

$$\boldsymbol{p}_{\mathrm{eff}} = 4\pi\epsilon_m K R^3 E_0 \hat{\boldsymbol{z}} \quad \text{with} \quad K\left(\epsilon_p, \epsilon_m\right) = \frac{\epsilon_p - \epsilon_m}{\epsilon_p + 2\epsilon_m} \tag{3.35}$$

where $K(\epsilon_p, \epsilon_m)$ is the Clausius-Mossotti (CM) factor, which is a measure of the strength of the effective polarization as a function of the permittivities. The sign of K determines whether the polarization is parallel or anti-parallel to the direction of the electric field. In this case, K is limited to $-0.5 \leq K \leq 1$ by considering the limit as either permittivity approaches zero.

EXAMPLE 3-4 Prove that $V_m\,(r, \theta)$ and $V_p\,(r, \theta)$ are of the forms

$$\left\{ \begin{aligned} V_m(r,\theta) &= -E_0 r\cos\theta + \frac{A\cos\theta}{r^2} \quad \text{for } r \geq R \text{ (in medium)} \\ V_p(r,\theta) &= -B\,r\cos\theta \quad \text{for } r \leq R \text{ (in particle)} \end{aligned} \right.$$

using the boundary conditions [Equations (3.27) and (3.31)], and the potential from the external electric field $\boldsymbol{E} = E_0\hat{\boldsymbol{z}}$ which can be expressed as

$$V_m(r \rightarrow \infty, \theta) = V_{\mathrm{external\ field}} = -E_0 z = -E_0 r\cos\theta \quad \text{(in medium)}$$

That is, the electric potential very far from the particle should be equal to the potential from the external electric field. To get the proof, first show that $\nabla^2 V = 0$ (Laplace's equation) using $\nabla \cdot \boldsymbol{D} = \rho_{\mathrm{free}}$ (Gauss's law in matter) where ρ_{free} is the free volume charge density. Then, use the general solution of Laplace's equation in spherical coordinates assuming azimuthal symmetry (i.e., V does not depend on the azimuthal angle φ):

$$\left\{ \begin{aligned} \nabla \cdot \boldsymbol{D} &= \rho_{\mathrm{free}} \\ \boldsymbol{E} &= -\nabla V \end{aligned} \right. \quad \Rightarrow \quad \nabla^2 V(r,\theta) = 0 \quad \Rightarrow \quad V(r,\theta) = \sum_{l=0}^{\infty}\left(B_l r^l + \frac{A_l}{r^{l+1}} \right) P_l(\cos\theta)$$

where B_l and A_l are constants and $P_l\,(\cos\theta)$ is the lth Legendre polynomial.

Solution   Gauss's law in matter is given by

$$\nabla \cdot \boldsymbol{D} = \nabla \cdot (\epsilon \boldsymbol{E}) = \epsilon \nabla \cdot \boldsymbol{E} = \rho_{\mathrm{free}}$$

Charges created through polarization are called "bound" charges, which by definition are not "free". Since there are no free volume charges, we have $\rho_{\mathrm{free}} = 0$. Thus, $\nabla \cdot \boldsymbol{E} = 0$ and

$$\boldsymbol{E} = -\nabla V \quad \Rightarrow \quad \nabla \cdot \boldsymbol{E} = \nabla \cdot (-\nabla V) = -\nabla \cdot \nabla V = -\nabla^2 V = 0$$

Thus, $\nabla^2 V = 0$. This is Laplace's equation. Assuming azimuthal symmetry (i.e., V does not depend on φ), the general solution in spherical coordinates is

$$\nabla^2 V(r,\theta) = 0 \Rightarrow \left\{ \begin{aligned} V_m(r,\theta) &= \sum_{l=0}^{\infty}\left(B_{m,l} r^l + \frac{A_{m,l}}{r^{l+1}} \right) P_l(\cos\theta) \quad \text{for } r \geq R \text{ (in medium)} \\ V_p(r,\theta) &= \sum_{l=0}^{\infty}\left(B_{p,l} r^l + \frac{A_{p,l}}{r^{l+1}} \right) P_l(\cos\theta) \quad \text{for } r \leq R \text{ (in particle)} \end{aligned} \right.$$

where $B_{m,l}$, $A_{m,l}$, $B_{p,l}$, and $A_{p,l}$ are constants and $P_l(\cos\theta)$ is the lth Legendre polynomial. Using the third boundary condition, we have

$$\text{For } r \geq R \text{ (in medium)}: \quad V_m(r \to \infty, \theta) = -E_0 z = -E_0 r \cos\theta = -E_0 r P_1(\cos\theta)$$

Thus, for $V_m(r,\theta)$, $B_{m,1} = -E_0 r$ and all other $B_{m,l} = 0$.

$$\text{For } r \geq R \text{ (in medium)}: \quad V_m(r,\theta) = -E_0 r P_1(\cos\theta) + \sum_{l=0}^{\infty} \frac{A_{m,l}}{r^{l+1}} P_l(\cos\theta)$$

For $r < R$, $V_p(r = 0, \theta)$ cannot diverge to infinity, so $A_{p,l} = 0$ for all l and

$$\text{For } r \leq R \text{ (in particle)}: \quad V_p(r,\theta) = \sum_{l=0}^{\infty} B_{p,l}\, r^l P_l(\cos\theta)$$

Using boundary condition [Equation (3.27)] and canceling out $P_l(\cos\theta)$ terms on both sides of the equation, we get

$$(\mathbf{1})\ V_m(R,\theta) = V_p(R,\theta)\quad (\text{at } r = R)\ \Rightarrow\ \begin{cases} -E_0 R + \dfrac{A_{m,1}}{R^2} = B_{p,1} R & (\text{for } l = 1) \\[3mm] \dfrac{A_{m,l}}{R^{l+1}} = B_{p,l} R^l & (\text{for } l \neq 1) \end{cases}$$

Using boundary condition [Equation (3.31)], we have

$$(\mathbf{2})\ \epsilon_m E_{r,m} = \epsilon_p E_{r,p}\quad (\text{at } r = R)\ \Rightarrow\ \epsilon_m \frac{-\partial V_m}{\partial r} = \epsilon_p \frac{-\partial V_p}{\partial r}\quad (\text{at } r = R)$$

$$\frac{\partial V_m}{\partial r} = -E_0 P_1(\cos\theta) + \sum_{l=0}^{\infty} -(l+1)\frac{A_{m,l}}{r^{l+2}} P_l(\cos\theta) \quad \text{and} \quad \frac{\partial V_p}{\partial r} = \sum_{l=0}^{\infty} l \cdot B_{p,l}\, r^{l-1} P_l(\cos\theta)$$

$$\frac{-\partial V_m}{\partial r} = \frac{-\epsilon_p}{\epsilon_m}\frac{\partial V_p}{\partial r}\quad (\text{at } r = R)\ \Rightarrow\ \begin{cases} E_0 + \dfrac{2A_{m,1}}{R^3} = \dfrac{-\epsilon_p}{\epsilon_m} B_{p,1} & (\text{for } l = 1) \\[3mm] (l+1)\dfrac{A_{m,l}}{R^{l+2}} = \dfrac{-\epsilon_p}{\epsilon_m} l\, B_{p,l}\, R^{l-1} & (\text{for } l \neq 1) \end{cases}$$

where again we cancelled out $P_l(\cos\theta)$ terms on both sides of the equation. Combining the above expressions for $l \neq 1$, we get

$$(l+1)\frac{A_{m,l}}{R^{l+2}} = \frac{-\epsilon_p}{\epsilon_m} l\, \frac{1}{R}\left(B_{p,l}\, R^l\right) = \frac{-\epsilon_p}{\epsilon_m} l\, \frac{1}{R}\left(\frac{A_{m,l}}{R^{l+1}}\right) = \frac{-\epsilon_p}{\epsilon_m} l\left(\frac{A_{m,l}}{R^{l+2}}\right)\quad (\text{for } l \neq 1)$$

The above equation has two general solutions:

$$(l+1) = \frac{-\epsilon_p}{\epsilon_m} l \quad \text{or} \quad A_{m,l} = 0 \quad (\text{for } l \neq 1)$$

Since in general $(l+1) \neq \dfrac{-\epsilon_p}{\epsilon_m} l$, we must have $A_{m,l} = 0$ for all $l \neq 1$. Thus,

$$\frac{A_{m,l}}{R^{l+1}} = B_{p,l}\, R^l = 0 \ (\text{for all } l \neq 1)\ \Rightarrow\ \begin{cases} A_{m,l} = 0 \\ B_{p,l} = 0 \end{cases} (\text{for all } l \neq 1)$$

With $A_{m,l} = B_{p,l} = 0$ for all $l \neq 1$, we obtain

$$\begin{cases} V_m(r,\theta) = -E_0 r P_1(\cos\theta) + \dfrac{A_{m,1}}{r^2} P_1(\cos\theta) & \text{for } r \geq R \text{ (in medium)} \\[3mm] V_p(r,\theta) = B_{p,1} r\, P_1(\cos\theta) & \text{for } r \leq R \text{ (in particle)} \end{cases}$$

Noting that $P_1(\cos\theta) = \cos\theta$, and letting $A = A_{m,1}$ and $-B = B_{p,1}$, we have

$$\left|\begin{array}{l} V_m(r,\theta) = -E_0 r\cos\theta + \dfrac{A\cos\theta}{r^2} \quad \text{for } r \geq R \text{ (in medium)} \\[3mm] \quad V_p(r,\theta) = -Br\cos\theta \quad \text{for } r \leq R \text{ (in particle)} \end{array}\right. \quad \blacktriangle$$

(E) Sphere with Loss in an AC Electric Field

In general, spherical particles (e.g., cells, nanoparticle, and metallic spheres) are conductive (non-insulating) and experience energy loss in an AC electric field. The dipole moment of such a particle, which provides a method for energy dissipation (loss)—such as via conduction—will lag behind a transient applied electric field signal. In other words, for an AC electric field signal, the phase of the dipole moment will lag behind the phase of the field. For an AC electric field E with angular frequency ω and amplitude E_0 directed in the z-direction, we have

$$E(t) = E_0\cos(\omega t)\hat{z} = \mathrm{Re}\left[E_0\exp(j\omega t)\right]\hat{z} \tag{3.36}$$

where $j = \sqrt{-1}$ is the imaginary unit, $\omega = 2\pi f$ is the angular frequency, f is the frequency, and $\bar{E}_0 = E_0$ is the applied AC electric field phasor because the phase angle is zero. Please refer to Appendix F for a review of complex numbers and phasors.

For this case, the solutions for the constants in the potential functions are assumed to be complex. Similar to the insulating sphere in Section 3.3.1(D), but with complex parameters $\tilde{A}$ and $\tilde{B}$, we have

$$\left|\begin{array}{l} \bar{V}_m = -E_0 r\cos\theta + \dfrac{\tilde{A}\cos\theta}{r^2} \quad \text{for } r \geq R \text{ (in medium)} \\[3mm] \quad \bar{V}_p = -\tilde{B}r\cos\theta \quad \text{for } r \leq R \text{ (in particle)} \end{array}\right. \tag{3.37}$$

$$\bar{V}_m = \bar{V}_p \text{ at } r = R \tag{3.38}$$

where $\bar{V}_m$ and $\bar{V}_p$ are electric potential phasors. Analogous to Equation (3.27), the electric potential phasor $\bar{V}$ must be continuous at $r = R$. The same boundary condition of Equation (3.29) can also be used here:

$$\bar{D}_{r,m} - \bar{D}_{r,p} = \epsilon_m\bar{E}_{r,m} - \epsilon_p\bar{E}_{r,p} = \sigma_{c(\text{free})} \text{ at } r = R \tag{3.39A}$$

$$\text{where}\left\{\begin{array}{l} \bar{D}_r = \bar{D}_{r,m} \text{ and } \bar{E}_r = \bar{E}_{r,m} = -\partial\bar{V}_m/\partial r \quad \text{for } r \geq R \text{ (in medium)} \\[3mm] \bar{D}_r = \bar{D}_{r,p} \text{ and } \bar{E}_r = \bar{E}_{r,p} = -\partial\bar{V}_p/\partial r \quad \text{for } r \leq R \text{ (in particle)} \end{array}\right. \tag{3.39B}$$

where $\bar{D}_r = \epsilon\bar{E}_r$ is the radial (r) component of the electric displacement phasor $\bar{D}$, while $\bar{E}_r$ is the radial (r) component of the electric field phasor $\bar{E}$ (please refer to Appendix F).

However, unlike the electrostatic case, the free surface charge density $\sigma_{c(\text{free})}$ is no longer zero because of loss in the form of conduction. Physically, it is difficult to express the amount of free charge contained in the particle. Instead, it is desirable to express this free charge in terms of other parameters. The instantaneous conservation of charge must be satisfied at the boundary and this can be used to find an expression for the free surface charge density $\sigma_{c(\text{free})}$. Using instantaneous conservation of charge and taking the derivative with respect to the surface area (Figure 3-9), we obtain another boundary condition.

$$J_{r,p} - J_{r,m} = \frac{\partial\sigma_{c(\text{free})}}{\partial t} \text{ at } r = R \tag{3.40}$$

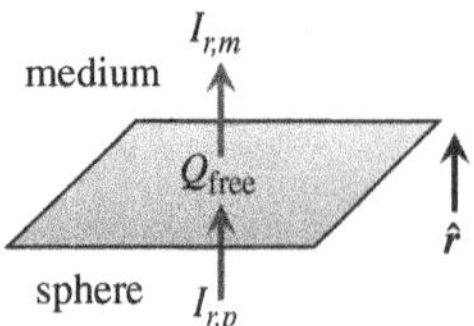

Figure 3-9 Instantaneous conservation of charge diagram for the derivation of Equation (3.40).

$$I_{r,p} - I_{r,m} = \frac{\partial Q_{\text{free}}}{\partial t} \quad \Rightarrow \quad \frac{\partial I_{r,p}}{\partial(\text{Area})} - \frac{\partial I_{r,m}}{\partial(\text{Area})} = \frac{\partial}{\partial t}\frac{\partial Q_{\text{free}}}{\partial(\text{Area})}$$

where $J_{r,p} = \sigma_p E_{r,p}$ and $J_{r,m} = \sigma_m E_{r,m}$ are the normal components of the current density outside and inside the sphere, respectively; $\sigma_{c(\text{free})}$ is the free electric surface charge density; σ_m and σ_p are the electrical conductivity of the medium and of the particle, respectively.

Converting J_r and E_r to phasor form ($\overline{J}_r$ and $\overline{E}_r$) such that all variables have the same exponential time dependence $e^{j\omega t}$, then $\partial/\partial t \to j\omega$ (please refer to Appendix F). Equation (3.40) becomes

$$\overline{J}_{r,p} - \overline{J}_{r,m} = \sigma_p \overline{E}_{r,p} - \sigma_m \overline{E}_{r,m} = j\omega\sigma_{c(\text{free})} \quad \text{at } r = R \tag{3.41}$$

Combining Equations (3.39) and (3.41), the boundary condition becomes

$$\sigma_{c(\text{free})} = \epsilon_m \overline{E}_{r,m} - \epsilon_p \overline{E}_{r,p} = \frac{\sigma_p}{j\omega}\overline{E}_{r,p} - \frac{\sigma_m}{j\omega}\overline{E}_{r,m} = \quad \Rightarrow \quad \left(\epsilon_m + \frac{\sigma_m}{j\omega}\right)\overline{E}_{r,m} = \left(\epsilon_p + \frac{\sigma_p}{j\omega}\right)\overline{E}_{r,p}$$

$$\overline{\epsilon}_m \overline{E}_{r,m} = \overline{\epsilon}_p \overline{E}_{r,p} \quad \text{at } r = R \quad \text{with} \quad \overline{\epsilon}_m = \epsilon_m + \frac{\sigma_m}{j\omega} \quad \text{and} \quad \overline{\epsilon}_p = \epsilon_p + \frac{\sigma_p}{j\omega} \tag{3.42}$$

where $\overline{\epsilon}_m$ and $\overline{\epsilon}_p$ are the complex permittivities. This is identical in form to Equation (3.31) for the electrostatic case, but now with complex parameters. The solution for the coefficients is

$$\tilde{A} = \frac{\overline{\epsilon}_p - \overline{\epsilon}_m}{\overline{\epsilon}_p + 2\overline{\epsilon}_m}R^3 E_0 \quad \text{and} \quad \tilde{B} = \frac{3\overline{\epsilon}_m}{\overline{\epsilon}_p + 2\overline{\epsilon}_m}E_0 \tag{3.43}$$

where scalar permittivities are replaced with complex values that incorporate the electrical conductivities σ_m (medium) and σ_p (particle). The (complex) dipole moment phasor $\overline{\boldsymbol{P}}_{\text{eff}}$ of the conductive sphere can be derived using the same method as the insulating sphere's (real) dipole moment $\boldsymbol{p}_{\text{eff}}$ from Section 3.3.1(D).

$$\overline{\boldsymbol{P}}_{\text{eff}} = 4\pi\epsilon_m \overline{K}(\omega)R^3 E_0\hat{\boldsymbol{z}} \quad \text{with} \quad \overline{K}(\omega) = \frac{\overline{\epsilon}_p - \overline{\epsilon}_m}{\overline{\epsilon}_p + 2\overline{\epsilon}_m} \quad \text{and} \quad \begin{cases} \overline{\epsilon}_m = \epsilon_m + \dfrac{\sigma_m}{j\omega} = \epsilon_m - j\dfrac{\sigma_m}{\omega} \\[2mm] \overline{\epsilon}_p = \epsilon_p + \dfrac{\sigma_p}{j\omega} = \epsilon_p - j\dfrac{\sigma_p}{\omega} \end{cases} \tag{3.44}$$

The phase difference from the electric field is contained in the complex Clausius-Mossotti (CM) factor $\overline{K}(\omega)$, which is frequency-dependent containing the permittivities and conductivities of the particle and medium. In the external AC electric field, the effective dipole moment $\boldsymbol{p}_{\text{eff}}(t)$ of the conductive sphere is the time varying real part of Equation (3.44) (please refer to Appendix F).

$$\boldsymbol{p}_{\text{eff}}(t) = \text{Re}\left[\overline{\boldsymbol{p}}_{\text{eff}}\exp(j\omega t)\right] = 4\pi\epsilon_m \text{Re}\left[\overline{K}(\omega)\exp(j\omega t)\right]R^3 E_0\hat{\boldsymbol{z}} \tag{3.45}$$

We can express the complex CM factor of $\overline{K}(\omega)$ in polar form as $\overline{K}(\omega) = |\overline{K}(\omega)|\exp(-j\varphi)$:

$$\boldsymbol{p}_{\text{eff}}(t) = 4\pi\epsilon_m \text{Re}\left\{|\overline{K}(\omega)|\exp(-j\varphi)\exp(j\omega t)\right\}R^3 E_0\hat{\boldsymbol{z}} = 4\pi\epsilon_m |\overline{K}(\omega)| \text{Re}\left\{\exp[j(\omega t - \varphi)]\right\} R^3 E_0\hat{\boldsymbol{z}}$$

$$\boldsymbol{p}_{\text{eff}}(t) = 4\pi\epsilon_m |\overline{K}(\omega)|\cos(\omega t - \varphi)R^3 E_0\hat{\boldsymbol{z}} \tag{3.46}$$

Equation (3.46) makes sense intuitively because $\boldsymbol{p}_{\text{eff}}(t)$ should lag behind in phase (in this case by φ) from the electric field $\boldsymbol{E}(t) = E_0 \cos(\omega t)\hat{\boldsymbol{z}}$. Next, we use the following vector identity

$$\nabla\left(\boldsymbol{p}_{\text{eff}} \cdot \boldsymbol{E}\right) = \boldsymbol{p}_{\text{eff}} \times \left(\nabla \times \boldsymbol{E}\right) + \boldsymbol{E} \times \left(\nabla \times \boldsymbol{p}_{\text{eff}}\right) + \left(\boldsymbol{p}_{\text{eff}} \cdot \nabla\right)\boldsymbol{E} + \left(\boldsymbol{E} \cdot \nabla\right)\boldsymbol{p}_{\text{eff}}$$

Since there are no time-varying magnetic fields, $\nabla \times \boldsymbol{E} = -\partial \boldsymbol{B}/\partial t = \boldsymbol{0}$ and

$$\nabla \times \boldsymbol{E} = \cos(\omega t)\left[\nabla \times \left(E_0 \hat{\boldsymbol{z}}\right)\right] = \boldsymbol{0} \quad \Rightarrow \quad \nabla \times \left(E_0 \hat{\boldsymbol{z}}\right) = \boldsymbol{0}$$

$$\nabla \times \boldsymbol{p}_{\text{eff}} = 4\pi\epsilon_m\left|\bar{K}(\omega)\right|\cos(\omega t - \varphi)R^3\left[\nabla \times \left(E_0 \hat{\boldsymbol{z}}\right)\right] = \boldsymbol{0}$$

$$\text{Thus,} \quad \nabla\left(\boldsymbol{p}_{\text{eff}} \cdot \boldsymbol{E}\right) = \left(\boldsymbol{p}_{\text{eff}} \cdot \nabla\right)\boldsymbol{E} + \left(\boldsymbol{E} \cdot \nabla\right)\boldsymbol{p}_{\text{eff}}$$

Using Equations (3.36) and (3.46), we have

$$\boldsymbol{E}(t) = E_0 \cos(\omega t)\hat{\boldsymbol{z}} \quad \text{and} \quad \boldsymbol{p}_{\text{eff}}(t) = 4\pi\epsilon_m\left|\bar{K}(\omega)\right|\cos(\omega t - \varphi)R^3 E_0 \hat{\boldsymbol{z}}$$

$$\left(\boldsymbol{p}_{\text{eff}} \cdot \nabla\right)\boldsymbol{E} = \left(\boldsymbol{E} \cdot \nabla\right)\boldsymbol{p}_{\text{eff}} = 4\pi\epsilon_m\left|\bar{K}(\omega)\right|\cos(\omega t)\cos(\omega t - \varphi)R^3\left[\left(E_0\hat{\boldsymbol{z}} \cdot \nabla\right)E_0\hat{\boldsymbol{z}}\right]$$

$$\text{Therefore,} \quad \nabla\left(\boldsymbol{p}_{\text{eff}} \cdot \boldsymbol{E}\right) = \left(\boldsymbol{p}_{\text{eff}} \cdot \nabla\right)\boldsymbol{E} + \left(\boldsymbol{E} \cdot \nabla\right)\boldsymbol{p}_{\text{eff}} = 2\left(\boldsymbol{p}_{\text{eff}} \cdot \nabla\right)\boldsymbol{E}$$

Finally, we can derive the DEP force $\boldsymbol{F}_{\text{DEP}}(t)$ as follows.

$$\boldsymbol{F}_{\text{DEP}}(t) = \boldsymbol{F}_{\text{dipole}} = \left(\boldsymbol{p}_{\text{eff}} \cdot \nabla\right)\boldsymbol{E} = \frac{1}{2}\nabla\left(\boldsymbol{p}_{\text{eff}} \cdot \boldsymbol{E}\right) = \frac{1}{2}\nabla\left[4\pi\epsilon_m\left|\bar{K}(\omega)\right|\cos(\omega t)\cos(\omega t - \varphi)R^3 E_0^2\right]$$

$$\boldsymbol{F}_{\text{DEP}}(t) = 2\pi\epsilon_m\left|\bar{K}(\omega)\right|\cos(\omega t)\cos(\omega t - \varphi)R^3\nabla\left(E_0^2\right) \tag{3.47}$$

Let $T = 2\pi/\omega$ be the period. The time-averaged value of the DEP force $\left\langle \boldsymbol{F}_{\text{DEP}}\right\rangle$ is

$$\left\langle \boldsymbol{F}_{\text{DEP}}\right\rangle = \frac{1}{T}\int_0^T \boldsymbol{F}_{\text{DEP}}(t)\,dt = \frac{2\pi\epsilon_m\left|\bar{K}(\omega)\right|R^3\nabla\left(E_0^2\right)}{T}\int_0^T \cos(\omega t)\cos(\omega t - \varphi)\,dt$$

$$\left\langle \boldsymbol{F}_{\text{DEP}}\right\rangle = \frac{2\pi\epsilon_m\left|\bar{K}(\omega)\right|R^3\nabla\left(E_0^2\right)}{T}\int_0^T \frac{1}{2}\left[\cos(\varphi) + \cos(2\omega t - \varphi)\right]dt$$

$$\left\langle \boldsymbol{F}_{\text{DEP}}\right\rangle = \frac{2\pi\epsilon_m\left|\bar{K}(\omega)\right|R^3\nabla\left(E_0^2\right)}{T} \cdot \frac{1}{2}\cos(\varphi)T = \pi\epsilon_m\left|\bar{K}(\omega)\right|\cos(\varphi)R^3\nabla\left(E_0^2\right)$$

$$\bar{K}(\omega) = \left|\bar{K}(\omega)\right|\exp(-j\varphi) = \left|\bar{K}(\omega)\right|\cos(\varphi) - j\left|\bar{K}(\omega)\right|\sin(\varphi) \quad \Rightarrow \quad \text{Re}\left[\bar{K}(\omega)\right] = \left|\bar{K}(\omega)\right|\cos(\varphi)$$

Finally, the time-averaged DEP force $\left\langle \boldsymbol{F}_{\text{DEP}}\right\rangle$ of a conductive sphere (with radius R) polarized by an external AC electric field $\boldsymbol{E}(t) = E_0 \cos(\omega t)\hat{\boldsymbol{z}}$ is

$$\left\langle \boldsymbol{F}_{\text{DEP}}\right\rangle = \pi\epsilon_m\text{Re}\left[\bar{K}(\omega)\right]R^3\nabla\left(E_0^2\right) \tag{3.48}$$

For a generic external AC electrical field $\boldsymbol{E}(\boldsymbol{r},\,t) = \boldsymbol{E}_0(\boldsymbol{r})\cos(\omega t)$, the time-averaged DEP force $\left\langle \boldsymbol{F}_{\text{DEP}}\right\rangle$ of a polarized conductive sphere (with radius R) is

$$\left\langle \boldsymbol{F}_{\text{DEP}}(\boldsymbol{r})\right\rangle = \pi\epsilon_m\text{Re}\left[\bar{K}(\omega)\right]R^3\nabla\left(\left|\boldsymbol{E}_0(\boldsymbol{r})\right|^2\right) \tag{3.49}$$

3.3.2 Electrical Properties of Microtubules

The aforementioned dipole moment has applications in biology. For example, since microtubules have a high dipole moment, their electrical properties are used for studying their biological functions. Microtubules are long cylindrical polymers composed of α-tubulin and β-tubulin subunits (both are globular proteins). They have hollow structures with a diameter of about 25 nm, and are tens of nanometers to hundreds of micrometers in length. [5] They form part of the cellular cytoskeleton and help provide the shape and rigidity of eukaryotic cells, as shown in Figure 3-10. Microtubules in neuronal systems are of key interest since their presence or absence has been linked to different brain diseases. A lack of microtubules in the brain has been linked to Alzheimer's disease, [6] whereas altered microtubule dynamics have been linked to a number of diseases including cancer. [7]

These microtubule polymer structures play important roles in a variety of intracellular functions. They can maintain the shape and rigidity of a cell via dynamic equilibrium achieved through simultaneous microtubule growth and shrinkage. They can form cilia and flagella for cell movement, or act as "rails" for macromolecular transport. The most important biological role of microtubules, however, is their function in the physical process of cell mitosis. All biological cells undergo mitosis, the division of a single cell into two daughter cells, as the host organism grows and ages. In this process, microtubules actively work to position and stabilize the mitotic spindle for the division. The purpose of the mitotic spindle, which is composed of microtubules, is to segregate chromosomes into the two daughter cells during cell division.

The biological roles of microtubules pertaining to their function in providing cellular structure and assisting in cell division are well-studied, but their electrical properties remain elusive. Due to the abundance of microtubules in neuron cells (as compared to non-neural cells), it has been hypothesized that microtubules may play a role in electrical signal transmission inside neurons. As biological analogs of carbon nanotubes, microtubules bear many similarities with carbon nanotubes in their shape and constituent distribution.

Microtubules are unique as biological components as they possess a very significant polarity. Each tubulin dimer (the protein building block of microtubules) has a negative external charge of $\sim 23e$. One of the main factors contributing to the academic interest in microtubules is the charge distribution on the tubulin protein. The majority of the tubulin's external charge resides on two tail-like structures, called the C-termini, that stem from the main protein body. Due to the small structural size of the C-termini, these structures have extremely high charge density. This is manifested in the tubulin protein which has an abnormally high dipole moment of 1750 debye. The

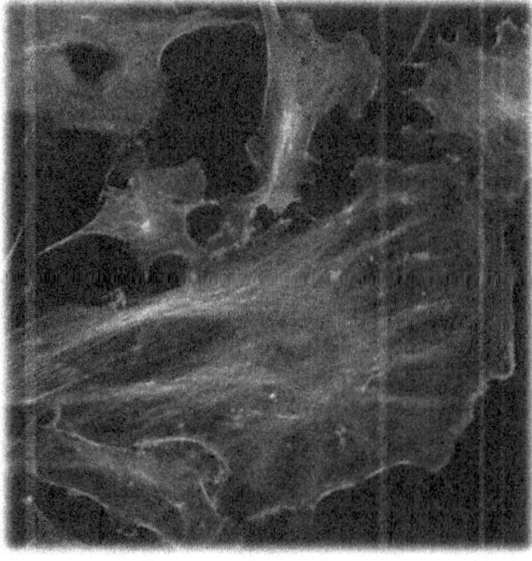

Figure 3-10   Microscope image of eukaryotic endothelial cells, with microtubules highlighted in green, cell nuclei stained blue, and actin filaments stained red. For a color version of this figure, please refer to https://imagej.nih.gov/ij/images/FluorescentCells.jpg. (*The microscope image is from the U.S. National Institutes of Health [NIH].*[4])

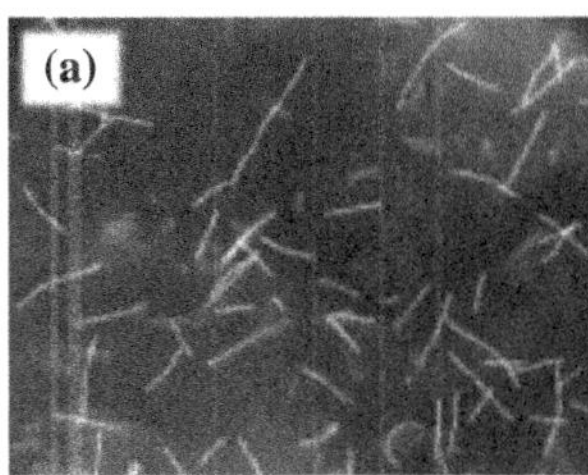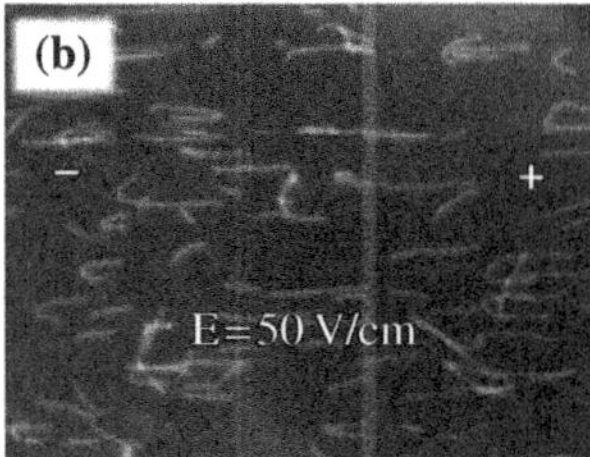

Figure 3-11 (a) Microtubules without an electric field. They are randomly oriented; (b) Under an applied electric field of 50 V/cm, the microtubules become aligned with the field and flow toward the positive electrode. (*The images are reprinted with permission from T. Kim et al.*[9])

tubulin protein stands out from other proteins in terms of charge and dipole moment. This extreme charge density is the primary reason scientists believe that microtubules are highly susceptible to electric fields, as shown in Figure 3-11. The unique tubulin sequence results in the characteristic polarity of a microtubule used in mitotic cell division, where structural support and chromosomal division are provided by electrostatic attraction and repulsion.[8]

The electrical properties of microtubules are predominantly exploited using DC fields. Let us take a look at how microtubules perform under AC fields. The abnormally high dipole moment of microtubules allows us to approximate microtubules as dipoles. Assuming that a cell is experiencing an external alternating electric field, the microtubules in the cell (representing dipoles) align with the electric field as the field inside a cell is relatively uniform as shown in Figure 3-12a. When the cell undergoes cellular division, the shape of the dividing cell starts to resemble a furrow-type shape as the cleavage furrow develops. The external electric field becomes non-uniform near the cleavage point in the cell. This non-uniform electric field leads the microtubules (the dipole) to experience DEP, as shown in Figure 3-12b. The DEP force leads to microtubule accumulation at the cell furrow, which significantly interferes with the cellular division process and prevents the tubulin dimers from binding to the microtubule. This process can lead to a mitotic delay in cell division. If the division process continues, the DEP forces created on the microtubules by cell cleavage will lead to abnormal cell division (i.e., improper exchange and separation of chromosomes), which can lead to cell death.

As shown in Figure 3-13, microtubules are densely located in the growth cone and dendritic regions because the information is received and sent by a cell in these regions.

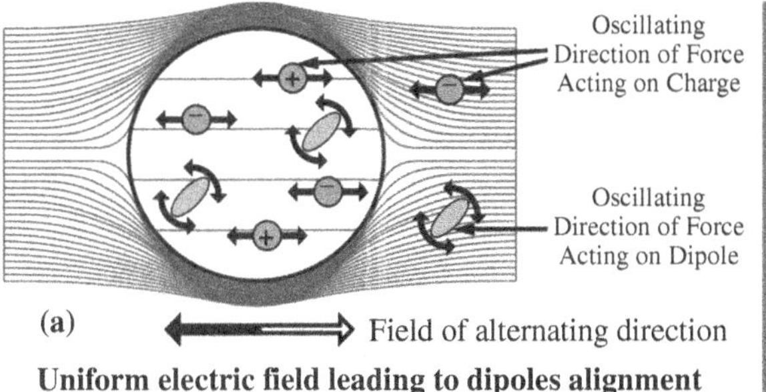

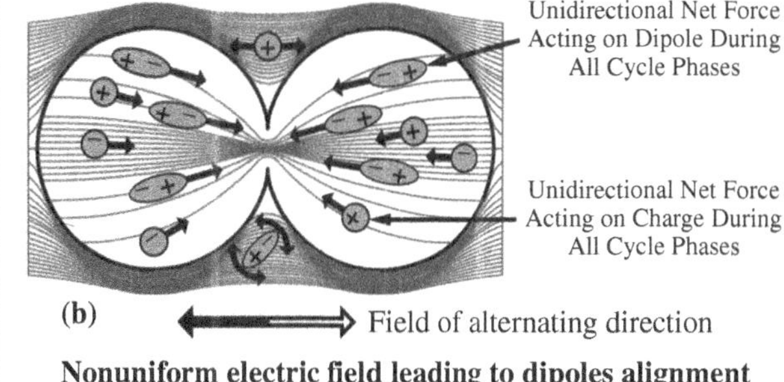

Figure 3-12 (a) A cell in an external electric field. Due to the uniform field inside the cell, the microtubules orient with the field. (b) A cell undergoes mitosis in an electric field. A non-uniform field is created at the cell furrow, which attracts microtubules due to a DEP force. (*The illustrations are reprinted with permission from A. F. Hottinger et al.*[10])

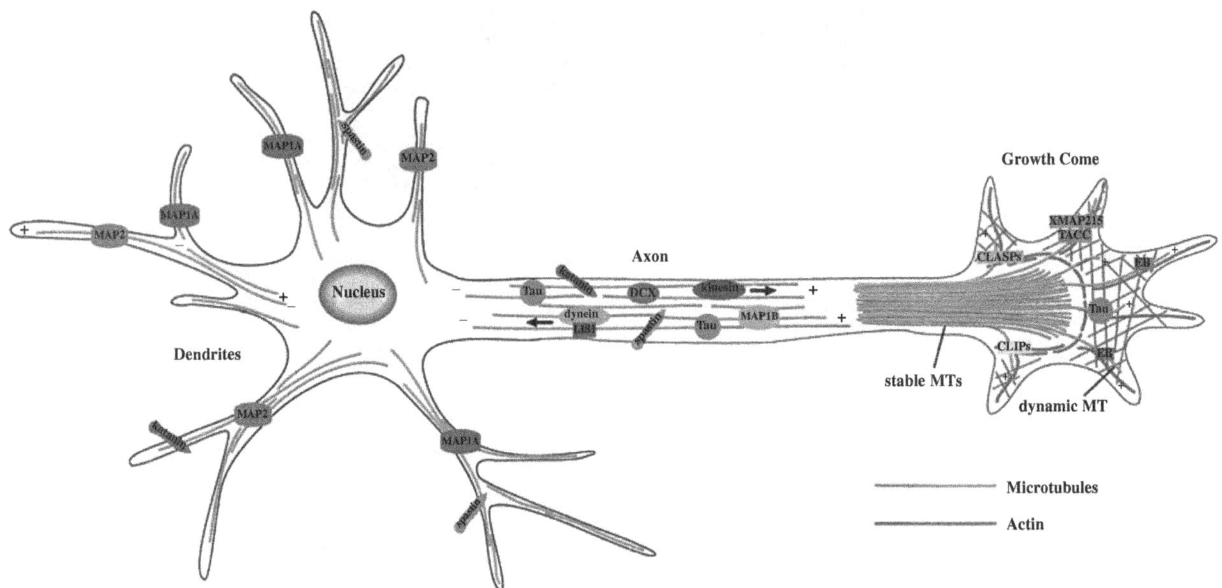

Figure 3-13   A schematic of the internal view of a neuron (*From M. Lasser et al.*[11])

Also, microtubules are arranged in a parallel fashion in the axon. This arrangement of microtubules acts as an efficient transportation network for macromolecules. The electrical properties of microtubules further allow the specialization of the roles of microtubules in ionic and/or electronic signal transport. Since "information" transfer in the brain occurs inside complex neural networks, this prompts the question of the signal transmission and information processing properties of microtubules. A few experiments have been conducted to determine the electrical modes and resonant frequencies of microtubules. The information helps identify the origins of brain waves. An AC signal was applied in a stepwise fashion to a microtubule bundle, and the bundle emitted an electrical signal at various resonant frequencies, but predominantly at 39 Hz.[12] This finding makes perfect sense because 40 Hz is within the neuronal γ frequency range. γ waves (30 to 100 Hz) are neural oscillations observed in humans, which are linked to mood and cognitive disorders (Alzheimer's disease, epilepsy, and even schizophrenia).[13] The findings above imply that microtubules play an important role in the development and progression of mental disorders.

3.4 COMPARISON OF FLUID TRANSPORT METHODS

We have presented a number of methods for transporting fluids in microsystems. For example, pressure, diffusion, or electric fields can be used to move and mix fluids through microfabricated channels. We have also seen how common methods for transporting fluids in large macroscopic systems can be ineffective in microscale systems.

Common fluid transport methods employed in microsystems are summarized in Table 3-2. Pressure can be used to fill capillaries and activate passive valves. Electrophoretic and electro-osmotic flow can be combined to move and separate charged species for detection. Diffusion is much more prominent in microsystems, but is not effective at mixing substances due to laminar flow. In microsystems, diffusion can be used for separation and should be accounted for in other applications.

TABLE 3-2   Overview of Fluid Transport Methods in Microfluidics

Method	Mechanism	What Moves?	Significance
Pressure-Driven Flow (PDF)	Forces generated by fluid pressure (e.g., force of gravity on vertical columns of fluid)	All of the fluid, but in a profile where it moves the most at the center and not at all at the edges	Far less significant in microsystems due to the small cross-sectional areas
Capillary Action	Surface interactions of liquid, gas, and solid interfaces	All of the fluid, depending on the relative strength of the adhesive and cohesive forces	Can be exploited to automatically fill capillaries and create passive valves
Electro-Osmotic Flow (EOF)	Electric potential between the charged surface and free charges in the fluid	All of the fluid sufficiently "far" from the wall, which is assumed to be all of it	Either very significant or insignificant depending on the systems' zeta potential
Diffusion	Molecules in the fluid spreading due to random motion	All molecules in the fluid at rates determined by the diffusion coefficients of the individual molecules	Far more significant in microsystems. Not effective at mixing substances under laminar flow
Electrophoretic Flow (EPF)	Electrostatic forces	Charged entities in the fluid	Can be highly significant. Commonly used to separate particles based on charge and size

3.5 APPLICATIONS

3.5.1 Separation by Diffusion

One way to separate two components in a fluid is through diffusion. We can use a microfluidic device called an H-filter to continuously extract components with relatively high diffusion coefficients from the rest of the fluid. Since smaller molecules and particles have significantly higher diffusion coefficients than larger molecules and particles, we can continuously extract smaller analytes from any given mixture. Assuming that we have a mixture (Mixture X) containing two different substances X1 and X2—where X1 has a much higher diffusion coefficient—the separation procedure is as follows.

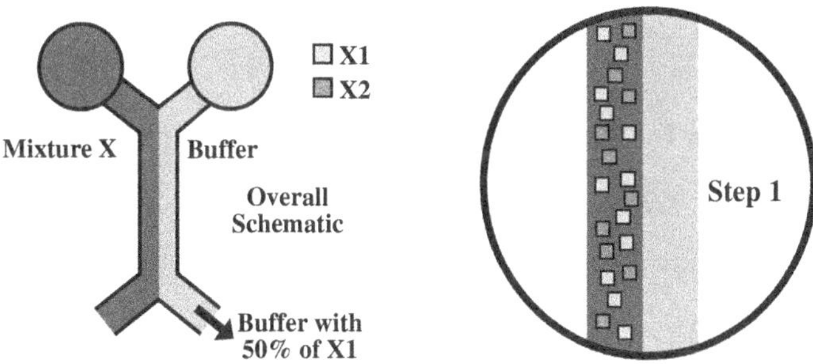

Step 1: Load mixture X and a buffer into the microsystem which is small enough to ensure fully laminar fluid flow. Separation by diffusion will not work if fluid flow is transitional or turbulent. The right insert is a zoomed-in image showing what happens in the microchannel.

Step 2: If X1 has a diffusion coefficient (D1) that is several orders of magnitude larger than that of X2 (D2), then with enough travel time, only X1 will be able to cross into the buffer.

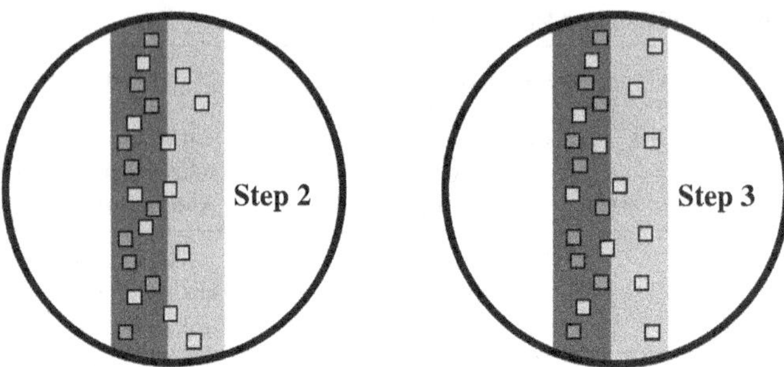

Step 3: If properly engineered, when the buffer is separated at the end, the buffer should contain 50% of X1 in the fluid without any X2 in it.

3.5.2 Cell Capture and Separation by Dielectrophoresis (DEP)

To manipulate cells using dielectrophoresis (DEP), we need to create a non-uniform electric field, like the one in the example shown in Figure 3-14. We can program the AC electric field frequency—which changes the CM factor $\bar{K}(\omega)$—to either capture (pDEP = positive DEP) or reject (nDEP = negative DEP) cells as well as other particles. If the capture voltage is too high, the electric field in a conductive medium can generate Joule heating, damaging the electrodes and causing cell death when the temperature exceeds 40°C. Note that the temperature rise is independent of the AC frequency because Joule heating depends

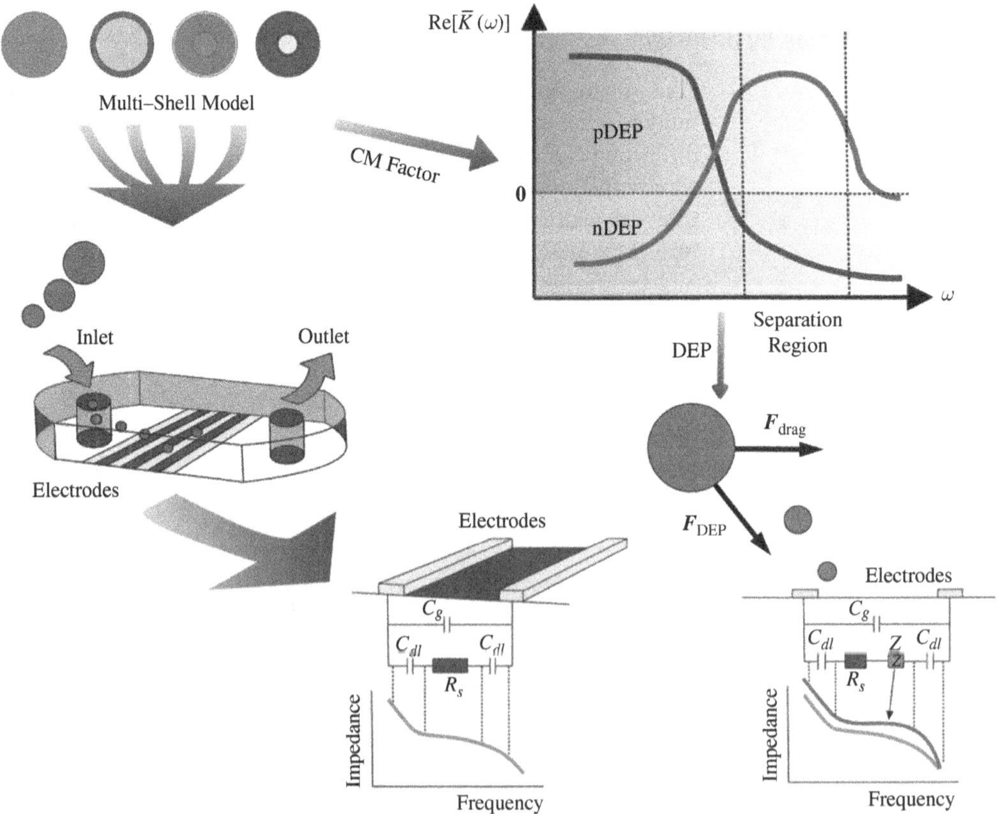

Figure 3-14   Using dielectrophoresis (DEP) powered by interdigitated electrodes (IDEs) to capture cells.

only on the root-mean-square (rms) electrical current and the electrical conductivity of the medium. On the other hand, the dielectric properties of the particles and the suspension media affect the magnitude of the DEP force. For example, the DEP force greatly increases with increasing polarizability of the particles immersed in a suspension medium.

(A) Spherical Multi-Layer Cellular Models

A double-layer spherical model (Figure 3-15, left) has been proposed to describe the cytoplasm and the membrane of a human embryonic kidney (HEK) 293 cell.[14] A triple-layer spherical model (Figure 3-15, right) has been used to simulate the nucleus, membrane, and cell wall of a yeast cell.[15] The geometric and dielectric parameters of a HEK 293 cell and yeast cells are listed in Table 3-3. With these models, living and dead yeast cells can be differentiated/separated according to their Clausius-Mossotti (CM) factor (refer to Figure 3-16).

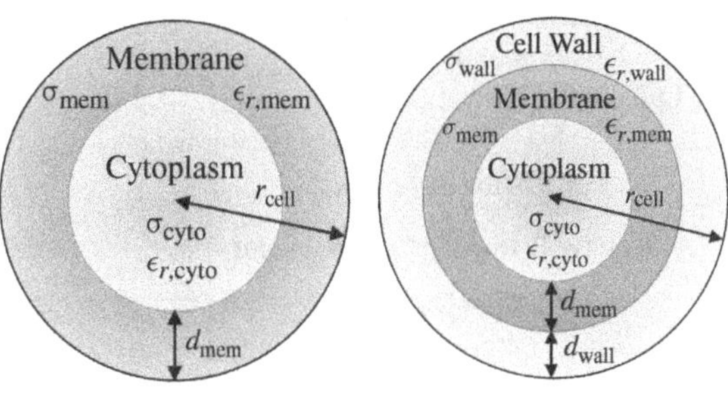

Figure 3-15   (Left) A double-layer model of an animal cell. (Right) A triple-layer model of a yeast cell.

TABLE 3-3   Geometric and Dielectric Parameters of a HEK 293 Cell and Yeast Cells[14,15]

Parameter	HEK 293 Cell	Live Yeast Cell	Dead Yeast Cell
Cell radius r_{cell}	6.25 μm	3.0 μm	2.5 μm
Cytoplasm conductivity σ_{cyto}	0.5 S/m	0.2 S/m	0.007 S/m
Cytoplasm relative permittivity $\epsilon_{r,cyto}$	60	50	50
Membrane thickness d_{mem}	7 nm	8 nm	8 nm
Membrane conductivity σ_{mem}	7×10^{-14} S/m	25×10^{-8} S/m	16×10^{-5} S/m
Membrane relative permittivity $\epsilon_{r,mem}$	9.5	6	6
Cell wall thickness d_{wall}	N/A	220 nm	250 nm
Cell wall conductivity σ_{wall}	N/A	14×10^{-3} S/m	1.5×10^{-3} S/m
Cell wall relative permittivity $\epsilon_{r,wall}$	N/A	60	60

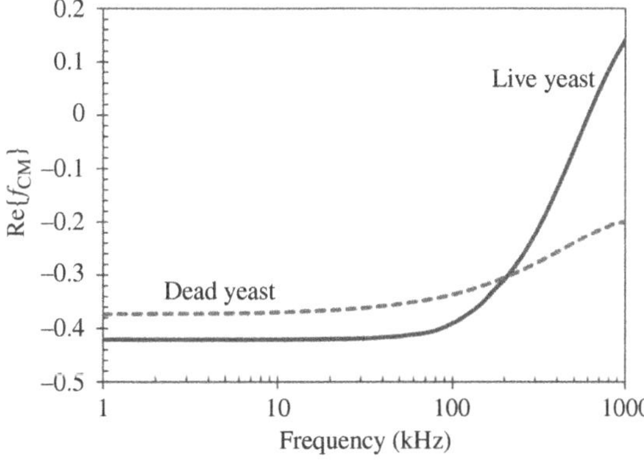

Figure 3-16   Clausius-Mossotti (CM) factors for dead yeast cells and live yeast cells. (*The figure is reprinted with permission from S. Patel et al.*[15])

EXAMPLE 3-5 A spherical insulating particle (such as a cell) of radius R_2 is in a uniform electric field $\mathbf{E} = E_0\hat{z}$. The particle has an inner sphere of radius R_1, which has a permittivity ϵ_1, and an outer concentric shell extending from radius R_1 to R_2, which has a permittivity ϵ_2. The particle is in a medium of permittivity ϵ_m. The figure on the right illustrates the concentric double-layer spherical particle.

As in Example 3-4, the potential $V(r,\theta)$ is the solution to Laplace's equation. Again, the general solution in spherical coordinates has the form:

$$\nabla^2 V(r,\theta) = 0 \quad \Rightarrow \quad V(r,\theta) = \sum_{l=0}^{\infty}\left(M_l r^l + \frac{N_l}{r^{l+1}} \right) P_l(\cos\theta) = \left(M_1 r + \frac{N_1}{r^2} \right)\cos\theta \quad \text{(for all } r)$$

where M_l and N_l are constants and $P_l(\cos\theta)$ is the lth Legendre polynomial. Due to the boundary conditions, only $l = 1$ is allowed. Let us define V_1, V_2, and V_m with the following boundary conditions from Equations (3.27) and (3.31):

$$\begin{cases} V_1 = V(r,\theta) \ \left(\text{for } 0 \leq r \leq R_1\right) \\ V_2 = V(r,\theta) \ \left(\text{for } R_1 \leq r \leq R_2\right) \\ V_m = V(r,\theta) \ \left(\text{for } r \geq R_2\right) \end{cases} \quad \text{and} \quad \begin{cases} V_1(r = R_1) = V_2(r = R_1) \\ \epsilon_1 E_{r,1}(r = R_1) = \epsilon_2 E_{r,2}(r = R_1) \\ V_2(r = R_2) = V_m(r = R_2) \\ \epsilon_2 E_{r,2}(r = R_2) = \epsilon_2 E_{r,m}(r = R_2) \end{cases}$$

Note that we must also have

$$V_m(r \to \infty, \theta) = V_{\text{external field}} = -E_0 z = -E_0 r\cos\theta \quad \text{(in medium)}$$

Show that the Clausius-Mossotti (CM) factor of the double-layer spherical particle can be given by

$$K = \frac{\epsilon_2' - \epsilon_m}{\epsilon_2' + 2\epsilon_m} \quad \text{where} \quad \epsilon_2' = \epsilon_2 \frac{\left[\left(\dfrac{R_2}{R_1}\right)^3 + 2\left(\dfrac{\epsilon_1 - \epsilon_2}{\epsilon_1 + 2\epsilon_2}\right) \right]}{\left[\left(\dfrac{R_2}{R_1}\right)^3 - \left(\dfrac{\epsilon_1 - \epsilon_2}{\epsilon_1 + 2\epsilon_2}\right) \right]}$$

Solution   We define V_1, V_2, and V_m as follows:

$$V_1 = Ar\cos\theta + \frac{N_1 \cos\theta}{r^2} = Ar\cos\theta \quad \left(\text{for } 0 \leq r \leq R_1\right)$$

$$V_2 = Br\cos\theta + \frac{C\cos\theta}{r^2} \quad \left(\text{for } R_1 \leq r \leq R_2\right) \qquad V_m = -E_0 r\cos\theta + \frac{D\cos\theta}{r^2} \quad \left(\text{for } r \geq R_2\right)$$

where we must have $N_1 = 0$ to prevent V_1 from diverging at $r = 0$. The form of V_m results from the condition that $V_m(r \to \infty, \theta) = -E_0 r\cos\theta$.

The boundary conditions of V_1 and V_2 at $r = R_1$ are

$$V_1(r = R_1) = V_2(r = R_1) \qquad \text{and} \qquad \epsilon_1 E_{r,1}(r = R_1) = \epsilon_2 E_{r,2}(r = R_1)$$

Solving $E_{r,1}$ and $E_{r,2}$ based on V_1 and V_2, we get

$$\begin{cases} E_{r,1} = -\dfrac{\partial V_1}{\partial r} = -A\cos\theta \quad \left(\text{for } 0 \leq r \leq R_1\right) \\[2mm] E_{r,2} = -\dfrac{\partial V_2}{\partial r} = -B\cos\theta + \dfrac{2C\cos\theta}{r^3} \quad \left(\text{for } R_1 \leq r \leq R_2\right) \end{cases}$$

Using the two boundary conditions of V_1 and V_2 at $r = R_1$, we obtain

$$\left\{ \begin{aligned} AR_1\cos\theta &= BR_1\cos\theta + \frac{C\cos\theta}{R_1^2} \quad \Rightarrow \quad A = B + \frac{C}{R_1^3} \\[2mm] \epsilon_1\left(-A\cos\theta\right) &= \epsilon_2\left(-B\cos\theta + \frac{2C\cos\theta}{R_1^3}\right) \quad \Rightarrow \quad -A\epsilon_1 = -B\epsilon_2 + \frac{2C\epsilon_2}{R_1^3} \end{aligned} \right.$$

We can relate variables B and C by removing variable A:

$$-B\epsilon_2 + \frac{2C\epsilon_2}{R_1^3} = -A\epsilon_1 = -B\epsilon_1 - \frac{C\epsilon_1}{R_1^3} \quad \Rightarrow \quad B\left(\epsilon_1 - \epsilon_2\right) = -\frac{C}{R_1^3}\left(\epsilon_1 + 2\epsilon_2\right)$$

$$C = -R_1^3\frac{B\left(\epsilon_1 - \epsilon_2\right)}{\left(\epsilon_1 + 2\epsilon_2\right)} = -BR_1^3 k_\epsilon \quad \text{with} \quad k_\epsilon \equiv \frac{\epsilon_1 - \epsilon_2}{\epsilon_1 + 2\epsilon_2}$$

where we defined k_ϵ for future simplicity. The boundary conditions of V_2 and V_m at $r = R_2$ are

$$V_2\left(r = R_2\right) = V_m\left(r = R_2\right) \quad \text{and} \quad \epsilon_2 E_{r,2}\left(r = R_2\right) = \epsilon_2 E_{r,m}\left(r = R_2\right)$$

Solving $E_{r,2}$ and $E_{r,m}$ based on V_2 and V_m, we get

$$\left\{ \begin{aligned} E_{r,2} &= -\frac{\partial V_2}{\partial r} = -B\cos\theta + \frac{2C\cos\theta}{r^3} \quad \left(\text{for } R_1 \leq r \leq R_2\right) \\[2mm] E_{r,m} &= -\frac{\partial V_m}{\partial r} = E_0\cos\theta + \frac{2D\cos\theta}{r^3} \quad \left(\text{for } r \geq R_2\right) \end{aligned} \right.$$

Using the two boundary conditions of V_2 and V_m at $r = R_2$, we obtain

$$\left\{ \begin{aligned} BR_2\cos\theta + \frac{C\cos\theta}{R_2^2} &= -E_0 R_2\cos\theta + \frac{D\cos\theta}{R_2^2} \quad \Rightarrow \quad -E_0 + \frac{D}{R_2^3} = B + \frac{C}{R_2^3} \\[2mm] \epsilon_2\left(-B\cos\theta + \frac{2C\cos\theta}{R_2^3}\right) &= \epsilon_m\left(E_0\cos\theta + \frac{2D\cos\theta}{R_2^3}\right) \quad \Rightarrow \quad -B\epsilon_2 + \frac{2C\epsilon_2}{R_2^3} = \epsilon_m E_0 + \frac{2D\epsilon_m}{R_2^3} \end{aligned} \right.$$

Substituting variable C into the equation above, we get

$$-E_0 + \frac{D}{R_2^3} = B + \frac{C}{R_2^3} = B + \frac{\left(-BR_1^3 k_\epsilon\right)}{R_2^3} = B\left(1 - \frac{R_1^3}{R_2^3}k_\epsilon\right)$$

$$\epsilon_m E_0 + \frac{2D\epsilon_m}{R_2^3} = -B\epsilon_2 + \frac{2C\epsilon_2}{R_2^3} = -B\epsilon_2 + \frac{2\left(-BR_1^3 k_\epsilon\right)\epsilon_2}{R_2^3} = -B\epsilon_2\left(1 + \frac{2R_1^3}{R_2^3}k_\epsilon\right)$$

Eliminating variable B by dividing the two expressions above, we have

$$\frac{-B\epsilon_2\left(1 + \dfrac{2R_1^3}{R_2^3}k_\epsilon\right)}{B\left(1 - \dfrac{R_1^3}{R_2^3}k_\epsilon\right)} = \frac{\epsilon_m E_0 + \dfrac{2D\epsilon_m}{R_2^3}}{-E_0 + \dfrac{D}{R_2^3}} \quad \Rightarrow \quad -\epsilon_2\frac{\left(\dfrac{R_2}{R_1}\right)^3 + 2k_\epsilon}{\left(\dfrac{R_2}{R_1}\right)^3 - k_\epsilon} = \epsilon_m\frac{R_2^3 E_0 + 2D}{-R_2^3 E_0 + D}$$

$$\epsilon_2' \equiv \epsilon_2\frac{\left(\dfrac{R_2}{R_1}\right)^3 + 2k_\epsilon}{\left(\dfrac{R_2}{R_1}\right)^3 - k_\epsilon} = -\epsilon_m\frac{R_2^3 E_0 + 2D}{-R_2^3 E_0 + D} \quad \Rightarrow \quad -\frac{\epsilon_2'}{\epsilon_m}\left(-R_2^3 E_0 + D\right) = \frac{\epsilon_2'}{\epsilon_m}R_2^3 E - \frac{\epsilon_2'}{\epsilon_m}D = R_2^3 E_0 + 2D$$

$$\left(\frac{\epsilon_2'}{\epsilon_m} - 1\right)R_2^3 E_0 = D\left(2 + \frac{\epsilon_2'}{\epsilon_m}\right) \quad \Rightarrow \quad D = R_2^3 E_0\left(\frac{\epsilon_2' - \epsilon_m}{\epsilon_2' + 2\epsilon_m}\right)$$

Similar to Equation (3.25), we can split $V_m(r, \theta)$ into two terms as follows.

$$V_m(r,\theta) = V_{\text{external field}} + V_{\text{dipole}} = -E_0 r \cos\theta + \frac{D\cos\theta}{r^2} \quad \text{for } r \geq R_2 \text{ (in medium)}$$

Because $V_{\text{dipole}} = \frac{p_{\text{eff}}\cos\theta}{4\pi\epsilon_m r^2} = \frac{D\cos\theta}{r^2}$, we have $p_{\text{eff}} = 4\pi\epsilon_m D = 4\pi\epsilon_m \left(\frac{\epsilon_2' - \epsilon_m}{\epsilon_2' + 2\epsilon_m}\right) R_2^3 E_0$

Similar to the previous discussion, we can define the CM factor as

$$K = \frac{\epsilon_2' - \epsilon_m}{\epsilon_2' + 2\epsilon_m} \quad \text{where} \quad \epsilon_2' = \epsilon_2 \frac{\left(\dfrac{R_2}{R_1}\right)^3 + 2k_\epsilon}{\left(\dfrac{R_2}{R_1}\right)^3 - k_\epsilon} = \epsilon_2 \frac{\left[\left(\dfrac{R_2}{R_1}\right)^3 + 2\left(\dfrac{\epsilon_1 - \epsilon_2}{\epsilon_1 + 2\epsilon_2}\right)\right]}{\left[\left(\dfrac{R_2}{R_1}\right)^3 - \left(\dfrac{\epsilon_1 - \epsilon_2}{\epsilon_1 + 2\epsilon_2}\right)\right]} \quad \blacktriangle$$

We can generalize the results of Example 3-5 to a concentric double-layer spherical particle with loss in an AC electric field $\boldsymbol{E}(t) = E_0\cos(\omega t)\hat{z} = \text{Re}\left[E_0 \exp(j\omega t)\right]\hat{z}$. The Clausius-Mossotti (CM) factor $\bar{K}(\omega)$ of such a double-layer spherical particle is

$$\bar{K}(\omega) = \frac{\bar{\epsilon}_{\text{particle}} - \bar{\epsilon}_m}{\bar{\epsilon}_{\text{particle}} + 2\bar{\epsilon}_m} \quad \text{with} \quad \bar{\epsilon}_{\text{particle}} = \bar{\epsilon}_2 \frac{\left[\left(\dfrac{R_2}{R_1}\right)^3 + 2\left(\dfrac{\bar{\epsilon}_1 - \bar{\epsilon}_2}{\bar{\epsilon}_1 + 2\bar{\epsilon}_2}\right)\right]}{\left[\left(\dfrac{R_2}{R_1}\right)^3 - \left(\dfrac{\bar{\epsilon}_1 - \bar{\epsilon}_2}{\bar{\epsilon}_1 + 2\bar{\epsilon}_2}\right)\right]} \quad \text{and} \quad \begin{cases} \bar{\epsilon}_1 = \epsilon_1 - j\dfrac{\sigma_1}{\omega} \\[2mm] \bar{\epsilon}_2 = \epsilon_2 - j\dfrac{\sigma_2}{\omega} \\[2mm] \bar{\epsilon}_m = \epsilon_m - j\dfrac{\sigma_m}{\omega} \end{cases} \quad (3.50)$$

where R_1 and $\bar{\epsilon}_1$ are respectively the radius and complex permittivity of the inner layer, R_2 and $\bar{\epsilon}_2$ are respectively the radius and complex permittivity of the outer layer, while $\bar{\epsilon}_m$ is the complex permittivity of the medium surrounding the particle. Again, $j = \sqrt{-1}$ is the imaginary unit.

We can apply this double-layer model of a spherical particle to obtain the CM factor $\bar{K}_{2\,\text{layer cell}}(\omega)$ of any sphere-shaped cell that can be modeled with two concentric layers (e.g., an animal cell).

$$\bar{K}_{2\,\text{layer cell}}(\omega) = \frac{\bar{\epsilon}_{\text{cell(2L)}} - \bar{\epsilon}_{\text{medium}}}{\bar{\epsilon}_{\text{cell(2L)}} + 2\bar{\epsilon}_{\text{medium}}} \quad \text{with} \quad \bar{\epsilon}_{\text{cell(2L)}} = \bar{\epsilon}_{\text{mem}} \frac{\left[\left(\dfrac{r_{\text{mem}}}{r_{\text{cyto}}}\right)^3 + 2\left(\dfrac{\bar{\epsilon}_{\text{cyto}} - \bar{\epsilon}_{\text{mem}}}{\bar{\epsilon}_{\text{cyto}} + 2\bar{\epsilon}_{\text{mem}}}\right)\right]}{\left[\left(\dfrac{r_{\text{mem}}}{r_{\text{cyto}}}\right)^3 - \left(\dfrac{\bar{\epsilon}_{\text{cyto}} - \bar{\epsilon}_{\text{mem}}}{\bar{\epsilon}_{\text{cyto}} + 2\bar{\epsilon}_{\text{mem}}}\right)\right]} \quad (3.51)$$

$$\text{with} \quad \bar{\epsilon}_{\text{cyto}} = \epsilon_{\text{cyto}} - j\frac{\sigma_{\text{cyto}}}{\omega} \qquad \bar{\epsilon}_{\text{mem}} = \epsilon_{\text{mem}} - j\frac{\sigma_{\text{mem}}}{\omega} \qquad \bar{\epsilon}_{\text{medium}} = \epsilon_{\text{medium}} - j\frac{\sigma_{\text{medium}}}{\omega}$$

where the model parameters are depicted in Figure 3-17 (left).

To derive the CM factor of a concentric triple-layer spherical cell (e.g., a yeast cell or a round bacterial cell), we treat the cytoplasm together with the cell membrane as a double-layer spherical particle with complex permittivity $\bar{\epsilon}'_{\text{inner}}$. The model parameters are shown in Figure 3-17 (right). We have

$$\bar{\epsilon}'_{\text{inner}} = \bar{\epsilon}_{\text{mem}} \frac{\left[\left(\dfrac{r_{\text{mem}}}{r_{\text{cyto}}}\right)^3 + 2\left(\dfrac{\bar{\epsilon}_{\text{cyto}} - \bar{\epsilon}_{\text{mem}}}{\bar{\epsilon}_{\text{cyto}} + 2\bar{\epsilon}_{\text{mem}}}\right)\right]}{\left[\left(\dfrac{r_{\text{mem}}}{r_{\text{cyto}}}\right)^3 - \left(\dfrac{\bar{\epsilon}_{\text{cyto}} - \bar{\epsilon}_{\text{mem}}}{\bar{\epsilon}_{\text{cyto}} + 2\bar{\epsilon}_{\text{mem}}}\right)\right]} \quad \text{with} \quad \begin{cases} \bar{\epsilon}_{\text{cyto}} = \epsilon_{\text{cyto}} - j\sigma_{\text{cyto}}/\omega \\[2mm] \bar{\epsilon}_{\text{mem}} = \epsilon_{\text{mem}} - j\sigma_{\text{mem}}/\omega \\[2mm] \bar{\epsilon}_{\text{wall}} = \epsilon_{\text{wall}} - j\sigma_{\text{wall}}/\omega \\[2mm] \bar{\epsilon}_{\text{medium}} = \epsilon_{\text{medium}} - j\sigma_{\text{medium}}/\omega \end{cases} \quad (3.52A)$$

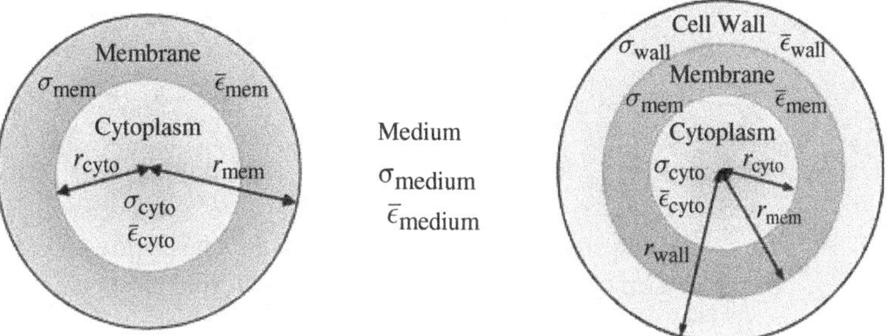

Figure 3-17   (Left) A double-layer cellular model. (Right) A triple-layer cellular model.

Next, we treat the inner portion of the cell containing both the cytoplasm and cell membrane as the inner layer of a double-layer particle, with the outer layer being the cell wall. Thus, the CM factor $\bar{K}_{3\,\text{layer cell}}(\omega)$ of a spherical three-layer cell is given by

$$\bar{K}_{3\,\text{layer cell}}(\omega) = \frac{\bar{\epsilon}_{\text{cell(3L)}} - \bar{\epsilon}_{\text{medium}}}{\bar{\epsilon}_{\text{cell(3L)}} + 2\bar{\epsilon}_{\text{medium}}} \quad \text{with} \quad \bar{\epsilon}_{\text{cell(3L)}} = \bar{\epsilon}_{\text{wall}} \left[\frac{\left(\dfrac{r_{\text{wall}}}{r_{\text{mem}}}\right)^3 + 2\left(\dfrac{\bar{\epsilon}'_{\text{inner}} - \bar{\epsilon}_{\text{wall}}}{\bar{\epsilon}'_{\text{inner}} + 2\bar{\epsilon}_{\text{wall}}}\right)}{\left(\dfrac{r_{\text{wall}}}{r_{\text{mem}}}\right)^3 - \left(\dfrac{\bar{\epsilon}'_{\text{inner}} - \bar{\epsilon}_{\text{wall}}}{\bar{\epsilon}'_{\text{inner}} + 2\bar{\epsilon}_{\text{wall}}}\right)} \right] \quad (3.52\text{B})$$

where $\bar{\epsilon}'_{\text{inner}}$, $\bar{\epsilon}_{\text{wall}}$, and $\bar{\epsilon}_{\text{medium}}$ are given in Equation (3.52A).

(B) DEP Force for Spherical and Ellipsoidal Particles

Suppose that we have a sinusoidal electric field $E(r,t) = E_0 \cos(\omega t)$. The rms electric field $E_{\text{rms}}(r)$ is

$$E(r,t) = E_0 \cos(\omega t) \quad \Rightarrow \quad E_{\text{rms}}(r) = \frac{1}{\sqrt{2}} E_0(r) \quad \Rightarrow \quad |E_{\text{rms}}(r)|^2 = \frac{1}{2}|E_0(r)|^2 \quad (3.53)$$

For a spherical particle having radius R in the sinusoidal electric field $E(r,t) = E_0 \cos(\omega t)$, the time-averaged DEP force $\langle F_{\text{DEP}}(r) \rangle_{\text{Sphere}}$ given by Equation (3.49) can be re-expressed as

$$\langle F_{\text{DEP}}(r) \rangle_{\text{Sphere}} = \pi \epsilon_m R^3 \, \text{Re}\left[\bar{K}_S(\omega)\right] \nabla\left(|E_0(r)|^2\right) = 2\pi \epsilon_m R^3 \, \text{Re}\left[\bar{K}_S(\omega)\right] \nabla\left(|E_{\text{rms}}(r)|^2\right) \quad (3.54\text{A})$$

$$\text{where} \quad \bar{K}_S(\omega) = \frac{\bar{\epsilon}_p - \bar{\epsilon}_m}{\bar{\epsilon}_p + 2\bar{\epsilon}_m} \quad \text{with} \quad \bar{\epsilon}_p = \epsilon_p - j\frac{\sigma_p}{\omega} \quad \text{and} \quad \bar{\epsilon}_m = \epsilon_m - j\frac{\sigma_m}{\omega} \quad (3.54\text{B})$$

For an ellipsoid with radius R (axes 1 and 2) and length $2L$ (axis 3) in a sinusoidal electric field again given by $E(r,t) = E_0 \cos(\omega t)$, the time-averaged DEP force $\langle F_{\text{DEP}}(r) \rangle_{\text{Ellipsoid}}$ is

$$\langle F_{\text{DEP}}(r) \rangle_{\text{Ellipsoid}} = \pi \epsilon_m L R^2 \, \text{Re}\left[\bar{K}_E(\omega)\right] \nabla\left(|E_0(r)|^2\right) = 2\pi \epsilon_m L R^2 \, \text{Re}\left[\bar{K}_E(\omega)\right] \nabla\left(|E_{\text{rms}}(r)|^2\right) \quad (3.55\text{A})$$

The equation for $\langle F_{\text{DEP}}(r) \rangle_{\text{Ellipsoid}}$ is similar to that of $\langle F_{\text{DEP}}(r) \rangle_{\text{Sphere}}$ since the axial half-length L of the ellipsoid corresponds to the radius R for a sphere. However, the Clausius-Mossotti (CM) factor is different:

$$\bar{K}_E(\omega, A_{\text{dp}}) = \frac{\bar{\epsilon}_p - \bar{\epsilon}_m}{3\left[\bar{\epsilon}_m + A_{\text{dp}}\left(\bar{\epsilon}_p - \bar{\epsilon}_m\right)\right]} \quad \text{with} \quad \bar{\epsilon}_p = \epsilon_p - j\frac{\sigma_p}{\omega} \quad \text{and} \quad \bar{\epsilon}_m = \epsilon_m - j\frac{\sigma_m}{\omega} \quad (3.55\text{B})$$

where A_{dp} is the depolarization factor (a dimensionless number) of the ellipsoid. A_{dp} is defined as

$$E_{\text{polarization}} = \frac{A_{dp}}{\epsilon_0} P = A_{dp}\left(\epsilon_r - 1\right)E_{\text{external}} \tag{3.56}$$

where $E_{\text{polarization}}$ is the induced electric field due to polarization of the particle, E_{external} is the external electric field, and $P = \chi_e \epsilon_0 E_{\text{external}} = \left(\epsilon_r - 1\right)\epsilon_0 E_{\text{external}}$ is the polarization density.[2]

An ellipsoid has three axes, and the depolarization factor A_{dp} varies depending on which axis is aligned with (i.e., parallel to) the external electric field E_{external}. There is a simple identity involving the three depolarization factors:

$$A_{dp(\text{axis 1})} + A_{dp(\text{axis 2})} + A_{dp(\text{axis 3})} = 1 \tag{3.57}$$

A sphere is a special case of an ellipsoid where all three axes are equivalent and symmetric, leading to

$$A_{dp(\text{sphere})} = A_{dp(\text{axis 1})} = A_{dp(\text{axis 2})} = A_{dp(\text{axis 3})} = 1/3 \quad \text{(for a sphere)} \tag{3.58}$$

Evidently, the depolarization factor for a sphere is $A_{dp(\text{sphere})} = 1/3$. When $A_{dp} = 1/3$, we have

$$\bar{K}_E\left(\omega, A_{dp} = 1/3\right) = \frac{\bar{\epsilon}_p - \bar{\epsilon}_m}{3\left[\bar{\epsilon}_m + \dfrac{1}{3}(\bar{\epsilon}_p - \bar{\epsilon}_m)\right]} = \frac{\bar{\epsilon}_p - \bar{\epsilon}_m}{\bar{\epsilon}_p + 2\bar{\epsilon}_m} = \bar{K}_S(\omega)$$

which matches the CM factor for a sphere, as desired.

Let us consider an ellipsoid with radius R and length $2L$ where two of the axes (called the radial axes) are equivalent and symmetric, but not the third axis (called the axial axis). We have

$$A_{dp(\text{axial})} + 2A_{dp(\text{radial})} = 1$$

When the axial (L) axis of the ellipsoid is aligned with the electric field E, the axial depolarization factor $A_{dp(\text{axial})}$ is as follows.[2,16]

Case 1: When $L \leq R$,

$$A_{dp(\text{axial})} = \left(1 + z_0^2\right)\left[1 - z_0 \text{arccot}(z_0)\right] \quad \text{where} \quad z_0 = \frac{1}{\sqrt{(L/R)^{-2} - 1}} \tag{3.59}$$

Case 2: When $L \geq R$,

$$A_{dp(\text{axial})} = \left(w_0^2 - 1\right)\left[\frac{1}{2}w_0 \ln\left(\frac{w_0 + 1}{w_0 - 1}\right) - 1\right] \quad \text{where} \quad w_0 = \frac{L/R}{\sqrt{(L/R)^2 - 1}} \tag{3.60}$$

When the radial (R) axis of the ellipsoid is aligned with the electric field E, the radial depolarization factor $A_{dp(\text{radial})}$ is

$$A_{dp(\text{radial})} = \frac{1}{2}\left(1 - A_{dp(\text{axial})}\right) \tag{3.61}$$

When $L < R$, the ellipsoid will generally be radially aligned with the fluid flow (i.e., aligned along the R axis) to minimize drag. Usually in this circumstance, the ellipsoid will also be radially aligned with the electric field E.

When $L > R$, the ellipsoid will generally be axially aligned with the fluid flow (i.e., aligned along the L axis) to minimize drag. Typically in this circumstance, the ellipsoid will also be axially aligned with the electric field E.

Aside from the sphere, there are two additional limiting cases. For a thin circular disk ($L \ll R$), $A_{dp(\text{axial})} = 1$ and $A_{dp(\text{radial})} = 0$. For a long rod ($L \gg R$), $A_{dp(\text{axial})} = 0$ and $A_{dp(\text{radial})} = 1/2$. The depolarization factors $A_{dp(\text{axial})}$ and $A_{dp(\text{radial})}$ of an ellipsoid are shown in Figure 3-18.

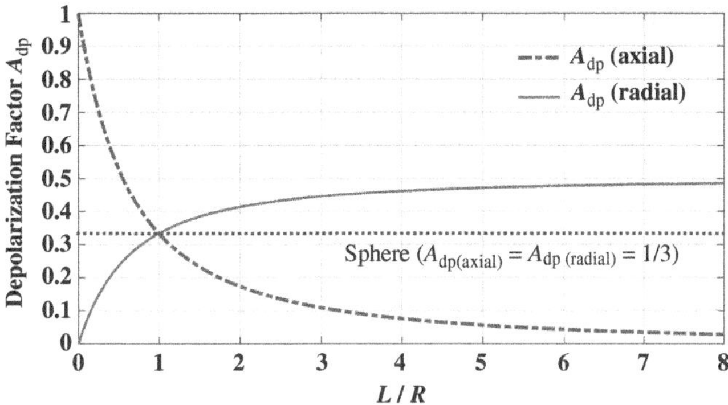

Figure 3-18   The depolarization factor A of an ellipsoid with length $2L$ and radius R.

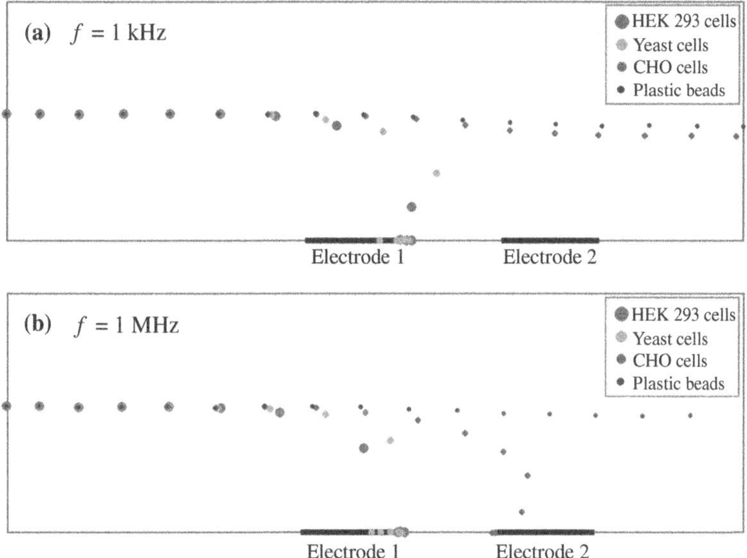

Figure 3-19   Simulation to trace particle movements in deionized water at (a) 1 kHz and (b) 1 MHz.

According to Equations (3.54) and (3.55), the direction or the type of the DEP force depends on the real part of the CM factor of a microparticle. As discussed previously, the real part of the CM factor is positive when the particle's polarizability is greater than the medium's polarizability. Therefore, it is very important to select the right medium. As a commonly used medium, deionized water has a relative permittivity (i.e., dielectric constant) of 78.5 and electrical conductivity between 1×10^{-5} S/m and 1×10^{-3} S/m.

Figure 3-19 shows the simulation results (from COMSOL Multiphysics® software) tracing the movements of four different types of microparticles in deionized water. The particles are HEK 293 cells, yeast cells, Chinese hamster ovary (CHO) cells, and plastic beads. At 1 kHz, only HEK-293 and yeast cells were captured. When the DEP frequency was increased to 1 MHz, CHO cells were captured as well because the magnitude of the DEP force increased with increasing frequency.

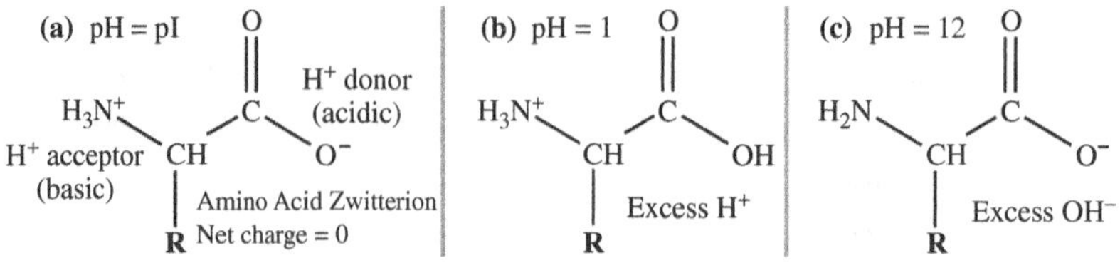

Figure 3-20   (a) A generic amino acid zwitterion in a pH = pI solution. A generic amino acid in (b) highly acidic (pH = 1) and (c) highly basic (pH = 12) solutions.

3.5.3 Isoelectric Point (pI)

(A) Isoelectric Point (pI)
The prefix "iso-" means "equal." The isoelectric point (pI) is the pH at which a molecule (e.g., amino acid or protein) has equal positive and negative charges (i.e., has no net charge). Let us look at the structure of a generic amino acid (Figure 3-20a). Ignoring the side chain (−R) for now, there is an amino group (−NH$_2$) and a carboxyl group (−COOH) in the structure of any amino acid. The amino group acts as a proton (H$^+$) acceptor, having a positive charge, and thus it is basic. On the other hand, the carboxyl group acts as a proton donor, having a negative charge, and thus it is acidic. At the isoelectric point, the net charge of the amino acid is zero, and it has a special name called "zwitterion" (meaning "hybrid").

If we put an amino acid in a highly acidic solution with pH = 1, which has lots of protons (H$^+$), the amino acid becomes protonated. The carboxyl group has gained a proton and lost its negative charge. The overall charge of the amino acid is +1 (Figure 3-20b).

On the other hand, if we put this amino acid in a highly basic solution with pH = 12, which has lots of hydroxide ions (OH$^-$), the amino acid becomes de-protonated. The amino group has lost a proton and lost its positive charge. The overall charge of the amino acid is −1 (Figure 3-20c).

The strength of an acid in a solution can be measured by its acid dissociation constant K$_a$ (also called the acidity constant), which is given by

$$HA_{aq} \rightleftharpoons A^-_{(aq)} + H^+_{(aq)} \quad \Rightarrow \quad K_a = \frac{[A^-][H^+]}{[HA]} \quad \text{and} \quad \begin{cases} pK_a = -\log_{10}(K_a) \\ pH = -\log_{10}[H^+] \end{cases} \tag{3.62}$$

where HA is a generic acid and A$^-$ is a conjugate base of the generic acid HA.

For amino acids, the pI value is dependent on the acid dissociation constants of amino and carboxyl groups. Figure 3-21 shows the status of a generic amino acid below, at, and above its pI. The isoelectric point is pI = $\left(pK_{a1} + pK_{a2}\right)/2$. However, if the side chain (−R) has its own pK$_a$, it also has to be considered when calculating the pI value of the amino acid.

The presence of charges on functional groups is determined by the pH of surrounding solution. At low pH values (pH < pI), the amino group adopts a positive charge. At high pH values (pH > pI), the carboxyl group adopts a negative charge. At pH = pI, the

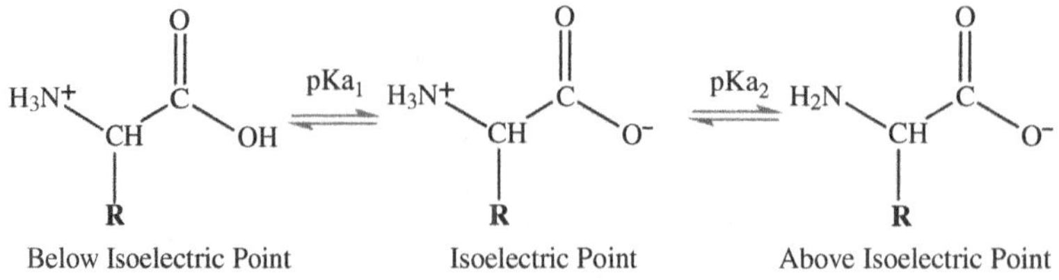

Figure 3-21   A generic amino acid below, at, and above its isoelectric point (pI).

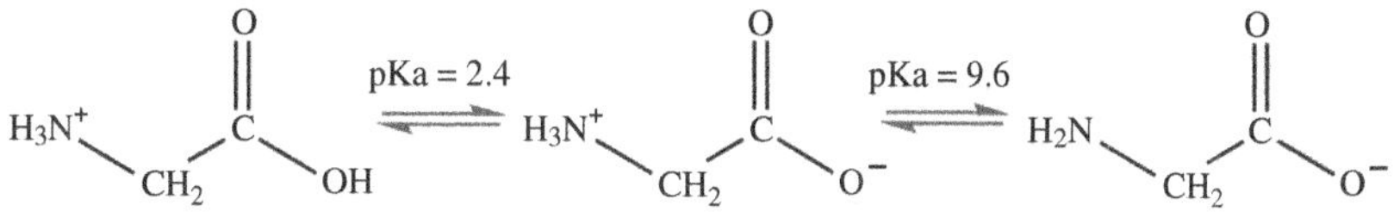

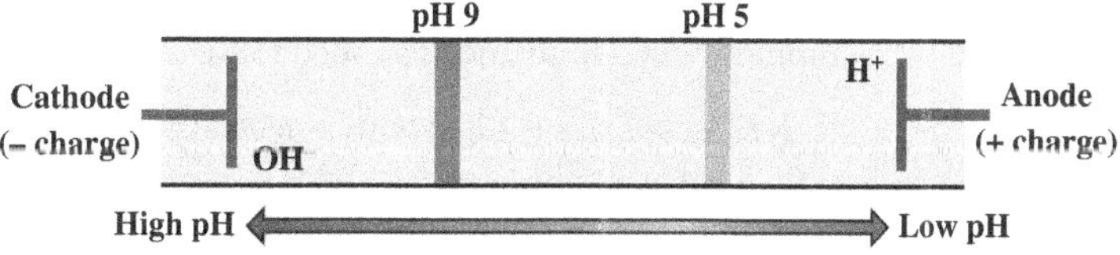

Figure 3-22   The three forms of glycine throughout the pH spectra.

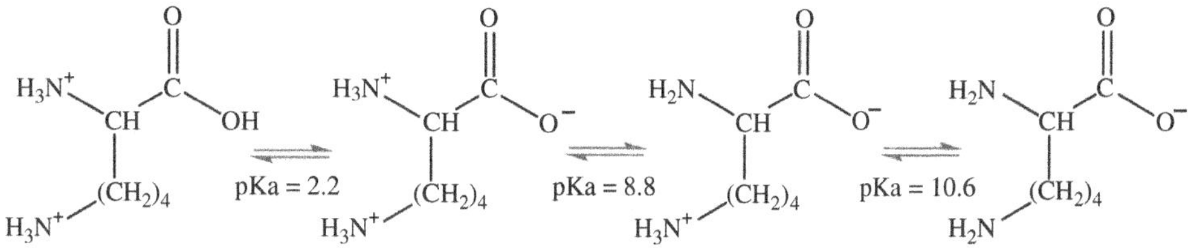

Figure 3-23   The four forms of lysine throughout the pH spectra.

molecule (or the surface of a macromolecule such as a protein) carries no net charge. At the isoelectric point, amino acids molecules are zwitterions having both H_3N^+ and COO^-. For a population of the same molecules, the sign and magnitude of the net charge depends on the composition at different pH values. At pH < pI, positively charged molecules coexist with neutrally charged zwitterions. When the pH is very low, only positively charged molecules exist. At pH > pI, negatively charged molecules coexist with neutrally charged zwitterions. When the pH is very high, only negatively charged molecules exist.

As an example, Figure 3-22 shows glycine, an amino acid which has two pK_a values. For glycine, the pK_a of the amino $(-NH_2)$ group is 9.6, while the pK_a of the carboxyl $(-COOH)$ group is 2.4. This leads to a pI value of

$$pI = \left(pK_{a1} + pK_{a2}\right) / 2 = (2.4 + 9.6) / 2 = 6.0$$

Another example is lysine (Figure 3-23). Due to the extra amino functional group in lysine, lysine has three pK_a values. For lysine, the pK_a of the two amino $(-NH_2)$ groups are 10.6 and 8.8, respectively, while the pK_a of the carboxyl $(-COOH)$ group is 2.2. The pI value of lysine is

$$pI = (pK_{a1} + pK_{a2})/2 = (8.8 + 10.6)/2 = 9.7$$

As illustrated above, for amino acids with basic side chains (e.g., lysine), their pI is the average of pK_a values from two amino groups. On the other hand, for amino acids with acidic side chains (e.g., aspartic acid), their pI is the average of pK_a values from two carboxyl groups.

(B) Isoelectric Focusing

Isoelectric focusing is a technique used to separate sample molecules based on differences in pI. To accomplish this task, a pH gradient is first set up across a gel. Next, a voltage is applied across the gel, with the positive terminal (anode) at the end with low pH and the negative terminal (cathode) at the end with high pH. Finally, a sample containing molecules with different pI values is added to the gel.

Molecules in a region of the gel that has a pH lower than their pI will adopt positive charges. Thus, the molecules will be repelled by the positive terminal (anode) and are attracted to the negative terminal (cathode).

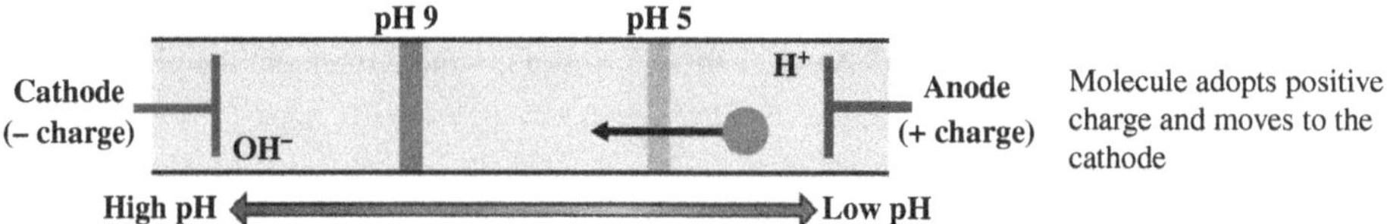

On the other hand, molecules in a region of the gel that has a pH higher than their pI will adopt negative charges. Therefore, they are repelled by the negative terminal (cathode) and attracted to the positive terminal (anode).

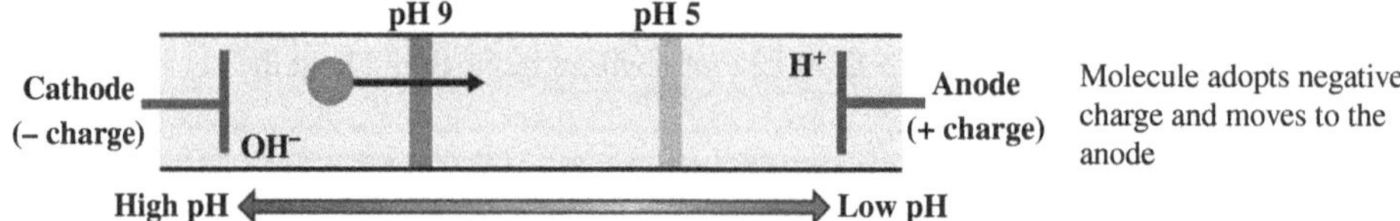

The result is that molecules will be pushed or pulled along the pH gradient until they have no net charge and thus accumulate in bands in the gel where the pH equals their respective pI values.

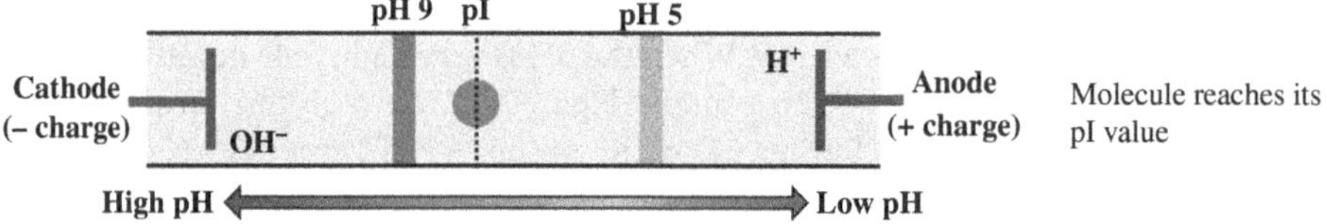

It is possible to combine isoelectric focusing with standard gel electrophoresis to separate molecules based on both their electrophoretic mobilities and pI values. This can be accomplished using 2D gel electrophoresis. The details are described in Section 3.5.4(B).

3.5.4 Gel Electrophoresis

In gel electrophoresis, charged samples (e.g., DNA) are propelled through a gel using electrophoretic flow (EPF) generated with an electric field. The two most commonly used gels are polyacrylamide and agarose gels. Polyacrylamide gel electrophoresis (PAGE) provides greater resolving power and is thus used for proteins and small DNA fragments ($\sim$5 to 1000 base pairs long). Agarose gels provide greater separation range and are hence used for medium to large DNA fragments. In the gel, samples are separated based on their electrophretic mobility μ_{EPF}, which depends on their size and charge. Fluid can be moved through a capillary using EOF while the differences in electrophoretic mobility μ_{EPF} separate species in the fluid.

(A) Capillary Electrophoresis Procedure

Capillary electrophoresis is used to separate molecules with different electrophoretic mobilities in a fluid and is applied following the procedure below.

Step 1: A capillary is filled with a neutral buffer using a combination of capillary action and EOF from an applied electric field. It is important that the buffer is loaded into the capillary from one side only to avoid air bubbles.

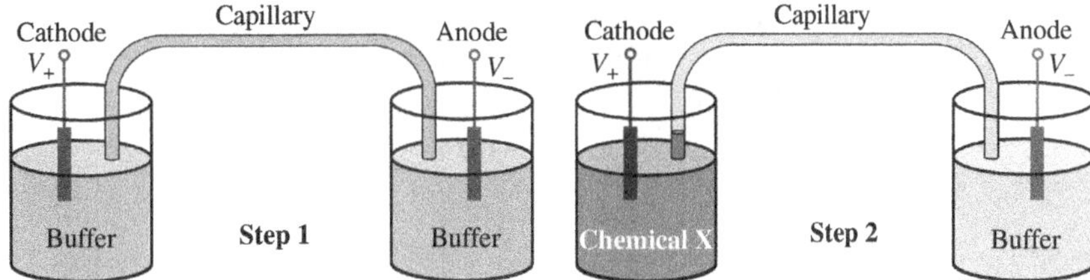

Step 2: After the buffer fills the capillary completely, the sample fluid containing the components to be separated (e.g., chemical mixture X to be separated into X1 and X2) is added into the capillary. About 5% of the total capillary volume is filled with chemical X.

Step 3: The original buffer is replaced, leaving a small pocket of chemical X in the capillary. The applied electric field carries the volume of chemical X to the other side of the capillary.

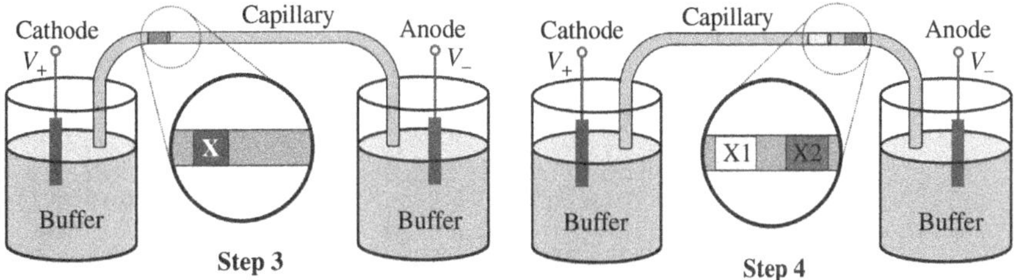

Step 4: The bulk of the fluid will move due to EOF, while charged molecules in the fluid will also be affected by EPF. If the electrophoretic mobilities of X1 and X2 are significantly different, they will travel at different speeds and become separated in the capillary.

Achieving high resolution separation is important in capillary electrophoresis. High resolution means that the separated sections are clear and distinctly separated with no cross-over between samples as shown in Figure 3-24. High resolution separation can be achieved by maximizing

- The difference in the electrophoretic mobility μ_{EPF} of the separated species.
- The amount of travel time to allow for more separation (e.g., a longer capillary).

Unfortunately, increasing travel time will also cause greater diffusion of all species within the fluid, so that the sections of "plug flow" can spread out in the capillary according to the diffusion distance $x_{\text{diffusion}} = \sqrt{2Dt}$ and eventually blend into each other.

Capillary electrophoresis can also be carried out on a microchip. In this case, it is called microchip electrophoresis (Figure 3-25).

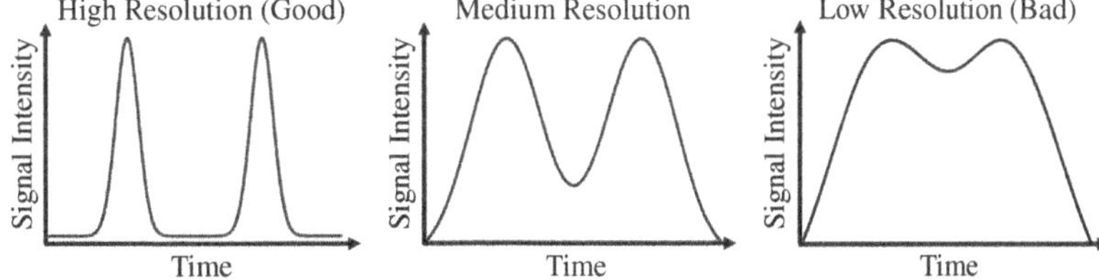

Figure 3-24 Signal intensity versus time for molecular separation by electrophoresis with high, medium, and low resolution. The two Gaussian peaks of each curve are due to the Gaussian distributions resulting from diffusion of the two molecular species.

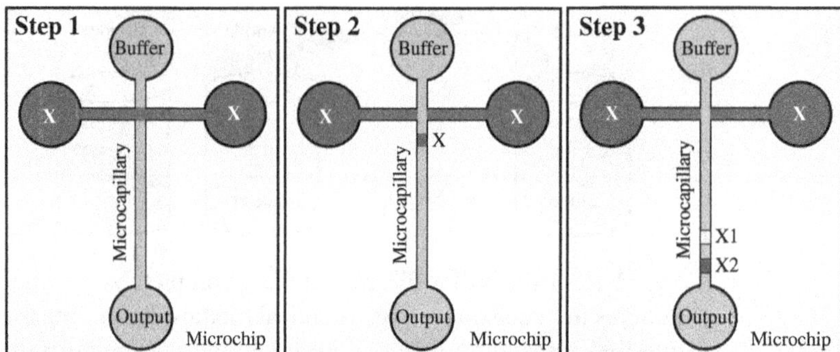

Figure 3-25   Microchip electrophoresis for separating chemical mixture X into X1 and X2.

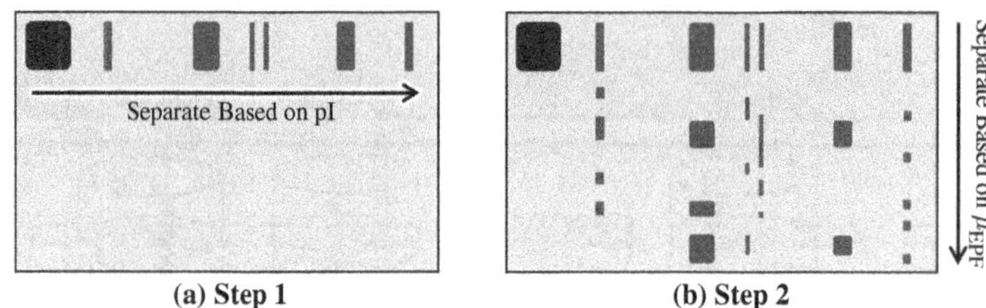

Figure 3-26   2D gel electrophoresis. (a) Step 1: Separation based on pI using isoelectric focusing. (b) Step 2: Separation based on electrophoretic mobility μ_{EPF} using electrophoresis.

(B) 2D Gel Electrophoresis

It is possible to separate species on the same gel based on their pI (by using isoelectric focusing) as well as their electrophoretic mobility μ_{EPF} (using gel electrophoresis). First, the surrounding buffer is replaced by a special gel solution with a pH gradient (large molecules do not get washed away as they do not diffuse easily), and isoelectric focusing is carried out along the gel. Next, the resulting strip is placed on the top of a 2D sheet of ordinary gel, and electrophoresis is performed to separate species based on their electrophoretic mobility μ_{EPF} (i.e., size and charge). As shown in Figure 3-26a, the sample is first separated based on pI (left to right). Then, the sample is further separated based on μ_{EPF} (top to bottom), as shown in Figure 3-26b. Note that the horizontal and vertical widths of the bands in Figure 3-26 result from diffusion and are thus correlated with the concentration, diffusion coefficient, and diffusion time of each species within the sample.

3.6 PROBLEMS

3-1 (Short-Answer). When carrying out 2D gel electrophoresis, is it necessary for isoelectric focusing to be done prior to electrophoresis?

3-2. In Section 3.3.1(D), we had an insulating sphere with radius R and permittivity ϵ_p in a medium of permittivity ϵ_m. An external uniform electric field $\mathbf{E} = E_0\hat{z}$ of magnitude E_0 is directed in the z-direction. We showed that the electric potential $V(r, \theta)$ is given by

$$\begin{cases} V_m = -E_0 r\cos\theta + \dfrac{A\cos\theta}{r^2} & \text{for } r \geq R \text{ (in medium)} \\[2ex] V_p = -Br\cos\theta & \text{for } r \leq R \text{ (in particle)} \end{cases}$$

In Section 3.3.1(E), we generalized the above expressions to a sphere with loss in an AC electric field.

(a) The electric field in the radial direction E_r can be found with the partial derivative of the electric potential V. Using $\boldsymbol{E} = -\boldsymbol{\nabla}V$, show in spherical coordinates (Appendix E) that $E_r = -\partial V/\partial r$.

(b) Provide a detailed derivation for the unknown constants A and B using the boundary conditions [Equations (3.27) and (3.31)] as shown below. This derivation will prove Equations (3.34) and (3.43).

$$V_m = V_p \;\; \text{at} \; r = R \qquad \text{and} \qquad \epsilon_m E_{r,m} = \epsilon_p E_{r,p} \;\; \text{at} \; r = R$$

3-3. For the insulating sphere with radius R in a uniform electric field from Section 3.3.1(D), we used the following boundary condition:

$$D_{r,m} - D_{r,p} = \sigma_{c(\text{free})} \;\; (\text{at} \; r = R) \quad \text{where} \quad \begin{cases} D_r = D_{r,m} & \text{for} \; r \ge R \; (\text{in medium}) \\ D_r = D_{r,p} & \text{for} \; r \le R \; (\text{in particle}) \end{cases}$$

where D_r is the radial (r) component of the electric displacement vector $\boldsymbol{D} = \epsilon\boldsymbol{E}$ and $\sigma_{c(\text{free})}$ is the free surface charge density. In Section 3.3.1(E), we generalized this boundary condition to a sphere with loss in an AC electric field.

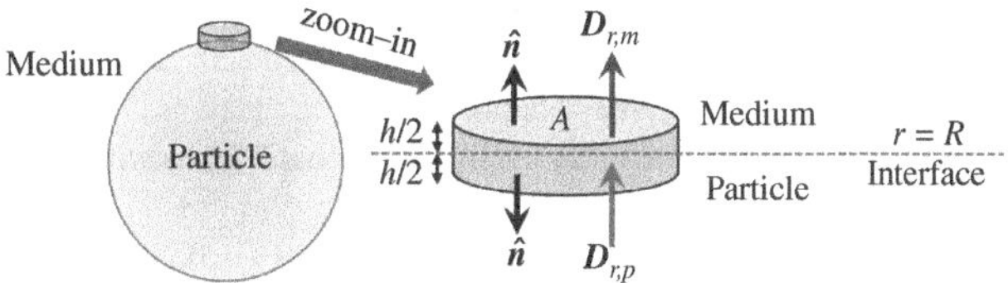

Derive this boundary condition from Gauss's law in integral form in terms of the enclosed free charge $Q_{\text{free,enclosed}}$, infinitesimal surface area element da, and unit vector normal to the surface $\hat{n}$.

$$\oiint \boldsymbol{D} \cdot d\boldsymbol{a} = \oiint \boldsymbol{D} \cdot \hat{n}\, da = Q_{\text{free, enclosed}} \quad (\text{Gauss's law})$$

Hint: Consider a "Gaussian pillbox," a tiny cylinder with cross-sectional area A and height $h \to 0$ across the particle-medium interface $(r = R)$ as shown in the figure above.

3-4. Within a microcapillary (refer to the figure below), the red (R) and blue (B) dyes both have the same diffusion coefficient of $D_1 = 10^{-7}\,\text{m}^2/\text{s}$, while the yellow (Y) dye has a diffusion coefficient of $D_2 - 10^{-9}\,\text{m}^2/\text{s}$. Initially, the center-to-center distance between the red (R) and yellow (Y) dye bands is 2.5 mm, while the center-to-center distance between the yellow (Y) and blue (B) dye bands is 7.5 mm. The initial width of each dye band (R, B, and Y) is 10 μm.

(a) Which dyes interact (i.e., meet) first, second, and third? How long after the initial state does the first interaction happen?

(b) Draw a picture of the microcapillary after the first interaction of the dyes with labeled distances.

3-5. Consider an amino acid (H_2N–R–$COOH$) with two pK_a values and three forms:

(a) Write down expressions for pK_{a1} and pK_{a2}.

(b) If $pK_{a1} = 2.34$ and $pH = 3.50$, find the concentration ratio $C_{\text{ratio X}}$ where

$$C_{\text{ratio X}} = \frac{\left[^+H_3N\text{–}R\text{–}COO^-\right]}{\left[^+H_3N\text{–}R\text{–}COOH\right]}$$

(c) Calculate the pH if the isoelectric point of the amino acid is $pI = 5.20$ and

$$C_{\text{ratio Y}} = \frac{\left[{}^{+}\text{H}_3\text{N}-\text{R}-\text{COO}^{-}\right]}{\left[\text{H}_2\text{N}-\text{R}-\text{COO}^{-}\right]} = \frac{1}{2}C_{\text{ratio X}}$$

3-6. A microchannel with a circular cross-section is filled with a buffer ($pH = 7$ and $T = 298$ K) containing 0.007M KCl and 0.003M NaCl. The channel is 3 cm long with a diameter of 15 μm. The inner wall of the chamber is conditioned such that it carries a surface charge of $\sigma_c = 10^{-8}$ C/cm². A voltage of 500 V is applied across the ends of the channel. For the buffer, $\epsilon = 80\,\epsilon_0$ and $\eta = 0.89 \times 10^{-3}$ Pa · s.
(a) What is the Debye length of this system?
(b) EOF causes all fluid *sufficiently far from the wall* to move at the same rate. This velocity profile is called plug flow.
    (i) What is the speed $|v_{\text{EOF}}|$ of the fluid located 1 nm away from the channel walls?
    (ii) What is the speed $|v_{\text{EOF}}|$ of the fluid at the center of the channel?
    (iii) Sketch a graph of fluid speed $|v_{\text{EOF}}|$ versus radial position across the channel.

3-7. We have a glass microchannel with a radius of 100 μm and a length of 10 cm that links two wells. The wells and the channel are filled with a buffer, and +5 kV is applied to the far well as shown below. The buffer is water-like and electrically neutral, with $\epsilon = 80\,\epsilon_0$ and $\eta = 0.89 \times 10^{-3}$ Pa · s. With this buffer, the zeta potential of the glass is $\zeta = -30$ mV. The grounded end of the channel has been loaded with a sample in a band that is 1 μm wide. The sample contains DNA that is 200 base pairs long and is marked using a red fluorescent dye. The DNA is negatively charged and has an electrophoretic mobility of $\mu_{\text{EPF}} = -5 \times 10^{-8}$ m²/(V · s). The diffusion coefficient of the DNA is 10^{-12} m²/s. As the DNA arrives at the right-hand well, it is detected optically.
(a) What is the velocity (speed and direction) of the buffer fluid in the channel?
(b) What is the velocity (speed and direction) of the center of the DNA band in the channel?
(c) What is the arrival time t of the center of the red DNA band at the other end? How wide will the band of DNA be as it arrives at the far well?

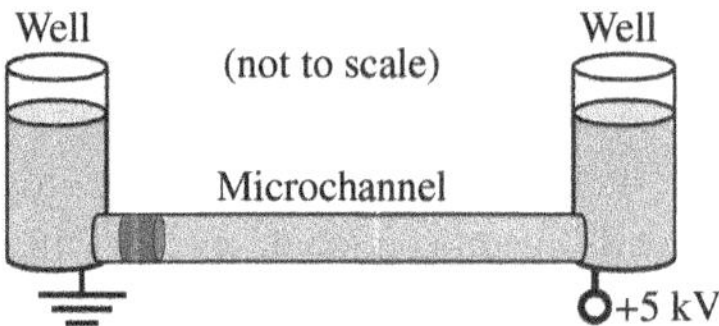

3-8. Many commercial microfluidic devices utilize H-filters to achieve diffusion-based separation. Provided that the H-filter is small enough to ensure fully laminar flow, we can continuously separate components with relatively high diffusion coefficients, such as small molecules. Assume that we have a chemical mixture X containing a uniformly distributed solute X0 with a diffusion coefficient of $D_0 = 2 \times 10^{-9}$ m²/s, along with other components with significantly lower diffusions coefficients (assumed to be zero for simplicity).

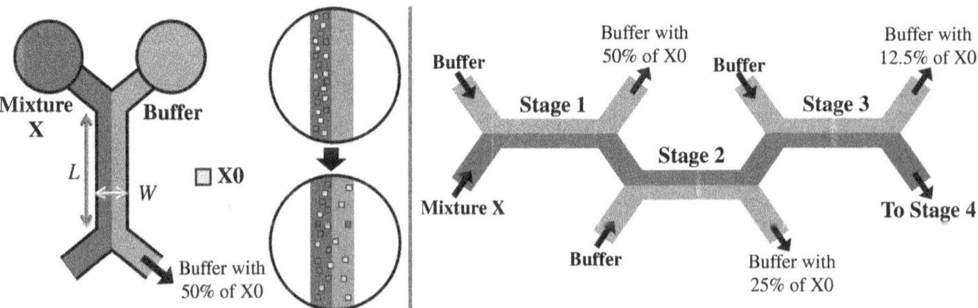

(a) We have a single-stage H-filter with a channel length of L and width of $W = 100$ μm (as shown in the figure on the left), and the average fluid velocity in the channel is $v_{\text{average}} = 1$ mm/s. To extract close to 50% of X0 from mixture X (the maximum possible) with the single-stage H-filter, how long should the channel be?

(b) By using a multi-stage setup with several H-filters connected together (as shown in the figure on the right), we can continuously extract more than 50% of the solute X0 from the chemical mixture X. If we extract 50% of X0 with each stage, how many stages do we need to extract 95% (or more) of the solute X0 from the chemical mixture X?

3-9. You have loaded a Y-shaped microchip with a red dye in well A and blue dye in well B, where both dyes are mixed with a water-based buffer. In contact with the buffer, the zeta potential of the glass is $+0.1$ V. The two branching channels connected to wells A and B each have a radius of 100 μm and half of the cross-sectional area of the main channel connected to well C. All three channels are cylindrical with circular cross-sections. One end of the main channel is grounded, while the other end is held at a potential of $V = +1000$ V. The main channel is 10 cm long, and both the blue and red dye molecules are uncharged and have a diffusion coefficient of 1.4×10^{-12} m²/s. For the buffer, the dynamic viscosity is $\eta = 0.89 \times 10^{-3}$ Pa · s and the permittivity is $\epsilon = 80\,\epsilon_0$. For the sign convention, please refer to Appendix D.

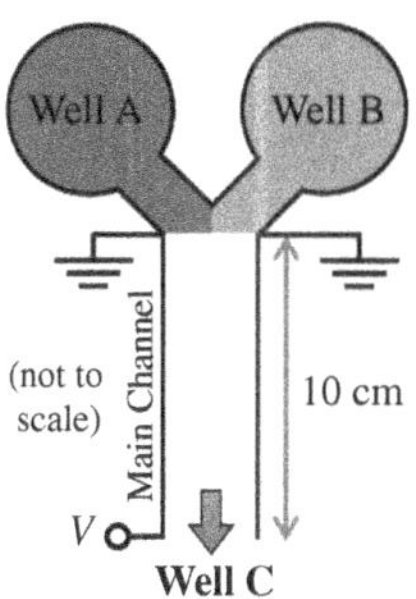

(a) If the main channel is initially filled with a clear buffer (the same as used for the dyes) and the dyes are added to wells A and B, how fast will the colored fronts move?

(b) If the two branching Y-channels are brought together to meet in such a way that the left side of the main channel cross-section is red and the right side is blue, what does a cross-section of the channel look like as the channel enters well C?

Hint: Imagine taking a cross-section of the channel just after the two smaller channels join at the Y-junction. You will have two semi-circles, one side red and the other side blue. What happens as they reach the end (bottom) of the 10-cm-long (joined) main channel?

(c) Repeating part (b), what would the cross-section look like if the applied potential is $V = +10$ V?

3-10. Capillary electrophoresis is used to separate a chemical mixture X (red) containing two different types of molecules X1 and X2 dissolved in a buffer. A 10-cm-long capillary is filled with the same buffer with a band of chemical mixture X which is initially $W_{\text{orig}} = 200$ μm wide. We can apply a potential difference (i.e., DC voltage) of $V = +60$ V or $V = -60$ V across the ends of the capillary. The zeta potential of the capillary with respect to the buffer is -35 mV. The buffer has a dynamic viscosity of 1.2×10^{-3} Pa · s and relative permittivity of 74. The electrophoretic mobilities and diffusion coefficients of X1 and X2 are $\mu_{\text{EPF(X1)}} = +2.1 \times 10^{-8}$ m²/(V · s), $\mu_{\text{EPF(X2)}} = +1.4 \times 10^{-9}$ m²/(V · s), $D_{X1} = 1.0 \times 10^{-9}$ m²/s, and $D_{X2} = 6.8 \times 10^{-10}$ m²/s.

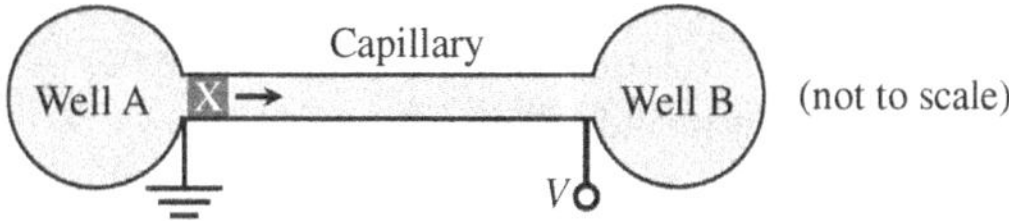

(a) If we want the center of the X1 and X2 bands to move from left to right across the capillary, should we apply $V = +60$ V or $V = -60$ V? What are the velocities of the center of the X1 and X2 bands?

(b) Accounting for diffusion, how long will it take for the X1 and X2 bands to be completely separated? Assume that the two bands are completely separated when the edges of the two bands (as defined by a diffusion distance of $\pm 1\sigma$) are more than $2\sigma_{X1} + 2\sigma_{X2}$ apart, where $\sigma = x_{\text{diffusion}} = \sqrt{2Dt}$.

(c) Is the capillary long enough to allow for the complete separation of the X1 and X2 bands?

3-11. We plan to create a 1:1 stoichiometric mixture of two substances A and B using diffusion. A 10-cm-long glass tube with a T-junction at the middle will be used to extract the mixture. High concentrations of substances A and B are placed in large wells on opposite sides of the glass tube. The glass tube has no (i.e., zero) zeta potential. The diffusion coefficients of substances A and B are $D_A = 10^{-6}$ m²/s and $D_B = 2 \times 10^{-5}$ m²/s, respectively. Substance A is composed of electrically neutral molecules. Substance B is composed of biomolecules each having an effective charge of $-6e$ and effective Stokes radius of 2.5 nm. The following buffers are available:

Buffer	Dynamic Viscosity $\left[\times 10^{-5} \text{kg}/(\text{m} \cdot \text{s})\right]$
I	0.08
II	0.3
III	5
IV	21

The lab bench power supply can output a DC voltage between 0 V and +50 V, with which we can maintain a potential difference between the two ends of the 10-cm glass tube. Which buffer should we use and what potential difference should we apply between the two ends of the tube to combine the two substances A and B, ensuring that they mix at the same rate (i.e., both substances A and B reach the center T-junction at the same time and with the same velocity)?

3-12. We wish to apply dielectrophoresis (DEP) to separate two types of blood cells using an applied electric field $\boldsymbol{E}(t) = E_0(z)\cos(\omega t)\,\hat{\boldsymbol{z}}$, where $\omega = 2\pi f$ and $E_0(z)$ is non-uniform. The four main components of human blood are plasma, red blood cells, white blood cells, and platelets. We have a filtered blood sample containing only red and white blood cells, which are kept alive in a PBS (phosphate-buffered saline) buffer solution. The properties of red and white blood cells are listed below.

Variable	Red Blood Cells	White Blood Cells
Cytoplasm Conductivity σ_{cyto}	0.5 S/m	0.5 S/m
Membrane Conductivity σ_{mem}	7×10^{-14} S/m	7×10^{-14} S/m
Cytoplasm Permittivity ϵ_{cyto}	$60\,\epsilon_0$	$60\,\epsilon_0$
Membrane Permittivity ϵ_{mem}	$9.5\,\epsilon_0$	$9.5\,\epsilon_0$
Membrane Thickness d_{mem}	8 nm	8 nm

The buffer solution has an electrical conductivity of 0.065 S/m and permittivity of $76\,\epsilon_0$. Each red blood cell can be treated as a disk-shaped ellipsoid with radius of $R_{RBC} = 3.8$ μm (axes 1 and 2) and thickness of $2L_{RBC} = 2.2$ μm (axis 3). Each white blood cell can be treated as a sphere with radius of $R_{WBC} = 7.5$ μm (all three axes). Both types of blood cells have two concentric layers consisting of the cytoplasm and cell membrane.

The spherical white blood cells are modeled with Equation (3.51), while the ellipsoidal red blood cells are modeled with the following complex permittivity $\overline{\epsilon}_{RBC}$ together with Equation (3.55):

$$\overline{\epsilon}_{RBC} = \overline{\epsilon}_{mem}\,\frac{k_d + 2\left(\dfrac{\overline{\epsilon}_{cyto} - \overline{\epsilon}_{mem}}{\overline{\epsilon}_{cyto} + 2\overline{\epsilon}_{mem}}\right)}{k_d - \left(\dfrac{\overline{\epsilon}_{cyto} - \overline{\epsilon}_{mem}}{\overline{\epsilon}_{cyto} + 2\overline{\epsilon}_{mem}}\right)} \quad \text{where } k_d = \frac{R_{RBC}^2 (L_{RBC}/2)}{(R_{RBC} - d_{mem})^2 (L_{RBC}/2 - d_{mem})}$$

(a) To minimize drag, the red blood cells are radially aligned with the applied electric field (i.e., aligned along the radial axis). Calculate k_d and the depolarization factor A_{dp} of a red blood cell.

(b) Use computer software to plot the real part of the CM factor $\mathrm{Re}\big[\bar{K}_{RBC}(f)\big]$ and $\mathrm{Re}\big[\bar{K}_{WBC}(f)\big]$ for red and white blood cells versus frequency f (logarithmic scale) from $f = 10^2$ Hz to $f = 10^{10}$ Hz.

(c) Using the plot obtained from part (b), what range of frequencies $f = \omega/(2\pi)$ would allow for DEP separation of red and white blood cells? Within this range, approximately what frequency $f_{optimal}$ would maximize $\big|\Delta\,\mathrm{Re}\big(\bar{K}\big)\big| = \big|\mathrm{Re}\big(\bar{K}_{RBC}\big) - \mathrm{Re}\big(\bar{K}_{WBC}\big)\big|$? Use a plot to justify your answer.

(d) Derive expressions for the time-averaged DEP force $\big\langle F_{DEP}(z)\big\rangle_{RBC}$ and $\big\langle F_{DEP}(z)\big\rangle_{WBC}$ of red blood cells and white blood cells in terms of $E_0(z)$, $\bar{K}_{RBC}(f)$, $\bar{K}_{WBC}(f)$, and the given parameters.

3-13. The figure below illustrates a portion of a microfluidic design, as found commonly on bioMEMS chips. Two wells (W_A and W_B) are connected by two smaller channels (C_A and C_B) both with channel lengths of 30 μm, which merge into a slightly bigger and cylindrical channel C_C with a length of 400 μm and radius of $r_0 = 25$ μm. C_C is connected to two smaller branches C_D and C_E on the far end of the channel. A voltage V is applied at the ends of channel C_C with the negative end applied between channels C_D and C_E.

Furthermore, C_C is equipped with temperature sensors located at half of the channel radius ($r = 0.5\,r_0$) as well as at the channel walls ($r = r_0$). The following table displays other characteristics of the system and the buffer solution used, which carries no net charge.

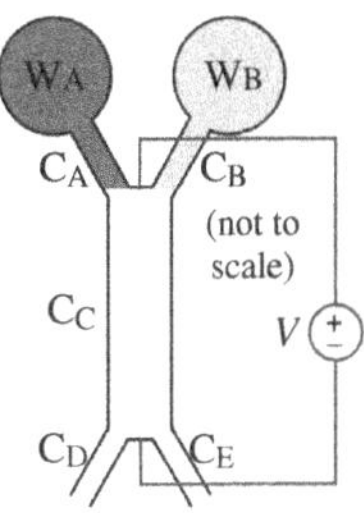

Parameter	η_{buffer}	ϵ_{buffer}	$\rho_{m(buffer)}$	n_{buffer}	$\rho_{c(buffer)}$	κ_{buffer}
Value	1.412 Pa · s	$42.5\,\epsilon_0$	1261 kg/m³	1.4746	160 Ω · m	0.8 W/(K · m)

Parameter	α_{dye}	β_{dye}	T_{min}	T_{opt}	T_{max}	ζ_{wall}
Value	40×10^{-15}	20×10^{-15}	$-50°C$	$63°C$	$150°C$	-20 mV

(a) The wells are initially filled with a clear buffer solution which flows through channels C_A and C_B into channel C_C. Assume that the channel wall is a perfect heat conductor and has the same temperature as the entire system. Note that the system heats up much more quickly than the movement of the fluid.

  If the system is operated at optimal conditions and the C_C temperature sensors measure a temperature of 72°C at half of the channel radius ($r = 0.5\,r_0$) as well as a temperature of $T_{opt} = 63°C$ at the channel walls ($r = r_0$), what is the applied voltage V across the ends of channel C_C? What is the temperature in the middle of channel C_C (at $r = 0$)?

(b) The central channel C_C is intended to be used to separate fluid components based on diffusion. Which condition(s) are required for the system to function this way and are they fulfilled for the buffer solution? Note that the system is still operated under optimal conditions.

(c) Now red dye is added to the buffer solution in well W_A, while yellow dye is added to the buffer solution in well W_B. The dye molecules are both uncharged, and both show a temperature-dependent diffusion behavior $D(T)$. Note that the dye molecules do not change any characteristics of the buffer solution. With respect to the flow in the channel, three distinct expressions can be obtained for $D(T)$:

$$D(T) \; [\text{m}^2/\text{s}] = \begin{cases} \alpha(T_0 - T)^2 + \beta T_0 & \text{(Laminar Flow)} \\ (\alpha + \beta)T^2 & \text{(Transitional Flow)} \\ (\alpha^2 \cdot \beta)^{1.5T} + \beta T_0 & \text{(Turbulent Flow)} \end{cases}$$

where $T_0 = T_{\text{opt}} = 63°\text{C}$. Generate a plot of the diffusion coefficient $D(T)$ versus temperature T from $55°\text{C}$ to $75°\text{C}$, if the system is operated at optimal conditions (include values for $r = 0$ and $r = r_0$).

(d) Assume that the diffusion coefficient of an individual molecule does not change if it moves to an area where the temperature is lower. Also assume that once the molecules are in the channel, they obtain the temperature related to their location instantly.
   (i) Generate a plot of diffusion length $x_{\text{diffusion}}(r)$ versus the radial position r in channel C_C, and include values for $r = 0$ and $r = r_0$.
   (ii) Sketch the circular cross-section at the end of channel C_C (where it branches out into channels C_D and C_E). How wide is the band where both dyes mix at the end of channel C_C at the cross-sectional center ($r = 0$) and at the top and bottom edges (where $|r| = r_0 = 25\ \mu\text{m}$)?

(e) In another experiment, a different yellow dye is used in well W_B. The expressions given before still apply. The diffusion coefficients for the dye in well W_A is the same as before, but the diffusion coefficients for the dye in well W_B change to $\alpha'_B = 20 \times 10^{-15}$ and $\beta'_B = 5 \times 10^{-15}$. Sketch the circular cross-section at the end of channel C_C (a qualitative sketch is sufficient).

3-14 (Challenging). Vesicles are biological structures that play an important role in a variety of cellular processes. Assume that the vesicles are spherical with radii of $R = 20$ nm and possess a surface charge density of $\sigma_c = -6 \times 10^{-5}\,\text{C/m}^2$. The buffer solution containing the vesicles is kept at room temperature (298 K). It has an effective univalent ion concentration of 0.35 mM, a relative permittivity of $\epsilon_r = 76$, and a dynamic viscosity of $\eta = 1.2 \times 10^{-4}$ Pa $\cdot$ s. Assume that the vesicles have a diffusion coefficient of $D = 5 \times 10^{-8}\,\text{m}^2/\text{s}$ within the buffer solution.

(a) Calculate the total charge q_{vesicle} of a vesicle and the Debye length λ_{DB} of the buffer solution.
(b) Derive an expression for the electric field $E(r)$ being a distance r away from the center of *a single* vesicle, where $r \geq 20$ nm.

Hint: Approximate the vesicle as a screened point charge and use the following equations:

$$\phi(r) = \frac{\psi_0}{r} \exp\left(\frac{-r}{\lambda_{DB}}\right) \quad \text{and} \quad \oiint D \cdot da = Q_{\text{free,enclosed}}$$

(c) A potential difference of 90 V is applied across a 12-cm-long horizontal capillary containing many of the aforementioned vesicles, with the left side of the capillary at a higher voltage. To determine the velocity of the vesicles in the buffer, what forces should we account for? Assume that there is no externally applied pressure and that the effect of capillary pressure is negligible.
(d) If the vesicles require 38 min to traverse the entire length of the capillary, what is the zeta potential of the buffer-glass interface? For the sign convention, please refer to Appendix D.

3-15 (Challenging). We stated previously that the solution to Fick's second law of diffusion in 1D for $t \geq 0$ is given by

$$\frac{\partial N}{\partial t} = D\frac{\partial^2 N}{\partial x^2} \quad \Rightarrow \quad N(x,t) = \frac{C_{\text{total}}}{2\sqrt{\pi D t}} \exp\left(\frac{(x - x_0)^2}{4Dt}\right) \quad \text{(1D Solution)}$$

Derive the 1D solution using the following four boundary conditions:

$$(1)\ \int_{-\infty}^{\infty} N(x,t)\,dx = C_{\text{total}} \qquad (2)\ N(x - x_0 = \pm\infty, t) = 0$$

$$(3)\ N(x, t = 0) = 0 \text{ for all } x \neq x_0 \qquad (4)\ N(x,t) \text{ is symmetric about } x = x_0$$

where $N(x, t)$ is the number density distribution centered about $x = x_0$, C_{total} is a constant proportional to the total number of the diffusing particles, and D is the diffusion coefficient.

Hint: Make use of the following Laplace transform (a linear transform) identities:

$$\mathcal{L}\left\{\frac{\partial f(x,t)}{\partial t}\right\} = sF(x,s) - f(x, t = 0) \qquad \mathcal{L}\{1\} = \frac{1}{s} \qquad \mathcal{L}^{-1}\left\{\frac{1}{\sqrt{s}}\exp\left(-a\sqrt{s}\right)\right\} = \frac{1}{\sqrt{\pi t}}\exp\left(-\frac{a^2}{4t}\right)$$

where $\mathcal{L}$ is the Laplace transform that converts from the time (t) domain into the s-domain, $\mathcal{L}^{-1}$ is the inverse Laplace transform that converts from the s-domain back to the t-domain, and a is a constant.

3-16 (Challenging). We have stated that the two depolarization factors A_{axial} and A_{radial} of an ellipsoid of length $2L$ and radius R are related via $A_{radial} = \frac{1}{2}(1 - A_{axial})$, where

$$\text{(For } L \leq R\text{):} \quad A_{axial} = \left(1 + z_0^2\right)\left[1 - z_0 \operatorname{arccot}(z_0)\right] \text{ where } z_0 = 1 / \sqrt{(L/R)^{-2} - 1}$$

$$\text{(For } L \geq R\text{):} \quad A_{axial} = \left(w_0^2 - 1\right)\left[\frac{1}{2}w_0 \ln\left(\frac{w_0 + 1}{w_0 - 1}\right) - 1\right] \text{ where } w_0 = \frac{L/R}{\sqrt{(L/R)^2 - 1}}$$

(a) Show that for a thin circular disk where $L \ll R$, $A_{axial} = 1$ and $A_{radial} = 0$.
(b) Show that for a long rod where $L \gg R$, $A_{axial} = 0$ and $A_{radial} = 1/2$.
(c) Using first equation, show that for a sphere $(L = R)$, $A_{axial} = A_{radial} = 1/3$.
(d) Using second equation, show that for a sphere $(L = R)$, $A_{axial} = A_{radial} = 1/3$.

Hint: Use the identity $\operatorname{arccot}(y) = \arctan(1/y)$ and the following Taylor series expansions:

$$\arctan(x) = x - \frac{1}{3}x^3 + \frac{1}{5}x^5 - \frac{1}{7}x^7 + \cdots \quad (\text{about } x = 0 \text{ where } |x| \leq 1)$$

$$\ln(x) = (x - 1) - \frac{1}{2}(x - 1)^2 + \frac{1}{3}(x - 1)^3 - \cdots \quad \left(\text{about } x = 1 \text{ where } |x - 1| < 1\right)$$

3-17 (Challenging). We wish to use dielectrophoresis (DEP) force to separate live and dead *E. coli* bacteria. An *E. coli* bacterium can be modeled as a rod-shaped ellipsoid with radius $R = 0.5$ μm (axes 1 and 2) and axial length $2L = 2.0$ μm (axis 3) and having no net electrical charge. Two wells A and B are connected by a cylindrical glass capillary with a radius of $r_0 = 200$ μm and length of $l = 0.15$ m. The zeta potential of the capillary is negligible, and the buffer used has an electrical conductivity of $\sigma_m = 0.002$ S/m, dynamic viscosity of $\eta = 9 \times 10^{-4}$ Pa · s, and permittivity of $\epsilon_m = 80\,\epsilon_0$. All the live and dead bacteria are placed in well A (the left well), and both wells plus the capillary are filled with the buffer. Assume that the bacteria are immobile and have negligible diffusion coefficients, and that there is no externally applied pressure.

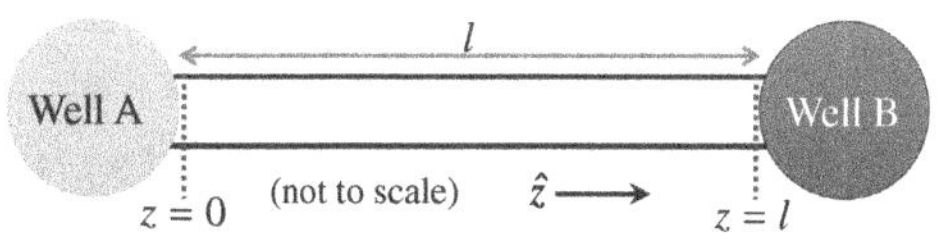

Variable	Live Bacteria	Dead Bacteria
Cytoplasm Conductivity σ_{cyto}	0.5 S/m	0.003 S/m
Membrane Conductivity σ_{mem}	5×10^{-5} S/m	0.01 S/m
Cytoplasm Permittivity ϵ_{cyto}	$50\,\epsilon_0$	$65\,\epsilon_0$
Membrane Permittivity ϵ_{mem}	$12.5\,\epsilon_0$	$12.5\,\epsilon_0$
Membrane Thickness d_{mem}	7 nm	7 nm

The following voltage is applied throughout the length of the capillary, where $\omega = 2\pi f$ is the angular frequency:

$$V(z) = C(z+D)^2 \cos(\omega t)\ [\text{V}] \quad \text{where} \quad \begin{cases} C = 3.5 \times 10^7 \\ D = 0.05 \end{cases} \quad (0 \le z\ [\text{m}] \le 0.15\ \text{m})$$

The complex permittivity $\bar{\epsilon}_{\text{bacteria}}$ of the double-layer ellipsoidal bacteria is given by

$$\bar{\epsilon}_{\text{bacteria}} = \bar{\epsilon}_{\text{mem}} \frac{k_d + 2\left(\dfrac{\bar{\epsilon}_{\text{cyto}} - \bar{\epsilon}_{\text{mem}}}{\bar{\epsilon}_{\text{cyto}} + 2\bar{\epsilon}_{\text{mem}}}\right)}{k_d - \left(\dfrac{\bar{\epsilon}_{\text{cyto}} - \bar{\epsilon}_{\text{mem}}}{\bar{\epsilon}_{\text{cyto}} + 2\bar{\epsilon}_{\text{mem}}}\right)} \quad \text{where} \quad k_d = \frac{R^2 L}{\left(R - d_{\text{mem}}\right)^2 \left(L - d_{\text{mem}}\right)}$$

where A_{dp} is the depolarization factor and $\bar{\epsilon} = \epsilon - j\sigma/\omega$ is the complex permittivity. We can model the ellipsoidal bacteria (both live and dead) using Equation (3.55).

(a) Given that the bacteria are axially aligned with the applied electric field to minimize drag, calculate the depolarization factor A_{dp}. Use computer software to plot the real part of the CM factor $\text{Re}\big[\bar{K}_{\text{bacteria}}(f)\big]$ for both live and dead bacteria versus frequency f (logarithmic scale) from $f = 10^2$ Hz to $f = 10^{10}$ Hz.

(b) Using the plot obtained from part (a), what would be an ideal frequency $f = \omega/(2\pi)$ to achieve successful DEP separation of live and dead bacteria? It is possible to tune the frequency of our voltage source to be $f_0 = 3 \times 10^x$ Hz, where $x = 1, 2, 3, 4, 5, 6, 7,$ or 8. Using computer software, calculate $\text{Re}\big[\bar{K}_{\text{bacteria}}(f_0)\big]$ at this frequency for live and dead bacteria.

(c) What is the time-averaged DEP force $\langle F_{\text{DEP}}(z)\rangle$ and resulting DEP velocities $v(z)$ experienced by the bacteria as functions of z and $\text{Re}\big[\bar{K}(f)\big] = \text{Re}\big[\bar{K}_{\text{bacteria}}(f)\big]$?

Note: Given the macroscale length of the capillary ($l = 0.15$ m), bacteria throughout virtually the entire capillary will move at a terminal velocity where the time-averaged DEP force $\langle F_{\text{DEP}}\rangle$ is balanced by Stokes' drag force F_{drag}. Assume an effective Stokes radius of $R_S = R = 0.5\ \mu\text{m}$.

(d) A mixture of live and dead bacteria is placed in well A. Can the dead bacteria cross the capillary and reach well B? Why or why not? Starting from well A ($z = 0$), how long does it take for the live bacteria to cross the capillary and reach well B ($z = l$)?

3-18 (Challenging). In a spatially non-uniform electric field, a neutral particle will become polarized and experience dielectrophoresis (DEP). We have a dielectric (i.e., insulating) spherical bead with radius a_{bead} and permittivity ϵ_{bead} serving as a simplified model of a cell. The spherical bead is immersed in a solution with permittivity ϵ_m inside a channel with length L and height h. To trap the bead with DEP force, we have a spherical electrode with radius r_0 at the bottom of the channel whose upper hemisphere is in contact with the solution. The electric potential $V(r)$ generated by the electrode is

$$V(r) = \frac{r_0 V_0 (h - r)}{rh} \quad (\text{where } r_0 < r \ll h)$$

where V_0 is a constant voltage applied on the electrode. The entire setup is shown in the figure below.

A linear pressure drop (i.e., applied pressure) of ΔP across the channel length L drives fluid flow in the channel toward the $\hat{x}$ direction. The dielectric bead is trapped in contact with the electrode by DEP force as shown in the figure below.

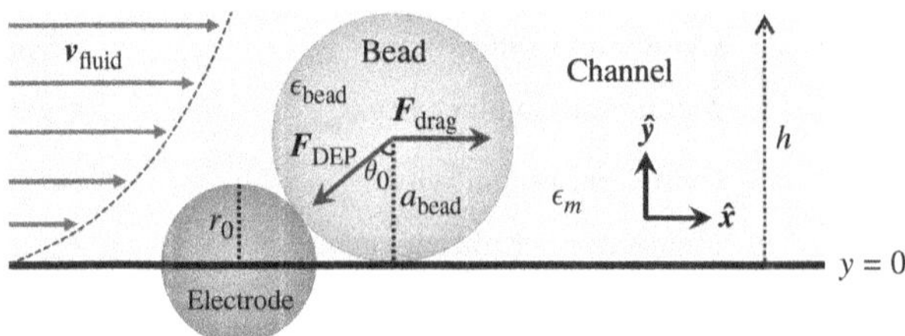

(a) Use the steady-state Navier-Stokes equation for incompressible fluids to derive an expression for the velocity profile $\mathbf{v}_{\text{fluid}} = v_{\text{fluid}}(y)\,\hat{\mathbf{x}}$ of the pressure-driven fluid flow and then use this result to derive the Stokes' drag force $\mathbf{F}_{\text{drag}}$ acting on the center of the dielectric spherical bead.

(b) Derive an expression for the DEP force $\mathbf{F}_{\text{DEP}}$ acting on the center of the dielectric spherical bead. To ensure that the trapped bead will not be carried away by fluid flow, find the maximum value of applied pressure $(\Delta P)_{\text{max}}$ across the channel that drives fluid flow.

Note: Make use of the following expression for the effective dipole moment $\mathbf{p}_{\text{eff}}$:

$$\mathbf{p}_{\text{eff}} = 4\pi\epsilon_m K a_{\text{bead}}^3 \mathbf{E} \quad \text{with} \quad \mathbf{E} = -\boldsymbol{\nabla}V \quad \text{and} \quad K = \frac{\epsilon_{\text{bead}} - \epsilon_m}{\epsilon_{\text{bead}} + 2\epsilon_m}$$

3.7 REFERENCES

[1] N. T. Nguyen and Z. G. Wu, "Micromixers: a review," *Journal of Micromechanics and Microengineering,* vol. 15, no. 2, pp. R1-R16, 2005.

[2] R. Pethig, *Dielectrophoresis: Theory, Methodology and Biological Applications.* Hoboken, NJ, USA; Chichester, UK: John Wiley & Sons, Ltd, 2017.

[3] T. B. Jones, *Electromechanics of Particles,* 1st ed. Cambridge, UK: Cambridge University Press, 1995.

[4] "Fluorescent cells", ImageJ Database, U.S. National Institutes of Health (U.S. NIH) [Online]. Available: https://imagej.nih.gov/ij/images/FluorescentCells.jpg, 2006.

[5] P. J. de Pablo, I. A. T. Schaap, F. C. MacKintosh, and C. F. Schmidt, "Deformation and collapse of microtubules on the nanometer scale," *Physical Review Letters,* vol. 91, no. 9, article 098101, 2003.

[6] T. O. Austin, L. Qiang, and P. W. Baas, "Chapter 4—Mechanisms of neuronal microtubule loss in Alzheimer's disease," in *Neuroprotection in Alzheimer's Disease,* I. Gozes, Ed., 1st ed. London, UK: Academic Press, 2017, pp. 59–71.

[7] L. Cirillo, M. Gotta, and P. Meraldi, "The elephant in the room: the role of microtubules in cancer," in *Cell Division Machinery and Disease,* M. Gotta and P. Meraldi, Eds., 1st ed. Cham, Switzerland: Springer International Publishing, 2017, pp. 93–124.

[8] A. P. Kalra, S. D. Patel, A. F. Bhuiyan, J. Preto, K. G. Scheuer, U. Mohammed, et al., "Investigation of the electrical properties of microtubule ensembles under cell-like conditions," *Nanomaterials,* vol. 10, no. 2, p. 19, 2020.

[9] T. Kim, M.-T. Kao, E. F. Hasselbrink, and E. Meyhöfer, "Nanomechanical model of microtubule translocation in the presence of electric fields," *Biophysical Journal,* vol. 94, no. 10, pp. 3880–3892, 2008.

[10] A. F. Hottinger, P. Pacheco, and R. Stupp, "Tumor treating fields: a novel treatment modality and its use in brain tumors," *NeuroOncology,* vol. 18, no. 10, pp. 1338–1349, 2016.

[11] M. Lasser, J. Tiber, and L. A. Lowery, "The role of the microtubule cytoskeleton in neurodevelopmental disorders," *Frontiers in Cellular Neuroscience,* vol. 12, p. 18, 2018.

[12] M. del Rocío Cantero, C. V. Etchegoyen, P. L. Perez, N. Scarinci, and H. F. Cantiello, "Bundles of brain microtubules generate electrical oscillations," *Scientific Reports,* vol. 8, no. 1, pp. 1–10, 2018.

[13] B. McDermott, E. Porter, D. Hughes, B. McGinley, M. Lang, M. O'Halloran, et al., "Gamma band neural stimulation in humans and the promise of a new modality to prevent and treat Alzheimer's disease," *Journal of Alzheimers Disease,* vol. 65, no. 2, pp. 363–392, 2018.

[14] R. Soffe, S. Baratchi, S. Tang, P. McIntyre, A. Mitchell, and K. Khoshmanesh, "Discontinuous dielectrophoresis: a technique for investigating the response of loosely adherent cells to high shear stress," in *Proceedings of the 9th International Joint Conference on Biomedical Engineering Systems and Technologies (BIOSTEC),* 2016, pp. 23–33.

[15] S. Patel, D. Showers, P. Vedantam, T.-R. Tzeng, S. Qian, and X. Xuan, "Microfluidic separation of live and dead yeast cells using reservoir-based dielectrophoresis," *Biomicrofluidics,* vol. 6, no. 3, article 034102, 2012.

[16] "Depolarization factor," Eric Weisstein's World of Physics [Online]. Available: http://scienceworld.wolfram.com/physics/DepolarizationFactor.html, 2007.

CHAPTER 4

Optical Detection and Quantum Dots

4.1 INTRODUCTION TO OPTICS

In previous chapters, we have focused on the transport and separation of compounds and fluids in bionanotechnological devices. We have learned about forces that prevail at small scales, how to manipulate forces to transport materials (i.e., molecules and particles) from one place to another, and how to separate different materials. In this chapter, we will focus on the optical detection of these materials once they have been transported and separated.

Before we start discussing optical detection, let us review the fundamentals of light. All light beams are composed of discrete particles called photons. Photons are particles that transmit electromagnetic waves, including light. The word "photon" originates from the Greek word for light, and was initially suggested to be a unit of illumination. The light sensed by our eyes consists of visible-wavelength photons. Photons are stable massless particles having no electric charge while carrying energy. Light pressure can be used to move and manipulate small molecules, such as via an optical tweezer. The electromagnetic wave frequency of a photon (i.e., light) is usually denoted by γ, and each photon has energy

$$E_{\text{photon}} = h\gamma = \frac{hc}{\lambda}\bigg|_{\text{vacuum}} = \frac{h v_n}{\lambda_n}\bigg|_{\text{medium }(n)} \tag{4.1}$$

where $h = 6.626 \times 10^{-34}$ J $\cdot$ s is the Planck constant, $c = 2.998 \times 10^8$ m/s $\cong 3 \times 10^8$ m/s is the speed of light in vacuum, λ is the wavelength of light in vacuum, $\gamma = c/\lambda = v_n/\lambda_n$ is the frequency of light, and n is the refractive index of the medium.

Both the photon energy E_{photon} and the frequency γ are *independent* of the medium the photon is traveling through. When traveling through a medium of refractive index n, the photon (i.e., light) has a speed of $v_n = c/n$ and a wavelength of $\lambda_n = \lambda/n$. The refractive index n of any medium depends on the vacuum wavelength λ of light traveling through the medium as well as the nature of the medium itself. The refractive index of vacuum is $n_{\text{vacuum}} = 1$ (exactly). For light with vacuum wavelengths of $\lambda = 100$ nm to 10 μm (which spans the UV, visible, and near-infrared ranges of light), the refractive index of air is given by $n_{\text{air}} = 1.0003 \cong 1$. Therefore, we may assume that in air,

$$\text{For } \lambda = 100 \text{ nm to } 10 \text{ } \mu\text{m:} \quad n_{\text{air}} = 1.0003 \cong 1 \quad \Rightarrow \quad \begin{cases} v_{n(\text{air})} \cong c \\ \lambda_{n(\text{air})} \cong \lambda \end{cases} \quad \Rightarrow \quad E_{\text{photon}} \cong \frac{hc}{\lambda_{n(\text{air})}} \tag{4.2}$$

Unless otherwise indicated, the wavelength of all light sources mentioned in this book refers to the wavelength of light in vacuum λ, which is approximately the same as the wavelength of light in air for $\lambda = 100$ nm to 10 μm.

EXAMPLE 4-1   How much energy is carried by a light pulse consisting of 2.14×10^{16} photons all having a (vacuum) wavelength of 600 nm?

Solution   The energy of a 600 nm photon is given by

$$E_{photon} = \frac{hc}{\lambda} = \frac{\left(6.626 \times 10^{-34}\ \text{J·s}\right)\left(3 \times 10^{8}\ \text{m/s}\right)}{600\ \text{nm}} = 3.313 \times 10^{-19}\ \text{J}$$

The total energy of $N_{photons} = 2.14 \times 10^{16}$ photons all having a wavelength of 600 nm is

$$E_{total} = N_{photons} \cdot E_{photon} = (2.14 \times 10^{16}) \cdot (3.313 \times 10^{-19}\ \text{J}) = 7.09\ \text{mJ} \quad \blacktriangle$$

The optical detection method is commonly used for detecting small amounts of sample. For the optical detection of most samples, quantitative analysis is based on the Beer-Lambert law. This law describes the absorption of light as it travels through a medium, as measured by light intensity. The Beer-Lambert law is

$$I = I_0 \cdot 10^{-\varepsilon_{BL} LC} = I_0 \cdot 10^{-A_\lambda} \quad (4.3) \qquad A_\lambda = -\log_{10}\left(\frac{I}{I_0}\right) = \varepsilon_{BL} LC \quad (4.4A)$$

where I_0 is the initial intensity of the light, ε_{BL} is the molar absorption (or molar extinction) coefficient, L is the optical depth, C is the molar concentration, and A_λ is the absorbance (also known as the optical density or OD) at wavelength λ. As shown in Figure 4-1, the optical depth L is the length of the path that light passes through, and I is the intensity of light after passing through the optical depth L.

When multiple light-absorbing species are involved (where i represents the ith light-absorbing species), the absorbance A_λ is

$$A_\lambda = L\sum_{i} C_i \varepsilon_{BL,\,i} \tag{4.4B}$$

The equations above are used in the design of optical detection devices. An application of the Beer-Lambert law is the oximeter device used to measure blood oxygen level (Figure 4-2).

Starting with $I_0 - I = I_0\left(1 - 10^{-\varepsilon_{BL} LC}\right)$, we have

$$10^{-\varepsilon_{BL} LC} = \exp\left[\ln\left(10^{-\varepsilon_{BL} LC}\right)\right] = \exp\left[-\varepsilon_{BL} LC(\ln 10)\right]$$

Therefore, $I_0 - I = I_0\left(1 - \exp\left[-\varepsilon_{BL} LC(\ln 10)\right]\right)$

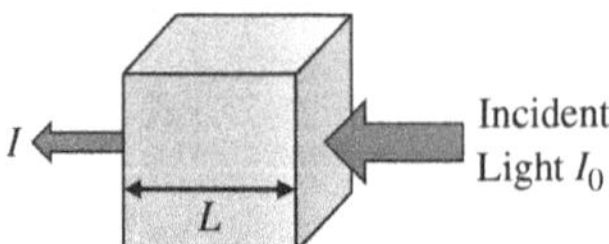

Figure 4-1   Illustration of the optical depth L in the Beer-Lambert law.

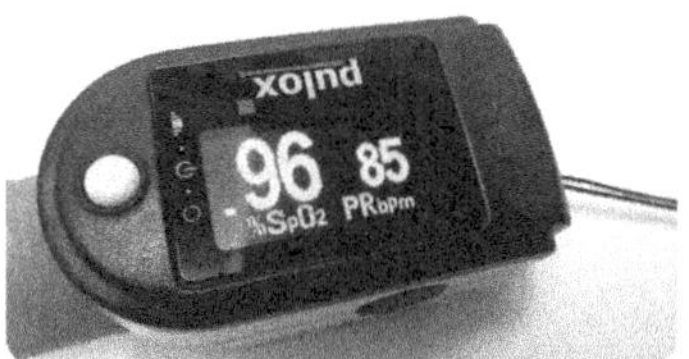

Figure 4-2   Fingertip pulse oximeter manufactured by Pulox. (*The image is by S. Bellini [Wikimedia Commons].*[1])

Using the Taylor expansion for small $\varepsilon_{BL}LC(\ln 10)$ and hence very small L:

$$\exp\left[-\varepsilon_{BL}LC(\ln 10)\right] \cong 1 - \varepsilon_{BL}LC(\ln 10)$$

$$I_0 - I \cong I_0\left(1 - \left[1 - \varepsilon_{BL}LC(\ln 10)\right]\right) = I_0(\ln 10)\varepsilon_{BL}LC$$

For optically thin situations where the optical depth L is very small, Equation (4.3) can be approximated as

$$I_0 - I = I_0\left(1 - 10^{-\varepsilon_{BL}LC}\right) \cong I_0(\ln 10)\varepsilon_{BL}LC \qquad (4.5)$$

The molar extinction coefficient value depends on a number of factors, including the material and the wavelength of incident light. Figure 4-3 is a graph of the molar extinction coefficient of oxygenated (HbO_2) and deoxygenated (Hb) hemoglobin at different wavelengths. Hemoglobin is an iron-containing protein within red blood cells whose primary function is to carry oxygen (O_2) from the lungs to the entire body. Red blood cells also utilize hemoglobin to carry a fraction of the waste carbon dioxide (CO_2) generated by the body to be expelled by the lungs.

Another application of the Beer-Lambert law is in spectrophotometers such as the one shown in Figure 4-4. Spectrophotometers measure a light beam's intensity as a function of its wavelength. This non-destructive equipment is commonly used in analytical chemistry for qualitatively or quantitatively characterizing different analytes, such as transition metal ions and highly conjugated organic compounds. In addition, the spectrophotometer can also be used for the detection and analysis of biological macromolecules, such as samples containing DNA, RNA, proteins, and/or enzymes. The spectrophotometer light source

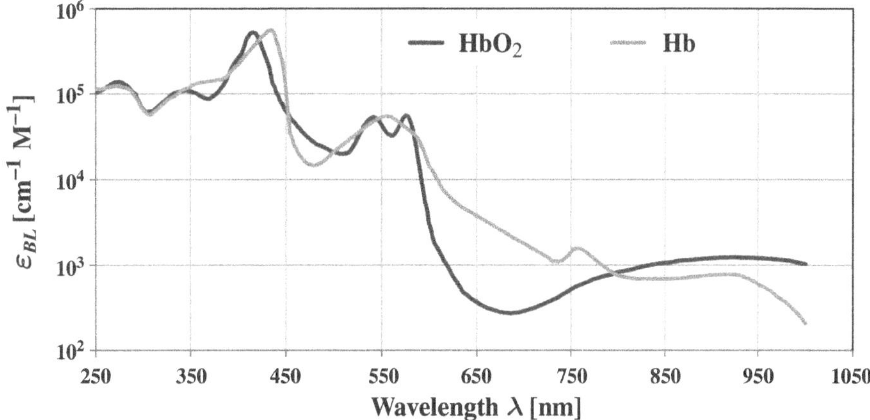

Figure 4-3   Molar absorption (or extinction) coefficient ε_{BL} of oxygenated (HbO_2) and deoxygenated (Hb) hemoglobin at different (vacuum) wavelengths of light λ. (*The graph is plotted with permission using data from S. Prahl [Oregon Medical Laser Center].*[2])

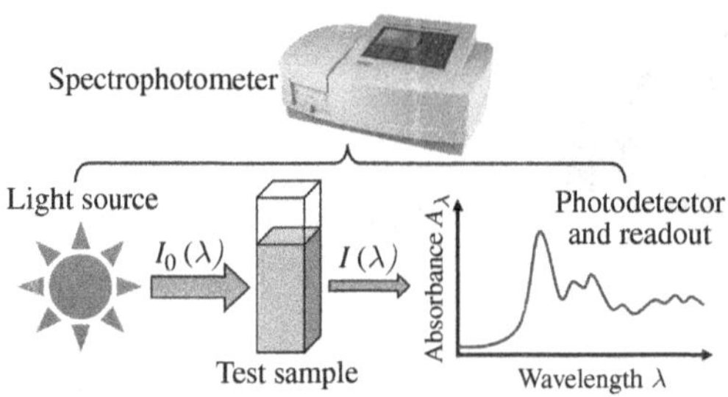

Figure 4-4   Schematic of a typical spectrophotometer. The readout usually consists of optical density (i.e., absorbance A_λ) values versus light (vacuum) wavelength λ.

covers the region of UV, visible light, and/or near-infrared. For example, protein measurements can be conducted at the wavelength of 280 nm (UV).

4.2 OPTICAL DETECTION AND FLUORESCENCE

Optical signals can be detected by photoabsorption. Different species can be identified and differentiated by comparing their optical absorption spectra, which is their absorbance A_λ (i.e., optical density) across many different wavelengths of light. For example, nucleic acids (DNA and RNA) absorb strongly at about 260 nm, while proteins absorb strongly at about 280 nm. By measuring the absorbance A_λ at these wavelengths, the concentration of nucleic acids and proteins in a sample can be determined.

Fluorescence is the emission of light by a molecule or a particle after absorbing light at a different (higher energy) wavelength. Optical signals can also be generated and detected by using fluorescence. For this purpose, fluorescent dyes or tags called fluorophores are commonly used in optical detection. These fluorescent dye (or tag) molecules are designed to absorb photons of one wavelength (the excitation wavelength) and use the absorbed photon energy to emit photons of another wavelength (the emission wavelength). For a fluorescent dye or tag, the emitted fluorescent photons have lower energy (i.e., a longer wavelength λ) than the absorbed photons, a phenomenon known as Stokes shift. Stokes shift is a consequence of the conservation of energy, and the difference between the absorbed light energy and the emitted light energy is mostly lost as heat. For instance, fluorophores can absorb UV photons and then re-emit lower energy photons in the visible range.

To tag molecules of interest for detection, fluorophores or fluorescent intercalators are commonly used. Fluorophores and fluorescent intercalators both exhibit fluorescence (i.e., absorb photons and then emit photons of a different wavelength). Ordinary fluorophores will usually fluoresce with similar or reduced intensities when the fluorophore is linked to another molecule. However, fluorescent intercalators will fluoresce with far greater intensities when they are linked to certain molecules, such as inside double-stranded DNA. An example is ethidium bromide (EtBr) which can fluoresce 20 times more when it is bound to DNA or RNA. EtBr binds in between the strands in double-stranded DNA or within folded regions of RNA.

Fluorophores such as fluorescent dyes also have specific quantum yields. The quantum yield (QY), also known as quantum efficiency (QE), is the probability that a photon absorbed by a fluorophore will result in an emitted photon. The number of photons absorbed is determined using the Beer-Lambert law. For example, a dye with $QY = 0.33$ will emit one photon for roughly every three photons absorbed. Table 4-1 shows the peak excitation wavelength, peak emission wavelength, quantum yield, and molar absorption coefficient for two commercial fluorescent dyes. In general, the absorption and emission characteristics of fluorophores depend on photon energy E_{photon} or equivalently photon frequency γ, which are both *independent* of the medium the photon is traveling through. The excitation and emission wavelengths of fluorophores are normally listed using the vacuum wavelength of light given by $\lambda = c/\gamma$, rather than the light wavelength in a medium such as a solution in which the fluorophore is used.

TABLE 4-1   Characteristics of Two Fluorescent Dyes from Invitrogen (by Thermo Fisher Scientific)[3]

Fluorophore	Excitation* [nm]	Emission* [nm]	QY	$\varepsilon_{BL}[cm^{-1}\,M^{-1}]$
Alexa Fluor® 488	496	519	0.92	7.1×10^4
Alexa Fluor® 647	650	665	0.33	2.4×10^5

*Wavelength λ of light in vacuum (or in air).

The emission of photons from fluorophores is omnidirectional. If a detector only takes up 1% of the surface area on the "sphere" of photons emitted, it will only be able to detect 1% of the photons. One problem in detecting fluorescence is the possible presence of native fluorescence. Native fluorescence, also called autofluorescence, occurs when some parts of the system other than the fluorophore labels are fluorescent. The presence of this extra fluorescence (which appears as noise) may overwhelm the desired fluorescence (i.e., the signal), making the detector ineffective. Note that some plastics have native fluorescence, so glass and quartz containers are better suited for optical detection using fluorescence as they have far less native fluorescence.

The excitation and detection of fluorescence can be achieved using confocal laser–induced fluorescence (LIF) as shown in Figure 4-5. This setup requires a dichroic mirror, a mirror which reflects light of some wavelengths while allowing light of other wavelengths to pass through. An excitation laser is reflected off the dichroic mirror, and is focused by the objective (a lens system) onto the sample. The sample fluoresces from the laser light excitation, and a fraction of the fluorescent light produced by the sample is captured by the objective. The captured fluorescent light passes through the dichroic mirror, past a pinhole and an optical bandpass filter, and finally enters the photodetector. Let us go through an example to illustrate how this setup works.

EXAMPLE 4-2 Alexa Fluor® 647 is bound to identical molecules at a picomolar concentration after carrying out separation. For optical detection of these molecules, an excitation laser with wavelength of 650 nm (in vacuum or in air) is used to uniformly illuminate a 300 μm (length) × 100 μm (width) × 100 μm (depth) section of a long microchannel that is 100 μm × 100 μm (square) in cross-section.

(a) Using the Beer-Lambert law and the value in Table 4-1 for the molar extinction coefficient, what transmission ratio do you obtain?

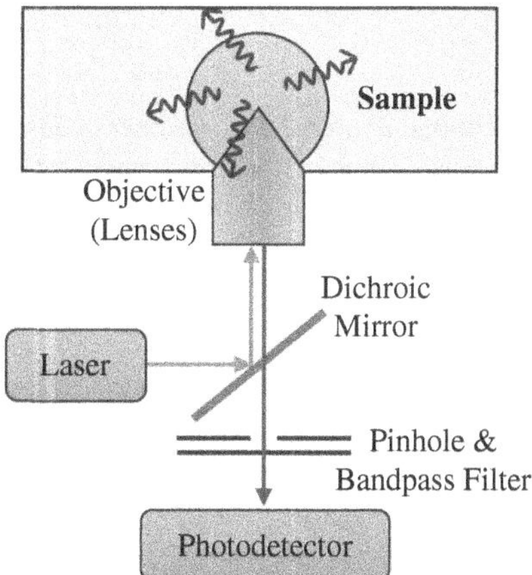

Figure 4-5 Optical detection with a confocal laser–induced fluorescence (LIF) setup.

(b) Assuming that the 5 mW laser is perfectly efficient in illuminating the 300 μm × 100 μm × 100 μm section of the microchannel (no light misses the microchannel), what is the intensity of light hitting the channel $\Phi_{incident}$ in terms of the number of incident photons per second?

(c) How many photons per second $\Phi_{absorbed}$ are absorbed by the fluorophore?

(d) Given the quantum yield of the fluorophore (Table 4-1), how many photons per second of fluorescence $\Phi_{objective}$ are collected by the objective? Assume that the circular objective acquires all light falling on it, and that it has a diameter of 0.5 mm and is located 3 mm away from the microchannel. Beyond this, the number of excitation photons (and incident photons for that matter) which reach the actual detector has to be addressed.

(e) If 1% of the incident photons are reflected or scattered back into the collection optics, and 10^{-10} of these manage to pass the optical filter and reach the detector. What is the rate of photons per second $\Phi_{baseline}$ from this excitation light? This is your baseline.

(f) Assume that 10% of all the fluorescence photons collected by the objective manage to pass through the filter and reach the detector. What is the rate of photons per second Φ_{signal} from this fluorescence? This is your signal. Is this setup acceptable for optical detection?

Solution

(a) Before computing the transmission ratio, we need the value of L used in the Beer-Lambert law. This concept is illustrated in Figure 4-1, where L is not the length of the microchannel, but is instead the length of the path that light passes through, which is 100 μm in this example. Hence, the transmission ratio is

$$I/I_0 = 10^{-\varepsilon_{BL}CL} = 10^{-\left(2.4\times10^5\,\frac{1}{\text{cm}\cdot\text{M}}\right)\left(10^{-12}\,\text{M}\right)\left(100\times10^{-4}\,\text{cm}\right)} = 0.99999999447$$

Although this number is very close to 1, we cannot make the approximation; otherwise, we cannot move on with the rest of the calculations. Thus, almost all the intensity of the excitation laser will pass right through the microchannel section. However, some of the intensity is still absorbed by the Alexa Fluor® 647.

(b) The number of incident photons per second $\Phi_{incident}$ is

$$\Phi_{incident} = \frac{\text{Power}}{E_{photon}} = \frac{P}{hc/\lambda} = \frac{P\lambda}{hc} = \frac{(5\text{ mW})(650\text{ nm})}{(6.626\times10^{-34}\text{ J}\cdot\text{s})(3\times10^8\text{ m/s})} = 1.63\times10^{16}\text{ photons/s}$$

(c) The total proportion of light absorbed is

$$1 - I/I_0 = 1 - 0.99999999447 = 5.53\times10^{-9}$$

$$\Phi_{absorbed} = \left(1 - \frac{I}{I_0}\right)\Phi_{incident} = (5.53\times10^{-9})(1.63\times10^{16}\text{ photons/s}) = 9.04\times10^7\text{ photons/s}$$

(d) The total number of emitted photons is the number of absorbed photons multiplied by the quantum yield (QY). Since the objective lens is sufficiently far away from the microchannel and is sufficiently large, the source of the emitted photons can be assumed to be a point source. Also, the lens can be thought of as being a section of the surface area of a sphere of radius 3 mm, with the center being the source of emitting photons. Due to energy conservation, the total intensity of emitted light must pass through the sphere's surface. Therefore,

$$\Phi_{objective} = \Phi_{absorbed}\cdot\text{QY}\cdot\frac{A_{lens}}{A_{sphere}} = (9.04\times10^7\text{ photons/s})(0.33)\frac{\pi(0.5\text{ mm}/2)^2}{4\pi(3\text{ mm})^2}$$

$$\Phi_{objective} = 5.18\times10^4\text{ photons/s}$$

(e) $\Phi_{\text{baseline}} = (1\%)(10^{-10})\Phi_{\text{incident}} = (0.01)(10^{-10})(1.63\times10^{16}\,\text{photons/s})$

$$\Phi_{\text{baseline}} = 1.63\times10^4\,\text{photons/s}$$

(f) $\Phi_{\text{signal}} = (10\%)\Phi_{\text{objective}} = (0.1)(5.18\times10^4\,\text{photons/s}) = 5.18\times10^3\,\text{photons/s}$

Given that the fluorescence signal Φ_{signal} is much weaker than the baseline signal Φ_{baseline}, this is not a good setup and would need to be adjusted (for instance, by increasing the molar concentration C of the fluorescent dye).   ▲

EXAMPLE 4-3
Optical Detection
of Bacteria

The setup illustrated in Figure 4-6 is used to optically detect bacteria. To do so, molecules sensitive to a particular wavelength are added to the solution containing the bacteria. These molecules are excited by a light source and fluoresce, meaning that they emit photons of another wavelength.

In this experiment, two different lasers are used. The wavelength of laser LX1 can be adjusted (Figure 4-7), and the (vacuum or air) wavelength of laser LX2 is kept constant at 478 nm. Furthermore, a list of different fictitious fluorophores is given in the following table. The chosen fluorophore is bound to identical bacteria with a resulting fluorophore concentration of 5.4×10^{-12} M. The illuminated microchannel is 275 μm long and is cylindrical with a radius of $r_{\text{channel}} = 60$ μm.

As shown in Figure 4-6, a special voltage-controlled prism is used to focus and merge two different laser beams LX1 and LX2. Note that the applied prism voltage V can only be positive. The DC current powering laser LX1 is set to a value of 37.5 mA. The transfer function of the prism is

$$\lambda_{\text{out}} = \frac{1}{n_{\text{medium}} \cdot n_{\text{prism}}}\lambda_{\text{LX1}} + \frac{1}{n^2_{\text{medium}}}\lambda_{\text{LX2}}$$

where $n_{\text{medium}} \cong 1$ is the refractive index of the medium surrounding the prism (which is assumed to be air), and λ_{out} is the (vacuum or air) wavelength of the output laser beam produced by the prism after merging laser beams LX1 and LX2. The refractive index of the prism n_{prism} is

$$n_{\text{prism}} = 0.6V^2 + 0.1V + 0.9$$

where V is the DC voltage applied to the prism.

Fluorophore	Excitation* [nm]	Emission* [nm]	QY	$\varepsilon_{BL}[\text{cm}^{-1}\,\text{M}^{-1}]$
A	658	687	0.23	5.4×10^6
B	713	725	0.82	4.8×10^5
C	749	763	0.82	9.5×10^6
D	813	856	0.44	5.6×10^5
E	854	887	0.64	9.5×10^6

*Wavelength λ of light in vacuum (or in air).

(a) Which fluorophore in the table gives the highest number of photons emitted by fluorescence and why?

(b) What DC voltage V should be applied to the prism in order to create the wavelength needed for this particular fluorophore?

(c) How many photons are absorbed each second by the fluorophore when the angle of incidence θ_1 is 30°? Note that the channel wall is infinitesimally thin and the refractive index of

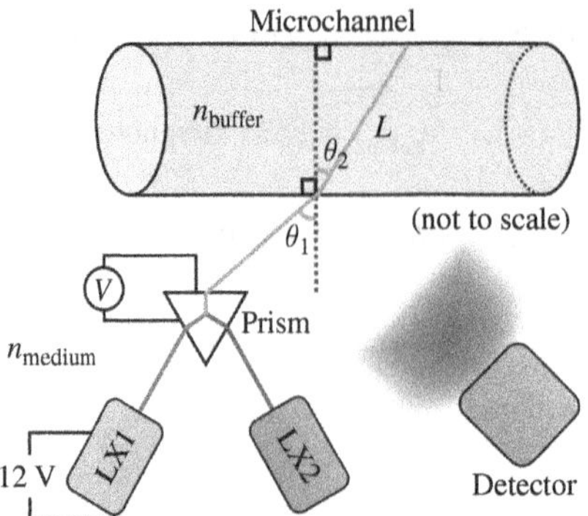

Figure 4-6   Experimental setup for optically detecting bacteria.

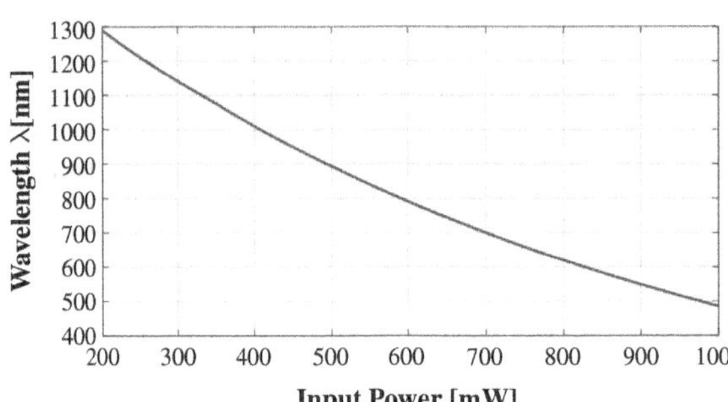

Figure 4-7   The (vacuum or air) wavelength λ of laser LX1 versus input power.

the buffer solution in the channel is $n_{\text{buffer}} = 3.2$. Assume that the output laser with wavelength λ_{out} leaving the prism is pulsed at a rate of 40 MHz with each pulse delivering 0.1 µJ of energy.

Hint: Make use of Snell's law given by $n_1 \sin \theta_1 = n_2 \sin \theta_2$.

(d) The objective lens collecting the photons emitted by fluorescence is located 5 mm away from the microchannel and has a square lens with a side length of 1 mm. How many photons are collected each second by the objective lens?

Solution

(a) To answer this question, we have to revisit the Beer-Lambert law: $I = I_0 \cdot 10^{-\varepsilon_{BL} LC}$

We want to have the highest ratio of light absorbed; that is, we want the absorbance $A_\lambda = \varepsilon_{BL} LC$ to be as large as possible. Thus, we prefer the highest molar extinction coefficient ε_{BL}.

The highest number of emitted fluorescence photons is given by fluorophore C because it has the highest quantum yield (QY) as well as the highest molar extinction coefficient ε_{BL}. The number of emitted fluorescence photons is proportional to the quantum yield, the molar extinction coefficient ε_{BL} (assuming that $A_\lambda = \varepsilon_{BL} LC$ is very small), and the number of incident photons at the excitation wavelength. However, the impacts of changes in the excitation wavelength $\lambda_{\text{excitation}}$ of the different fluorophores are minimal compared with the differences in quantum yield and molar extinction coefficient.

(b) Figure 4-6 shows that laser LX1 is connected to 12V DC, and thus the power of the laser can be calculated for the given current rating of 37.5 mA DC as follows.

$$P_{\text{LX1}} = (12 \text{ V})(37.5 \text{ mA}) = 450 \text{ mW}$$

The corresponding wavelength of laser LX1 can be obtained from Figure 4-7 and is approximately 950 nm. Using the equation provided and given that the refractive index of the medium surrounding the prism is $n_{\text{medium}} \cong 1$, n_{prism} and hence V can be obtained. To maximize the fluorescence intensity, we want to set the output laser wavelength λ_{out} leaving the prism to be equal to the excitation wavelength $\lambda_{\text{excitation}}$ of fluorophore C (i.e., 749 nm).

$$\lambda_{\text{excitation}} = \lambda_{\text{out}} = \frac{1}{n_{\text{medium}} \cdot n_{\text{prism}}} \lambda_{\text{LX1}} + \frac{1}{n_{\text{medium}}^2} \lambda_{\text{LX2}} = \frac{1}{n_{\text{prism}}} \lambda_{\text{LX1}} + \lambda_{\text{LX2}}$$

$$749 \text{ nm} = \frac{1}{n_{\text{prism}}} \cdot 950 \text{ nm} + 478 \text{ nm} \quad \Rightarrow \quad n_{\text{prism}} = 3.506$$

$$n_{\text{prism}} = 3.506 = 0.6V^2 + 0.1V + 0.9 \quad \Rightarrow \quad 0.6V^2 + 0.1V - 2.606 = 0$$

Using the quadratic formula, we obtain

$$V = -2.17 \text{ V} \quad \text{or} \quad +2.00 \text{ V}$$

The applied voltage for the prism cannot be negative, so $V = +2.00$ V.

(c) Using Snell's law, the angle of refraction θ_2 can be obtained as follows.

$$n_1 \sin\theta_1 = n_2 \sin\theta_2 \quad \Rightarrow \quad n_{\text{medium}} \sin\theta_1 = n_{\text{buffer}} \sin\theta_2$$

$$\theta_2 = \arcsin\left(\frac{n_{\text{medium}}}{n_{\text{buffer}}} \cdot \sin\theta_1\right) = \arcsin\left(\frac{1}{3.2} \cdot \sin 30°\right) = 8.99°$$

Now the optical depth L can be obtained as follows:

$$L = \frac{2r_{\text{channel}}}{\cos(\theta_2)} = \frac{2(60 \text{ μm})}{\cos(8.99°)} = 121.5 \text{ μm}$$

Using the Beer-Lambert law, the transmission ratio can be calculated as follows:

$$I/I_0 = 10^{-\varepsilon_{BL}CL} = 10^{-\left(9.5\times10^6 \frac{1}{\text{cm}\cdot\text{M}}\right)\left(5.4\times10^{-12}\text{ M}\right)\left(121.5\times10^{-4}\text{ cm}\right)} = 0.999998565$$

The average power P_{avg} of the laser beam (with wavelength λ_{out}) leaving the prism is

$$P_{\text{avg}} = (40 \text{ MHz})(0.1 \text{ μJ}) = 4.00 \text{ W}$$

The number of incident photons per second Φ_{incident} is

$$\Phi_{\text{incident}} = \frac{P_{\text{avg}}}{hc/\lambda_{\text{out}}} = \frac{P_{\text{avg}}\lambda_{\text{out}}}{hc} = \frac{(4.00 \text{ W})(749 \text{ nm})}{(6.626\times10^{-34}\text{ J}\cdot\text{s})(3\times10^8 \text{ m/s})} = 1.51\times10^{19} \text{ photons/s}$$

The number of photons absorbed each second by the fluorophore Φ_{absorbed} is

$$\Phi_{\text{absorbed}} = \left(1 - \frac{I}{I_0}\right)\Phi_{\text{incident}} = (1 - 0.999998565)(1.51\times10^{19} \text{ photons/s})$$

$$\Phi_{\text{absorbed}} = 2.16\times10^{13} \text{ photons/s}$$

(d) The number of photons collected by the objective lens each second $\Phi_{\text{collected}}$ is given by

$$\Phi_{\text{collected}} = \Phi_{\text{absorbed}} \cdot \text{QY} \cdot \frac{A_{\text{lens}}}{A_{\text{sphere}}} = (2.16\times10^{13} \text{ photons/s})(0.82)\frac{(1 \text{ mm})^2}{4\pi(5 \text{ mm})^2}$$

$$\Phi_{\text{collected}} = 5.65\times10^{10} \text{ photons/s} \quad \blacktriangle$$

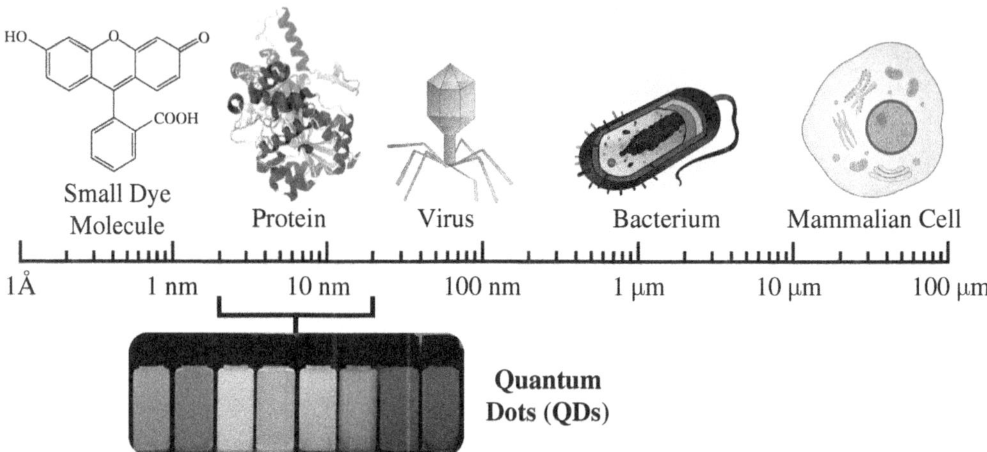

Figure 4-8   The size of quantum dots (QDs) compared with common biological entities. QDs of different structures and sizes can emit different wavelengths. (*The photograph of QDs is from the U.S. National Institutes of Health [NIH].*[4])

4.3 QUANTUM DOTS

Quantum dots (QDs) are a new class of fluorescent probes (fluorophores). While conventional organic fluorescent dyes are composed of small organic molecules on the order of 1 nm in size, QDs are composed of inorganic semiconductor nanocrystals. QDs are highly luminescent colloidal semiconductor nanocrystals with sizes typically in the range of 2 to 20 nm.[5] Soon after their synthesis was first reported in the early 1990s, QDs were used as biological fluorescent probes beginning in 1998. Compared with organic fluorescent dyes, QDs have superior optical properties. For example, the emission wavelength of QD fluorescent probes can be continuously tuned within a wide range by varying the size or composition of the semiconductor nanocrystals.[6] Figure 4-8 illustrates the physical size as well as the different emission colors of QDs.

4.3.1 Theory of Quantum Dot Fluorescence

(A) QD Band Structure and Quantum Confinement

For bulk semiconductor crystals, the conduction band (CB) and valence band (VB) are effectively continuous due to the sheer number of electrons and the Pauli exclusion principle (i.e., no two electrons may share the same quantum state). There are two types of charge carriers in any semiconductor material that contribute to the electric current: electrons and holes. A hole is an electron vacancy with a positive electric charge of $+e$. Because every one of the innumerous electrons and holes occupies a distinct quantum state, the different energy states of all the electrons and holes together form two continuous bands: the VB and CB. Between the VB and the CB of a semiconductor, there is a forbidden region of energy states called the bandgap that electrons and holes cannot occupy (Figure 4-9). The bandgap energy E_g is the energy difference between the bottom of the CB and the top of the VB. In a semiconductor, only the conduction band electrons and valence band holes can move freely and conduct electricity.

Unlike bulk semiconductor crystals, a quantum dot (QD) has a much more limited number of electrons and holes. For a QD, this causes the CB and VB to become discrete. The electronic and optical properties of QDs, such as the discrete CB and VB, all result from a phenomenon known as quantum confinement. Quantum confinement occurs when electrons and holes are spatially confined, and the electrons and holes of QDs are confined in all three dimensions.[7]

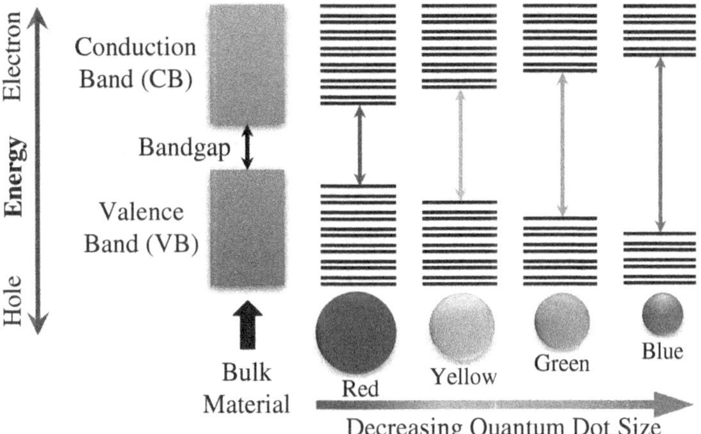

Figure 4-9 The conduction band (CB), valence band (VB), and bandgap for bulk semiconductor crystals and quantum dots (QDs).

The electrons and holes of a spherical or somewhat spherical QD can be treated as being confined in an infinite spherical quantum well. From classical mechanics, the kinetic energy of a particle is

$$E_{\text{kinetic}} = \frac{1}{2}mv^2 = \frac{(mv)^2}{2m} = \frac{p^2}{2m} \tag{4.6}$$

where p is the momentum, m is the mass, and v is the speed of the particle.

The classical kinetic energy E_{kinetic} is somewhat analogous to the kinetic energy of particles in an infinite quantum well, but the kinetic energy of particles in a quantum well is quantized into discrete levels. Using $p = \hbar k$ (the de Broglie equation for matter waves), the allowed kinetic energy levels $E_{n,l}$ for a particle trapped within an infinite spherical quantum well are given by

$$E_{n,l} = \frac{p^2}{2m^*} = \frac{(\hbar k)^2}{2m^*} = \frac{\hbar^2\left(\dfrac{z_{n,l}}{r_0}\right)^2}{2m^*} = \frac{\hbar^2 z_{n,l}^{\,2}}{2m^* r_0^2} \quad \text{where} \quad \begin{cases} p = \hbar k \\ k = \dfrac{z_{n,l}}{r_0} \end{cases} \text{and} \begin{cases} n = 1,2,3,4,\ldots \\ l = 0,1,2,3,\ldots \end{cases} \tag{4.7}$$

where $\hbar = h/2\pi$ is the reduced Planck constant, p is the particle's momentum, m^* is the particle's effective mass, and k is the particle's wavenumber. r_0 is the radius of the spherical quantum well which represents the radius of a spherical QD, while $z_{n,l}$ is the nth zero of $j_l(x)$, the lth spherical Bessel function of the first kind (Figure 4-10 and Table 4-2). Here, n and l are independent quantum numbers.[7]

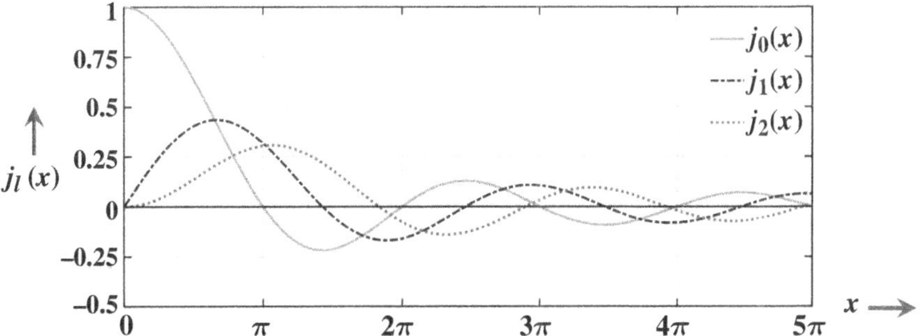

Figure 4-10 The first three spherical Bessel functions of the first kind $j_l(x)$.

TABLE 4-2   The First Few Zeros $z_{n,l}$ of the Spherical Bessel Function $j_l(x)$

$z_{n,l}$	$n=1$	$n=2$	$n=3$	$n=4$	$n=5$
$l=0$	π	2π	3π	4π	5π
$l=1$	4.493	7.725	10.904	14.066	17.221
$l=2$	5.763	9.095	12.323	15.515	18.689
$l=3$	6.988	10.417	13.698	16.924	20.122
$l=4$	8.183	11.705	15.040	18.301	21.525

Notice that there is a minimum allowed value for $z_{n,l}$ ($z_{min} = z_{1,0} = \pi$) corresponding to the quantum numbers $n, l = 1, 0$. Thus, there is a minimum allowed kinetic energy (called the ground state) for particles in an infinite spherical quantum well (such as a QD) given by

$$\text{KE}_{min} = E_{1,0} = \frac{\hbar^2 z_{1,0}^2}{2m^* r_0^2} = \frac{\left(\dfrac{h}{2\pi}\right)^2 \pi^2}{2m^* r_0^2} = \frac{h^2}{8m^* r_0^2} \tag{4.8}$$

(B) Bandgap of Quantum Dots

In a semiconductor, the only free charge carriers are the excited CB electrons and excited VB holes. VB electrons and CB holes are not free as they are unexcited and thus they cannot conduct electricity. In intraband transitions, excited electrons transition from one energy level in the CB to another (for instance, from $n, l = 1,1$ to $n, l = 2,0$), while excited holes transition from one energy level in the VB to another level. As shown in Figure 4-11, the CB electron energy is measured *upward* from the bottom of the CB, while the VB hole energy is measured *downward* from the top of the VB. When a VB hole gains energy, it drops to a lower energy level within the VB.

Since there is a minimum allowed kinetic energy $\text{KE}_{min} = E_{1,0}$ for all electrons and holes within the QD, the bandgap $E_{g,QD}$ of the QD is usually significantly greater than the

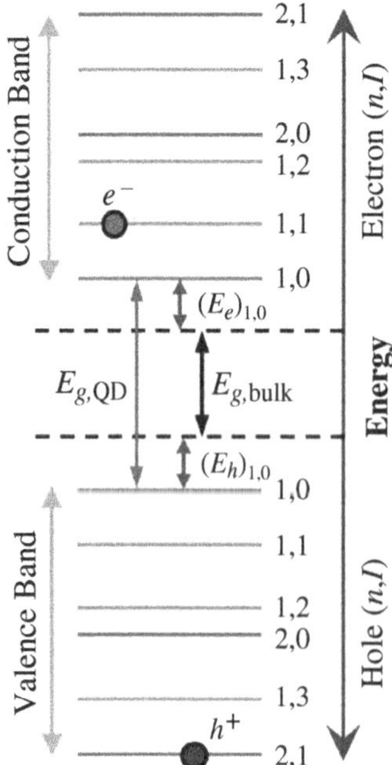

Figure 4-11   Energy-level diagram of a quantum dot (QD).

bandgap of the bulk semiconductor $E_{g,\text{bulk}}$.[8] In addition to the minimum kinetic energies of the electron $\text{KE}_{e,\text{min}}$ and hole $\text{KE}_{h,\text{min}}$, there is also electric potential energy $\text{PE}_{e/h}$ between the electron and hole. From the conservation of energy, we have

$$E_{g,\text{QD}} = E_{g,\text{bulk}} + \text{KE}_{e,\text{min}} + \text{KE}_{h,\text{min}} + \text{PE}_{e/h} \tag{4.9}$$

Furthermore, we have

$$\text{PE}_{e/h} = \frac{1}{4\pi\epsilon}\frac{-e^2}{\Delta s} \quad \Rightarrow \quad E_{g,\text{QD}} = E_{g,\text{bulk}} + \left(E_e\right)_{1,0} + \left(E_h\right)_{1,0} + \frac{1}{4\pi\epsilon}\frac{-e^2}{\Delta s}$$

where $\epsilon = \epsilon_r\epsilon_0$ is the permittivity of the *bulk* semiconductor material of which the QD is composed, e is the elementary charge, $\Delta s \cong r_0/1.8$ is the distance between the electron and hole from theoretical calculations of electron-hole wavefunction overlap, and r_0 is the radius of the spherical quantum dot. The potential energy $\text{PE}_{e/h}$, which is typically much lower than the combined minimum kinetic energy $\text{KE}_{e,\text{min}} + \text{KE}_{h,\text{min}}$, is negative because the electron and hole are oppositely charged.[9]

Note that there are also higher order terms due to polarization which we will ignore as they are usually insignificant. Hence, for spherical quantum dots with radius r_0, we obtain the Brus equation which governs their optical absorption and emission behavior[10]:

$$E_{g,\text{QD}} = E_{g,\text{bulk}} + \frac{h^2}{8m_e^*r_0^2} + \frac{h^2}{8m_h^*r_0^2} - \frac{1}{4\pi\epsilon_r\epsilon_0}\frac{1.8e^2}{r_0}$$

$$E_{g,\text{QD}} = E_{g,\text{bulk}} + \frac{h^2}{8r_0^2}\left(\frac{1}{m_e^*} + \frac{1}{m_h^*}\right) - \frac{1.8e^2}{4\pi\epsilon_r\epsilon_0 r_0} \tag{4.10}$$

In the equations above, m_e^* and m_h^* are the effective masses of the electron and hole, respectively. The effective mass is the apparent mass of an electron or a hole within the periodic potential of a crystal lattice, as opposed to the real mass which accurately describes the behavior in free space. The effective mass is sometimes given as the ratio m^*/m_0, where $m_0 = 9.11 \times 10^{-31}$ kg is the rest mass of the electron. For both electrons and holes, m^*/m_0 usually varies between 0.01 and 10. The smaller the size r_0 of the QD, the larger the bandgap energy $E_{g,\text{QD}}$ of the QD. When the size of the quantum dot approaches a very large value ($r_0 \to \infty$), the bandgap of the QD approaches that of the bulk semiconductor:

$$\text{When } r_0 \to \infty: \quad E_{g,\text{QD}} \to E_{g,\text{bulk}} \tag{4.11}$$

(C) Quantum Dot Fluorescence

Interband transitions occur when electrons and holes jump between the CB and the VB as shown in Figure 4-12. Interband transitions mainly take place between electrons and holes having the same quantum numbers n and l.[11] When a QD absorbs a photon of sufficiently high energy, a VB electron is excited into the CB, leaving behind a VB hole. For this excitation to happen, the photon must have more energy than the bandgap energy $E_{g,\text{QD}}$ of the QD:

$$E_{\text{photon}} = \frac{hc}{\lambda} \geq E_{g,\text{QD}} = E_{g,\text{bulk}} + \frac{h^2}{8r_0^2}\left(\frac{1}{m_e^*} + \frac{1}{m_h^*}\right) - \frac{1.8e^2}{4\pi\epsilon_r\epsilon_0 r_0}$$

$$\lambda \leq \frac{hc}{E_{g,\text{bulk}} + \dfrac{h^2}{8r_0^2}\left(\dfrac{1}{m_e^*} + \dfrac{1}{m_h^*}\right) - \dfrac{1.8e^2}{4\pi\epsilon_r\epsilon_0 r_0}} = \lambda_0 \tag{4.12}$$

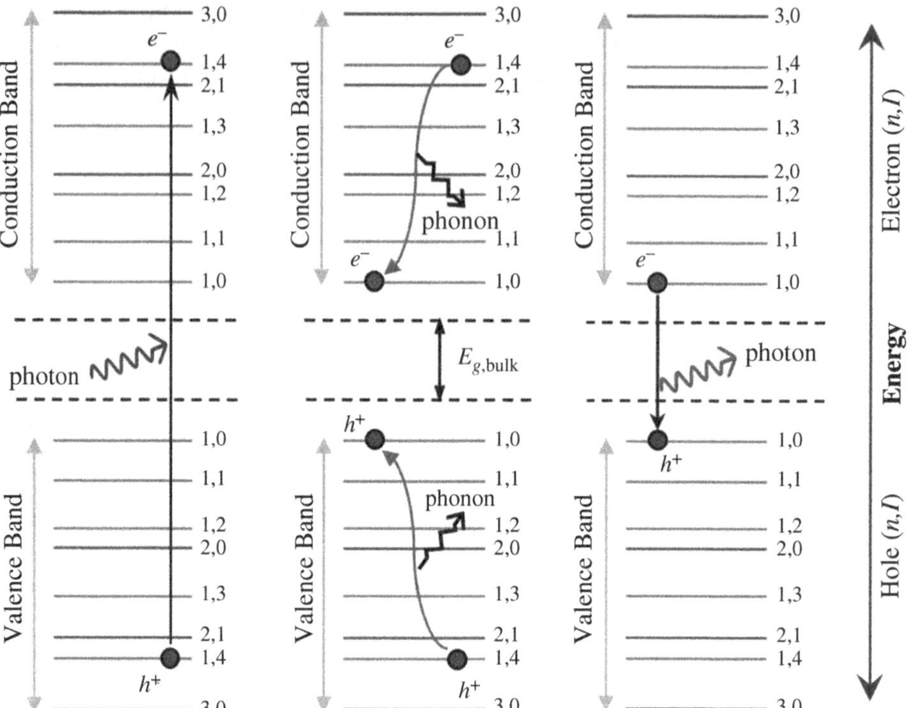

Figure 4-12   (Left) A high-energy photon excites a VB electron into the CB, producing a high-energy electron-hole pair. (Center) The high-energy electron-hole pair relaxes to the ground (1,0) state, emitting two phonons. (Right) The ground (1,0) state electron-hole pair recombine, emitting a lower energy photon with wavelength λ_0.

where λ and λ_0 refer to the photon (i.e., light) wavelength in vacuum. To obtain the photon wavelength in a medium with refractive index n, we can use $\lambda_n = \lambda/n$ and $\lambda_{0,n} = \lambda_0/n$. In such a medium, the speed of light is $v_n = c/n$. Note that the absorption and emission characteristics of QDs depend on photon energy E_{photon} or equivalently photon frequency γ, which are both *independent* of the medium the photon is traveling through. For QDs, the excitation and emission wavelengths are normally listed using the vacuum wavelength of light given by $\lambda = c/\gamma$, rather than the light wavelength in a medium such as a buffer solution.

Thus, QDs can absorb light of all wavelengths shorter than or equal to λ_0. If the absorbed photon has a very short wavelength (i.e., has high energy), an electron in the lower portion of the VB jumps to a high-energy level in the CB, leaving behind a high-energy electron-hole pair. Conversely, an excited CB electron can recombine with a hole in the VB, emitting a photon. In this case, the kinetic energies of both the electron and hole, plus the *bulk* bandgap energy $E_{g,\text{bulk}}$, and plus the *negative* electric potential energy $PE_{e/h}$, are transferred to the emitted photon. Due to energy conservation, the emitted photon will have at least as much energy as the QD bandgap energy $E_{g,\text{QD}}$. Therefore, the light emitted by a QD via fluorescence must have wavelengths which are shorter than or equal to λ_0.[11]

Excited CB electrons (and VB holes) in high-energy levels are highly unstable and will quickly relax to a low energy level at or close to the ground state ($n, l = 1,0$) within the *same* band, emitting phonons. Phonons are quasi-particles that are quantized crystal lattice vibrations. Phonons are thermal energy carriers, so the excess electron and hole energy in intraband transitions is eventually lost as heat. For intraband transitions, phonons rather than photons are emitted or absorbed to satisfy the conservation of both momentum and energy. Note that interband transitions are associated with the emission and absorption of photons.[12,13] Therefore, most interband transitions involving the recombination of electron-hole pairs occur between electrons and holes in low energy levels at or close to the ground $(n, l = 1,0)$ state. The transitions result in the emission of photons with wavelengths of λ_0 or slightly shorter than λ_0.[12] This emission produces the narrow emission spectra of QDs that are uniform in size. The entire process is depicted in Figure 4-12.

In summary, quantum dots can absorb all light of wavelengths $\lambda \leq \lambda_0$, but will only emit light of wavelengths of λ_0 or slightly shorter than λ_0. The value of λ_0 for a QD depends on the size (radius r_0) of the QD, as well as properties of the semiconductor material of which the QD is composed. Each semiconductor material will have a different bulk bandgap $E_{g,\text{bulk}}$, relative permittivity ϵ_r, and effective electron and hole masses m_e^*/m_0 and m_h^*/m_0. Light of shorter wavelengths is emitted by smaller QDs, as well as by QDs composed of semiconductors that exhibit higher bandgap, lower effective electron and hole masses, and/or higher permittivity (dielectric constant).

EXAMPLE 4-4 In a simplified one-dimensional model of an intrinsic semiconductor, the energy E_C of the bottom of the conduction band (relative to the bottom of the valence band) is

$$E_C = \frac{\hbar^2 k_1^2}{3m_0} \quad \text{where} \quad k_1 = \frac{\pi}{a}$$

where $a = 4.27$ Å is the crystal lattice spacing, m_0 is the electron rest mass, and the Fermi energy level is at 0.86 eV. Assuming that the Fermi level lies halfway between the valence and conduction bands, calculate the bandgap energy E_g.

Note: The Fermi level is an important concept in semiconductor physics. Due to the Pauli exclusion principle, every energy level can only accommodate a finite number of electrons. The Fermi level is the energy level having a 50% probability of being occupied by an electron. Energy levels below the Fermi level have greater than 50% chance of being occupied by an electron, while energy levels above the Fermi level have less than 50% chance of being occupied by an electron.

Solution We calculate the energy E_C of the bottom of the conduction band (relative to the bottom of the valence band) as follows:

$$E_C = \frac{\hbar^2 k_1^2}{3m_0} = \frac{(h/2\pi)^2 (\pi/a)^2}{3m_0} = \frac{h^2}{12m_0 a^2} = \frac{(6.626 \times 10^{-34} \text{ J}\cdot\text{s})^2}{12(9.11 \times 10^{-31} \text{ kg})(0.427 \text{ nm})^2} = 2.20 \times 10^{-19} \text{ J}$$

$$E_C = \frac{2.20 \times 10^{-19} \text{ J}}{1.6 \times 10^{-19} \text{ J/eV}} = 1.38 \text{ eV}$$

Hence, the bandgap energy is $E_g = 2(1.38 - 0.86) \text{ eV} = 1.04 \text{ eV}$ because the Fermi level is at the middle of the energy gap.

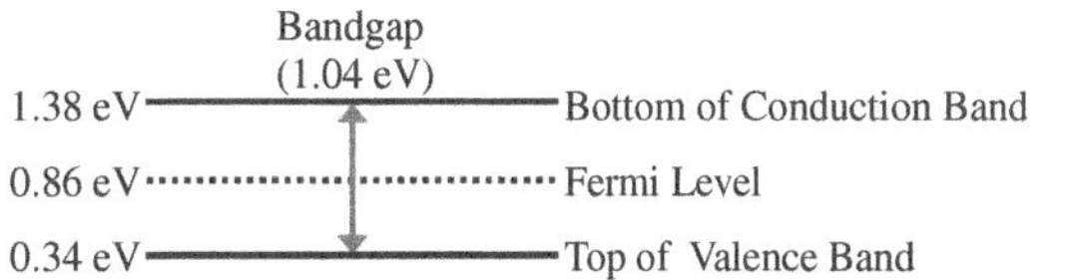

4.3.2 Structure of Quantum Dots

Fluorescent quantum dot (QD) probes typically have multilayered structures. The formation of such structures takes a number of steps. After synthesis of QD nanoparticles, hydrophobic QDs can be modified to become hydrophilic by coating with amphiphilic polymers (i.e., polymers with both hydrophobic and hydrophilic parts in the molecular structure). Fluorescent QD probes can be used in biological settings by conjugating (i.e., binding) polymer-coated QDs to biomolecules. Based on their structures, QDs can be classified as follows.[14]

(1) *Core QDs:* Core QDs have uniform (i.e., not layered) internal compositions. They can be composed of singular (e.g., Si or Ge), binary (e.g., CdSe, CdS, or InAs), or ternary (e.g., Cd_2SSe) semiconductor compounds. Typically, the optical properties of multilayered QDs are primarily determined by their cores. Core QDs cannot be used directly as biological probes because they have poor stability and low quantum yield as well as being hydrophobic.

(2) *Core-Shell QDs:* A core-shell QD is composed of a nanocrystal core surrounded by an inorganic crystalline shell. For instance, a CdSe core is commonly coated with either ZnS or CdS to obtain core-shell QDs. Currently, multi-shell (e.g., core/shell/shell) QDs such as CdSe/CdS/ZnS QDs are being studied to improve the optical properties of QDs. Unlike core QDs, core-shell QDs have high stability and high quantum yield. Since they are hydrophobic, core-shell QDs cannot be used directly as biological probes.

(3) *Water-Soluble QDs:* These QDs are made by polymer-coating core-shell QDs. These QDs are hydrophilic, so they are soluble in water and biological buffers. Water-soluble QDs can be used as biological probes.

(4) *QD Bioconjugates:* QD bioconjugates are made by conjugating (i.e., binding) water-soluble QDs to bioaffinity molecules (Figure 4-13). Bioaffinity molecules—such as antibodies, peptides, and proteins—are biomolecules that can easily bind to QDs. The binding can be accomplished through coupling, cross-linking, or other methods. By attaching bioconjugate molecules, the cellular- and tissue-targeting specificity of QDs can be significantly improved. For instance, QD bioconjugates can be designed to be delivered into cancerous cells to allow for optical identification and imaging of tumors.

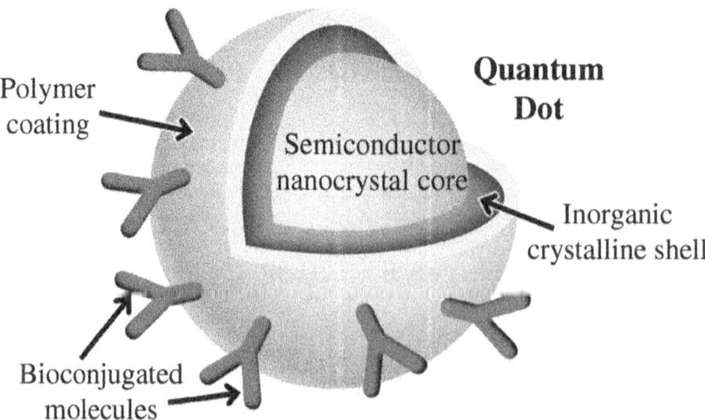

Figure 4-13   The structure of a quantum dot (QD) bioconjugate designed for biomedical applications. The antibodies conjugated to the surface of this water-soluble QD allows for QD uptake into specific cells and tissues.

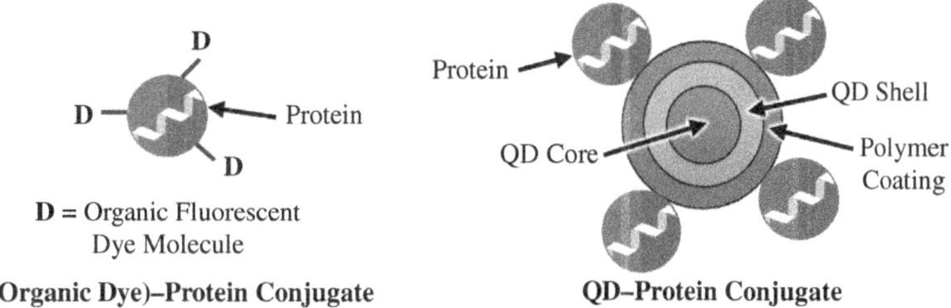

Figure 4-14   An (organic fluorescent dye)–protein conjugate (left) and a QD-protein conjugate (right).

Figure 4-14 shows a comparison of a QD-protein conjugate with an (organic fluorescent dye)–protein conjugate. The QD shown (~10 to 20 nm in diameter) is coated with an amphiphilic polymer and is an order of magnitude larger than the organic fluorescent dye molecules (~1 nm in size). Owing to its large size, each QD can conjugate to multiple biomolecules such as proteins and small bioaffinity molecules. On the other hand, due to its small size and dim light emission, each organic fluorescent dye molecule can only conjugate to a single small biomolecule, and a large biomolecule such as a protein needs to be conjugated with several organic dye molecules to be effectively labeled.[14]

4.3.3 Properties of Quantum Dots

The properties of QDs are dependent on many factors including QD particle size, shape, crystallinity, and the presence of defects and impurities. Improving QD synthesis methods can produce QDs with uniform sizes and shapes so that the QDs will have narrow emission spectra.

(A) Optical Absorption and Emission Characteristics

QDs and conventional organic fluorescent dyes absorb light differently. For organic fluorescent dyes, their absorption bands are shorter than those of QDs but closer to the emission bands. Therefore, the Stokes shift (i.e., wavelength difference between maximum absorbance and maximum emission) for organic fluorophores is significantly less than that of QDs. This characteristic is advantageous for the selective excitation of a fluorophore, but it is disadvantageous for the excitation of multiple fluorophores where each fluorescent dye has to be excited with a separate light source. Due to the small Stokes shift, the presence of light scattering and autofluorescence can make it difficult to collect the emitted light efficiently and thus precise optical filters or other instrumentation are needed. In contrast, QDs can absorb light of all wavelengths which are shorter than those of the emitted light.[6] As an example, Figure 4-15 compares the normalized absorption and emission spectra for commercial (organic dye)–protein and QD-protein conjugates.

There are a number of advantages of QD photoabsorption. First, the effective Stokes shift for QDs can be as large as 100 to 400 nm, which is substantially larger than that of organic dyes (~15 to 30 nm). The dramatically larger Stokes shift helps improve the detection sensitivity of QD probes as the signal is easier to distinguish from the autofluorescence background. Second, QDs have much higher extinction coefficients (~0.5 to 5×10^6 M^{-1} cm^{-1}) than fluorescent dyes (~5 to 10×10^4 M^{-1} cm^{-1}). Therefore, QDs can absorb light much more efficiently than fluorescent dyes. Finally, since multiple colors of QDs can be effectively excited by a single light source using short-wavelength light far from the emission of any color, multicolor QD probes can be visualized simultaneously (multiplexing).[15]

The emission spectrum of QDs is formed by the summation of the emissions from many individual QD nanocrystals whose sizes are slightly different. The width of the emission

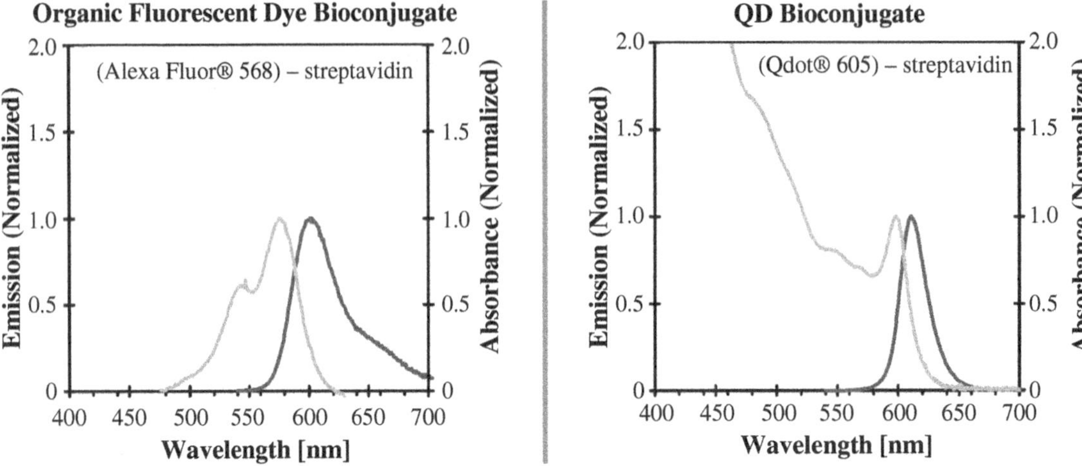

Figure 4-15   Comparison of normalized absorption and emission spectra. (Left) Organic fluorescent dye (Alexa Fluor® 568)–protein (streptavidin) bioconjugate; (right) QD (Qdot® 605)–protein (streptavidin) bioconjugate. (*The figures are reprinted with permission from C. Z. Hotz.*[16])

spectrum is therefore determined by the uniformity of the size distribution of QDs. QDs with a uniform size distribution will have a narrow emission spectrum. Usually, the size distribution of QDs follows a normal (i.e., Gaussian) distribution. Commercial batches of QDs typically have narrow emission spectra with FWHM (full width at half maximum) of 20 to 35 nm, which is significantly narrower than that of organic dyes. Figure 4-16 shows a comparison of the unnormalized emission and absorption spectra for commercial organic fluorophore-protein conjugates compared with QD-protein conjugates.

Aside from controlling the uniformity of QD size, the emission wavelengths of QD probes can be easily tuned by changing the size and/or chemical composition of the QDs. Consequently, many different fluorescent probes can be prepared from the same QD material.

Compared with conventional organic dyes, QDs have significantly higher emission intensities as well as higher quantum yields. Recall that fluorescent quantum yield is the

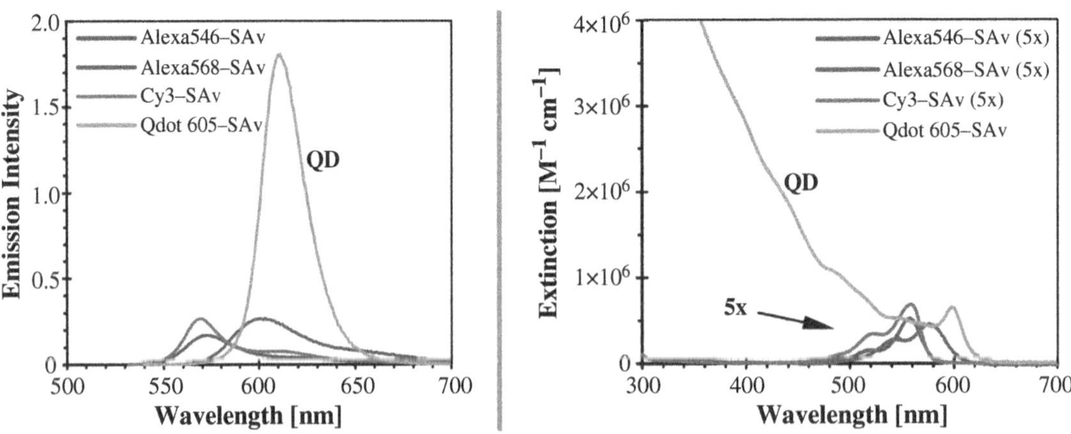

Figure 4-16   Comparison of (left) unnormalized emission and (right) absorption (i.e., ε_{BL}) spectra of streptavidin (SAv) protein conjugated with Alexa Fluor® 546 (organic dye), Alexa Fluor® 568 (organic dye), Cy3® (organic dye), and Qdot® 605 (quantum dot). For clarity, the absorption spectra of the three organic fluorescent dyes have been increased fivefold (5×). (*The figures are reprinted with permission from C. Z. Hotz.*[16])

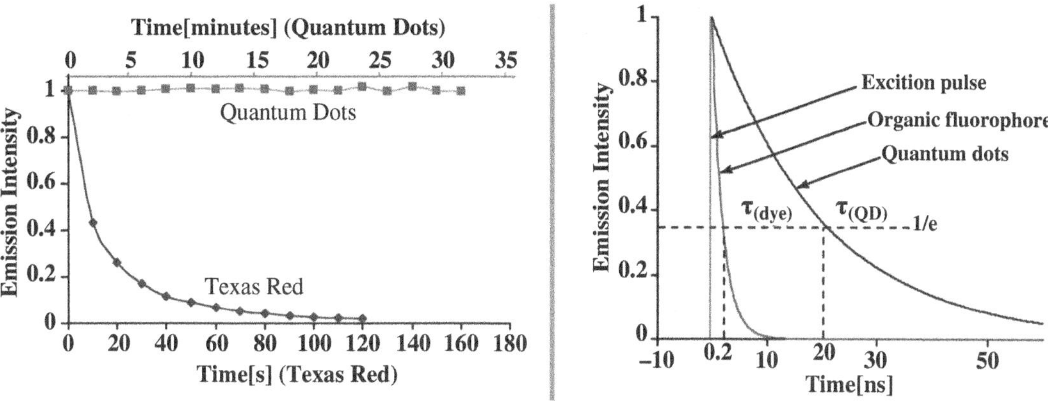

Figure 4-17   (Left) Comparison of the photostability of QDs and Texas Red (an organic fluorescent dye) under the same optical excitation conditions. (Right) Comparison of the emission intensity decay curves and fluorescence lifetimes of QDs and organic fluorescent dyes. (*The figures are reprinted with permission from X. H. Gao et al.*[15])

ratio of photons emitted to photons absorbed by a fluorescent material, and that the brightness of a fluorophore is positively correlated with both the extinction coefficient and the quantum yield. Since QDs have a higher extinction coefficient and higher quantum yield than organic dyes, they are typically 10 to 20 times brighter than organic dyes. Moreover, (organic dye)-biomolecule conjugates usually have a significantly lower quantum yield than the organic dyes by themselves (i.e., unconjugated organic dyes). In contrast, QDs retain their quantum yield after conjugating to bioaffinity molecules.[6]

(B) Photostability and Fluorescence Lifetime
Conventional organic fluorescent dyes gradually degrade when excited by light and emit less light progressively over time. Unlike organic dye molecules, QDs have exceptional photostability against photobleaching even under intense illumination. This property makes QDs well-suited for continuous observation of the target probe over long periods of time, such as cell/tissue tracking studies and some imaging applications. A comparison of photostability under the same optical excitation conditions is given in Figure 4-17 (left), which shows that QDs are several orders of magnitude more photostable than organic fluorescent dyes.[16]

Fluorescence lifetime is the time that a fluorophore remains in the excited state before emitting a photon and relaxing to the ground state. More precisely, the fluorescence lifetime is the time between excitation of the fluorophore (by an infinitesimally-brief light pulse) and the time when the fluorophore emission intensity has decayed to $1/e$ (roughly 37%) of the original value. QDs have significantly longer fluorescence lifetimes (20 to 50 ns) than typical organic fluorophores (less than 5 ns). That means the excited states of QDs decay much more slowly than those of organic dyes. The time delay between excitation and collection of the emitted light allows the fluorescence signal to be more easily distinguished from background autofluorescence via time-domain imaging, effectively mitigating sources of background fluorescence (e.g., polymeric substrates, blood) during the collection of QD-emitted light.[6] Figure 4-17 (right) illustrates the emission intensity decay curves and fluorescence lifetimes of QDs compared with organic dyes.

4.3.4 Applications and Challenges of Quantum Dots

While QD fluorophores offer many advantages over organic fluorescent dyes, there are a few challenges that need to be considered in any application of QDs. Table 4-3 lists the

TABLE 4-3   The Advantages and Challenges of Quantum Dots

Advantages of Quantum Dots	Challenges of Quantum Dots	
☑ Exceptional photostability	Toxicity and bioaccumulation issues	☒
☑ Superb brightness mainly due to very high molar absorption coefficient	Large size limiting uptake	☒
☑ Relatively long fluorescence lifetime	Intermittent fluorescence	☒
☑ Tunable emission wavelength and narrow emission spectra	Expensive to purchase	☒
☑ Large effective Stokes shift	Complicated fabrication process	☒

advantages of QDs compared with organic dyes (as described in Section 4.3.3) together with the main challenges of QDs.

The first issue is the toxicity and non-biodegradability of many QDs. QDs without a stable polymer coating can be toxic, especially if the QDs contain heavy metals such as cadmium (Cd) and/or poisonous metalloids such as arsenic (As). Polymer-coated QDs are in general nontoxic to cells and animals. However, owing to the high chemical stability of polymer-coated QDs, these QDs tend to be non-biodegradable and may bioaccumulate within cells and tissues. A second issue is the large size of water-soluble QDs (as is evident in Figure 4-14) relative to organic fluorescent dyes and proteins. The relatively large size of QDs limits their uptake within cells, tissues, and organs. For instance, it is extremely difficult to get QDs to cross the blood-brain barrier for imaging the brain. Another potential difficulty is that QDs can exhibit intermittent fluorescence (sometimes called "blinking") under continuous excitation, which can render time-averaged intensity measurements non-reproducible. Intermittent fluorescence is caused by quantum effects such as charge trapping which are beyond the scope of this book.[17,18]

Since QD bioconjugates suitable for biomedical applications have complex structures and surface chemistry, their fabrication process is both complicated and expensive compared with organic fluorescent dyes. Thus, QD probes are far more expensive to purchase than organic fluorescent probes.

The applications of QDs in cell and tissue staining, as well as *ex vivo* and *in vivo* targeting and imaging have received considerable interest. The advancement of QD bioconjugation research opens up prospects for future clinical applications. We present a few examples of their biomedical applications here.

Figure 4-18 shows fluorescent images of QD-stained cells and tissues, as well as mouse *in vivo* targeting and imaging with QDs. Due to their super high brightness and photostability, QDs can image detailed cellular structures, as well as molecular and cellular movements in real time for an extended period. Since multicolor QD probes can be visualized simultaneously with a single light source, QDs are used to assist the *in vivo* targeting and imaging of blood vessels, lymph nodes, cancer cells, and tumors.[15]

EXAMPLE 4-5   A spherical quantum dot (QD) with a radius of 3 nm emits yellow light with a (vacuum or air) wavelength of $\lambda_0 = 600$ nm. The effective electron mass m_e^*/m_0 and effective hole mass m_h^*/m_0 are both 0.2. The QD is composed of an intrinsic semiconductor with a relative permittivity of

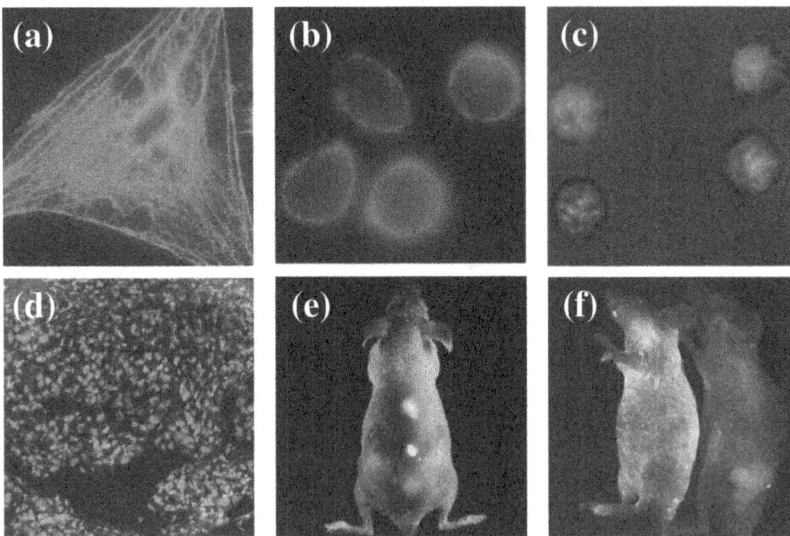

Figure 4-18 Fluorescent micrographs of QD-stained cells and tissues, and *in vivo* targeting and imaging with QDs. (a) 3T3 fibroblast cells labeled with QD-actin conjugates; (b) live breast tumor cells labeled with QD-antibody conjugates; (c) live mammalian cells labeled with intracellular QD-(TAT peptide) conjugates; (d) frozen tissue specimens labeled with QDs and a nuclear dye; (e) *in vivo* and simultaneous imaging of multicolor QD-encoded microbeads in a live mouse; (f) *in vivo* imaging and molecular targeting of mouse prostate tumor using QD-antibody conjugates. (*All images are reprinted with permission from X. H. Gao et al.*[16,19])

$\epsilon_r = 11.7$. Use the Brus equation and the following simplified one-dimensional model for an intrinsic semiconductor:

$$E_{C,\text{bulk}} = \frac{\hbar^2 k_1^2}{3m_0} \quad \text{with} \quad k_1 = \frac{\pi}{a}$$

where $E_{C,\text{bulk}}$ is the energy at the bottom of the conduction band of the bulk semiconductor. Find the Fermi level $E_{F,\text{bulk}}$ and the energy at the top of the valence band $E_{V,\text{bulk}}$ of the *bulk* semiconductor. Assume that the crystal lattice spacing is $a = 3$ Å and that the Fermi level lies halfway between the valence and conduction bands. Please refer to Example 4-4 for a description of the Fermi level.

Solution   Noting that 1 eV $= 1.60 \times 10^{-19}$ J, the energy E_{photon} of each photon emitted by the QD is

$$E_{\text{photon}} = \frac{hc}{\lambda} = \frac{\left(6.626 \times 10^{-34} \ \text{J} \cdot \text{s}\right)\left(3 \times 10^8 \ \text{m/s}\right)}{600 \ \text{nm}} = 2.07 \ \text{eV}$$

The emitted photon energy E_{photon} is approximately equal to the QD bandgap energy $E_{g,\text{QD}}$:

$$E_{\text{photon}} \cong E_{g,\text{QD}} = E_{g,\text{bulk}} + \text{KE}_{e,\text{min}} + \text{KE}_{h,\text{min}} + \text{PE}_{e/h}$$

$$\text{KE}_{e,\text{min}} = \text{KE}_{h,\text{min}} = \frac{h^2}{8m^* r_0^2} = \frac{h^2}{8\left(0.2m_0\right)r_0^2} = \frac{\left(6.626 \times 10^{-34} \ \text{J} \cdot \text{s}\right)^2}{8(0.2)\left(9.11 \times 10^{-31} \ \text{kg}\right)(3 \ \text{nm})^2} = 0.209 \ \text{eV}$$

$$\text{PE}_{e/h} = -\frac{1.8e^2}{4\pi\epsilon_r\epsilon_0 r_0} = -\frac{1.8\left(1.6 \times 10^{-19} \ \text{C}\right)^2}{4\pi(11.7)\left(8.854 \times 10^{-12} \ \text{F/m}\right)(3 \ \text{nm})} = -0.074 \ \text{eV}$$

$$E_{g,\text{bulk}} \cong E_{\text{photon}} - \text{KE}_{e,\min} - \text{KE}_{h,\min} - \text{PE}_{e/h}$$

$$E_{g,\text{bulk}} \cong 2.07 \text{ eV} - 0.209 \text{ eV} - 0.209 \text{ eV} + 0.074 \text{ eV} = 1.73 \text{ eV}$$

Hence, the CB, VB, and Fermi level energies of the bulk semiconductor are

$$E_{C,\text{bulk}} = \frac{\hbar^2 k_1^2}{3m_0} = \frac{\left(\frac{h}{2\pi}\right)^2 \left(\frac{\pi}{a}\right)^2}{3m_0} = \frac{h^2}{12 m_0 a^2} = \frac{\left(6.626 \times 10^{-34} \text{ J}\cdot\text{s}\right)^2}{12\left(9.11 \times 10^{-31} \text{ kg}\right)\left(3 \times 10^{-10} \text{ m}\right)^2} = 2.79 \text{ eV}$$

$$E_{V,\text{bulk}} = E_{C,\text{bulk}} - E_{g,\text{bulk}} = 2.79 \text{ eV} - 1.73 \text{ eV} = 1.06 \text{ eV}$$

$$E_{F,\text{bulk}} = E_{C,\text{bulk}} - \left(E_{g,\text{bulk}}\right)/2 = 2.79 \text{ eV} - (1.73 \text{ eV})/2 = 1.93 \text{ eV} \quad \blacktriangle$$

4.4 PROBLEMS

4-1 (Short-Answer). **(a)** State the main applications and limitations of the Beer-Lambert law.

(b) Compare the size of a quantum dot (QD) emitting red light with the size of a QD emitting blue light both within the same medium. Assume that both QDs have the same shape and are composed of the same semiconductor material. Which QD should be larger?

4-2. The concentration of bacterial DNA with a molar mass of 4.6×10^5 g/mol in an aqueous solution is 15 µg/mL. The absorbance $A_\lambda = -\log_{10}(I/I_0)$ was 0.310 when the solution was placed in a 1 cm square cuvette and 260 nm (in air) UV light was passed through it.

(a) Calculate the molar absorption coefficient ε_{BL} of the bacterial DNA.

(b) What will be the new absorbance A_λ if the concentration is reduced to 10 µg/mL?

4-3. We have a solution containing a fluorophore-labeled DNA sample (concentration of a picomolar), which can tolerate a maximum absorbed optical power of 7 mW without denaturing. The DNA sample has a molar absorption coefficient of 3.9×10^5 cm^{-1} M^{-1}, and is loaded in a microchannel with a square cross-section of 100 µm $\times$ 100 µm. An excitation laser with wavelength of 600 nm (in vacuum or in air) is used to illuminate the channel. A continuous stream of 5.4×10^{24} photons were emitted by the laser over a 2-second period. Will the DNA sample denature if the laser is 100% efficient in illuminating the microchannel?.

4-4. The detection of biomolecules (such as proteins and DNA) is frequently achieved by labeling them with fluorescent probes. Figure 4-5 shows a confocal laser–induced fluorescence (LIF) system. Assume that a 15 mW laser uniformly illuminates a 200 µm (length) $\times$ 100 µm (width) $\times$ 100 µm (depth) section of a long microchannel that is 100 µm $\times$ 100 µm (square) in cross-section. After separation, the sample contains a 2×10^{-12} M concentration of identical molecules that are each labeled with the fluorophore Alexa Fluor® 488. Characteristics of the fluorescent dye are shown in Table 4-1.

(a) Assuming that you can get a laser with any desired wavelength, what wavelength should it be?

(b) Assuming that the laser is perfectly efficient in illuminating the microchannel section (no light misses the microchannel), what is the intensity Φ_{incident} (photons per second) of light hitting the channel? How many photons Φ_{absorbed} are absorbed each second by the fluorophore?

(c) How many photons per second of fluorescence $\Phi_{\text{objective}}$ are collected by the objective? Assume that the circular objective acquires all light falling on it, and that it has a diameter of 1 mm and is located 3 mm away from the microchannel.

(d) The fraction of incident photons f_Φ that are reflected or scattered back into the collection optics is

$$f_\Phi = 1 - \exp\left[-\left(\frac{100 \text{ nm}}{\lambda}\right)^4\right]$$

where λ is the (vacuum or air) wavelength of the incident photons. Assume that 10^{-9} of these photons manage to pass the optical filter and reach the detector. What is the rate of photons per second Φ_{baseline} from this excitation light? This is your baseline (i.e., noise floor).

(e) Assume that 40% of all the fluorescence photons collected by the objective manage to pass through the optical filter and reach the detector. What is the rate of photons per second Φ_{signal} from this fluorescence? This is your signal. Calculate the signal-to-noise ratio (SNR) of this setup. Is this setup acceptable for optical detection?

4-5. You are tasked with studying a prototype quantum dot (QD)-based fluorescent probe. To do this, you decide to shine laser light with a wavelength of $\lambda_{excitation} = 480$ nm at the QD probe and observe that the spherical QDs re-emit light with a wavelength of $\lambda_{emission} = 538$ nm. Electrons and holes within the crystal lattice of the QD have effective masses of $m_e^* = m_h^* = 0.24\, m_0$ and particle wave numbers of $k = 1.31 \times 10^9$ m^{-1}. The QD probes are comprised of a semiconductor material having a relative permittivity of $\epsilon_r = 12.4$. Assume that all given wavelengths are in vacuum or in air.

(a) Calculate the energy lost E_{lost} between the incident photon and the emitted photon. What causes this energy loss?

(b) Assume that $E_{photon}(\lambda_{emission}) = E_{g,QD}$. Is this assumption reasonable? Find the radius r_0 of the spherical QDs and the bandgap energy $E_{g,bulk}$ of the bulk semiconductor comprising the QDs.

4-6. Consider light with incident intensity I_0 and wavelength λ hitting a slab with thickness L. Assume that the slab is composed of a liquid solution with many light-absorbing species. Recall Equation (4.4B) for the absorbance A_λ given by

$$A_\lambda = L \sum_i C_i \cdot \varepsilon_{BL,i}(\lambda)$$

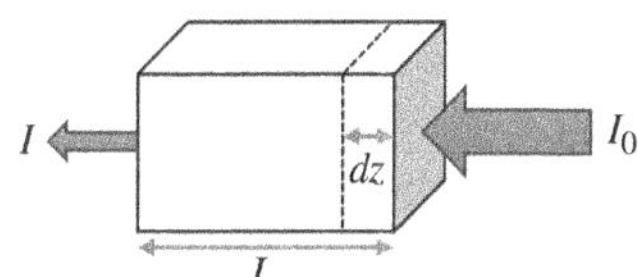

(a) Derive the Beer-Lambert law $I(z) = I_0 \exp[-\mu(\lambda)\, z]$, where z is the optical depth and $\mu(\lambda)$ is a wavelength-dependent proportionality constant.

(b) Express $\mu(\lambda)$ in terms of the molar absorption coefficient $\varepsilon_{BL,i}(\lambda)$ and the molar concentration C_i of each light-absorbing species.

4-7. We have spherical quantum dots (QDs) comprised of ZnO (a semiconductor material). The radii of the QDs follow a Gaussian distribution centered about 5.6 nm. Due to the O^{2-}/O^- surface defect, there is a trap energy level between the valence band (VB) and conduction band (CB) that can trap electrons and holes. An electron from the CB can recombine with a hole in the trap energy level, emitting a photon. Likewise, an electron in the trap energy level can recombine with a hole in the VB, also emitting a photon. Therefore, ZnO QDs with the surface defect exhibit three emission peaks. For ZnO, the relative permittivity is $\epsilon_r = 9.4$, the bandgap is $E_{g,bulk} = 3.4$ eV, the effective electron mass is $m_e^*/m_0 = 0.24$, and the effective hole mass is $m_h^*/m_0 = 0.45$. Assume that all given wavelengths are in vacuum or in air.

(a) Estimate the emission wavelength $\lambda_{primary}$ corresponding to the primary emission peak, which corresponds to photons emitted from electrons in the CB recombining with holes in the VB.

(b) The secondary emission peak corresponds to photons emitted from electrons in the CB recombining with holes in the trap energy level. The wavelength of the secondary emission peak is $\lambda_{secondary} = 520$ nm. Calculate the energy of the trap energy level relative to the CB and VB of the QDs.

(c) Estimate the emission wavelength $\lambda_{tertiary}$ of the tertiary emission peak, which corresponds to photons emitted from electrons in the trap energy level recombining with holes in the VB.

(d) Sketch the (relative) emission intensity of the QDs as a function of wavelength λ. A qualitative sketch is sufficient.

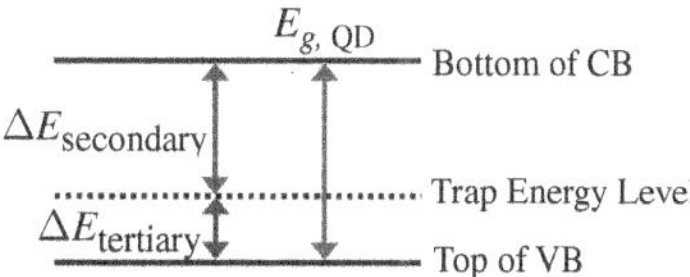

4-8. You are asked to design an experiment for a molecular detection application. You have a square 4 mm × 4 mm cuvette, and access to two dyes and two lasers with the following properties:

Fluorophore	Excitation* [nm]	Emission* [nm]	QY	ε_{BL} [cm^{-1} M^{-1}]
X (Organic-based)	650 to 675	700	0.50	1.5×10^5
Y (Quantum Dot–based)	N/A	700	0.85	8.0×10^6

Laser	Power [mW]	Emission Wavelength* [nm]
A	25	660
B	180	450

*Wavelength λ of light in vacuum (or in air).

Assume that the laser is perfectly efficient in illuminating the sample in the cuvette, and that 1% of the emitted fluorescence photons are collected by the detector (this is your signal). The proportion of photons that are backscattered into the collection optics and manage to reach the detector is given by (this is your noise or baseline)

$$\frac{I_{scatter}}{I_0} = \frac{160 \text{ nm}^4}{\lambda^4}$$

where λ is the (vacuum or air) photon wavelength, I_0 is the incident intensity, and $I_{scatter}$ is the backscatter intensity. The factor of $1/\lambda^4$ comes from Rayleigh scattering.

(a) Derive expressions for the number of detected signal photons per second Φ_{signal} and the number of detected noise photons per second Φ_{noise}. What is the signal-to-noise ratio (SNR)?

(b) With a fluorophore concentration of one picomolar ($C = 1$ pM), select a single fluorophore and a single laser that would be best suited for a molecular detection experiment. That is, what choice of fluorophore and laser would maximize the signal-to-noise ratio?

(c) If you want to achieve a signal-to-noise ratio of at least 100 using the fluorophore and laser combination from part (b), what is the minimum required fluorophore molar concentration C?

4-9. We require spherical QDs that emit monochromatic fluorescent photons with (vacuum or air) wavelengths of λ_0. Assume that the energy of each emitted photon is equal to the QD bandgap energy: $E_{photon}(\lambda_0) = E_{g,QD}$. In reality, $E_{photon}(\lambda_0)$ will be equal to or slightly larger than $E_{g,QD}$.

(a) Find an expression for r_0 in terms of the photon emission wavelength λ_0. Namely, find $r_0(\lambda_0)$.

(b) For silicon, the bandgap is $E_{g,bulk} = 1.12$ eV, the effective electron mass is $m_e^*/m_0 = 0.20$, the effective hole mass is $m_h^*/m_0 = 0.29$, and the relative permittivity is $\epsilon_r = 11.7$. Evaluate $r_0(\lambda_0)$ and the inverse function $\lambda_0(r_0)$ for spherical silicon QDs.

(c) Is it possible to obtain a photon emission wavelength of 1200 nm using spherical silicon QDs? Why or why not? Using computer software, generate a plot of $\lambda_0(r_0)$ vs. r_0 from $r_0 = 1$ nm to $r_0 = 11$ nm.

4-10 (Challenging). We are interested in the full width at half maximum (FWHM) of the emission spectra (i.e., emission intensity vs. wavelength) for QDs. Realistically, a batch of QDs will have a distribution of sizes and will emit fluorescence photons with a distribution of wavelengths. For CdSe, the relative permittivity is $\epsilon_r = 10.6$, the bandgap is $E_{g,bulk} = 1.84$ eV, the effective electron mass is $m_e^*/m_0 = 0.13$, and the effective hole mass is $m_h^*/m_0 = 0.30$. Assume that the energy of each emitted photon is equal to the QD bandgap energy: $E_{photon}(\lambda) = E_{g,QD}$. In reality, $E_{photon}(\lambda)$ will be equal to or slightly larger than $E_{g,QD}$. Assume that all given wavelengths are in vacuum or in air.

(a) We have CdSe QDs with a distribution of radii centered about r_0. What radius r_0 will produce an emission wavelength distribution with a peak of $\lambda_0 = 550$ nm?

(b) The radii r of the spherical CdSe QDs follow a Gaussian distribution $f(r)$ with mean r_0 and standard deviation σ_r as given below. Derive the expression given below for the FWHM of this distribution.

$$f(r) = \frac{1}{\sigma_r \sqrt{2\pi}} \exp\left(-\frac{(r - r_0)^2}{2\sigma_r^2}\right) \quad \Rightarrow \quad \text{FWHM}_r = 2\sqrt{2\ln(2)}\,\sigma_r$$

(c) The (relative) intensity distribution $I_{\text{emission}}(\lambda)$ versus emitted fluorescent photon wavelength λ for a batch of CdSe QDs is given below. We want the peak of $I_{\text{emission}}(\lambda)$ to be narrow enough such that its FWHM is 20 nm or smaller. What condition must σ_r satisfy to achieve $\text{FWHM}_\lambda \leq 20$ nm?

$$I_{\text{emission}}(\lambda) = \frac{\sigma_r \sqrt{2\pi}}{\lambda_0} f(r)\lambda(r)$$

Hint: Assume that $I_{\text{emission}}(\lambda)$ is approximately symmetric about λ_0, and use the result from part (b).

(d) Using software, generate a plot of (relative) emission intensity $I_{\text{emission}}(\lambda)$ versus wavelength λ for spherical CdSe QDs. Is $I_{\text{relative}}(\lambda)$ symmetric about λ_0 as we assumed?

4-11 (Challenging). A fluorescent dye conjugate is used in an experiment to test its photostability. The fluorescent dye has an excitation wavelength of 500 nm and an emission wavelength of 530 nm. The conjugate is continuously exposed to a 500 nm laser, and the fluorescence intensity over time is measured by a square 2.5 mm $\times$ 2.5 mm photodetector which captures 0.7% of the fluorescence photons. Assume that noise due to reflected and backscattered incident photons is negligible, and that all given photon wavelengths are in vacuum or in air. The measured fluorescence intensity $I_{\text{measured}}(t)$ as a function of time t is given by the following sigmoid function:

$$I_{\text{measured}}(t) = \frac{P_{\text{measured}}(t)}{A} = \frac{D}{1 + \exp[B(t-C)]} \ [\text{W/m}^2] \qquad (t \geq 0)$$

where $P_{\text{measured}}(t)$ is the optical power measured by the photodetector over the detector area of A, and the three constants are $D = 65$ W/m^2, $B = 0.002$ s^{-1}, and $C = 1300$ s.

(a) The fluorescent dye conjugate is considered effectively degraded when the fluorescence intensity drops below 5% of its initial intensity at $t = 0$. How long does the dye conjugate last until it is effectively degraded at $t = T_f$?

(b) Assume that the fluorescent dye conjugate initially (at $t = 0$) has a quantum yield of 0.58 and that the optical power output of the 500 nm laser P_{laser} is constant. Calculate P_{laser} assuming that the laser is perfectly efficient in illuminating the dye conjugate. Derive an expression for the quantum yield of the dye conjugate as a function of time.

(c) Calculate the total fluorescence energy emitted by the dye conjugate (whatever amount is exposed to the laser) throughout its entire useful lifespan from $t = 0$ to $t = T_f$.

4-12 (Challenging). A biosample in a microchannel is labeled with quantum dots (QDs) with emission wavelengths of 650 nm for molecular detection. The QD has a fluorescence lifetime of $\tau = 20$ ns, quantum yield of QY $= 0.95$, and molar absorption coefficient of $\varepsilon_{BL} = 6.2 \times 10^5$ cm^{-1}M^{-1}. The molar concentration of the QDs in the channel is $C = 5 \times 10^{-9}$ M. The channel has a square cross-section with edge length of 200 μm. The QDs in the channel are excited by a 510 nm InGaN laser pulse, and the optical power output of the laser pulse $P_{\text{laser}}(t)$ can be described by the following equation:

$$P_{\text{laser}}(t) = \begin{cases} 300(-t^2 + 2t) \ [\text{mW}] & (0 \leq t \ [\text{ns}] \leq 2) \\ 0 & (t \ [\text{ns}] \geq 2) \end{cases}$$

where t represents time in nanoseconds. Assume that the laser is perfectly efficient in illuminating the channel, and that all given wavelengths are in vacuum or in air.

(a) Derive an expression for the number of photons absorbed by the QDs per nanosecond $\Phi_{\text{absorbed}}(t)$. Use this result to calculate the total number of photons N_{absorbed} absorbed by the QDs from the laser.

(b) Suppose that we excite the QDs with a single infinitesimally short laser pulse at time $t = 0$. Derive an expression for the number of photons per second $\Phi_{\text{emis(impulse)}}(t)$ emitted by the QDs in response to this impulse. Letting N_{absorbed} be the total number of photons absorbed by the QDs, we can obtain the impulse response $h_{\text{emission}}(t)$ of the QD emissions as follows:

$$h_{\text{emission}}(t) = \frac{\Phi_{\text{emis(impulse)}}(t)}{N_{\text{absorbed}}}$$

Hint: Consider the total number of photons N_{emitted} emitted by the QDs from time $t = 0$ to $t = \infty$.

(c) For optical detection, our signal is the number of fluorescent photons emitted per unit time $\Phi_{\text{emission}}(t)$ by the QDs. Derive an expression for $\Phi_{\text{emission}}(t)$ and use computer software to plot $\Phi_{\text{emission}}(t)$ versus time t.

Note: The light emission of the QDs in response to the input laser light is given by the convolution of $h_{\text{emission}}(t)$ and $\Phi_{\text{absorbed}}(t)$ as follows:

$$\Phi_{\text{emission}}(t) = h_{\text{emission}}(t) * \Phi_{\text{absorbed}}(t) = \int_{v=0}^{v=t} h_{\text{emission}}(t-v)\Phi_{\text{absorbed}}(v)\, dv$$

Do not evaluate this convolution by hand. Instead, use computer software to numerically evaluate $\Phi_{\text{emission}}(t)$ to generate the plot.

4.5 REFERENCES

[1]   S. Bellini. "Pulox Pulse Oximeter," Wikimedia Commons [Online]. Available: https://commons.wikimedia.org/wiki/File:Pulox_Pulse_Oximeter.JPG#filelinks, 2014.

[2]   S. Prahl. "Optical Absorption of Hemoglobin", Oregon Medical Laser Center [Online]. Available: https://omlc.org/spectra/hemoglobin/, 1999.

[3]   "Alexa Fluor Dyes—Across the Spectrum," ThermoFisher Scientific [Online]. Available: https://www.thermofisher.com/ca/en/home/brands/molecular-probes/key-molecular-probes-products/alexa-fluor/alexa-fluor-dyes-across-the-spectrum.html, 2021.

[4]   "What are Quantum Dots?", U.S. National Institute of Biomedical Imaging and Bioengineering [Online]. Available: https://www.nibib.nih.gov/news-events/multimedia/video-gallery, 2015.

[5]   J. Drbohlavova, V. Adam, R. Kizek, and J. Hubalek, "Quantum Dots: Characterization, preparation and usage in biological systems," *International Journal of Molecular Sciences*, vol. 10, no. 2, pp. 656-673, 2009.

[6]   C. Z. Hotz, "Applications of Quantum Dots in Biology: An Overview," in *Nanobiotechnology Protocols*. vol. 303, S. J. Rosenthal and D. W. Wright, Eds., 2nd ed. Totowa, NJ, USA: Humana Press, 2005, pp. 1-17.

[7]   M. Ventra, S. Evoy, and J. R. Heflin, Eds., *Introduction to Nanoscale Science and Technology*, 1st ed. Boston, MA, USA: Springer Science & Business Media, 2004.

[8]   J. R. Zurita-Sánchez and L. Novotny, "Multipolar interband absorption in a semiconductor quantum dot. I. Electric quadrupole enhancement," *Journal of the Optical Society of America B*, vol. 19, no. 6, pp. 1355-1362, 2002.

[9]   E. O. Chukwuocha, M. C. Onyeaju, and T. S. T. Harry, "Theoretical studies on the effect of confinement on quantum dots using the Brus equation," *World Journal of Condensed Matter Physics*, vol. 2, no. 2, pp. 96-100, 2012.

[10] L. E. Brus, "Electron-electron and electron-hole interactions in small semiconductor crystallites: The size dependence of the lowest excited electronic state.," *The Journal of Chemical Physics*, vol. 80, no. 9, pp. 4403-4409, 1984.

[11] R. J. D. Tilley, *Colour and the Optical Properties of Materials*, 2nd ed. Chichester, UK: John Wiley & Sons, Ltd., 2011.

[12] A. Assadihaghi, H. Teimoori, and T. J. Hall, "SOA-Based Optical Switches," in *Optical Switches: Materials and Design*, B. Li and S. J. Chua, Eds., 1st ed. Cambridge, UK: Woodhead Publishing Ltd., 2010, pp. 158-180.

[13] "ECE 5330 Semiconductor Optoelectronics," Cornell University [Online]. Available: https://courses.cit.cornell.edu/ece533/Lectures/Lectures.htm, 2020.

[14] D. Bera, L. Qian, T. K. Tseng, and P. H. Holloway, "Quantum dots and their multimodal applications: A review," *Materials*, vol. 3, no. 4, pp. 2260-2345, 2010.

[15] X. H. Gao, L. L. Yang, J. A. Petros, F. F. Marshal, J. W. Simons, and S. M. Nie, "In vivo molecular and cellular imaging with quantum dots," *Current Opinion in Biotechnology*, vol. 16, no. 1, pp. 63-72, 2005.

[16] C. Z. Hotz, "Quantum Dots," in *Molecular Biomethods Handbook*, J. M. Walker and R. Rapley, Eds., 2nd ed. Totowa, NJ, USA: Humana Press, 2008, pp. 697-710.

[17] R. Hardman, "A toxicologic review of quantum dots: Toxicity depends on physicochemical and environmental factors," *Environmental Health Perspectives*, vol. 114, no. 2, pp. 165-172, 2006.

[18] R. Bilan, F. Fleury, I. Nabiey, and A. Sukhanova, "Quantum dot surface chemistry and functionalization for cell targeting and imaging," *Bioconjugate Chemistry*, vol. 26, no. 4, pp. 609-624, 2015.

[19] X. H. Gao, Y. Y. Cui, R. M. Levenson, L. W. K. Chung, and S. M. Nie, "In vivo cancer targeting and imaging with semiconductor quantum dots," *Nature Biotechnology*, vol. 22, no. 8, pp. 969-976, 2004.

CHAPTER 5

DNA and RNA Bionanotechnology

Deoxyribonucleic acid (DNA) and ribonucleic acid (RNA) are nucleic acids found in all cellular life, and contain the blueprints for synthesizing proteins which in turn form the building blocks of living organisms along with the processes needed to keep them alive. DNA (normally double-stranded) consists of a sequence of nucleotide base pairs held together by a sugar-phosphate backbone in a double helix (Figure 5-1).

5.1 INTRODUCTION TO DNA AND RNA

The molecular structure of DNA, which is normally double-stranded, is shown in Figure 5-2. A closer examination shows that DNA is made up of two parallel strands of nucleotides held together by hydrogen bonds. Any strand of double-helix DNA is composed of matching nucleotide base pairs covalently bonded to two sugar-phosphate backbones. The sugar-phosphate backbones forming the two sides of the DNA "ladder" are composed of deoxyribose sugars together with phosphate groups. The "steps" or "rungs" of the DNA "ladder" are composed of matching nucleotide base pairs. Nucleotides of opposite strands match up in pairs—adenine (A) pairing with thymine (T), and cytosine (C) pairing with guanine (G). The sequence of nucleotides along a strand of DNA or RNA is important since it determines the shape, amino acid sequence, and functions of proteins in addition to how the processes in living organisms are regulated. The nucleotide sequence of a very long strand of DNA, such as the DNA sequence of a chromosome, can be grouped into genes. The combination of all of the genes of an organism forms its genome.

Let us take genomics—the study of genomes—as an example. Figure 5-3 shows a segment of the genome of *Salmonella* Typhimurium, a species of bacteria that can cause diarrhea and food poisoning. As with all gene sequences, this gene sequence is composed of four nucleotide bases—A, T, C, and G. Although these genetic codes are challenging to

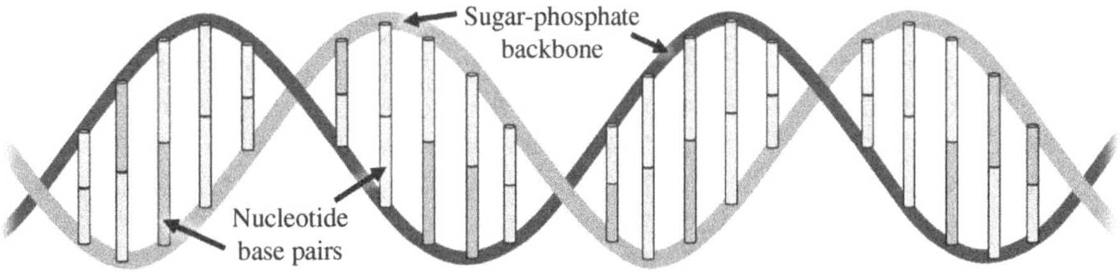

Figure 5-1   Double-stranded DNA has a double helix structure, like a spiral staircase.

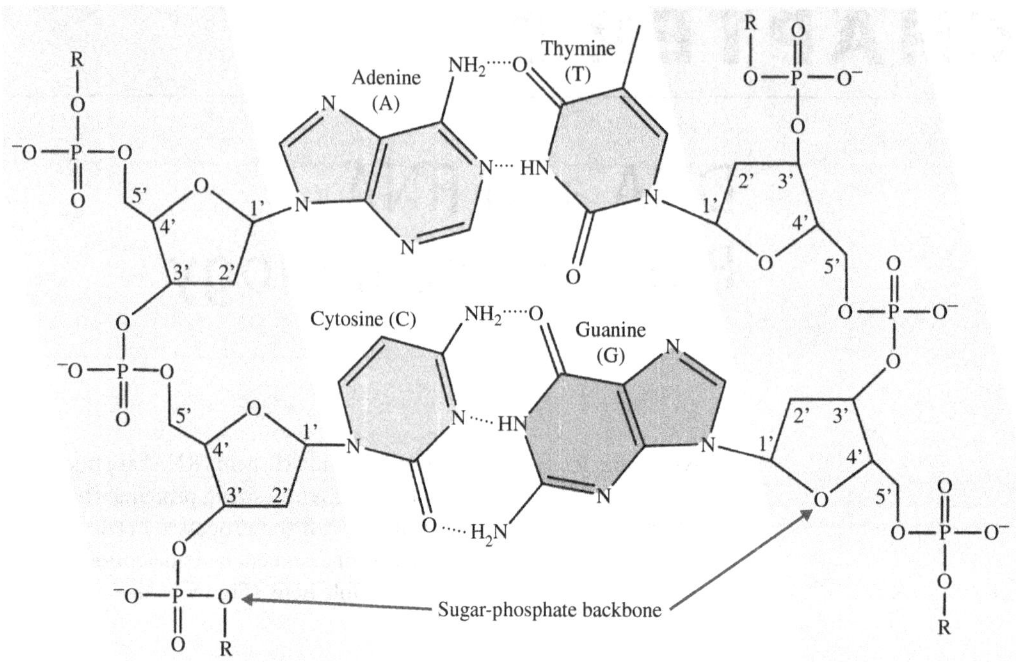

Figure 5-2 Molecular structure of double-stranded DNA. The dotted lines represent hydrogen bonds.

understand, they control the fate of all organisms, including humans. Abnormal genes can dramatically increase the likelihood of a person getting cancer and many other crippling diseases. For instance, Angelina Jolie—a Hollywood star—was detected to carry the breast cancer gene, an abnormal *BRCA1* gene (the normal *BRCA1* gene suppresses breast and ovarian cancers). Her mother, grandmother, and aunt all died from breast cancer. With the abnormal gene, her chance of getting breast cancer was greater than 87%. To avoid getting cancer, she underwent surgery to remove both of her breasts, which reduced her chances of getting breast cancer to less than 5%. Another example is former U.S. president Jimmy

```
ORIGIN   1 TTTTTGCTGG GATCGAACGC CTTAGTGGAG TAGCGCTGTA AGGCGACAGA AACGATATCC
        61 ATAAATGCTC CTGGTTGGTT TAGTACCCTT TTGTATCAGC AGGGTACCGG GTTATCGGTA
       121 AAAAGATAAG GGAGGAAAAT GCGGAAACGG TTATTGCATC AGCGCGGCCG CAGGCGCAGT
       181 TGCTCTCTTT TAGGCAGCCC GTCTACGACC AGATTCCATG AGTCATTTAT CAAATCGTTG
       241 AGTAGCGAGA CGGTGATATC CTCGCCCGCA TAGACTGAAA TCCAGTGTTT CTTATTCATG
       301 TGATAGCCAG GCGCAATGCT GGGGTAAATT TGTTGATTTA CCAGGGACTT TTGGGGATCT
       361 GACTTCAGGT TCACCACTGG GCGACAGTGA TGTTCAGTGA ACAGCATGAA TATTTTGCCC
       421 GCCGACTTTA AACACATCGT ACTGTGGGCC GAAAACGGCA GTGTTCGGTA AAAGGCAGTT
       481 CCAGCGCAAA GCTTTTGCCC AGGCGTGCAG TGTTTGACCG TCCATTATTG CTCCTCGCGA
       541 GTCAGCGGCG GCCCACATGG CTTCGAATCC CAGCGCAATA TATTCGCCAG CGCGACGGGA
       601 TCGGCCGCGG GCGAAATCCA TTGTTGTTTC AGTCAGCGCC AGAAAAAGGC CGTGCGAAGG
       661 CGGCGGTATT CATCCGACAT AAACACCATC AAAACGGAAC GATGACATAA ATCGCGCAAT
       721 TCGGGGAACA TATCGTCGGC CCGTTGTTCC GTCTCTTTGG TGAGCTTTTC GCTGACAGCC
       781 AGTTGACGGA TGCCCGATGG GCGCGCGGGA TGGTTCAGAC CCCAACTGAT GTAACTGTTC
       841 CAGATAAAAC GAGTCATCAT TTTGGCATCG GTAATGGATC GATCCAGCTC CATTATCATT
```

Figure 5-3 The first 900 nucleotides of the rox-A gene for *Salmonella* Typhimurium. [*Source: GenBank (Accession Number AF288225).*[1,2]]

Carter, who has an extensive family history of cancer and inherited genes that predisposed him to cancer. In August 2015, he was diagnosed with melanoma, and the cancer had spread to his liver and even his brain. By using the targeted cancer treatment drug pembrolizumab, he was cancer-free in 2018.

The advancement of "omics" biology disciplines and biotechnologies (e.g., genomics, proteomics, and metabolomics) can help us prevent and predict the onset of diseases. Dr. Michael Snyder, a molecular geneticist and a professor at Stanford University, provided us a good example for this advancement. In 2009, his genetic test showed that he had an increased risk for diabetes. Dr. Snyder treated this information seriously although his family had no known history of diabetes and he was not overweight. Within the following two and half years, he had regularly taken his blood and performed self check-ups by tracing 40,000 different types of molecules, including hormones, blood sugar levels, immunoproteins, and gene mutations. After the examination, he predicted that he would get diabetes in the coming years. In 2011, he was diagnosed with diabetes. Dr. Snyder correctly predicted his disease and he published his studies in the prestigious journal *Cell* in 2012.[3]

Determining DNA sequences has become a central tool in the biological and medical sciences. Some important applications of DNA sequencing include (1) detecting pathogens and microbes (e.g., bacteria, viruses, fungi, and parasites) in the human body, food, and the environment; (2) screening of genetic diseases (e.g., cancer, sickle cell disease, cystic fibrosis, and glaucoma) to help with preventative treatments; (3) identifying the type of cancer and potential treatments with cancer genome sequencing; (4) identifying crime suspects by sequencing forensic DNA; (5) detection of anti-microbial resistance such as antibiotic-resistant bacteria; (6) identification of disease-causing target genes for drug discovery and precision medicine; (7) assisting the study of human ancestry and evolutionary biology; and (8) helping us understand how DNA determines cellular and protein function.

5.1.1 DNA: An Overview

Modern genetics originated from the Mendelian inheritance theory established by Gregor Mendel between 1856 and 1866 from his famous pea plant breeding experiments. Later, scientists discovered the basic patterns of genetic inheritance and developed the field of genetics. Genetics is the study of heredity at the molecular, cellular, and organismal levels, and is concerned with genes and genetic variation. A gene is a segment of double-stranded DNA which encodes the instructions necessary to synthesize important biomolecules such as RNA and proteins. The genes in eukaryotic organisms (e.g., mammals) are found in chromosomes, which are long molecules of double-stranded DNA each containing many genes. All human genes are found in 46 chromosomes (i.e., 23 pairs of chromosomes), with half inherited from the mother and the other half from the father. When a sperm cell and an egg cell combine to produce a zygote, cell division and DNA replication begin, eventually producing a new human being.[4]

Let us review the history of genetics and DNA first. By the early 20th century, scientists knew that chromosomes consisted of DNA, RNA, and proteins, but they were not sure whether DNA, RNA, or protein is the heritable genetic material. To clarify this, Avery, MacLeod, and McCarty designed a landmark experiment in 1944 by using two strains of *Streptococcus pneumoniae* bacteria: S-strain and R-strain. The S-strain is deadly, as it has a bacterial shell that protects it from being destroyed by the immune system. However, the toxicity of S-strains can be eliminated by heating. The R-strain is nonvirulent as it lacks a protective shell. Earlier experiments in the 1920s by Frederick Griffith had shown that an unknown heritable material in the deadly S-strain bacteria—even when killed by heat—can be absorbed by nonvirulent R-strain bacteria, transforming R-strain bacteria into S-strain bacteria.[5,6]

In their experiment (1944), Avery et al. first deactivated a culture of S-strain bacteria by heating. The resulting solution was homogenized and filtered to produce killed S-strain filtrate. Next, the filtrate was split into three separate samples, and a different type of enzyme (protease to destroy proteins, DNase to destroy DNA, and RNase to destroy RNA) was added to each sample. Each of the three samples was added to cultured live R-strain bacteria. After waiting, the two samples where protease or RNase was added contained R-strain as well as transformed S-strain bacteria. The third sample where DNase was added contained only R-strain bacteria. The results confirmed that DNA from virulent S-strain bacteria was the unknown heritable material which can be absorbed by nonvirulent R-strain bacteria, transforming them into S-strain bacteria. The procedure for Avery, MacLeod, and McCarty's experiment (1944) is shown in Figure 5-4.[6,7]

Despite Avery, MacLeod, and McCarty's milestone experiment (1944), scientists at the time were not convinced that DNA was the heritable material. Many scientists still believed that proteins were the heritable material since proteins are in general much more chemically complex than DNA or RNA. Furthermore, since bacterial cells are different from eukaryotic cells (such as mammalian cells), it was not clear if bacteria had DNA. In 1952, Alfred Hershey and Martha Chase designed and conducted another set of pivotal experiments to further prove that DNA, not protein, is the heritable genetic material. At the time, it was known that bacteriophages, which are viruses that target bacteria, can transfer heritable material into bacteria to replicate. The lifecycle of bacteriophages is shown in Figure 5-5.[6,8]

Hershey and Chase labeled two phage samples with different radioactive labels—one with ^{32}P and the other with ^{35}S. It was known that P (phosphorus) is found in DNA but not in proteins, while S (sulfur) is found in proteins but not in DNA. The two radioisotope-labeled phage samples were mixed with bacteria, where the viruses infected

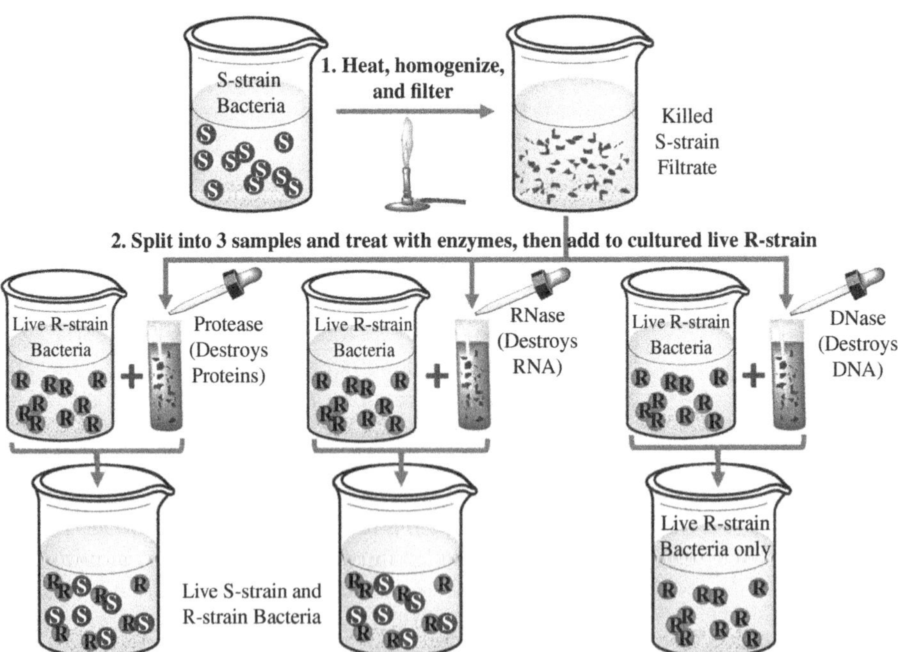

Figure 5-4 An illustration of Avery, MacLeod, and McCarty's landmark experiment (1944). The results verified that DNA from S-strain bacteria was the unknown heritable material that can be absorbed by nonvirulent R-strain bacteria, transforming them into deadly S-strain bacteria.[6,7]

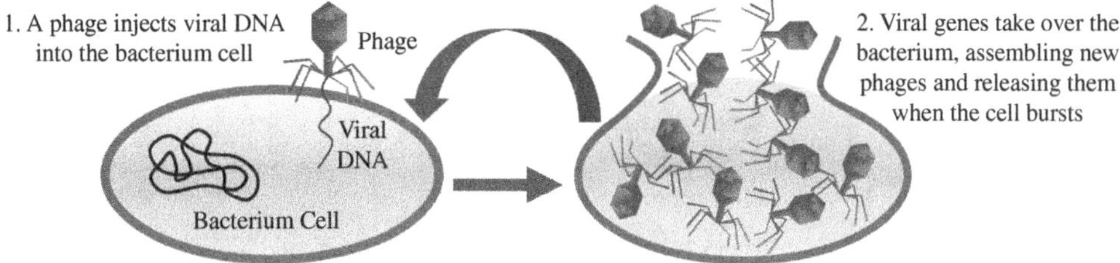

Figure 5-5   An illustration of the lifecycle of bacteriophages (also known as phages).

the bacteria and replicated as expected. After a while, the two samples were thoroughly agitated in a blender and then centrifuged to separate the bacteria from the replicated viruses. In the two resulting centrifuge tubes, the bacteria settled on the bottom as the pellet, while the viruses remained in the supernatant fluid at the top. The majority of the ^{32}P was found in the pellet with the bacteria, while nearly all of the ^{35}S were found in the supernatant fluid with the phages. The results suggest that viral proteins labeled with ^{35}S did not enter bacteria, while viral DNA labeled with ^{32}P entered and remained in bacteria. The procedure for Hershey and Chase's experiment (1952) is illustrated in Figure 5-6.[6,8]

Avery, MacLeod, and McCarty's experiment (1944) plus Hershey and Chase's experiment (1952) together showed that DNA was the heritable material in both bacteria and viruses. Since it was known at the time that some viruses inject heritable material into eukaryotic cells to replicate, scientists reasoned that perhaps DNA was the heritable material of eukaryotic cells as well. Later experiments in the 1950s showed that eukaryotic cells were transformed by DNA, and conclusively demonstrated that DNA was in fact the heritable material of eukaryotic cells. Today, it is believed that DNA is the heritable material of all living organisms on Earth.[9]

In the 1950s, Rosalind Franklin experimentally obtained X-ray diffraction images of DNA, which led to the discovery of the DNA double helix structure by Francis Crick and James Watson who studied the DNA structure with model-building. Meanwhile, Erwin Chargaff discovered that in the four nucleotide bases of DNA—adenine (A), thymine (T),

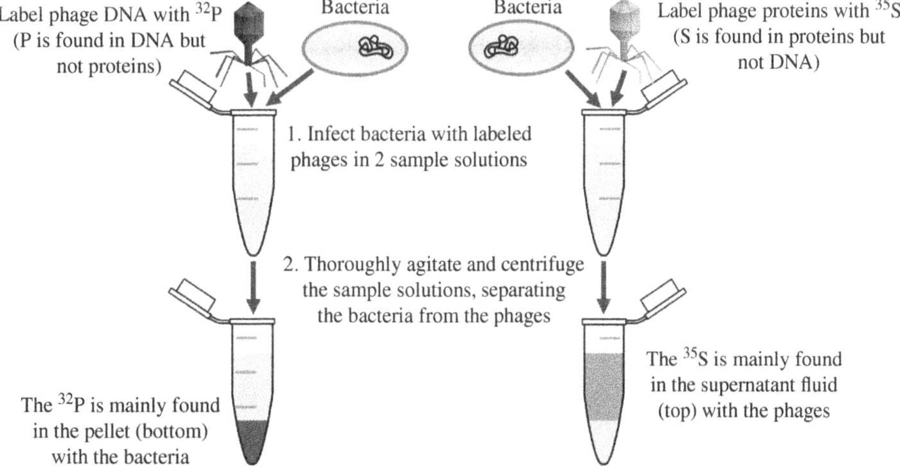

Figure 5-6   An illustration of Hershey and Chase's pivotal experiment (1952). The results indicate that DNA is the heritable material that phages inject into bacteria to replicate.[6,8]

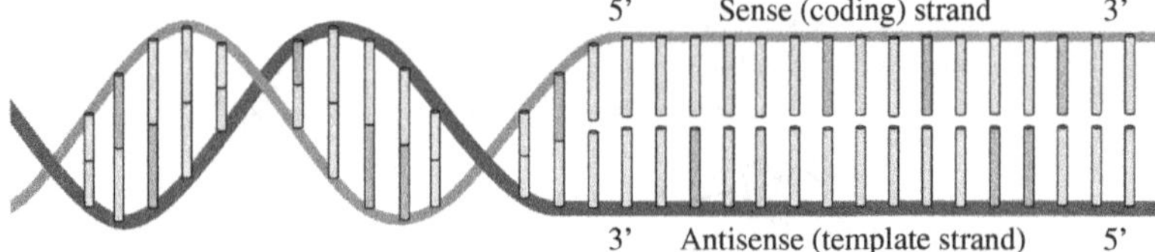

Figure 5-7   The sense and antisense strands of double-stranded DNA.

cytosine (C), and guanine (G), the amount of A equals the amount of T, and the amount of C equals the amount of G.[10]

Now let us focus on the molecular structure of DNA. As shown in Figure 5-2, carbon atoms in the deoxyribose sugar forming the DNA backbone are labeled 1', 2', 3', 4', and 5'. In addition, DNA has directionality. All single strands of DNA have a 5' end and a 3' end. Double-stranded DNA is composed of a sense strand (also known as coding strand) which carries translatable code from 5' to 3' and an antisense strand (also known as template strand) which carries translatable code from 3' to 5'. The sense strand has the same sequence as the transcribed RNA (e.g., messenger RNA which encodes proteins and is read during protein synthesis), while the antisense strand is used as a complementary template for the transcription of RNA. In double-stranded DNA, the 5' end of the sense strand aligns with the 3' end on the antisense strand (Figure 5-7).

By convention, the nucleotide sequence of DNA or RNA is always written from 5' to 3'. Every strand of single-stranded DNA has a complementary strand, where the nucleotide base A corresponds with T, and C corresponds with G. For instance, the complementary strand of ACCGGTATG (5' to 3') is TGGCCATAC (3' to 5'). However, since DNA sequence is written from 5' to 3', the complementary strand of ACCGGTATG is CATACCGGT (both 5' to 3').

EXAMPLE 5-1   What is the difference between the 5' and 3' carbons in DNA?

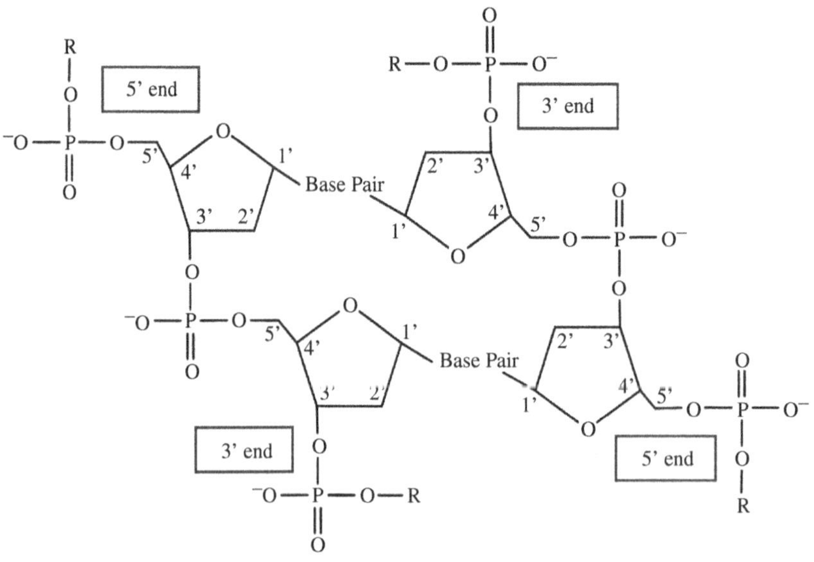

Figure 5-8   Molecular structure of DNA backbone with labeled carbon atoms.

Solution In DNA, the sugar-phosphate backbone chain is formed by phosphate groups attached to the 5' and 3' carbon atoms of each deoxyribose sugar (Figure 5-8). The 3' carbons are on the sugar rings of the DNA backbone, while the 5' carbons are not on the sugar rings. The 5' carbons are from hydroxymethyl groups ($-CH_2OH$) which are linked to the 4' carbons on the sugar ring. In other words, phosphate groups are attached to the 3' carbons through hydroxyl groups ($-OH$), whereas they are attached to the 5' carbons through hydroxymethyl groups ($-CH_2OH$). ▲

5.1.2 RNA: An Introduction

There are three main differences between deoxyribonucleic acid (DNA) and ribonucleic acid (RNA). Both DNA and RNA are supported by a sugar-phosphate backbone, but DNA contains deoxyribose sugars while RNA contains ribose sugars. Both DNA and RNA contain adenine (A), cytosine (C), and guanine (G) nucleotide bases. DNA contains thymine (T), while RNA contains uracil (U) instead. In addition, stable RNA is typically single-stranded while stable DNA is typically double-stranded. Every single-stranded RNA sequence has a corresponding DNA sequence, where all the bases are identical but with uracil (U) being replaced with thymine (T). During transcription when cells read a DNA sequence and translates it into a single-stranded RNA sequence, the resulting RNA has the same sequence as the sense strand of the DNA, but with thymine (T) replaced with uracil (U). There are two main categories of RNA produced through transcription: mRNA (messenger RNA) and ncRNA (non-coding RNA). mRNA contain the instructions for synthesizing proteins. Although ncRNA do not code for proteins, they play important roles in protein synthesis, gene regulation, and in many diseases.

The differences in molecular structure between RNA and DNA are illustrated in Figure 5-9. While ribose has a hydroxyl ($-OH$) group at the 2' carbon, deoxyribose lacks

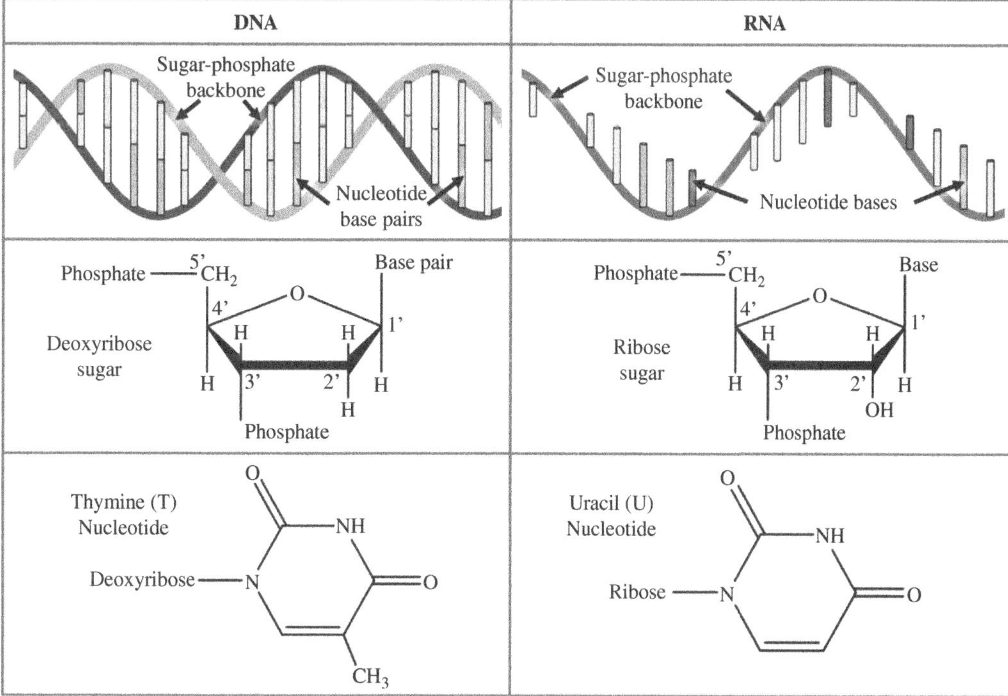

Figure 5-9 Comparison of the molecular structures of DNA with RNA. While stable DNA is usually double-stranded, stable RNA is usually single-stranded.

the 2' hydroxyl group—as suggested by the "deoxy-" prefix. The thymine (T) nucleotide base in DNA is analogous to the uracil (U) nucleotide base in RNA.

5.1.3 DNA Dissociation

The double helix structure of DNA can be broken using heat. A parameter describing the change is the melting temperature (T_m). DNA melting temperature T_m is defined as the temperature at which 50% of double-stranded DNA (dsDNA) is changed to single-stranded DNA (ssDNA) by breaking the hydrogen bonds between all base pairs—a process called dissociation or denaturation. For DNA contained in any buffer solution, T_m is affected by the salt concentration of the buffer through Debye shielding, as well as the presence of denaturants in the buffer such as formamide or dimethyl sulfoxide (DMSO), which disrupts hydrogen bonds. The approximate T_m for a strand of DNA can be calculated using the following empirical formula:[11]

$$T_m[°C] = 81.5 - \frac{600}{N} + 16.6\log_{10}\left(M_{salt}\right) + 0.41(\%GC) - 0.65(\%denaturant) - (\%mismatch)$$

$$\text{applicable when } \left(\text{roughly}\right) 10 \leq N \leq 1000 \tag{5.1}$$

where N is the number of base pairs in the dsDNA or equivalently the number of nucleotides in *one strand* of ssDNA, M_{salt} is the univalent salt concentration in [mol/L], (%GC) is the percentage G−C (and C−G) base-pair content in the dsDNA, (%denaturant) is the total percentage of formamide and DMSO in the buffer solution by volume, and (%mismatch) is the percentage of mismatched base pairs in the dsDNA. (%GC), (%denaturant), and (%mismatch) are percentages, not fractions. For instance, 60% is 60, *not* 0.60 in this formula.

Very Short DNA Strands   The two complementary ssDNA strands comprising any segment of dsDNA are held together by the hydrogen bonds within each base pair. The two strands of ssDNA comprising a very short piece of dsDNA are held together by very few hydrogen bonds. This makes the melting temperature T_m of very short strands of DNA highly sensitive to even minor changes in the buffer solution containing the DNA. For these very short strands of DNA where $N < 10$, many properties of the buffer solution are not included in Equation (5.1) (such as pH, composition, and concentrations of ionic species and solvents), and the presence (or absence) of other biomolecules can significantly affect the melting temperature T_m. Thus, Equation (5.1) is not applicable to very short strands of DNA where $N < 10$.

Long DNA Strands   For long strands of DNA where $N > 1000$, both dsDNA and (especially) ssDNA will self-fold into 3D structures causing Equation (5.1) to become highly inaccurate. For long strands of dsDNA, the total bond strength holding together the two strands of ssDNA depends not only on the hydrogen bonds holding together each base pair, but also on the strength of the van der Waals forces created by the geometry of the self-folded 3D structures.

Although Equation (5.1) for the melting temperature T_m of DNA is an empirical rather than theoretical equation, the six terms in the equation do make intuitive sense.

$$T_m[°C] = \underbrace{81.5}_{\text{Intercept}} - \underbrace{\frac{600}{N}}_{\text{Length}} + \underbrace{16.6\log_{10}\left(M_{salt}\right)}_{\text{Dissolved Ions}} + \underbrace{0.41(\%GC)}_{\text{G−C Content}} - \underbrace{0.65(\%denaturant)}_{\text{Denaturants}} - \underbrace{(\%mismatch)}_{\text{Mismatched Bases}}$$

Intercept   This term is the intercept of the equation for the DNA melting temperature T_m, which is 81.5°C. It is reasonable that the temperature corresponding to this term is significantly higher than room temperature (about 20°C), as well as human body temperature (about 37°C). If this term were theoretically much lower (e.g., 20°C), DNA would be too thermally unstable to be a reliable carrier of hereditary information, which is clearly not true.

(Strand) Length   The two complementary ssDNA strands comprising any segment of dsDNA are held together by hydrogen bonds. Because longer strands of dsDNA are held together more strongly (i.e., by more hydrogen bonds), they should have higher melting temperatures T_m than shorter strands. Therefore, the dsDNA strand length N (i.e., the number of base pairs) should be positively correlated with the melting temperature T_m.

Dissolved Ions   As shown in Figures 5-2 and 5-8, each phosphate group in the sugar-phosphate backbone of DNA is negatively charged with a valence of −1. When salt is dissolved into the buffer solution, the positively charged ions (i.e., cations) from the salt electrically screen the negatively charged phosphate in the DNA backbone via Debye screening. While the two ssDNA strands comprising a segment of dsDNA are held together mainly by hydrogen bonding, there is an opposing repulsive force between the two complementary strands of ssDNA generated by electrostatic repulsion between negatively charged phosphate groups. Electrical screening by any present salt cations significantly reduces the repulsive electrostatic forces between negatively charged phosphate groups, thereby increasing the bond strength between the two complementary ssDNA strands and increasing the melting temperature T_m.

G–C Content   G–C (and C–G) base pairs are held together by three hydrogen bonds, while A–T (and T–A) base pairs are held together by only two hydrogen bonds. Therefore, G–C (and C–G) base pairs are held together significantly more strongly than A–T (and T–A) base pairs. Thus, increasing (%GC) should also increase the melting temperature T_m of dsDNA.

Denaturants   DMSO and formamide denature dsDNA by weakening the hydrogen bonds between the two complementary ssDNA strands comprising the segment of dsDNA. Therefore, the addition of one or both of the denaturants should weaken the bonds holding dsDNA together, thereby decreasing the melting temperature T_m of dsDNA.

Mismatched Bases   The presence of mismatched bases in a strand of dsDNA will definitely decrease the melting temperature T_m of the dsDNA strand. Correctly matched base pairs are held together by either two or three hydrogen bonds. Due to differences in molecular geometries, mismatched base pairs are not properly held together by hydrogen bonds, resulting in physical deformations in the dsDNA at the location of each mismatched base pair. Therefore, the presence of mismatched base pairs weakens the bond strength holding together the dsDNA strand, especially in comparison to correctly matched base pairs. The more mismatched bases in the dsDNA strand, the lower the DNA melting temperature T_m.

Equation (5.1) allows us to calculate the DNA melting temperature T_m, which is defined as the temperature at which 50% of dsDNA is changed to ssDNA. In reality, the fraction $f_m(T)$ of dsDNA changed to ssDNA versus temperature T follows an S-shaped (or sigmoid) curve, starting at close to zero for temperatures well below T_m and approaching one for temperatures well above T_m (Figure 5-10). $f_m(T)$ is commonly called the dissociation fraction

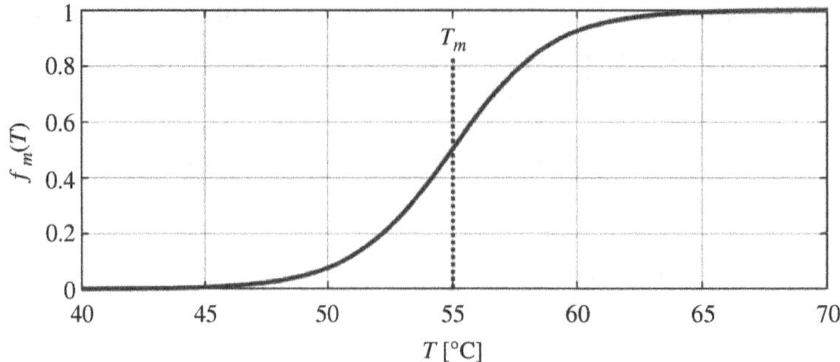

Figure 5-10   The dissociation fraction (or melted fraction) $f_m(T)$ of DNA versus temperature T.

(or melted fraction) of DNA. The simplest and most commonly used model for $f_m(T)$ as a function of temperature T of the buffer solution containing the DNA is the single-parameter logistic function as given in Equation (5.2) below.[12]

$$f_m(T) = \frac{1}{1 + \exp\left[-A\left(T - T_m\right)\right]} \quad \text{where } A\left[1/°C\right] > 0 \tag{5.2}$$

where $A\ [1/°C]$ is a *positive* fitting constant that depends mainly on the properties of the DNA-containing buffer solution, the DNA strand length, and the presence of any mismatched bases in the dsDNA. T_m is the DNA melting temperature at which 50% of dsDNA becomes ssDNA, as given by Equation (5.1).

Other important characteristics for both ssDNA and dsDNA are molecular mass (mass per molecule) and molar mass (mass per mole of molecules). A commonly used unit for the molecular mass of large biomolecules such as DNA is the dalton (Da). Strictly speaking, the dalton (Da) is a unit of mass with 1 Da $\cong 1.6605 \times 10^{-27}$ kg. However, the dalton is also frequently used as a unit of molar mass with 1 Da $= 1$ g/mol (exactly). We have

$$1\,\text{Da} = 1\,\text{g/mol} \cong 1.6605 \times 10^{-27}\,\text{kg} \tag{5.3}$$

In addition, there is a relationship between the dalton (Da) unit and Avogadro's number N_A given by

$$(1\,\text{Da})\,(N_A) = (1.6605 \times 10^{-27}\,\text{kg})\,(6.0221 \times 10^{23}\,\text{mol}^{-1}) = 1\,\text{g/mol} \tag{5.4}$$

The molecular or molar mass m_{ssDNA} of ssDNA with N_{bases} as the number of nucleotides is

$$m_{ssDNA} \cong (325\,\text{Da})\,N_{bases} \tag{5.5A} \qquad\qquad m_{dsDNA} \cong (650\,\text{Da})\,N_{bps} \tag{5.5B}$$

Therefore, 1 mol of ssDNA strands that are each 10 nucleotides long would weigh 3.25 kg. The molecular or molar mass m_{dsDNA} of dsDNA is obtained by simply doubling the formula for ssDNA, where N_{bps} is the number of base pairs in the dsDNA.[13]

One useful way to represent and visualize dsDNA dissociating into ssDNA and ssDNA recombining back to dsDNA is through energy diagrams. For systems of complementary

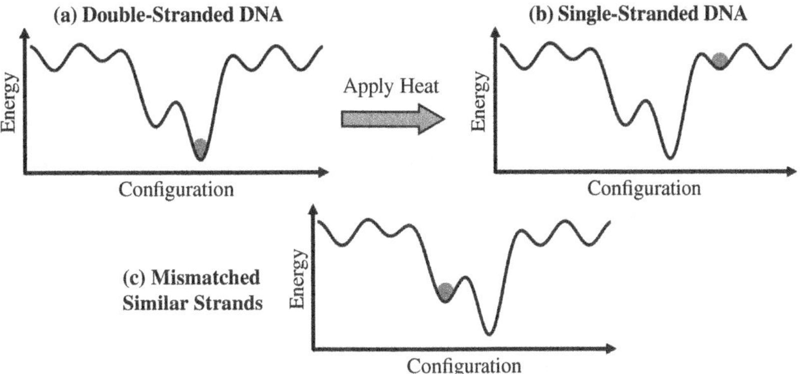

Figure 5-11   Energy configuration diagrams of DNA.

single strands of DNA, the minimum energy configuration is for the DNA to be double-stranded with its complement (Figure 5-11a). By adding heat (energy) to the system, the higher energy single-stranded states become accessible (Figure 5-11b). In systems with similar but not exactly complementary strands, two single DNA strands can join together in a double-stranded state with lower energy than single-stranded DNA, but still higher energy than a perfect match (Figure 5-11c). This is the basis of heteroduplex analysis (refer to Section 5.3.1).

5.2 POLYMERASE CHAIN REACTION (PCR)

Polymerase chain reaction (PCR) is a standard procedure used for amplifying (i.e., making many identical copies of) a sample of DNA *in vitro* (i.e., outside of a living organism). The goal of PCR is to produce enough copies of the desired target DNA sample for DNA sequencing or other applications. The sample of target DNA to be amplified using PCR is called the PCR product. PCR is a cyclical process which amplifies the desired PCR product exponentially with each passing cycle. Each PCR cycle consists of three main steps carried out at different temperatures: denaturing, annealing, and extension/elongation. Hence, the lab equipment for carrying out PCR is called a thermal cycler (or thermocycler).

Quantitative real-time PCR (qPCR) is a PCR variant designed specifically for quantifying the initial target DNA concentration. The most common applications of qPCR include gene expression analysis, gene mutation detection, and cancer phenotyping. There are several major differences between (regular) PCR and qPCR. The analysis step for (regular) PCR, which is typically gel electrophoresis, is carried out at the end once enough copies of the PCR product have been produced. For qPCR, fluorescent probes (i.e., fluorophores) such as organic fluorescent dyes or fluorescent intercalators that bind to DNA are added to the PCR buffer solution at the beginning. During qPCR, optical detection of the fluorescence intensity is carried out in real time to track the number of copies of the target DNA (i.e., PCR product). Once enough copies of the target DNA have been produced, the initial target DNA concentration can be calculated. Therefore, the thermal cycler for qPCR must contain an optical detection system consisting of light sources to excite the fluorophores and photodetectors to measure the fluorescence intensity in real time.[14]

5.2.1 Polymerase Chain Reaction (PCR) Procedure

(1) *Reagents*: PCR requires the following:
- ➤ The desired DNA sample (PCR product) that we want to amplify.
- ➤ Free nucleotide bases (A, T, C, and G) in the form of deoxynucleotide triphosphates (dNTPs).
- ➤ DNA polymerase enzyme.
  - Since there are numerous types of DNA polymerase, the chosen DNA polymerase enzyme must have a suitable active temperature range.
- ➤ Forward and reverse primers.
  - Primers are short sections (about 20 nucleotides long) of *single-stranded* DNA which mark the beginning and the end of the copied section of DNA during PCR. The forward primer has the same sequence of bases as the beginning of the sense strand (always written from 5' to 3'). The base sequence of the reverse primer is complementary to the bases at the end of the sense strand.
- ➤ Buffer solution with ions to control pH and charge concentration, and (**qPCR only**) fluorescent probes such as organic fluorescent dyes or fluorescent intercalators.

(2) *Denaturing*: The DNA sample is heated above its melting temperature T_m. The double-stranded DNA become single-stranded.

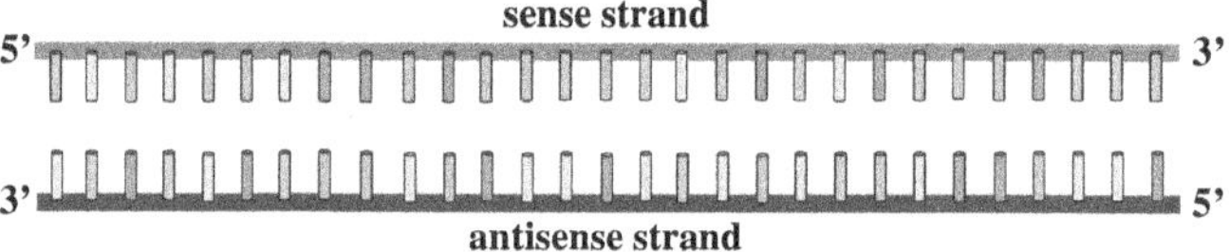

(3) *Annealing*: The sample is cooled quickly (via annealing) in the presence of the primers, such that the primers will bind with the complementary sections of DNA.

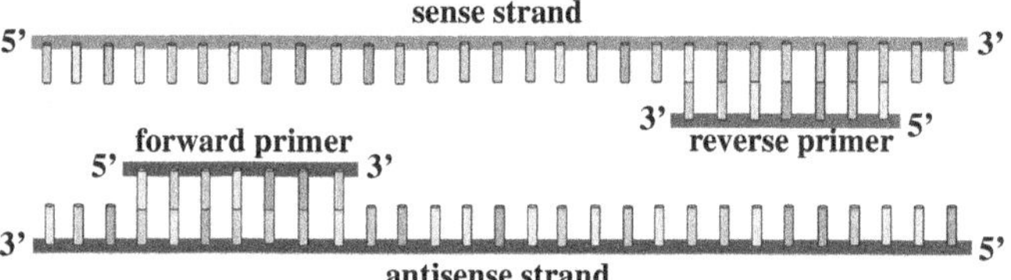

(4) *Extension/Elongation*: DNA polymerase moves along the strands starting at the primers, building complementary strands (from 5' to 3') using the extra nucleotide bases (i.e., dNTPs) in the solution.

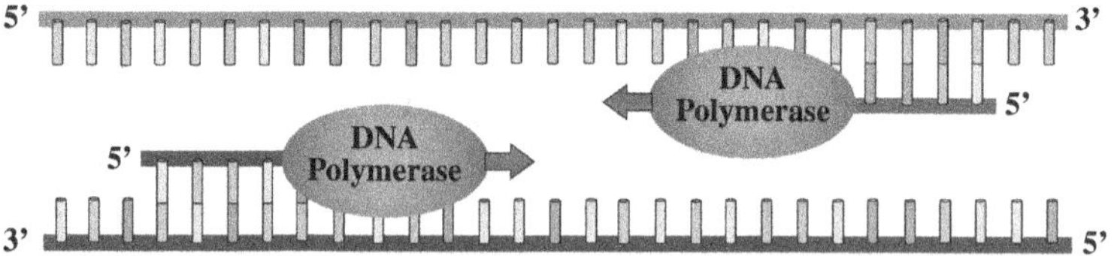

(5) *Extension/Elongation*: DNA polymerase will continue to build DNA until the process is stopped through temperature control, making arbitrarily long strands.

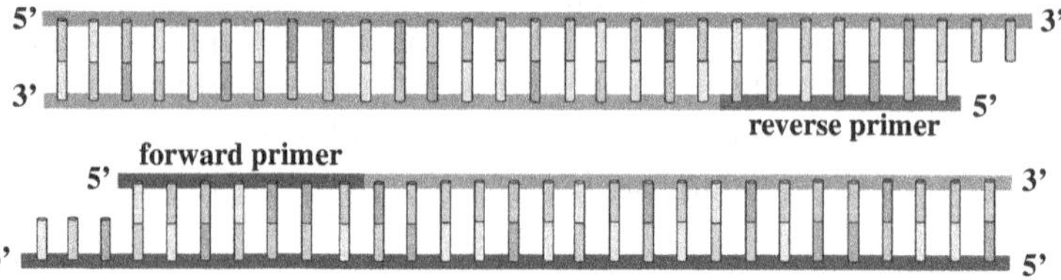

(6) *Denaturing:* The temperature is increased above T_m to denature the double-stranded DNA into single-stranded DNA, and the process shown previously is then repeated.

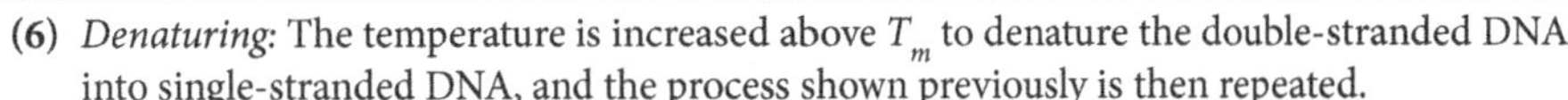

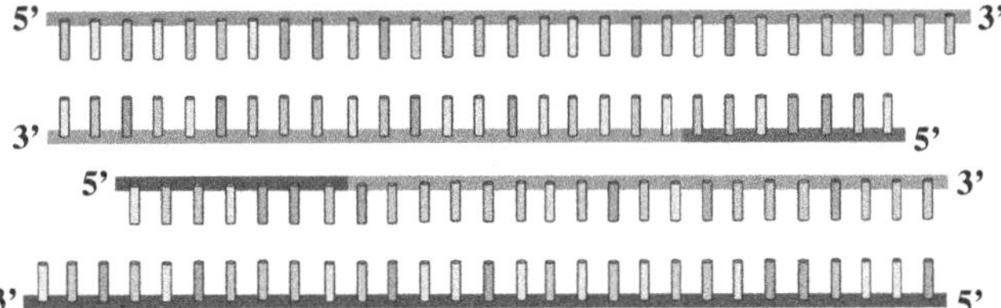

(7) *Annealing:* When the primers are annealed onto the strands, they also attach to the newly created strands.

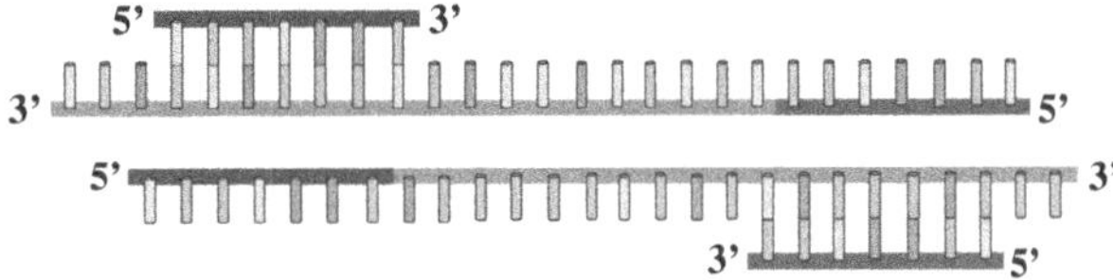

(8) *Extension/Elongation:* When the new strands are elongated, they can only be built up to one end of each previous strand, which limits the length of the synthesized DNA to be in between (and including) the two primers.

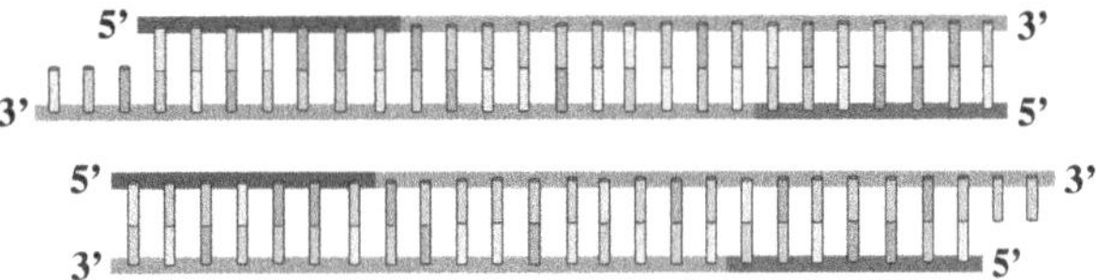

(9) *Result:* After repeating the PCR cycle many times, there is exponential growth of the replicated DNA segments with the selected sequence. Once enough copies of the target DNA (i.e., PCR product) have been produced, the target DNA can be sequenced or used for other applications.

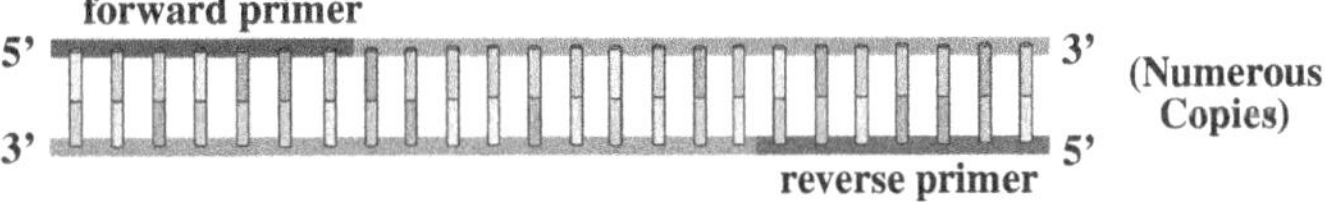

(qPCR Only) The fluorescence intensity increases with every PCR cycle due to the fluorescent probes in the solution attaching to the DNA strands. Hence, the fluorescence intensity can be used to quantify the concentration of the target DNA in real time, and determine the initial target DNA concentration.

EXAMPLE 5-2 You plan to design a test that will be used to manage an outbreak of *Salmonella* Typhimurium. A segment of the *Salmonella* Typhimurium genome is shown in Figure 5-3. Assume that you want a PCR product with a length of 140 bps (base pairs) and that you have chosen, as your forward primer, the 20 nts (nucleotides) starting at base number 300. Obtained from Figure 5-3, the DNA sequence from 300 to 319 is "G TGATAGCCAG GCGCAATGC", while the DNA sequence from 420 to 439 is "C GCCGACTTTA AACACATCG". Both sequences are written from 5' to 3'.

    (a) What is the sequence of your forward primer?

    (b) What is the sequence of your reverse primer (also 20 nts long)?

    (c) The PCR buffer has a salt concentration of [NaCl] = 160 mM and no chemical denaturants. What are the melting temperatures T_m of the forward and reverse primers?

Solution

    (a) The sequence of the forward primer is just the first 20 nts of the PCR sequence.

        Forward primer = G TGATAGCCAG GCGCAATGC (5' to 3')

(**b**) The reverse primer will be the complement of the last 20 nts of the PCR sequence (i.e., the DNA sequence from 420 to 439). As with all DNA and RNA, the convention is to write sequences from 5' to 3', so the sequence must start from the end of the PCR sequence.

Reverse primer = CGATGTGTT TAAAGTCGGC G (5' to 3')

(**c**) With [NaCl] = 160 mM, the monovalent salt concentration is $M = 0.160$ M. In addition, $N = 20$ (nts) for both primers and there are no denaturants or mismatched base pairs. Using Equation (5.1) and letting (%denaturant) = (%mismatch) = 0, we have

$$T_m\,[^\circ\text{C}] = 81.5 - 600/N + 16.6\log_{10}(M_{\text{salt}}) + 0.41(\%\text{GC})$$

Forward primer (%GC = 12/20 = 60%):

$$T_m\,[^\circ\text{C}] = 81.5 - 600/20 + 16.6\log_{10}(0.160) + 0.41 \times (60) = 62.9^\circ\text{C}$$

Reverse primer (%GC = 10/20 = 50%):

$$T_m\,[^\circ\text{C}] = 81.5 - 600/20 + 16.6\log_{10}(0.160) + 0.41 \times (50) = 58.8^\circ\text{C}$$

The melting temperatures T_m of primers is an important consideration when performing PCR and determining a PCR procedure. There must not be too much of a disparity between the melting temperatures T_m of forward and reverse primers.   ▲

5.2.2 Modeling the Polymerase Chain Reaction (PCR)

Each PCR cycle consists of three steps: (1) denaturing, (2) annealing, and (3) extension/elongation. Suppose that we are using DNA polymerase which can elongate ssDNA at a rate of $R_{\text{polymerase}}$ nucleotide bases per second, and that we are starting with C_0 copies of *double-stranded* DNA—which we want to amplify—in the PCR buffer solution. Our desired PCR product to be amplified has a length of N_{product} nucleotides, and both forward and reverse primers have a length of N_{primer} nucleotides. The total time τ_{cycle} required for every PCR cycle is given by

$$\tau_{\text{cycle}} = t_{\text{denaturing}} + t_{\text{annealing}} + t_{\text{extension}} + t_{T\,\text{ramping}} \tag{5.6}$$

where $t_{\text{denaturing}}$ is the time required for the denaturing step to dissociate the dsDNA PCR product into ssDNA strands, $t_{\text{annealing}}$ is the time required for the annealing step, $t_{\text{extension}}$ is the time required for the extension step, and $t_{T\,\text{ramping}}$ is the time required for temperature ramping; that is, $t_{T\,\text{ramping}}$ is the time needed for the temperature to rise or drop to the desired level before and after the denaturing, annealing, and extension steps.

In every PCR cycle, the purpose of the extension/elongation step is to allow DNA polymerase to elongate the forward and reverse primers which have (respectively) attached to the antisense ssDNA strand and sense ssDNA strand of the PCR product during the annealing step. Therefore, the minimum time $t_{\text{extension}}$ required for the extension/elongation step of every PCR cycle can be calculated as follows.

$$t_{\text{extension}} \geq \frac{N_{\text{product}} - N_{\text{primer}}}{R_{\text{polymerase}}} \tag{5.7}$$

The goal of the denaturing step is to dissociate dsDNA into ssDNA. Thus, we can reasonably assume that the fraction $f_m(T)$ of dsDNA dissociated to ssDNA depends purely on the temperature $T_{\text{denaturing}}$ of the denaturing step. Using Equation (5.2) and letting $T = T_{\text{denaturing}}$, we have

$$f_m = f_m\left(T = T_{\text{denaturing}}\right) = \frac{1}{1 + \exp\left[-A\left(T_{\text{denaturing}} - T_m\right)\right]} \tag{5.8}$$

where $A[1/°C]$ is a *positive* fitting constant, and T_m is the DNA melting temperature (at which 50% of dsDNA becomes ssDNA) as given in Equation (5.1).

For the first PCR cycle, we start with C_0 copies of *double-stranded* DNA in the PCR buffer solution. Out of the C_0 dsDNA copies, $f_m \cdot C_0$ dsDNA copies will be denatured into ssDNA, and $(1 - f_m) \cdot C_0$ copies will remain as dsDNA. During the extension step, the $f_m \cdot C_0$ copies of dsDNA that have been denatured will be doubled into $2f_m \cdot C_0$ copies of dsDNA. Therefore, we now have C_1 copies in total of the *double-stranded* DNA PCR product given by

$$C_1 = 2f_m \cdot C_0 + \left(1 - f_m\right) \cdot C_0 = C_0 \cdot \left(1 + f_m\right)$$

For the second PCR cycle, we start with C_1 copies of dsDNA, with $f_m \cdot C_1$ dsDNA copies denatured into ssDNA, and $(1 - f_m) \cdot C_1$ copies remaining as dsDNA. During the extension step, the $f_m \cdot C_1$ copies of denatured dsDNA are doubled to $2f_m \cdot C_1$ copies of dsDNA. Therefore, we now have C_2 copies in total of the dsDNA PCR product given by

$$C_2 = 2f_m \cdot C_1 + \left(1 - f_m\right) \cdot C_1 = C_1 \cdot \left(1 + f_m\right) = C_0 \cdot \left(1 + f_m\right)^2$$

Now let us generalize the above expressions and arguments. After the Kth PCR cycle, we will have C_K copies of the dsDNA PCR product given by

$$C_K = C_{K-1} \cdot \left(1 + f_m\right)$$

where C_{K-1} is the copies of the dsDNA product after the $(K-1)$th PCR cycle. The above recursive relation can be solved as follows:

$$C_K = C_{K-1} \cdot \left(1 + f_m\right) = C_{K-2} \cdot \left(1 + f_m\right)^2 = \cdots = C_0 \cdot \left(1 + f_m\right)^K \text{ with } K = \left\lfloor \frac{t}{\tau_{\text{cycle}}} \right\rfloor_{\text{floor}} \tag{5.9}$$

where t represents time and $K = \left\lfloor t/\tau_{\text{cycle}} \right\rfloor_{\text{floor}}$ is the number of elapsed PCR cycles, which is t/τ_{cycle} rounded *down* to the nearest integer. Since the extension/elongation step is the *final step* of each PCR cycle, and the full extension time of $t_{\text{extension}}$ is required to completely elongate the primers up to the PCR product length, any period of time less than τ_{cycle} will not result in successfully amplified PCR products. Putting everything together, we have

$$C_K = C_0 \cdot \left(1 + f_m\right)^K = C_0 \left(1 + \frac{1}{1 + \exp\left[-A\left(T_{\text{denaturing}} - T_m\right)\right]}\right)^K \text{ with } K = \left\lfloor \frac{t}{\tau_{\text{cycle}}} \right\rfloor_{\text{floor}} \tag{5.10A}$$

$$\text{where } \begin{cases} \tau_{\text{cycle}} = t_{\text{denaturing}} + t_{\text{annealing}} + t_{\text{extension}} + t_{T \text{ ramping}} \\ \text{with } t_{\text{extension}} \geq \left(N_{\text{product}} - N_{\text{primer}}\right)/R_{\text{polymerase}} \end{cases} \tag{5.10B}$$

where C_0 is the starting copies of the *double-stranded* DNA PCR product, and C_K is the number of copies of the *double-stranded* DNA PCR product after K full PCR cycles.

5.2.3 Primer Selection with GenBank and BLAST

The NCBI Genomes database (i.e., GenBank) and associated Basic Local Alignment Search Tools (BLAST) are useful tools to assist the design of PCR tests. Suppose that we want to design a PCR test to detect the presence or absence of the viral genome of the macaque simian foamy virus. For assistance, we use GenBank and associated BLAST tools. A short tutorial on the use of GenBank, Primer-BLAST, and Nucleotide-BLAST is as follows.[1]

---

1. Access GenBank via Google or the following link: https://www.ncbi.nlm.nih.gov/genome/. Then, search for the macaque simian foamy virus in GenBank.

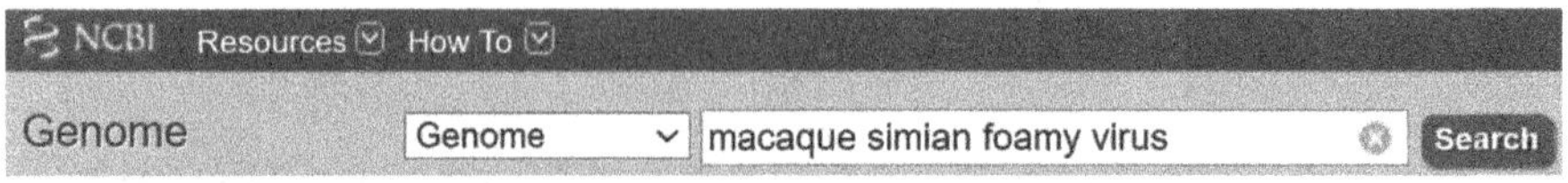

---

2. Next, click on the Accession Number (X54482.1) in the search results.

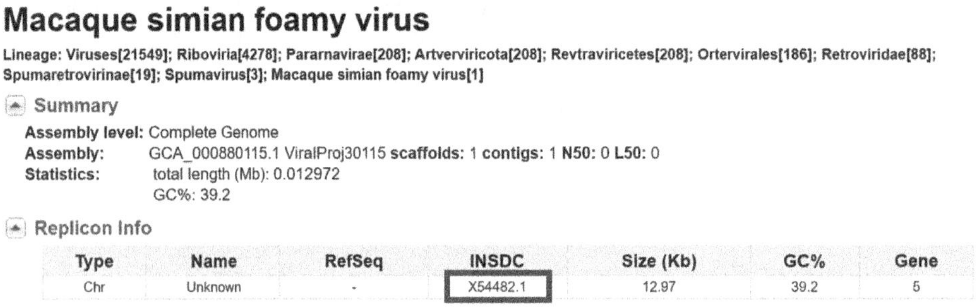

Macaque simian foamy virus

Lineage: Viruses[21549]; Riboviria[4278]; Pararnavirae[208]; Artverviricota[208]; Revtraviricetes[208]; Ortervirales[186]; Retroviridae[88]; Spumaretrovirinae[19]; Spumavirus[3]; Macaque simian foamy virus[1]

▲ Summary

Assembly level: Complete Genome
Assembly: GCA_000880115.1 ViralProj30115 scaffolds: 1 contigs: 1 N50: 0 L50: 0
Statistics: total length (Mb): 0.012972
                GC%: 39.2

▲ Replicon Info

Type	Name	RefSeq	INSDC	Size (Kb)	GC%	Gene
Chr	Unknown	-	X54482.1	12.97	39.2	5

---

3. To select the forward and reverse primer ranges, click "Pick Primers."

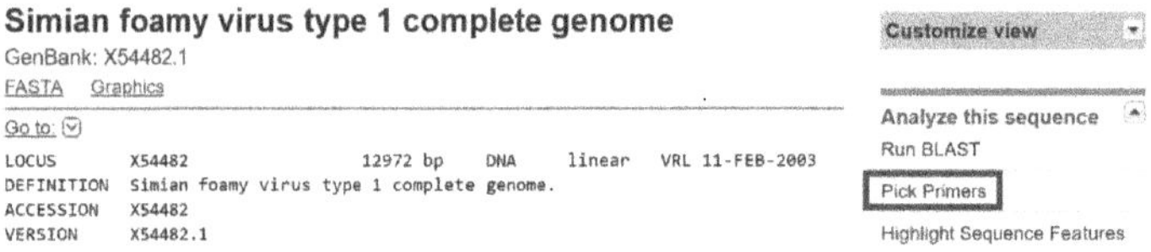

Simian foamy virus type 1 complete genome

GenBank: X54482.1
FASTA Graphics
Go to: ▽

```
LOCUS       X54482              12972 bp    DNA     linear   VRL 11-FEB-2003
DEFINITION  Simian foamy virus type 1 complete genome.
ACCESSION   X54482
VERSION     X54482.1
```

Customize view

Analyze this sequence
Run BLAST
Pick Primers
Highlight Sequence Features

Tip: Under "Primer Parameters" in the Primer-BLAST search, you can choose a range for the desired PCR product size. If necessary, you can also loosen the tolerances for the melting temperatures of the primers. When Primer-BLAST finds primers, it considers factors such as the desired PCR product length, nucleotide sequence region, melting temperatures, and if the primers will attach to each other or any other undesired areas of the DNA.

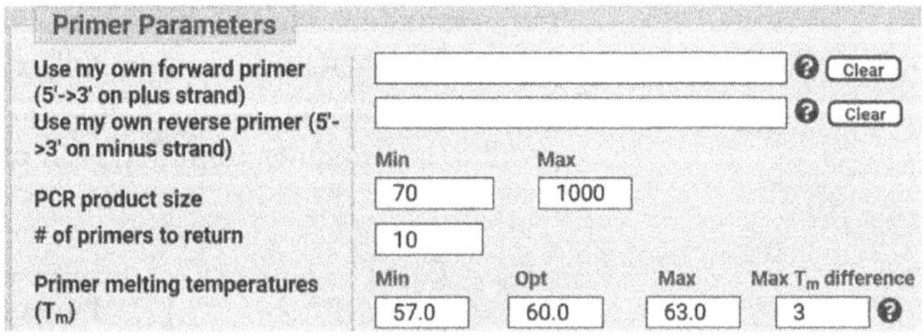

Primer Parameters

Use my own forward primer (5'->3' on plus strand)
Use my own reverse primer (5'->3' on minus strand)

	Min	Max	
PCR product size	70	1000	
# of primers to return	10		

Primer melting temperatures (T_m)	Min	Opt	Max	Max T_m difference
	57.0	60.0	63.0	3

---

4. Select "nr" as the Database and leave all other settings unchanged. Finally, click "Get Primers" to get the primers using Primer-BLAST.

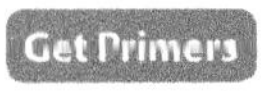

Get Primers

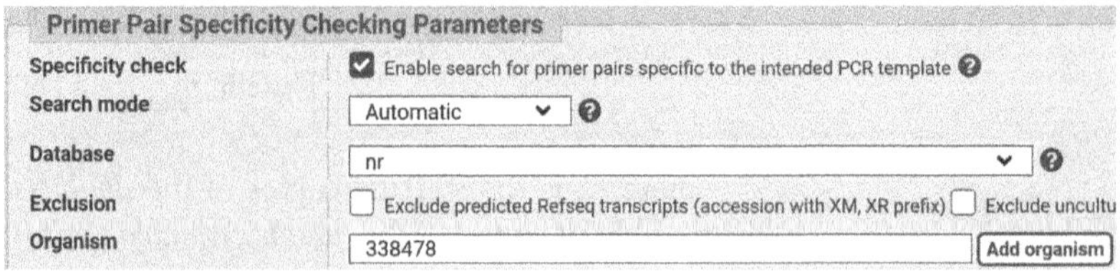

Primer Pair Specificity Checking Parameters

Specificity check   ☑ Enable search for primer pairs specific to the intended PCR template
Search mode   Automatic
Database   nr
Exclusion   ☐ Exclude predicted Refseq transcripts (accession with XM, XR prefix) ☐ Exclude uncultu
Organism   338478   Add organism

---

5. To check how unique the product sequences are, do a BLAST search. Access the Nucleotide-BLAST search via the following link and click on Nucleotide BLAST:

https://blast.ncbi.nlm.nih.gov/Blast.cgi

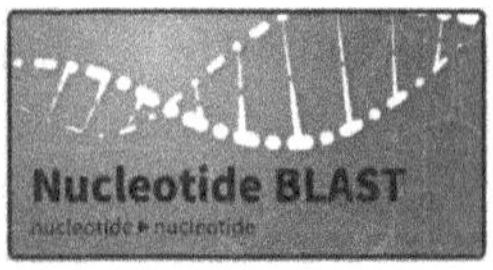

6. Enter the nucleotide sequence with the shown settings and click

BLAST

to run the BLAST search in the viral database.

EXAMPLE 5-3
Primer Selection
for Virus PCR
Follow the instructions of the GenBank and BLAST tutorial for the macaque simian foamy virus. Please aim for a PCR product size of 200 to 300 base pairs for your primers. For simplicity, it is assumed that the viral genome is encoded by DNA (rather than RNA) and can hence be detected by standard PCR.

(a) What portion of the viral genome have you chosen for the PCR product? State the start and stop nucleotide numbers, the size of the PCR product, and the sequence itself.

(b) What are the forward and reverse primers you have chosen? Show where these primers match the genome. What are the melting temperatures T_m of these two primers?

(c) How much would the (unlabeled) primers cost from Integrated DNA Technologies (IDT), Mr. Gene, Invitrogen, or elsewhere? How many guaranteed yield copies of each primer are there for the chosen amount of primers?

(d) How unique are the product sequences? Do a Nucleotide-BLAST search in the viral database for the nucleotide sequences of the primers and the PCR product. Primers are considered acceptable if the query cover (i.e., the percentage nucleotide sequence overlap) with other species is less than 90%. PCR products are okay if there is no significant nucleotide sequence overlap with other species.

Solution

(a) Found from the NCBI Genomes database (GenBank), a segment of the macaque simian foamy virus genome is shown in Figure 5-12 (top). Obtained using the "Get Primers" search, the length of the PCR product is 250 nucleotides, and is from nucleotide numbers 7851 to 8100 (Figure 5-12, top and bottom).

(b) The chosen forward and reverse primers are as follows.

$$\text{Forward primer (7851-7870)} = \texttt{TTCGGCCAGA AGGATGGAAC} \quad (5' \text{ to } 3')$$

$$\text{Reverse primer (8100-8081)} = \texttt{TCCCATTCAG CTGGCATAGC} \quad (5' \text{ to } 3')$$

The locations where these primers match the genome are highlighted in Figure 5-12 (top). From the above screenshot, the melting temperatures of the primers are

$$\text{Forward primer: } T_m = 60.04°C \qquad \text{Reverse primer: } T_m = 60.18°C$$

It is important that the primer melting temperatures T_m are high enough not to become detached during the elongation phase. Also, the two melting temperatures should be relatively close to one another.

```
7801 ACAATATGCA CATCAAAATA TATGGGATTA TTATGTCCCC TTTGAACAAA TTCGGCCAGA
7861 AGGATGGAAC TCAAAAAGTT ATTATGAAGA TGCTAGAATA GGAGGGTTTT ATATACCAAA
7921 ATGGTTACGA AATAATTCCT ATACCCATGT CTTATTTTGT TCTGATCAAA TTTATGGAAA
7981 ATGGTATAAT ATTGATCTCA CAGCCCAGGA GAGGGAAAAT TTATTAGTCC GAAAATTAAT
8041 TAATTTAGCT AAAGGAAATT CATCACAATT AAAAGATAGA GCTATGCCAG CTGAATGGGA
8101 TAAACAAGGA AAAGCTGATC TATTTAGACA AATTAATACT TTAGATGTTT GTAATAGACC
```

Primer pair 1

	Sequence (5'->3')	Template strand	Length	Start	Stop	Tm	GC%
Forward primer	TTCGGCCAGAAGGATGGAAC	Plus	20	7851	7870	60.04	55.00
Reverse primer	TCCCATTCAGCTGGCATAGC	Minus	20	8100	8081	60.18	55.00
Product length	250						

Products on intended targets

>X54482.1 Simian foamy virus type 1 complete genome

Figure 5-12   (Top) A segment of the macaque simian foamy virus genome. (Bottom) A screenshot of the Prime-BLAST search results. [*Source: GenBank (Accession Number X54482).*[1,15]]

(c) From the website of IDT (https://www.idtdna.com/order/OrderEntry.aspx?type=dna), the costs of the forward and reverse primers are (not including shipping):

Forward primer: $7.40 USD for 25 nmol with a guaranteed yield of 12 nmol (or 74.3 μg)

Reverse primer: $7.40 USD for 25 nmol with a guaranteed yield of 12 nmol (or 72.6 μg)

To calculate the number of copies N of the forward and reverse primers based on the guaranteed yield, we use Equation (5.5) as follows:

$$m_{ssDNA} \cong (325 \text{ Da}) \, N_{bases} = (325)(1.66 \times 10^{-27} \text{ kg})(20) = 1.079 \times 10^{-23} \text{ kg}$$

$$N_{forward \, primer} = (74.3 \text{ μg})/(1.079 \times 10^{-23} \text{ kg}) = 6.89 \times 10^{15} \text{ copies}$$

$$N_{reverse \, primer} = (72.6 \text{ μg})/(1.079 \times 10^{-23} \text{ kg}) = 6.73 \times 10^{15} \text{ copies}$$

Alternatively, one can use the given guaranteed yield of 12 nmol as follows:

$$N_{forward \, primer} = N_{reverse \, primer} = (12 \text{ nmol})(6.022 \times 10^{23} \text{ mol}^{-1}) = 7.23 \times 10^{15} \text{ copies}$$

(d) Shown below are the results of the Nucleotide-BLAST search for the forward primer sequence. The top three results, all with query covers of 100%, belong to the same species that we are targeting (i.e., simian foamy virus). For all other results, the query cover is below 90%, so the forward primer is acceptable.

Description	Scientific Name	Max Score	Total Score	Query Cover	E value	Per. Ident	Acc. Len	Accession
Taiwanese macaque simian foamy virus strain SFVmcy_FV21, co...	Taiwanes...	40.1	40.1	100%	0.029	100.00%	12972	MN585198.1
Simian foamy virus type 1 polymerase (pol) gene, 3' end; and enve...	Simian fo...	40.1	40.1	100%	0.029	100.00%	3534	M33561.1
Simian foamy virus type 1 complete genome	Macaque ...	40.1	40.1	100%	0.029	100.00%	12972	X54482.1
Nylanderia fulva virus 1 isolate SinvNfC03 polyprotein gene, partial...	Nylanderi...	32.2	32.2	80%	7.2	100.00%	10904	MG696806.1
Nylanderia fulva virus 1 isolate SinvNfB02 polyprotein gene, compl...	Nylanderi...	32.2	32.2	80%	7.2	100.00%	10918	MG696805.1
Nylanderia fulva virus 1 isolate SinvNfA01 polyprotein gene, compl...	Nylanderi...	32.2	32.2	80%	7.2	100.00%	10909	MG696804.1
Nylanderia fulva virus 1 polyprotein gene, complete cds	Nylanderi...	32.2	32.2	80%	7.2	100.00%	10887	KX580898.1
Nylanderia fulva virus 1 isolate Florida initial polyprotein gene, com...	Nylanderi...	32.2	32.2	80%	7.2	100.00%	10913	KX024775.1
Hepatitis C virus NS5B gene for NS5 protein, partial cds, strain: H...	Hepacivir...	32.2	32.2	80%	7.2	100.00%	542	AB989413.1

For the reverse primer, there are many other viral species for which the query cover is 90% or higher, such as the porcine reproductive and respiratory syndrome virus. If we use the PCR test in a setting where these other viral species are unlikely to appear, the reverse primer will still be acceptable. A Nucleotide-BLAST search of the entire PCR product (250 nts in length) returns results that are all from the same viral species (i.e., simian foamy virus). Hence, the entire PCR product is workable. ▲

5.2.4 Reverse Transcription–Polymerase Chain Reaction (RT-PCR)

The first step of RNA sequencing is typically reverse transcription–PCR (RT-PCR), a PCR variant. RT-qPCR (quantitative real-time RT-PCR) is the standard technique for quantifying the concentration of a specific target RNA, which can be used to determine RNA viral loads (e.g., blood HIV concentration), assist the screening of RNA biomarkers, and analyze gene expressions.

RT-PCR first converts the target RNA strands into cDNA (complementary DNA) strands, which are ssDNA strands with sequences complementary to those of the target RNA—but with uracil (U) replaced with thymine (T). Next, RT-PCR amplifies the cDNA strands, creating enough copies to allow the cDNA to be sequenced. Since every cDNA strand is complementary to the target RNA strand, the cDNA sequence can be used to determine the target RNA sequence. Because the amplified concentration of cDNA strands depends directly on the initial concentration of the target RNA strand, we can use RT-qPCR to quantify the concentration of target RNA in the original sample.

RT-PCR relies on the use of reverse transcriptase (RT) enzyme, which uses each target RNA strand as a template to generate a cDNA strand, a process known as reverse transcription. There are different types of reverse transcriptase with different optimal reaction temperature ranges and RNase H activities. RNase H activity is the highly undesirable tendency of the reverse transcriptase to degrade the target RNA strand. Hence, we desire reverse transcriptase that have low RNase H activity.

Another complication of RT-PCR is the required reverse transcription primers. Reverse transcription (RT) primers are short sections of *single-stranded* DNA complementary to a part of the target RNA strand. There are three categories of reverse transcription primers used for RT-PCR: sequence-specific primers, oligo(dT) primers, and random hexamers. Each type of reverse transcription primer (as listed below) is usually used independently. However, oligo(dT) primers and random primers are often used together in a combination that is typically more effective than either oligo(dT) primers or random primers alone.[16]

- **Sequence-specific primers** are short ssDNA strands (roughly 20 nucleotides long), which are complementary to the 3' end of the desired portion of the target RNA strand. As the name suggests, sequence-specific primers are specific to the sequence of the target RNA strand, and their selection requires preliminary knowledge of a small portion of the target RNA sequence.

- **Oligo(dT) primers** are short ssDNA strands (about 12 to 18 nucleotides long) comprised of only thymine (T) bases (i.e., the sequence "TTTTT..."). Oligo(dT) primers are designed to bind to the 3' poly(A) tails of mRNA (messenger RNA). The 3' poly(A) tails are single-stranded RNA sequences containing only adenine (A) bases (i.e., the sequence "AAAAA...") commonly found at the 3' end of mRNA. mRNA strands contain the instructions for synthesizing proteins, and are created when cells transcribe ssDNA templates into complementary strands of mRNA. Poly(A) tails are used to control the stability of the mRNA strands in cellular organisms, and are hence almost universally found in eukaryotic mRNA. Oligo(dT) primers are not suitable for RNA strands that lack poly(A) tails.

- **Random primers**, also called random hexamers, are random sequences of ssDNA that are around six nucleotides long. Random primers bind to random parts of the target RNA strand, and are especially useful if the target RNA sequence is unknown and/or if the target RNA strands are degraded.

The procedure for RT-PCR (and RT-qPCR) is as follows.

<table>
<tr><td>

(1) *Reagents:* RT-PCR requires the following:
- ➤ The desired target RNA sample, which is purified to remove contaminating DNA as well as RNase enzymes (which degrade RNA).
- ➤ Free nucleotide bases (A, T, C, and G) in the form of deoxynucleotide triphosphates (dNTPs).
- ➤ Reverse transcriptase (RT) enzyme.
- ➤ Reverse transcription primers.
- ➤ Buffer solution with ions to control pH and charge concentration, and (**RT-qPCR only**) fluorescent probes such as organic fluorescent dyes or fluorescent intercalators.
- ➤ RT-PCR also requires additional reagents needed for regular PCR (or regular qPCR), which include
  - DNA polymerase enzyme.
  - Forward and reverse primers (about 20 nucleotides long) marking the beginning and end of the cDNA strands

</td></tr>
<tr><td>

(2) *Incubation:* The RNA sample in buffer solution is heated to uncoil the target RNA strands into a more linear form to allow the reverse transcription primers to attach.

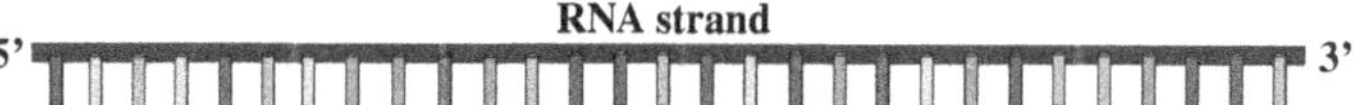

</td></tr>
<tr><td>

(3) *Annealing:* The sample is cooled quickly (via annealing) in the presence of the ssDNA reverse transcription primers, such that the primers will bind with the complementary sections of RNA.

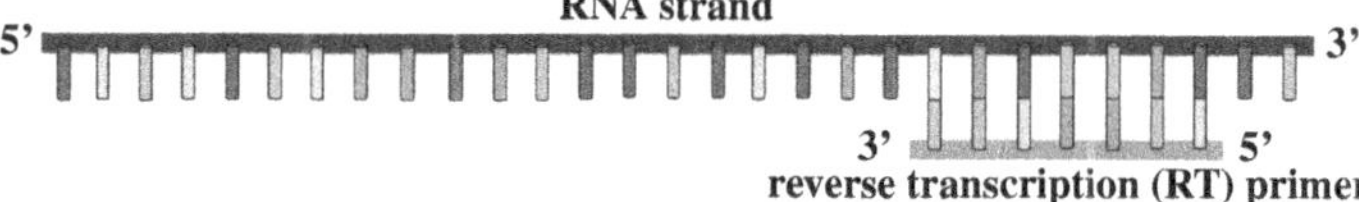

</td></tr>
<tr><td>

(4) *Reverse Transcription:* Reverse transcriptase moves along the strands starting at each primer, building complementary strands (from 5' to 3') of cDNA using the extra nucleotide bases (i.e., dNTPs) in the solution. The cDNA is complementary to the target RNA strand, but with uracil (U) replaced with thymine (T).

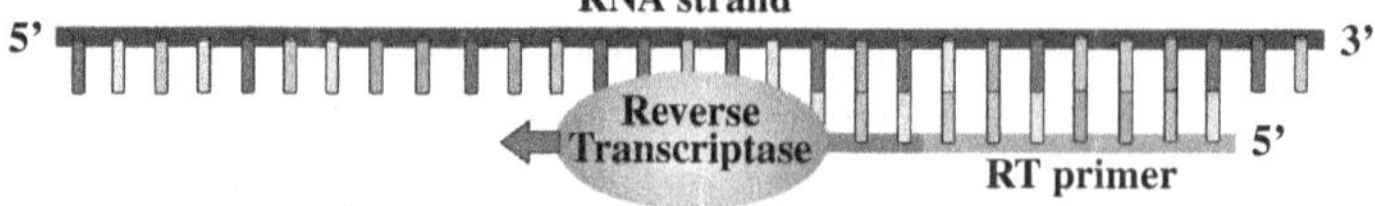

</td></tr>
<tr><td>

(5) *Dissociation and Enzyme Inactivation:* The buffer solution is heated to dissociate the target RNA strands from the cDNA strands. Because reverse transcriptase could interfere with the next step (i.e., cDNA amplification), it is usually necessary to heat-inactivate the reverse transcriptase enzymes in the solution with further heating.

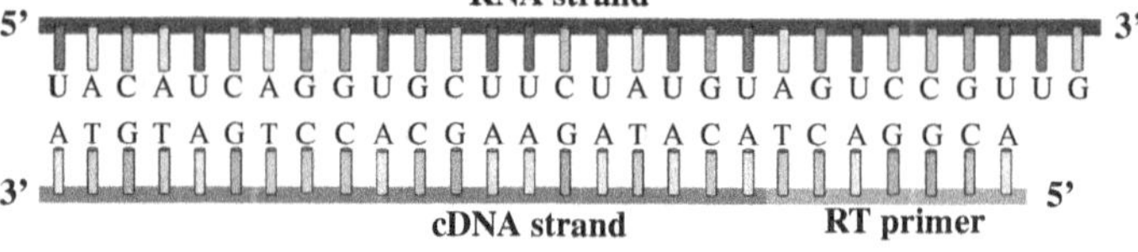

</td></tr>
</table>

(**6**) *cDNA Amplification:* The resulting strands of cDNA are amplified using regular PCR (or regular qPCR). Once enough copies of the cDNA have been produced, the cDNA can be sequenced using any DNA sequencing technique to determine the target RNA sequence.

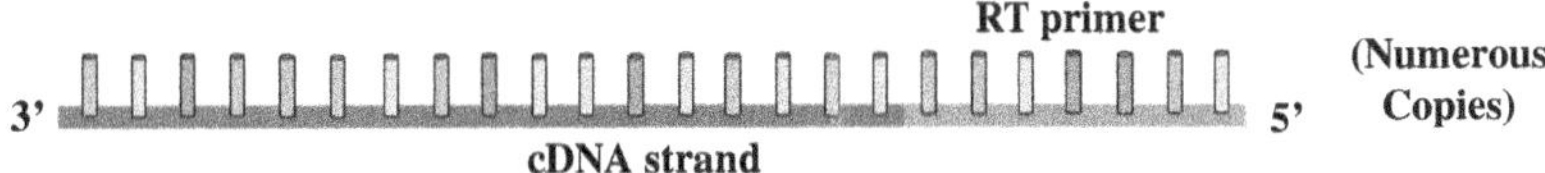

(**RT-qPCR Only**) The fluorescence intensity increases with every PCR cycle due to the fluorescent probes in the buffer solution attaching to the cDNA strands and their complementary ssDNA strands. Thus, the fluorescence intensity can be used to quantify the concentration of the cDNA product, and determine the initial target RNA concentration.

RT-PCR (and RT-qPCR) can be classified as one-step or two-step RT-(q)PCR. For one-step RT-(q)PCR, the DNA polymerase, forward primers, and reverse primers are all mixed into the initial buffer solution, allowing all of the steps of RT-(q)PCR to be completed in a single-reaction vessel. For two-step RT-(q)PCR, the cDNA created from reverse transcription is transferred to a secondary reaction vessel where cDNA amplification by regular PCR (or qPCR) is carried out. The one-step method is simpler, faster, and less prone to contamination, while the two-step method is more sensitive and more flexible.[17]

5.3 DETECTION OF DNA MUTATIONS

5.3.1 Heteroduplex Analysis (HA)

Heteroduplex analysis (HA) is a technique for determining the presence of mutations in selected DNA. HA is done by comparing the suspect DNA segment with a reference sample of the un-mutated DNA segment. The overall procedure for HA is as follows.

(**1**) The reference DNA sample (with sense strand "A" and antisense strand "a") and the suspect DNA sample ("B" and "b") are amplified using PCR.

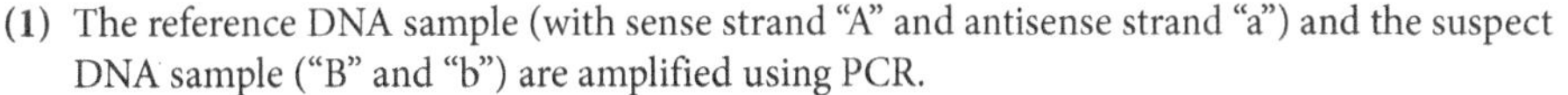

(**2**) The dsDNA samples are heated above their melting temperatures T_m to denature (i.e., dissociate) them into separate single strands of ssDNA.

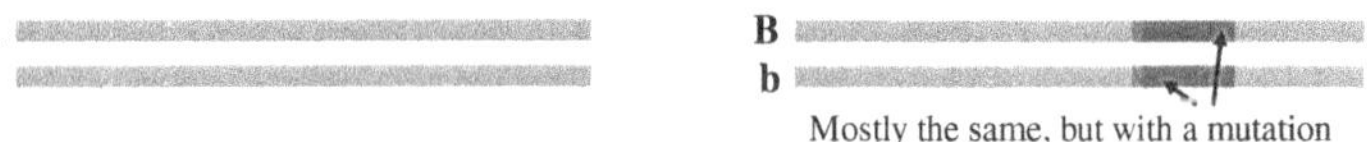

(**3**) The single strands of ssDNA are then cooled. This can result in the lowest energy configuration (Aa, Bb), but since the DNA samples are similar, some strands with the mutation can bond with the reference strands (Ab, Ba).

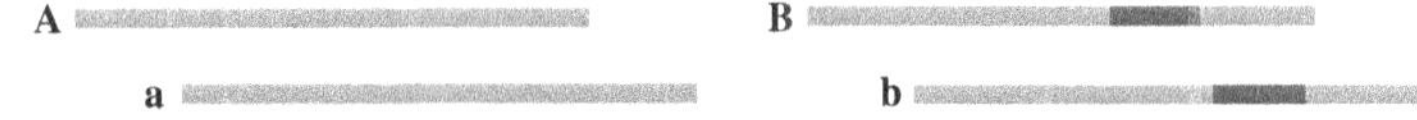

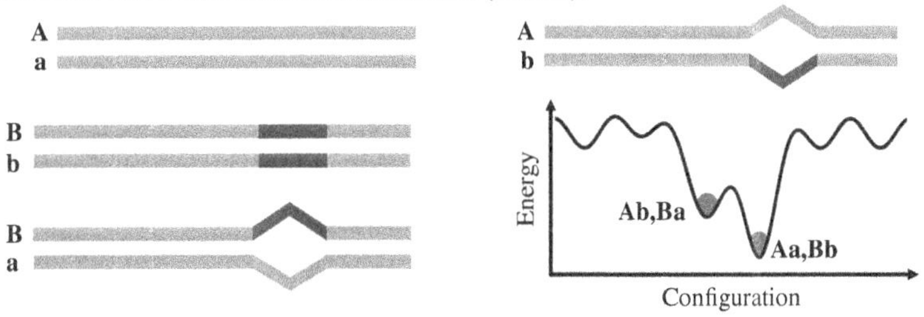

(**4**) The resulting dsDNA samples are analyzed using gel electrophoresis. In mismatched dsDNA (e.g., Ab, Ba), the mismatched sections consisting of wrongly paired bases will cause physical deformations in the DNA. The mismatches result in a lower electrophoretic mobility for dsDNA traveling through the gel during electrophoresis, and thus mismatched dsDNA (e.g., Ab, Ba) will arrive later than correctly matched dsDNA (e.g., Aa, Bb).

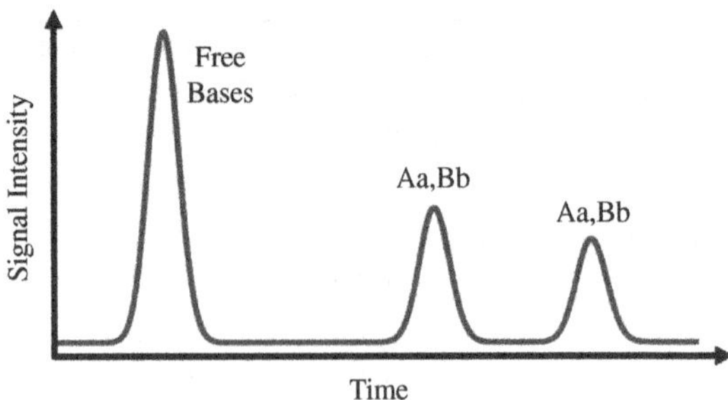

Figure 5-13 An example signal intensity versus time plot for heteroduplex analysis (HA). The presence of three peaks indicates that there are mutations detected in the DNA.

Figure 5-13 shows an example of the results of HA. The first peak is due to the remaining free nucleotide bases (i.e., dNTPs) from PCR. Since free nucleotide bases are small in comparison to strands of ssDNA, they travel significantly faster than ssDNA through the gel and show up as the first peak. As the concentration of free nucleotide bases is much higher than the concentration of ssDNA, the first peak due to the free bases is also the largest peak. The second peak is from the correctly matched dsDNA (e.g., Aa, Bb). Due to physical deformations in the mismatched dsDNA resulting in lower electrophoretic mobility, any mismatched dsDNA (e.g., Ab, Ba) will show up as a third peak. If there are only two peaks, no mutations are detected; if there are three peaks, as illustrated in Figure 5-13, there are mutations in the DNA.

While HA is easy to perform, there are a few disadvantages. First, HA requires a reference sample of DNA that is known not to contain the mutation. Second, HA can only detect the presence of a mutation, but not what the mutation is. Determining the exact nature of the mutation would require sequencing the DNA samples.

5.3.2 Single-Strand Conformation Polymorphism (SSCP)

Single-strand conformation polymorphism (SSCP) is a technique that is similar to heteroduplex analysis (HA). SSCP can be used to identify whether there are differences in DNA with similar lengths. The SSCP process is the same as that of HA, but instead of a final slow cooling (to bond Aa, Bb, Ab, and Ba), the system is snap cooled so that the DNA stays single-stranded. Single-stranded DNA will fold in on itself and take different shapes (3D geometries) through self-bonding. Different shapes of ssDNA have different electrophoretic mobilities and thus have different arrival times when analyzed with gel electrophoresis. As with HA, SSCP can only detect the presence or absence of a DNA mutation, but not the DNA sequence corresponding to the mutation.

5.4 DNA SEQUENCING

So far, we have discussed how to determine the presence or absence of mutations and whether there are differences in the nucleotide sequences of DNA samples. Now we move on to DNA sequencing. DNA sequencing is a process used to determine the exact order of nucleotide bases in a DNA sequence. There are a number of techniques for sequencing DNA, each having advantages and disadvantages.

5.4.1 Sanger DNA Sequencing

The Sanger DNA sequencing method (initially called "chain-termination" sequencing) was developed in 1977 by Frederick Sanger and his colleagues based on earlier work by Arthur

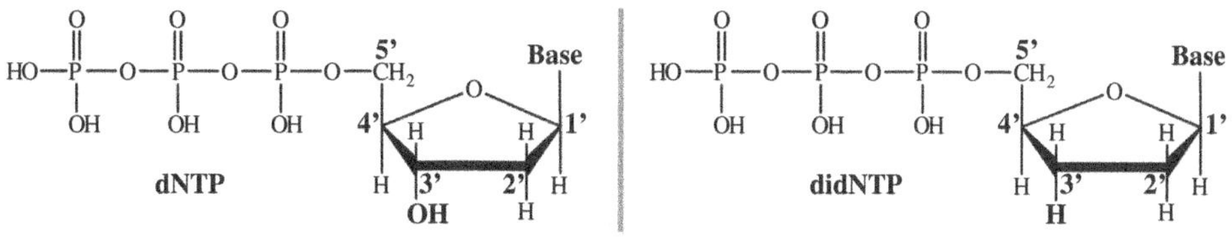

Figure 5-14   Molecular structure of dNTP (left) versus didNTP (right).

Kornberg on DNA replication.[18] Sanger sequencing is a useful and highly flexible process that can read long DNA sequences (>500 nucleotides), and avoids the use of hazardous chemicals, unlike the Maxam-Gilbert DNA sequencing method which will be discussed later. The Human Genome Project (1990 to 2003), which aimed to sequence all 3.2 billion base pairs of the entire human genome for the first time ever, used Sanger sequencing at a cost of ~$1 to $2 USD (inflation-adjusted) per base pair sequenced.[19] The Sanger sequencing process relies upon reading the DNA sequence from many copies (i.e., at least billions of copies) of a DNA fragment created either using a cloning vector (i.e., a bacterial plasmid or virus used to replicate the DNA fragment) or PCR. The sequences of many DNA fragments composing the desired section of DNA are then stitched together to produce the desired sequence. The disadvantage of the Sanger method is that a known primer is required for every DNA fragment to start the reaction.

Sanger sequencing relies on the use of di-deoxynucleotide triphosphates (didNTPs) together with deoxynucleotide triphosphates (dNTPs) as free nucleotide bases. As shown in Figure 5-14, the only difference between didNTPs and dNTPs is that dNTPs have a hydroxyl (−OH) functional group at the 3' carbon. Since DNA polymerase does not distinguish between didNTPs and dNTPs, the lack of a 3' hydroxyl functional group allows didNTPs to act as DNA chain terminators during DNA elongation by DNA polymerase.

During DNA synthesis by DNA polymerase, a new complementary DNA strand is synthesized using an existing ssDNA strand as a template and free nucleotide bases in the form of dNTPs and didNTPs. The hydroxyl (−OH) functional group at the 3' carbon of a dNTP forms an ester linkage (− O −) between two adjacent nucleotides. As with dNTPs, didNTPs are also able to attach to the newly formed single strands of DNA as they grow. However, as soon as a didNTP is incorporated, DNA polymerase is unable to add further bases to the existing nucleotides. Lacking the 3' hydroxyl group, a didNTP incorporated into the ssDNA chain cannot form an ester linkage with an incoming nucleotide. Therefore, ssDNA elongation by DNA polymerase is terminated as soon as a didNTP is incorporated, which is shown in Figure 5-15. The result is a series of terminated ssDNA sequences, each with a specific length and being terminated with a didNTP.

Initially, radioactively labeled didNTPs were used for Sanger sequencing, which required four separate reactions. Typical radioactive labels used are ^{33}P, ^{32}P, or ^{35}S. Both ^{33}P and ^{32}P are suitable radioactive labels because phosphorus (P) is found within the sugar-phosphate backbones of DNA as well as the triphosphate groups of didNTPs and dNTPs. Although sulfur (S) is not normally found in DNA or in free nucleotide bases (i.e., didNTPs and dNTPs), radioactive ^{35}S can replace oxygen (O) atoms within phosphate groups.

Sanger sequencing was greatly improved in 1986 by Lloyd Smith et al., who developed four different-colored fluorophores for fluorescently labeling every type of didNTP.[20] Fluorescently labeled didNTPs allow for single-reaction Sanger sequencing, enabling

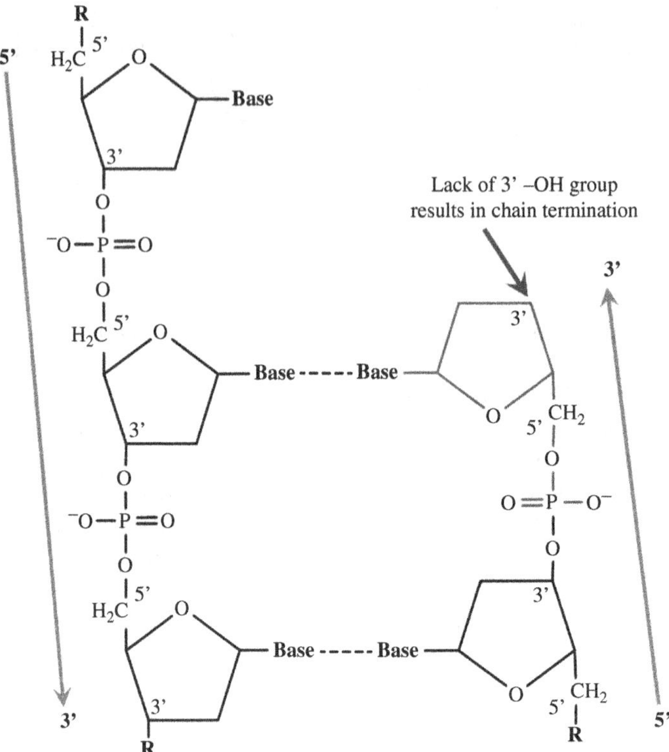

Figure 5-15   Lacking a 3' hydroxyl (–OH) group, a didNTP terminates the ssDNA chain.

high-throughput and automated DNA sequencing. The procedure for Sanger DNA sequencing is as follows.

---

(1) Sanger DNA sequencing requires the following:
➤ Many copies (at least billions) of the DNA template (i.e., fragment) to be sequenced, which can be created with a cloning vector or PCR.
➤ Many copies (at least billions) of a sequencing primer (a short ssDNA about 20 nucleotides long), which is complementary to the 3' end of either the sense strand or antisense strand of the DNA template.
➤ DNA polymerase and free nucleotide bases (A, T, C, and G) in the form of dNTPs and didNTPs. The didNTPs are either radioactively labeled or fluorescently labeled.

(2, Fluorescently Labeled Variant) Only a single reaction is required, containing
➤ Copies of the DNA template to be sequenced, copies of the sequencing primer (ssDNA about 20 nucleotides long), and DNA polymerase.
➤ Free nucleotide bases (A, T, C, and G) in the form of dNTPs.
➤ Four types of didNTPs (A, T, C, and G), each type being labeled with a different colored fluorophore.

(2, Radioactively Labeled Variant) Since there are four types of nucleotide base (A, T, C, and G), four separate reactions are required. Each reaction contains
➤ Copies of the DNA template to be sequenced, copies of the sequencing primer (ssDNA about 20 nucleotides long), and DNA polymerase.
➤ Free nucleotide bases (A, T, C, and G) in the form of dNTPs.

➤ One type of didNTP (A, T, C, or G) is added to each of the four reactions. The didNTPs are radioactively labeled.

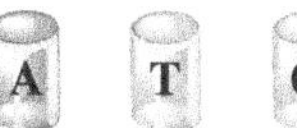

(3) Similar to PCR, the DNA sample is heated above its melting temperature to turn dsDNA into ssDNA. The sample is then cooled quickly (i.e., annealed), allowing the sequencing primers to bind with the complementary sections of ssDNA.

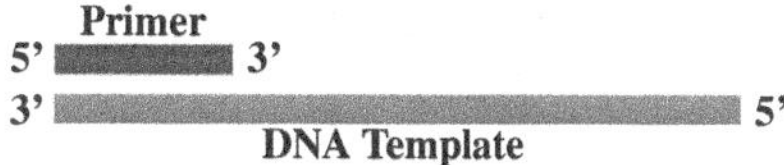

(4) DNA polymerase moves along the DNA strands from 5' to 3', building complementary strands using the extra nucleotide bases (dNTPs and didNTPs). Since DNA polymerase does not distinguish between dNTPs and didNTPs, the DNA synthesis reaction is terminated as soon as a didNTP is incorporated into an ssDNA strand.

(5) With billions of sample DNA molecules and sequencing primers present, the elongation reaction can be terminated at any position along the DNA sequence. If this DNA synthesis process runs for long enough and with the right ratio of dNTPs/didNTPs, the sample solution will eventually contain DNA segments that terminate at every base along the same sample DNA sequence.

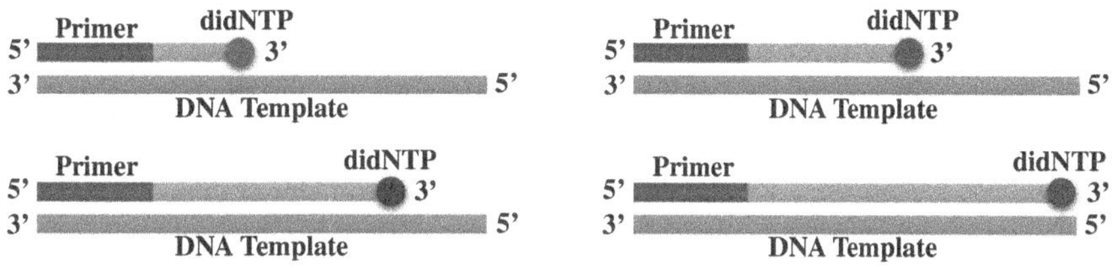

(6) Using polyacrylamide-urea gel, polyacrylamide gel electrophoresis (PAGE) is prepared. The urea prevents single-stranded DNA samples from recombining with each other (i.e., renaturing). As DNA molecules are negatively charged, they will migrate toward the positive electrode with electrophoretic mobilities dependent on molecular size. Shorter strands of ssDNA will move more quickly through the gel than longer strands of ssDNA.

(7, Fluorescently Labeled Variant) To perform gel electrophoresis, the reaction is loaded onto a single lane of polyacrylamide-urea gel. To visualize the resulting ssDNA bands, the single-lane gel is exposed to UV light. The four types of different fluorophore-labeled didNTPs will emit different colors of light corresponding to ssDNA segments with different termination didNTPs.

(7, Radioactively Labeled Variant) For gel electrophoresis, each of the four reactions is loaded onto a separate lane of polyacrylamide-urea gel. To keep track of ssDNA movement progress across the gel, a negatively charged visible dye that migrates slightly faster than smaller segments of ssDNA is added to all lanes. To visualize the ssDNA bands, X-ray film is exposed to the gel. The resulting dark bands in the X-ray film represent ssDNA segments of different lengths. The template DNA sequence is given by the sequence of bands in the four lanes.

(8) The resulting ssDNA sequence bands from gel electrophoresis (i.e., PAGE) are read from the positive (+) electrode toward the negative (−) electrode (Figure 5-16). A sequence consisting of up to ~800 base pairs can be read in one iteration of Sanger DNA sequencing. The Sanger sequencing method sequences ssDNA in the 5' to 3' direction, starting at the first nucleotide past the 3' end of the primer. Note that the sequencing primers are *never* sequenced, since the primers do not contain any didNTP.

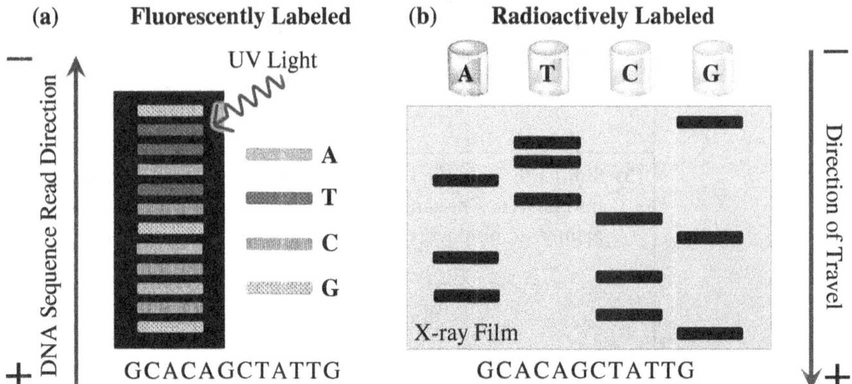

Figure 5-16 Reading the DNA sequence generated by the Sanger sequencing method from (a) visible light emissions from UV-illuminated gel containing fluorescently labeled didNTPs and (b) X-ray film exposed by gel containing radioactively labeled didNTPs. The negative (−) electrode is located at the top, while the positive (+) electrode is located at the bottom. Hence, the negatively charged ssDNA strands travel from top to bottom, while the DNA sequence is read from bottom to top.

5.4.2 Maxam-Gilbert DNA Sequencing

The Maxam-Gilbert DNA sequencing method was developed by Walter Gilbert and Allan Maxam in 1977.[21] It is a chemical cleavage method, which directly "chops up" the DNA at specific bases based on the chemical cleavers used. Unlike Sanger sequencing, Maxam-Gilbert sequencing acts on copies of the purified DNA samples alone and does not require any primers, DNA polymerase, or free nucleotide bases (i.e., no dNTPs or didNTPs). Hence, Maxam-Gilbert sequencing was initially more popular than Sanger sequencing. However, the Maxam-Gilbert sequencing method is labor-intensive (i.e., technically complex); it uses hazardous chemicals extensively; it can only sequence short DNA sequences; it is slow, and it requires a large amount of sample DNA. Owing to these weaknesses, Maxam-Gilbert sequencing was eventually replaced by Sanger sequencing in most applications after improvements for the Sanger sequencing method were established. Today, Maxam-Gilbert sequencing is only used in specialized applications such as studies of DNA-protein interactions (DNA footprinting), nucleic acid structure, and epigenetic modifications to DNA. For their contributions on the determination of base sequences in nucleic acids, Frederick Sanger and Walter Gilbert were awarded the Nobel Prize in Chemistry in 1980.

Maxam-Gilbert sequencing relies on the chemical cleavage of ssDNA at specific nucleotide bases, as shown in Figure 5-17. The ssDNA chemical cleavage process consists of two steps. In the first step, the glycosidic bond linking a nucleotide base with the sugar-phosphate backbone is cleaved (i.e., broken), removing the base from the ssDNA. In the second step, the phosphodiester linkage exposed by the removed base is cleaved. As a result, the initial ssDNA strand is cleaved into two strands. Since the initial ssDNA strand is labeled only at one end (the 5' end), only one of the two resulting ssDNA strands from the cleavage will be labeled.

Depending on the chemical mixture used for DNA cleavage, the specificity of the process can be controlled because the chemical mixture used determines the type of nucleotide base (or bases) at which ssDNA cleavage occurs. Commonly used chemical mixtures and

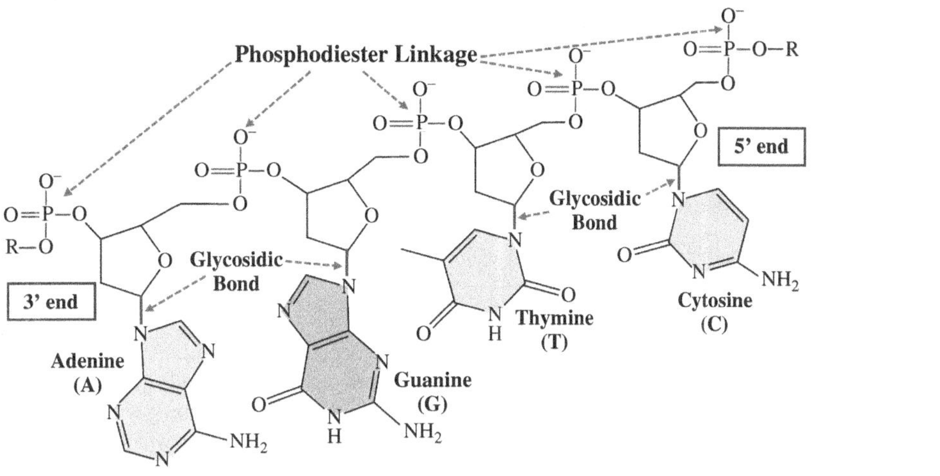

Figure 5-17   The molecular structure of ssDNA illustrating the glycosidic bonds and phosphodiester linkages cleaved during Maxam-Gilbert sequencing.

TABLE 5-1   Chemical Mixtures and Their Base-Specific ssDNA Cleavage[21]

Chemical Mixture	Base Specificity during ssDNA Cleavage
DMS (dimethyl sulfate) + Piperidine	Guanine (G)
DMS (dimethyl sulfate) + Piperidine in formic acid	Adenine (A) and Guanine (G)
Hydrazine + Piperidine	Cytosine (C) and Thymine (T)
Hydrazine + Piperidine in 2M NaCl	Cytosine (C)

their base-specific cleavage are shown in Table 5-1. For instance, hydrazine plus piperidine will cleave ssDNA at both cytosine (C) and thymine (T) nucleotide base sites, while DMS plus piperidine will cleave ssDNA only at guanine (G) nucleotide base sites. The procedure for Maxam-Gilbert DNA sequencing is as follows.

(1) Maxam-Gilbert DNA sequencing requires the following:
- ➤ Many copies (at least billions) of the DNA template (i.e., fragment) to be sequenced, which can be created with a cloning vector or PCR. The desired ssDNA template to be sequenced, which can either be the sense strand or antisense strand of the dsDNA template, is radioactively labeled with ^{32}P at the 5' end.
- ➤ Four different chemical mixtures (Table 5-1) with different base specificity during ssDNA cleavage.

(2) The DNA sample is heated above its melting temperature to turn dsDNA into ssDNA. Next, four separate reactions are prepared, with each reaction containing at least billions of copies of the labeled ssDNA template and one of the four chemical mixtures.

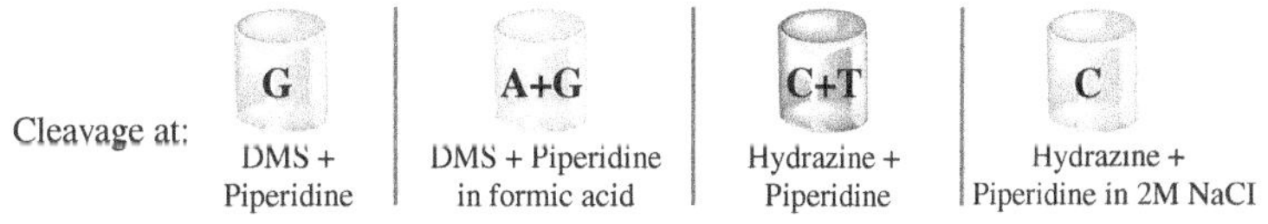

Cleavage at:

G	A+G	C+T	C
DMS + Piperidine	DMS + Piperidine in formic acid	Hydrazine + Piperidine	Hydrazine + Piperidine in 2M NaCl

(3) With billions of ssDNA template molecules present in each one of the four reactions, the ssDNA template will be cleaved at every possible nucleotide base allowed by each chemical mixture. Since only one end (the 5' end) of the ssDNA template molecules are labeled, only one of the two resulting ssDNA strands from each cleavage will be labeled.

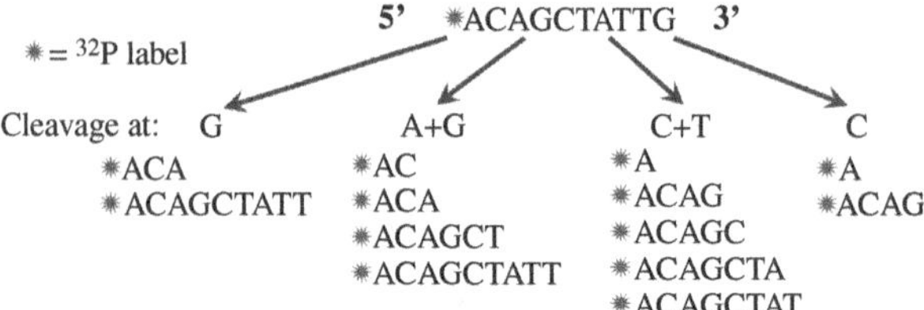

(4) Using polyacrylamide-urea gel, polyacrylamide gel electrophoresis (PAGE) is prepared. The urea prevents ssDNA samples from recombining with each other (i.e., renaturing). As DNA molecules are always negatively charged, they will migrate toward the positive electrode with electrophoretic mobilities dependent on molecular size. Shorter strands of ssDNA will move more quickly through the gel than longer strands of ssDNA.

(5) For gel electrophoresis, each of the four reactions is loaded onto a separate lane of polyacrylamide-urea gel. To keep track of ssDNA movement progress across the gel, a negatively charged visible dye that migrates slightly faster than smaller fragments of ssDNA can be added to all lanes. To visualize the ssDNA bands, X-ray film is exposed to the gel. The resulting dark bands in the X-ray film represent ssDNA fragments of different lengths. The template DNA sequence is given by the sequence of bands in the four lanes.

(6) The resulting ssDNA sequence bands from gel electrophoresis (i.e., PAGE) are read from the positive (+) electrode toward the negative (−) electrode (Figure 5-18). A DNA sequence consisting of up to ~500 base pairs can be read in one iteration of Maxam-Gilbert sequencing. The Maxam-Gilbert sequencing method sequences ssDNA in the 5' to 3' direction because the ssDNA strands that produce bands are radioactively labeled at the 5' end.

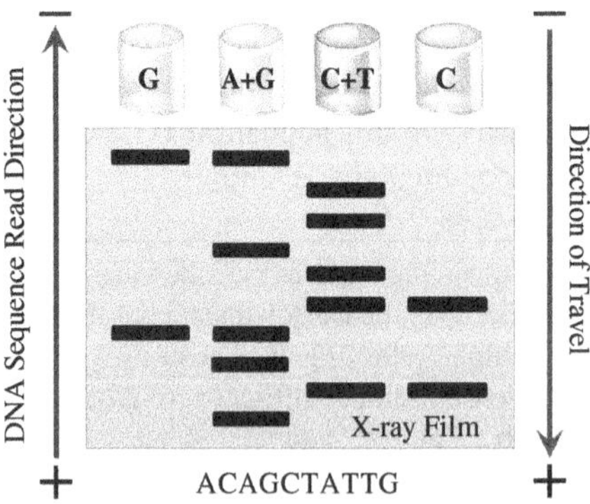

Figure 5-18   Reading the DNA sequence generated using the Maxam-Gilbert sequencing method from X-ray film exposed by gel containing radioactively (^{32}P)-labeled ssDNA. The negative (−) electrode is located at the top, while the positive (+) electrode is located at the bottom. Hence, the negatively charged ssDNA strands travel from top to bottom, while the DNA sequence is read from bottom to top.

In summary, Maxam-Gilbert DNA sequencing allows us to break (i.e., cleave) copies of an ssDNA strand at specific nucleotide bases using base-specific chemical reagents and conditions. The labeled ssDNA fragments then undergo four-lane electrophoresis in a polyacrylamide-urea gel with autoradiography to determine the DNA sequence. After gel electrophoresis, the locations of ssDNA fragments correspond to their molecular size as well as the nucleotide base at which chemical cleavage occurred, allowing the DNA template to be sequenced.

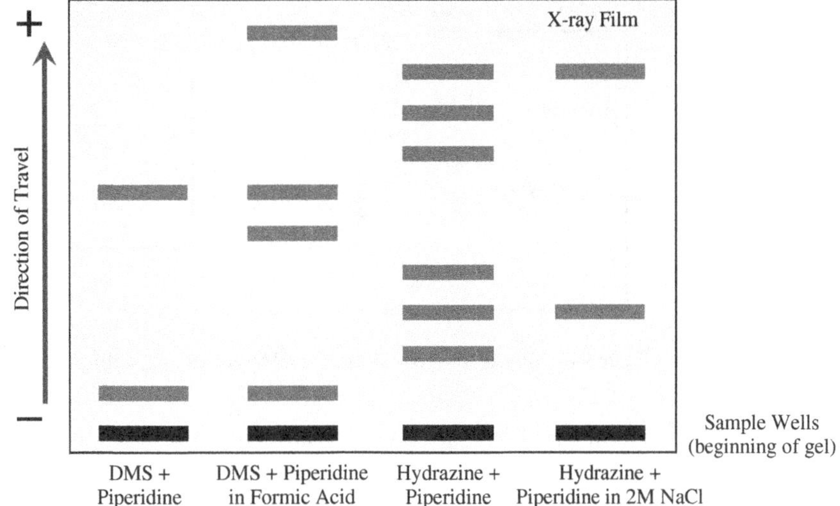

Figure 5-19   Four-lane gel electrophoresis results generated from Maxam-Gilbert sequencing.

EXAMPLE 5-4
Maxam-Gilbert
Sequencing

Using the Maxam-Gilbert method, one 10-nts-(nucleotides)-long section of ssDNA was sequenced. The four-lane gel electrophoresis results are shown in Figure 5-19, where each lane corresponds to one type of ssDNA reaction (i.e., cleavage) with a different chemical mixture (Table 5-1). The ssDNA samples are originally placed at the bottom and migrate upward through the gel. What is the ssDNA sequence?

Solution

Cleavage at:

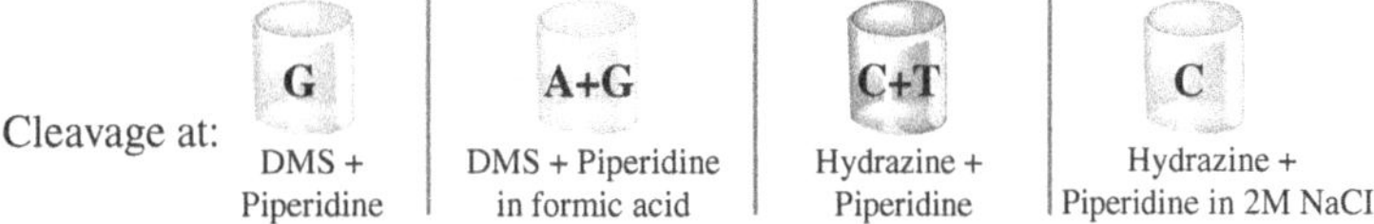

During gel electrophoresis for Maxam-Gilbert sequencing, the shortest strands of ssDNA travel the furthest through the gel. Therefore, to determine the sequence, the gel is read in a direction opposite to the direction of travel. In this case, the sequence is read from top to bottom. Note that the four bands of the bottom row are the DNA sample wells. The first ssDNA band must correspond to A as it appears in the A+G column, but not in the G column. The next band must correspond to C, since it appears in both the C+T and C columns. Repeating this procedure, the final sequence is "ACTTGATCTG" (5′ to 3′).   ▲

5.4.3 Second and Third Generation DNA Sequencing

Sanger sequencing and Maxam-Gilbert sequencing belong to the first-generation of DNA sequencing methods. Second-generation DNA sequencing, sometimes referred to as next-generation DNA sequencing, differs from first-generation sequencing in several key aspects. Second-generation DNA sequencing utilizes automated, miniaturized, and parallelized platforms to sequence DNA, reducing the cost and time required for DNA sequencing by many orders of magnitude compared to first-generation sequencing. In second-generation sequencing, the DNA to be sequenced is broken into DNA fragments of 50 to 400 bases each, and these DNA fragments are simultaneously sequenced allowing millions to billions of nucleotide bases to be sequenced in a single run.

Recently, third-generation DNA sequencing methods have been developed. Compared with the second-generation methods, third-generation methods can handle DNA sequences that are several orders of magnitude longer. The increased read length is the key

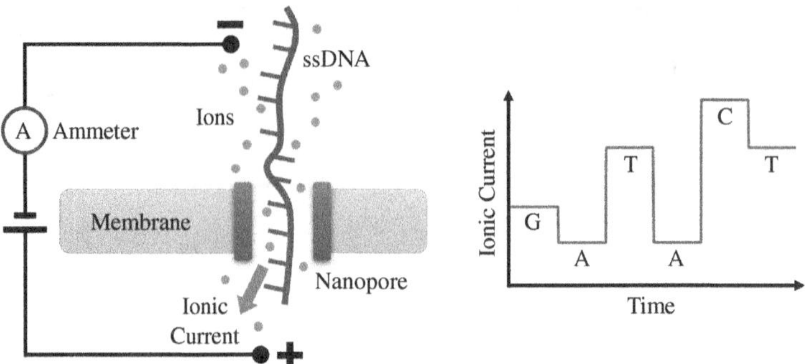

Figure 5-20   Illustration of nanopore DNA sequencing, a third-generation DNA sequencing method.

advantage of third-generation sequencing. Moreover, third-generation sequencing is more sensitive. It is able to sequence DNA more quickly than second-generation sequencing, and it can be carried out with smaller and more portable equipment. The additional sensitivity may allow epigenetic markers (i.e., biomolecules that regulate the expression of genes) to be detected in addition to DNA nucleotide bases.[22]

An example of a third-generation DNA sequencing method is nanopore DNA sequencing, as shown in Figure 5-20. Nanopore sequencing can sequence both DNA and RNA without requiring labeling or DNA/RNA amplification. Nanopores are pores (i.e., holes/orifices) that are nanometers in size, and can be created as holes in a metal alloy or a semiconductor, or with pore-forming proteins. Nanopore sequencing relies on electrophoresis to transport single-stranded DNA or RNA samples along with a steady supply of ions through a nanopore. The movement of each nucleotide in the sample through the orifice creates a distinct electric signal by disrupting the flow of the ion supply in a unique fashion, allowing the DNA or RNA sequence to be determined. Thus, nanopores can be used as molecular transducers, and nanopore sequencing technology could potentially replace current sequencing technologies in the future. As with other third-generation sequencing methods, nanopore sequencing technology could significantly reduce the time and expense involved in current sequencing methods, especially for large sequences such as the human genome.[23]

Early nanopore sequencing work by Vercoutere et al. involved the use of α-hemolysin nanopores in a lipid bilayer to detect single base pair (bp) differences in hairpin DNA molecules. A hairpin DNA molecule is an ssDNA molecule with complimentary ends, so that its two ends bind together (i.e., folds on itself) like a hairpin. As the hairpin DNA travels through the narrow 1.5 nm diameter portion of the nanopore, the ssDNA unfolds, creating ion current change that is detected. This allows different DNA sequences to be discriminated down to one base pair resolution by reading the changes in ionic current as the ssDNA moves through the pore.[24]

5.5 RNA SEQUENCING AND SYNTHESIS

RNA Sequencing   RNA sequencing is used to determine the exact order of nucleotide bases in an RNA strand. Applications of RNA sequencing include—but are not limited to—studying gene expressions, determining the genomes and mutations of RNA viruses (e.g., coronaviruses, influenza, rabies, HIV, and hepatitis C), and screening for RNA biomarkers resulting from diseases such as cancer and diabetes.

The first step of RNA sequencing is usually RT-PCR (refer to Section 5.2.4). RT-PCR first converts the target RNA strands into cDNA strands, which are ssDNA strands with sequences complementary to that of the target RNA—but with uracil (U) replaced with thymine (T). Then, RT-PCR amplifies the cDNA strands, creating enough copies to allow the cDNA to be sequenced. The cDNA can be sequenced with any DNA sequencing method, but is most commonly sequenced with next-generation DNA sequencing methods. Since every cDNA strand is complementary to the target RNA strand, the cDNA sequence is used to determine the target RNA sequence.

As an example, assume that the cDNA sequence was determined to be:

$$\text{cDNA sequence} = \text{ACCGA TCTAT CTGAT} \ (5' \text{ to } 3')$$

The complementary ssDNA sequence is ATCAG ATAGA TCGGT (5' to 3')

To obtain the target RNA sequence, we simply replace thymine (T) with uracil (U):

$$\text{target RNA sequence} = \text{AUCAG AUAGA UCGGU} \ (5' \text{ to } 3')$$

RNA Synthesis   Aside from RNA sequencing and quantifying the concentration of target RNA, there are applications where we want to synthesize numerous copies of RNA with a specific sequence. Common applications of RNA synthesis include creating sufficient copies of guide RNA for CRISPR gene editing, or synthesizing RNA therapeutics such as cancer immunotherapy treatments and mRNA-based vaccines. There are two popular methods for synthesizing numerous copies of RNA. Both methods involve the use of RNA polymerase, which uses an ssDNA template to transcribe (i.e., generate) a complementary single-stranded RNA sequence. In all living cellular organisms, RNA polymerase enzymes are used to transcribe ssDNA templates into RNA strands (e.g., mRNA which contain the blueprints for synthesizing proteins essential for survival). Hence, there are numerous different kinds of RNA polymerase, which are naturally found in all living cellular organisms (including humans) and even in many viruses.

While DNA polymerase and reverse transcriptase enzymes require primers to initiate ssDNA extension/elongation, RNA polymerase instead requires the ssDNA template to have a promoter region (i.e., a specific ssDNA sequence) located at the upstream end of the transcription-initiation site. RNA polymerase binds to the promoter portion of the ssDNA template, and transcribes the complementary RNA strand from 5' to 3'. Different RNA polymerase enzymes require different promoter sequences. In cellular organisms, promoter regions are found upstream of RNA-coding sequences in a gene and signal the starting site at which RNA should be transcribed (Figure 5-21). To synthesize sufficient copies of the desired RNA sequence, we require enough copies of the complementary ssDNA sequence, which must each contain a promoter region with a sequence compatible with the type of RNA polymerase used. The chosen type of RNA polymerase must also have a suitable active temperature range.[25]

Plasmid Vector-Based RNA Synthesis   The first method is to clone the complementary ssDNA sequence corresponding to the desired RNA sequence into plasmid vectors, which are small extrachromosomal DNA commonly found in bacteria. The ssDNA sequence must have a suitable promoter at the upstream end. Then, the plasmids are introduced into

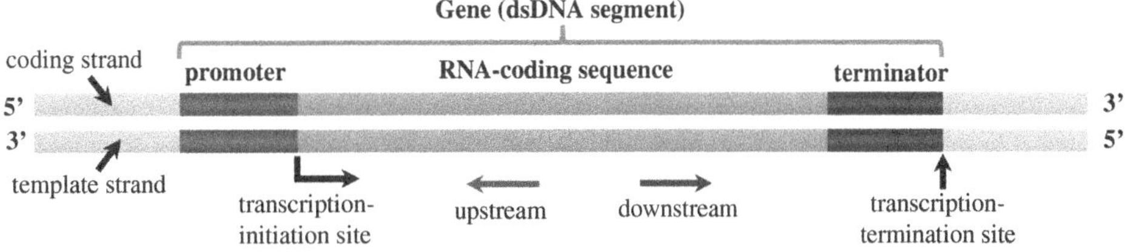

Figure 5-21   A gene (a segment of dsDNA) consists of a promoter at the upstream end where transcription begins, an RNA-coding sequence, and a terminator at the downstream end where transcription ends. The coding (sense) strand of the gene has the same sequence as the transcribed RNA, while the template (antisense) strand of the gene is used as a complementary template for the transcription of RNA.

bacterial cells. When the bacterial cells replicate, the inserted DNA sequence will also replicate "naturally." Using RNA polymerase, multiplied copies of the inserted DNA sequence is used to transcribe many copies of the desired RNA sequence. Some commercial plasmid vector transcription kits contain multiple phage polymerase promoters to allow the use of different phage-derived RNA polymerase. The downside of this method is that it requires 1 to 2 weeks to complete; the longer period results in a higher likelihood of off-target effects and integration of the plasmid DNA into the bacterial cells may cause cell death.

In Vitro *RNA Synthesis*   The second method uses *in vitro* transcription. This method requires designing an ssDNA template complementary to the desired RNA sequence (but with nucleotide base U replaced with T) with a suitable promoter at the upstream end. Next, PCR (as described in Section 5.2) is used to create many copies of the ssDNA template. Finally, RNA polymerase is used to transcribe many copies of the desired RNA sequence from copies of the ssDNA template. *In vitro* RNA synthesis generates copies of the desired RNA sequence outside of the cell and takes 1 to 3 days to complete. However, this method can sometimes be difficult to use and is potentially more prone to errors. Commercial lab kits are available for carrying out *in vitro* RNA synthesis.

5.6 DNA SELF-ASSEMBLY

The complementary sections of a single strand of DNA or RNA can bind together to reach a lower energy configuration, resulting in self-folded structures. The final conformation (i.e., shape and structure) of the strand is completely determined by the nucleotide base sequence. Therefore, it is possible to create extended structures with controlled 3D configurations. This self-folding is not just limited to single strands of DNA or RNA, and multiple strands can be combined to form more complex structures. Complementary sections of strands (either self-folded or from two separate strands) bind together without any defects, but mismatched bases in sequences that bind together may cause defects which change the shape of the extended structure (Figure 5-22).

Different strategies can be employed to make complex DNA nanostructures. To start the fabrication process, a short ssDNA segment protruding from a dsDNA strand, known as a sticky end, can be used to bond to other sticky ends. Each sticky end may be attached to a longer double helix chain of dsDNA to make longer chains or junctions. Four-armed DNA junctions composed of four dsDNA arms which are joined together, known as Holliday junctions, can be used to make 2D DNA sheets known as DNA tiles. The DNA tiles have a number of free sticky ends and can be used to make 2D or 3D structures referred to as DNA lattices. DNA can also be shaped into pre-defined geometric structures (e.g., templates or scaffolds) which can arrange target molecules (both inorganic and organic) into a desired shape, enabling applications such as molecular transporters, biosensors, and drug delivery vehicles.[26-28]

A specific form of DNA nanotechnology is DNA origami. The process begins by shaping viral ssDNA into a scaffold to create a backbone which is held together by shorter segments of DNA called staples. Each staple supports the 2D or 3D DNA structure by binding to a specific region of the DNA structure following DNA base pairing rules. The scaffold

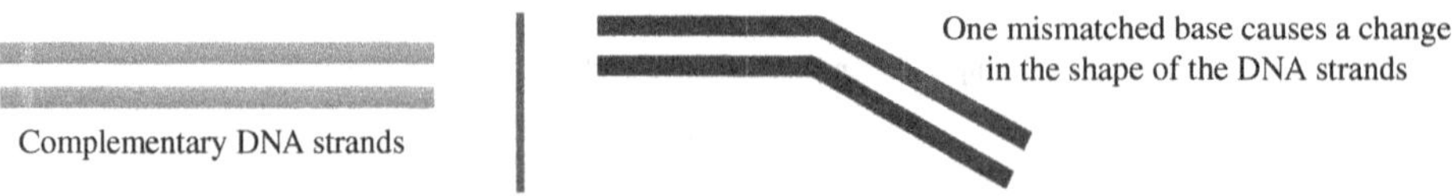

Figure 5-22   By utilizing mismatched bases, DNA nanostructures with predefined shapes and geometries can be self-assembled.

and staples are heated and then slowly cooled to ensure proper bonding. The methods for creating 2D and 3D DNA origami in increasingly complicated shapes are detailed as follows.

2D DNA Origami: The scaffold is formed from a single ssDNA strand. DNA staples, with free sticky ends, are used to define the shape. Heating the structure finalizes the shape of the origami. The figures are reprinted with permission from P. W. K. Rothemund.[29]

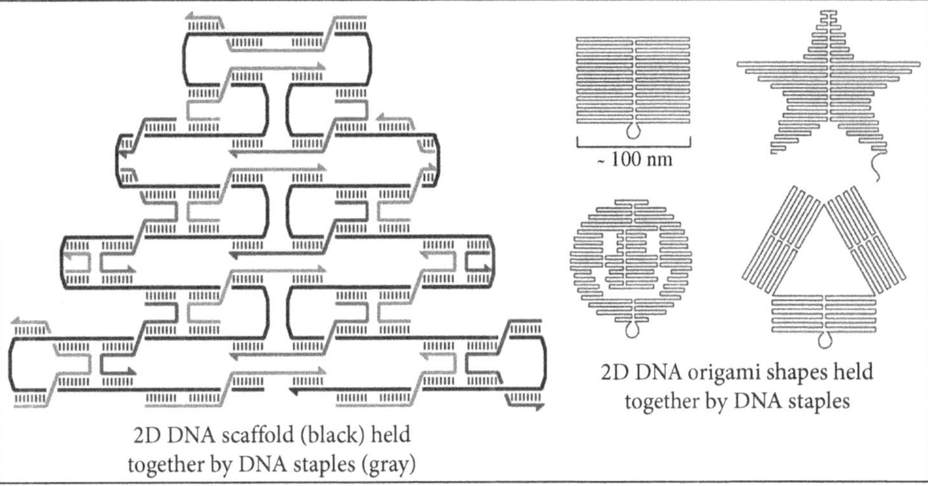

~ 100 nm

2D DNA origami shapes held together by DNA staples

2D DNA scaffold (black) held together by DNA staples (gray)

3D DNA Origami: Multiple layers of 2D DNA origami shapes can be assembled to form 3D structures. Commonly used shapes are square or honeycomb shapes. Each cylinder shown below is comprised of a double-stranded DNA sequence. The figures are reprinted with permission from C. E. Castro et al.[30]

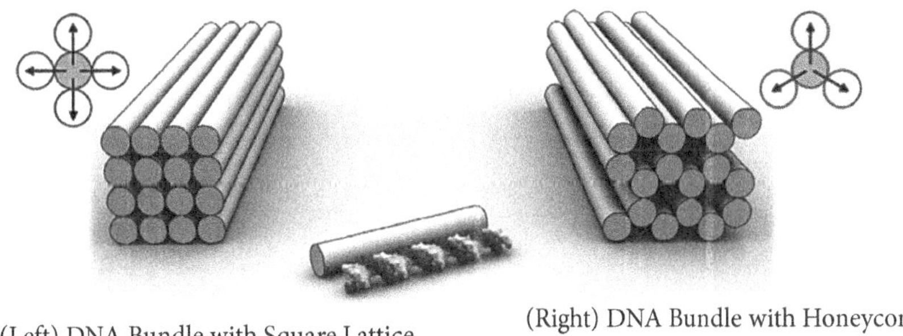

(Left) DNA Bundle with Square Lattice

(Right) DNA Bundle with Honeycomb Lattice

Curved DNA Structures: Curved DNA structures can be created by inserting or deleting nucleotides in the double-stranded DNA "cylinders" shown above. As shown below on the left, the orange cylinders have fewer bases than the blue cylinders, making their curvature more noticeable. The figures are reprinted with permission from H. Dietz et al.[31]

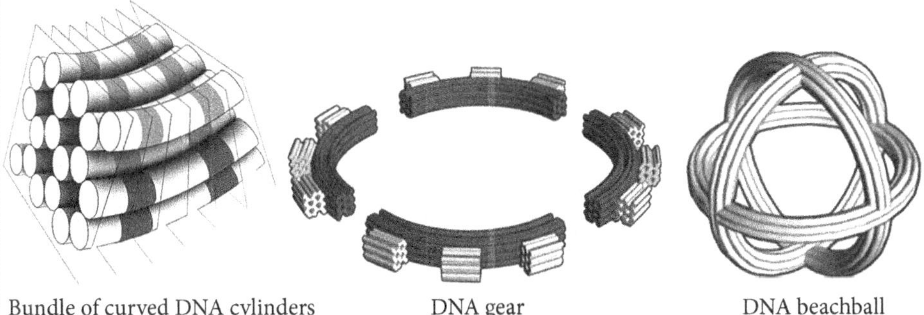

Bundle of curved DNA cylinders   DNA gear   DNA beachball

DNA Bricks: DNA bricks can be formed using small scaffolds. The bricks can then be assembled without the need for additional scaffolds, permitting the formation of more complex shapes. The figures are reprinted with permission from Y. Ke et al.[32]

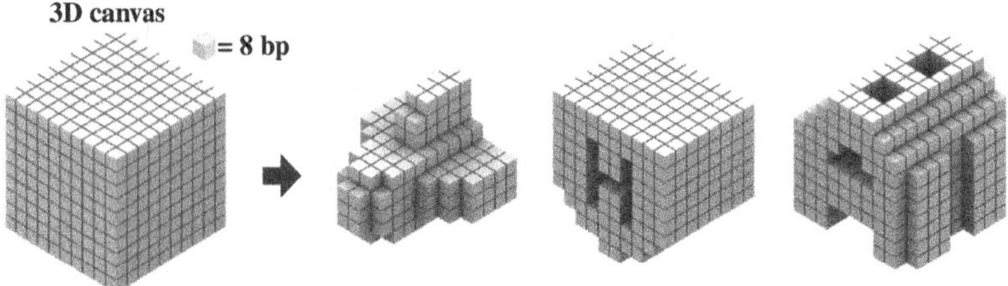

LEGO®-like nano-shapes formed from DNA bricks

DNA Gridirons: DNA Holliday junctions can be used to create vertices and enclose more complex 3D shapes, known as DNA gridirons. The vertices of a DNA gridiron are bound together by multiple scaffold strands. The figures are reprinted with permission from D. Han et al.[33]

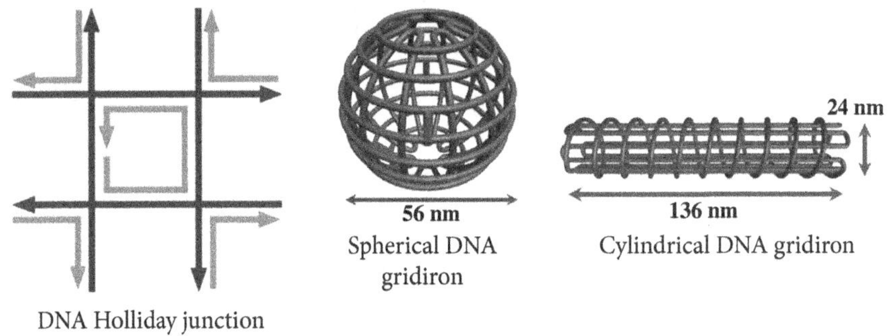

DNA Holliday junction   Spherical DNA gridiron   Cylindrical DNA gridiron

Complex DNA Structures: More complex DNA scaffolds can be manufactured by mapping a 3D polyhedral mesh designed with the assistance of computer software to actual DNA. As with 2D DNA origami, staples are then added and the structure is heated to form a DNA nanostructure. The figures are reprinted with permission from E. Benson et al.[34]

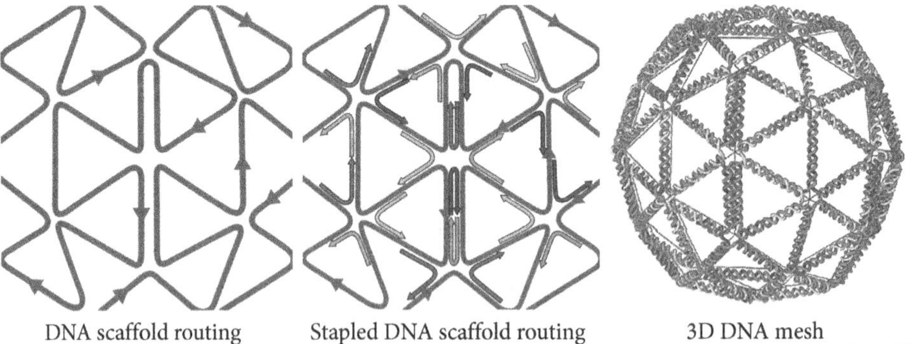

DNA scaffold routing   Stapled DNA scaffold routing   3D DNA mesh

Using any combination of the strategies above, 2D or 3D DNA nanostructures of a designated shape or form can be fabricated. These engineered DNA nanostructures can be used as drug delivery vehicles, which are used to minimize toxicity, increase drug solubility, and add cell-targeting capabilities. To use DNA nanostructures in this context, the DNA must be constructed into pre-defined shapes such as boxes or other hollow geometries into which genes, drugs, or nanoparticles can be loaded. The advantage of using DNA nanostructures is that they are inherently biocompatible, and can overcome biological barriers such as the immune response. Furthermore, DNA nanostructures can facilitate the uptake of cancer-targeting agents that would otherwise not pass into the cell.

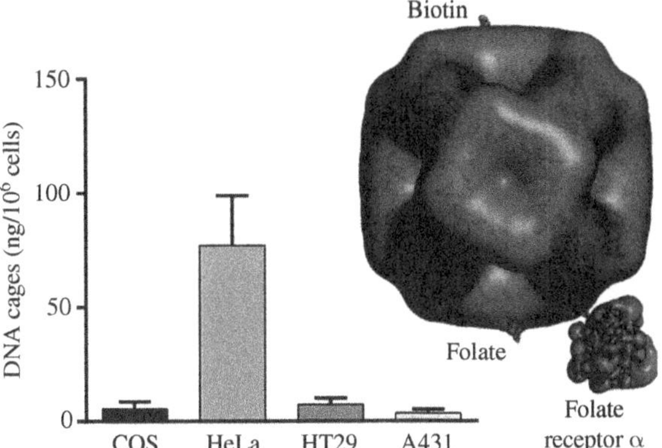

Figure 5-23 DNA nanocages for targeted cancer drug delivery. (Left) Histogram of DNA nanocage concentration in different cell type populations. (Right) Electrostatic potential distribution of a DNA nanocage containing doxorubicin as it binds to the folate receptor α, the target molecule used to identify cancer cells. (*The images are reprinted with permission from S. Raniolo et al.*[35])

The shape programmability of DNA nanostructures allows them to be carefully designed for the biological environments they will encounter *in vitro* and *in vivo*. For example, even though DNA nanostructures may be promising for drug delivery or cancer detection, they may be rendered useless if they are unable to survive the chemical or physical conditions in biological environments, such as variable pH levels. Furthermore, the physical and chemical properties of a given DNA nanostructure may be modified when specific loads (e.g., drugs) are carried, such as the increased stimulatory activity of DNA tetrahedral nanostructures with larger payloads.

Crucially, DNA nanostructures designed for drug delivery must also effectively transport and release therapeutic agents. DNA nanostructures can be designed to gradually release their contents over a lifetime of a 12- to 62-hour period within cell-like environments.[26] Whether the contents are toxic cancer drugs such as doxorubicin or gene suppressants such as specifically designed RNA strands, the nanostructure must be able to protect its contents from the body's defense mechanisms (e.g., the immune response) and harsh conditions. Moreover, the drug-carrying nanostructures must also protect the body's healthy cells and tissues from the impact of the carried drugs. The drugs carried by the nanostructures should not be released until they have reached the targeted cancer sites. To deliver these payloads for providing therapeutic treatment of cancer, DNA nanostructures must be able to sense cancer cells. Effectively identifying and targeting cancer cells usually rely on biochemical signals. Once reaching the targeted cells, the nanostructures should either freely enter or penetrate the targeted cells. This problem involves either designing a way to forcefully create an entry through cancer cells or killing them from the outside.

Figure 5-23 shows a DNA nanocage design for targeted doxorubicin (a cancer medication) delivery. Because HeLa cells—a cancerous cell line—have overexpressed (i.e., far more copies than normal) folate receptor α, they absorb up to 40 times more folate-functionalized DNA nanocages than cells without folate receptor α. Once the DNA nanocages are absorbed by the cancerous cells, the nanocages automatically disintegrate to release doxorubicin. This process occurs without any additional stimuli to the DNA nanocages since the pH conditions found within the cellular cytoplasm degrade the nanocages naturally.[35]

5.7 DNA TWEEZERS

DNA tweezers were invented at Bell Laboratories in the year 2000, and could be potentially applied in targeted drug/gene delivery, microsurgery, and molecular/nanoscale device assembly. They can be opened or closed by changing the configuration of the DNA. The main structure of DNA tweezers is made of three single-stranded DNA segments, namely A, B and C, as shown in Figure 5-24.[36]

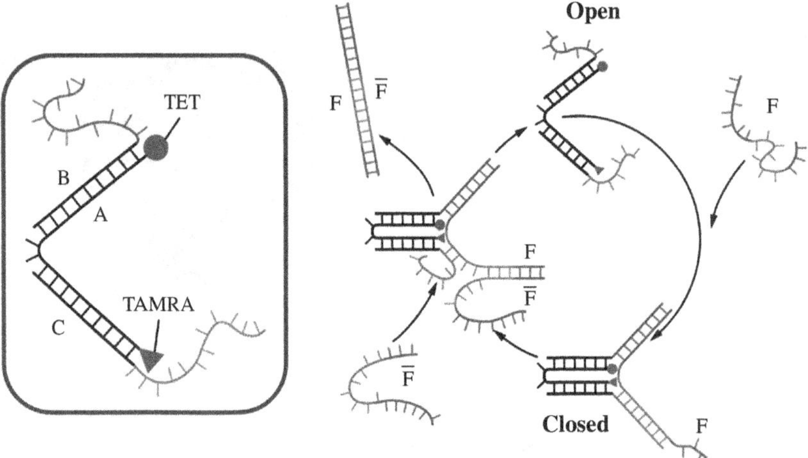

Figure 5-24 DNA tweezers. (*The illustration is reprinted with permission from B. Yurke et al.*[36])

In Figure 5-24, A, B, C, F, and F̄ are ssDNA segments. Segment A is labeled with fluorescent tags (TET and TAMRA) on both ends and attaches to both segments B and C at the "opening" of the tweezers. After attaching to A, both B and C have free-hanging single-stranded segments. Hence, the resulting "opened" DNA tweezers have free-hanging single-stranded segments on either side of the opening. The tweezers are "closed" by adding the single-stranded sequence segment F. F binds to the free ends on both strand B and strand C, forcing the ends of A closed and closing the tweezers. The tweezers are reopened by adding segment F̄ (the complement of F), which has a dramatically higher affinity for F than the free ends of B or C. Thus, F̄ attaches to F and reopens the tweezers.

Whether the tweezers are in the "open" or "closed" state is tracked using the fluorescent tags (TET and TAMRA) on the ends of A. When the fluorophore TET and fluorescent quencher TAMRA are brought together (i.e., the tweezers are closed), the fluorescence is quenched. When the tweezers are open, the fluorophore TET emits a fluorescence signal.

Like other self-assembled systems, DNA tweezers are created through energy minimization. How they "open" and "close" is also controlled by energy minimization. Adding the F or F̄ strand changes the energy landscape of the system by creating a new system which includes F or both F and F̄. The following energy configuration diagrams explain how the DNA tweezer works.

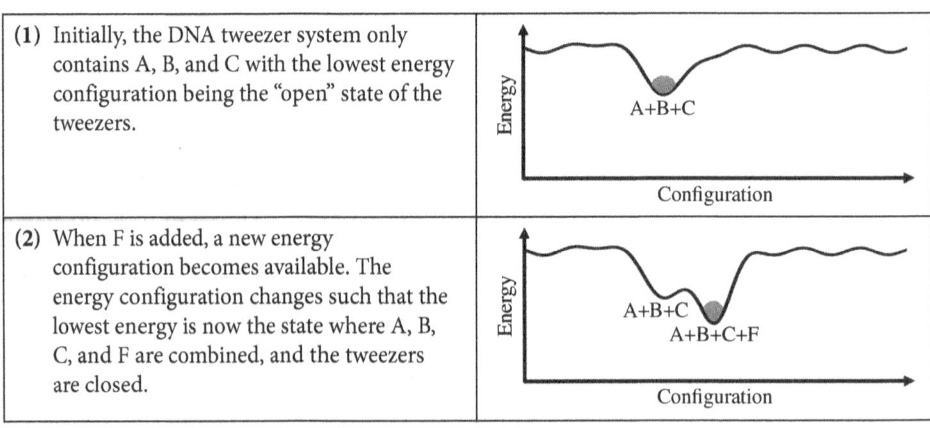

(1) Initially, the DNA tweezer system only contains A, B, and C with the lowest energy configuration being the "open" state of the tweezers.	
(2) When F is added, a new energy configuration becomes available. The energy configuration changes such that the lowest energy is now the state where A, B, C, and F are combined, and the tweezers are closed.	

(3) When $\bar{F}$ is added, the system becomes A, B, C, F, and $\bar{F}$. There is now a lower state where F and $\bar{F}$ are together with A, B, and C, and the tweezers are reopened. Removal of F and $\bar{F}$ returns the DNA tweezers to state (1).

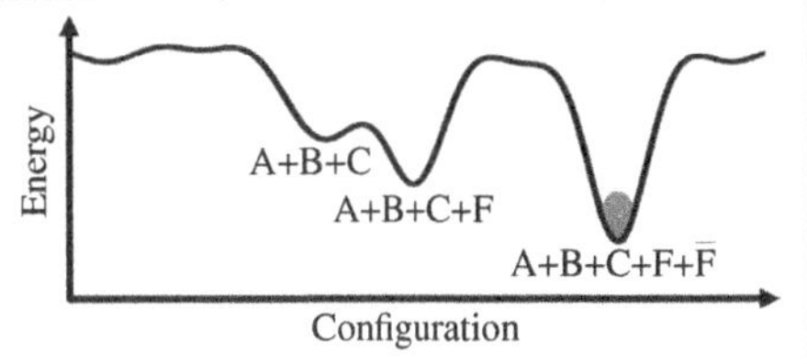

5.8 CRISPR GENE EDITING

Just as we vaccinate ourselves against deadly viruses and their associated diseases, micro-organisms have also evolved their own defense mechanisms against viruses. Viruses called bacteriophages, or simply just phages, infect and replicate themselves within bacteria and archaea (both single-celled organisms). To protect against bacteriophages, bacteria and archaea have evolved an adaptive immune system. Bacteria that survive the initial infection store parts of the phage's viral DNA to protect themselves against subsequent attacks by that particular virus. The mechanisms behind this immune system allow the bacteria and archaea to selectively target specific DNA sequences. The mechanisms for targeting specific DNA sequences can be exploited to insert, remove, replace, activate, or suppress genes in other types of cells, such as those belonging to a human or a mouse.[37]

Clustered regularly interspaced short palindromic repeats (CRISPR) is a family of DNA sequences characterized by a specific pattern. While analyzing microbial genomes, researchers observed a pattern composed of a particular DNA sequence, followed by the same sequence in reverse, then followed by a string of random bases (called spacers). This pattern repeats multiple times (with varying sequences) and is found in more than 40% of bacteria and 90% of archaea. Later, scientists discovered the same spacer DNA sequences in bacteriophages, indicating that the spacers were fragments of foreign phage DNA and that CRISPR was the key component of the microbes' (i.e., bacterial and archaeal) adaptive immune systems. The overall DNA sequence is called the CRISPR locus. There are different possible sequences for the locus, and CRISPR refers to the family of sequences that the loci belong to.[38,39]

5.8.1 CRISPR-Cas Systems

While spacers help the microbes identify foreign DNA (such as from phages), there is a separate mechanism for cleaving (and inactivating) the foreign DNA. This task is given to enzymes called CRISPR-associated proteins (also known as Cas proteins). The CRISPR locus DNA sequence can be copied into RNA (i.e., transcribed) by the microbes to generate CRISPR RNA (crRNA). The resulting crRNA combines with Cas proteins and allows the protein to recognize and subsequently cleave foreign DNA. Figure 5-25 illustrates an overview of the CRISPR-Cas invader DNA silencing mechanism used by microbes to defend against phages. The process of cleaving DNA and hence disabling genes is called "knocking out," while the process of inserting genes is called "knocking in." CRISPR facilitates knocking out, and other methods are used for knocking in.[39]

A particular CRISPR Cas protein named CRISPR-Cas9 has sparked worldwide interest due to its simplicity and ease of use. CRISPR-Cas9 is a nuclease, which is a specialty enzyme designed for cutting DNA and is derived from the bacteria species *Streptococcus pyogenes* and *Staphylococcus aureus*. By replacing CRISPR RNA (crRNA) along with an associated RNA called trans-activating CRISPR RNA (tracrRNA) with an artificial guide RNA (gRNA), Cas9 can be used to target and cut any desired and specific DNA sequences. This is contrasted with previous methods used in genetic engineering such as Zinc-finger nucleases (ZFNs) or transcription activator-like effector nucleases (TALENs), which require a

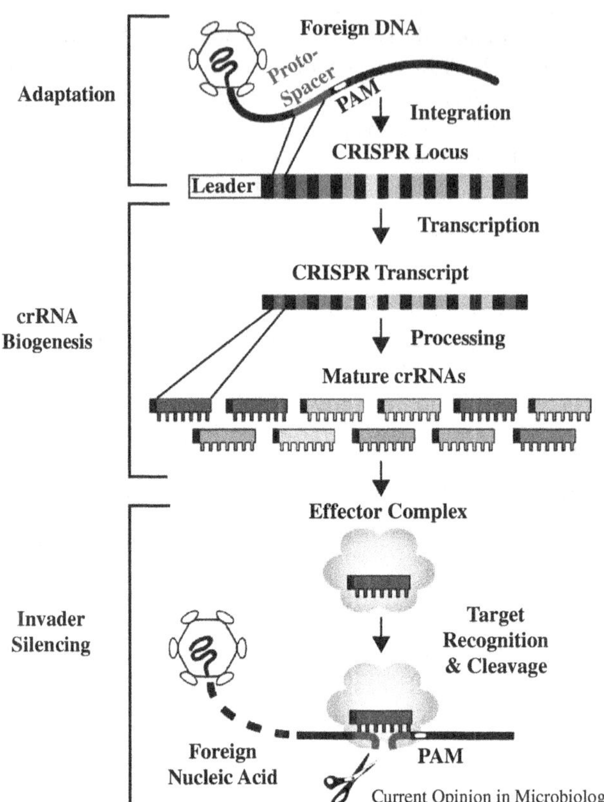

Figure 5-25 Overview of invader DNA silencing by CRISPR-Cas. (*The illustration is reprinted with permission from M. P. Terns and R. M. Terns.*[38])

new protein to be engineered and created for each target DNA sequence. CRISPR-Cas9 is a reusable enzyme that allows one to utilize a guide RNA to target a specific DNA sequence, which requires significantly less effort than previous genetic engineering methods. Moreover, Cas9 can be used for multiple targets if multiple guide RNAs are provided.[40] For these reasons, CRISPR-Cas9 has become extremely popular for genetic studies and gene editing. In 2020, the Nobel Prize in Chemistry was awarded to Emmanuelle Charpentier and Jennifer Doudna for their discovery of CRISPR-Cas9 genetic scissors.

5.8.2 CRISPR-Cas9 Procedure

CRISPR-Cas9 is a sophisticated tool, but we can simplify its use into a few key steps. The first step is to identify the target DNA site that we would like to cut. Target sites are approximately 23 bases long, including a ~3 base-long protospacer adjacent motif (PAM) at the end, which prevents the Cas9 nuclease from cutting the host's own DNA. This ensures that Cas9 cleaves foreign phage DNA rather than the microbe host's own DNA. The ~20 base-long guide RNA is the complement of the target sequence minus the PAM. Many tools, such as the MIT CRISPR tool, E-CRISP, and Harvard's CHOPCHOP tool, are available online and can automatically identify suitable guide RNA using some scoring criteria.

With the DNA target site being identified, the next step is to synthesize the guide RNA. As described in Section 5.5, there are two methods for the guide RNA synthesis. For both RNA synthesis methods, commercial lab kits are available for synthesizing many copies of guide RNA. The first method is plasmid vector-based RNA synthesis, which uses bacteria to clone plasmid vectors containing the complementary ssDNA sequence corresponding to the desired RNA sequence. RNA polymerase is then used to transcribe many copies of the guide RNA. The downside of this method is that it requires 1 to 2 weeks to complete, resulting in a higher likelihood of off-target effects. Also, integration of the plasmid DNA into bacteria cells may cause cell death.

Another method is to use *in vitro* RNA synthesis. This method requires designing an ssDNA template complementary to the desired RNA sequence with a suitable promoter at the upstream end. PCR is used to create many copies of the DNA template, and RNA polymerase is used to transcribe many copies of the guide RNA from the DNA template. This generates guide RNA outside of the cell and takes 1 to 3 days to complete. However, this method can be difficult to use and is more prone to errors.

The last step of using CRISPR Cas9 is to deliver the system to the target. In general, it is necessary to deliver both the Cas9 protein and the guide RNA. There are several options, such as using engineered viruses in the form of viral vectors to deliver Cas9 protein and guide RNA. Different delivery mechanisms have varying degrees of effectiveness and targeting precision. Since the Cas9 protein does not need to be modified for specific experiments, CRISPR-Cas9 gene editing kits can be purchased commercially. Note that what we covered here is a general overview of using CRISPR-Cas9. There are many customization options for using the CRISPR system, from the guide RNA to the delivery mechanism, and even choosing among the different Cas proteins which are available.

5.8.3 Applications and Challenges of CRISPR Gene Editing

Applications   The flexibility of being able to efficiently cleave any chosen arbitrary sections of DNA opens up new doors in genetic engineering. For example, mouse models of human diseases can be created within a few weeks instead of years, accelerating the pace of disease research. CRISPR gene editing provides researchers the opportunity to study individual genes or change multiple genes at once. The faster pace of research enabled by CRISPR also leads to a positive feedback loop, in that they motivate other researchers to invest in CRISPR research, further contributing to the accelerating pace of research. Synthesizing guide RNA is extremely streamlined; licenses for guide RNA design software, as well as pre-built lab kits, are available at low cost. Other possible applications include improving disease resistance in crops or as a means of gene therapy in humans.[39]

CRISPR-Cas9 can also be used as a possible tool in cancer gene therapy. Certain types of cancers are treated by suppressing oncogenes, which are genes with the potential to cause cancer. Traditionally, this was done using RNA interference (RNAi) technology, which suppresses gene expression by damaging targeted mRNA transcribed by the oncogenes. However, RNAi is limited by its inability to remove oncogenes; copies of the original oncogene are left intact after the RNAi treatment. Chen et al. proposed CRISPR-Cas9 as a potential successor to RNAi as CRISPR-Cas9 permanently removes the targeted genes due to its knock out properties.[41]

Limitations and Challenges   Unfortunately, CRISPR-Cas9 is still a new technology with limitations. The precision of CRISPR-Cas9 is not guaranteed. Off-target effects, such as deleting or modifying the wrong gene, may result in severe, irreversible consequences for the organism.

The two most common methods to obtain Cas9 proteins are from the bacteria species *Staphylococcus aureus* and *Streptococcus pyogenes*. Both bacteria species cause diseases in humans, namely methicillin-resistant *Staphylococcus aureus* (MRSA) infections and strep throat. As such, our bodies have naturally evolved an immune response against such diseases. The corresponding antibodies have been discovered in over 80% of healthy individuals, complicating the use of CRISPR-Cas9 in humans.[42]

Human antibodies against the two bacteria species do not necessarily respond to and kill CRISPR-edited cells, since these intracellular responses are meant to coat bacteria and viruses with antibodies to deny them entry into cells or to mark them for destruction by the immune system. However, human antibodies can also mark cancerous or infected cells within the host body, and the existence of T cells (a type of white blood cell) which can detect Cas proteins suggests the possibility of CRISPR edited cells being destroyed by the body. This hypothesis is based on speculation that the interferon-γ secreted by T cells may cause the T cells to kill CRISPR edited cells. In summary, antibodies that respond to Cas9 systems have been discovered, but researchers do not yet know whether or not the immune system will destroy CRISPR-edited cells.[42]

Ethics   The ethics of using CRISPR gene editing boils down to the ethics of editing the human genome. Is it essential to edit the human genome to create super-humans? Should this technology only be used to cure diseases? We can use gene editing as a cancer treatment or as a means to cure muscular dystrophy. Similarly, we can use it to achieve taller, stronger, and smarter humans. Along this train of thought, where do we draw the line between creating super-humans and curing diseases? In the end, CRISPR gene editing represents a flexible and potentially dangerous technology with a large, morally gray zone.

5.9 PROBLEMS

5-1 (Short-Answer). **(a)** In a dsDNA molecule with no mismatched bases, 38% of the nucleotide bases consist of guanine (G). One of the ssDNA strands of the dsDNA molecule contains 5% of the thymine (T) nucleotide bases in the dsDNA molecule. What percentage of thymine (T) nucleotide bases are found in the other (complementary) ssDNA strand?

(b) Starting with a single copy of mother dsDNA, two full PCR (or qPCR) cycles were completed. Both strands of the mother DNA are shown in black, the first copies of the DNA strands are shown in white, and the second copies of the DNS strands are shown in gray. Out of the four choices below, which one represents the PCR products?

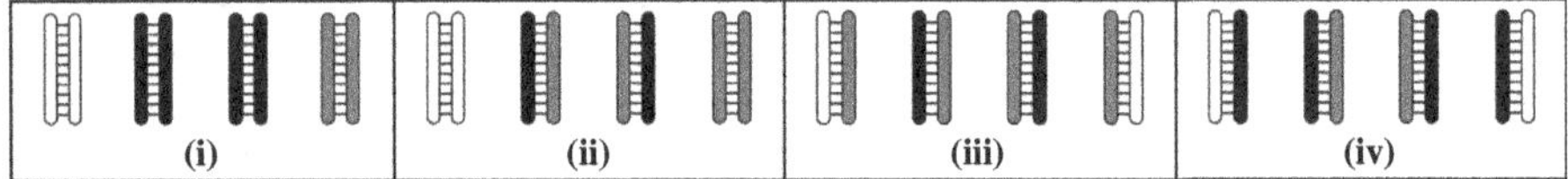

(c) If we want to use first-generation DNA sequencing to sequence a DNA PCR product, are both ssDNA strands comprising the dsDNA PCR product useful? Can the forward or reverse primers used during PCR (or qPCR) also be used as the primer for Sanger sequencing?

5-2. The template strand of a bacterial gene has the following sequence:

template strand = AGATC TAGAG – (226 nucleotide bases) – GTCAT CGATG TATAT AA (5' to 3')

One end of the template strand is the promoter (7 nucleotides long), while the other end is the terminator (also 7 nucleotides long).

Recall that an mRNA contains the blueprint for synthesizing a protein, which consists of a chain of amino acids. The process of using an mRNA template to synthesize a protein is called translation. Every mRNA sequence can be broken down into a sequence of consecutive codons. In mRNA, a codon is a three nucleotides long sequence of RNA that either codes for a specific amino acid or terminates protein translation. The sequence "AUG" is a start codon which signals the beginning of protein translation while simultaneously coding for the amino acid methionine. The codons "UAA", "UGA", and "UAG" are stop codons which do not code for any amino acid but instead signal the end of protein translation.

(a) Which end of the template strand is the promoter and which end is the terminator? What is the mRNA sequence transcribed from this gene?

Hint: Please refer to Figure 5-21 for more details about gene transcription.

(b) In total, how many combinations of codons are there?

(c) How many amino acids are in the protein translated by the mRNA obtained from part (a)? This is the protein that the bacterial gene codes for. Assume that the 226 nucleotide bases in the middle do not contain any stop codons.

5-3. You have selected the following 600 base-pairs long PCR product from a segment of the *Salmonella* genome (nucleotides 601 to 1200 from 5' to 3', as shown below). For carrying out PCR, you have the DNA sample in a PCR buffer solution with an excess number of free bases, a salt concentration of $[MgSO_4] = 220$ mM, no chemical denaturants, and an excess of forward and reverse primers.

```
 601 TCGGCCGCGG   GCGAAATCCA   TTGTTGTTTC   AGTCAGCGCC   AGAAAAAGGC   CGTGCGAAGG
 661 CGGCGGTATT   CATCCGACAT   AAACACCATC   AAAACGGAAC   GATGACATAA   ATCGCGCAAT
 721 TCGGGGAACA   TATCGTCGGC   CCGTTGTTCC   GTCTCTTTGG   TGAGCTTTTC   CGTGACAGCC
 781 AGTTGACGGA   TGCCCGATGG   GCGCGCGGGA   TGGTTCAGAC   CCCAACTGAT   GTAACTGTTC
 841 CAGATAAAAC   GAGTCATCAT   TTTGGCATCG   GTAATGGATC   GATCCAGCTC   CATTATCATT
 901 GACTGGCAGA   GATCCTGCTT   TAAATGCAAA   TACAACGTGT   TAATCAGCTC   ATCTTTGGTC
 961 GCGAAATAGC   GAAACAATGT   TCCTTCTGCA   ACACCTGCGT   TACGCGCAAT   CACCGCCGTT
1021 GAGGCGATAC   CGGATTGCGC   TATCGCCTGG   GTGCCGCTTC   AGTAATGCTT   GTTTTTTGTC
1081 TTCACTCTTC   GGACGAGCCA   CTACACGTTA   CCTATGTCTG   GAAAACTATT   GAATCATGCC
1141 GTTGTGCGTC   GCAACGGTGA   ATGTCAACCT   TGAAAAGTAC   CTTGACGGCG   TATCTTTGCT
```

(a) What is the sequence of your forward primer and reverse primers (both 25 nucleotides long)?

(b) What is the melting temperature T_m of the forward and reverse primers?

(c) For our PCR protocol, we require the melting temperatures T_m of all primers to be $T_m \leq 65°C$. To accomplish this reduction in T_m, what changes to the PCR buffer solution can we make?

(d) Is this a good primer pair for PCR? Why or why not?

5-4. We wish to amplify a DNA PCR product to be used for DNA sequencing. The PCR product is 500 nts (nucleotides) long, and our forward and reverse primers are all 20 nts long. The DNA polymerase we are using has an ssDNA elongation rate of 18 nts per second. The PCR cycle time of our thermal cycler is 70 s, excluding the time required for the extension/elongation step. The equivalent univalent salt concentration in the PCR buffer is 230 mM, no chemical denaturants are used, and the %GC content in the PCR product is 38%. For this PCR setup, the dissociation fraction f_m as given in Equation (5.2) can be modeled with a single-parameter logistic function with a fitting constant of $A = 0.18 \, [1/°C]$.

(a) If we set a denaturing temperature of $92°C$ in every PCR cycle, and starting with just 1000 copies of the double-stranded PCR product, how much time is required for PCR amplification to create at least 4 billion copies of the double-stranded PCR product?

(b) If the PCR cycle time is $\tau_{cycle} = 100$ s, and starting with 3000 copies of the double-stranded PCR product, can we obtain at least 5 billion copies of the double-stranded PCR product in 34 min?

5-5. We want to sequence the middle 602 nucleotides (nts) of the following mouse gene (written 5' to 3'):

GATCT ATGTG TAAGC TGCCA – (602 nts) – ACTTT CCCGT TTGAC AGTTT CTATT CCAAT

where the sequence of the middle 602 nts is unknown. We have dsDNA fragments each containing the entire gene, and want to apply PCR to create at least 3 billion copies of the unknown sequence for DNA sequencing.

(a) Provide the sequences of a suitable set of primers for PCR, with consideration of the melting temperatures T_m.

(b) In our starting sample, the exact number of copies of the dsDNA fragments is unknown, but there should be at least 10^4 copies. If our thermal cycler has a cycle time of 80 s, how long must we run the PCR reaction to obtain at least 3 billion copies of the unknown sequence? Assume that in the denaturing step of each PCR cycle, the dissociation fraction of the dsDNA product is $f_m \geq 95\%$.

(c) We want to purchase the required primers online. At minimum, how many moles and what mass (in picograms) of each primer do we require?

(d) We do *not* want to break the DNA strands of the unknown sequence generated by PCR into DNA fragments. Given this constraint, which DNA sequencing methods are suitable?

5-6. To sequence an 870 nts (nucleotides) long strand of mRNA, nanopore sequencing (a third-generation sequencing method) was performed. A buffer solution filled with ions is passed through the nanopore at a constant rate yielding an unblocked ion current of 120 pA. The mRNA enters the nanopore at its 5' end and passes through at a constant speed of 50 nts per second. Each of the nucleotides blocks a certain percentage of the ions passing through the nanopore, as given in the table below. The figure below shows the ion current I_{ion} versus time t results from nanopore sequencing for the first 24 nts.

Nucleotide	Adenine (A)	Cytosine (C)	Guanine (G)	Uracil (U)
% of Ion Current Blocked	70	40	80	50

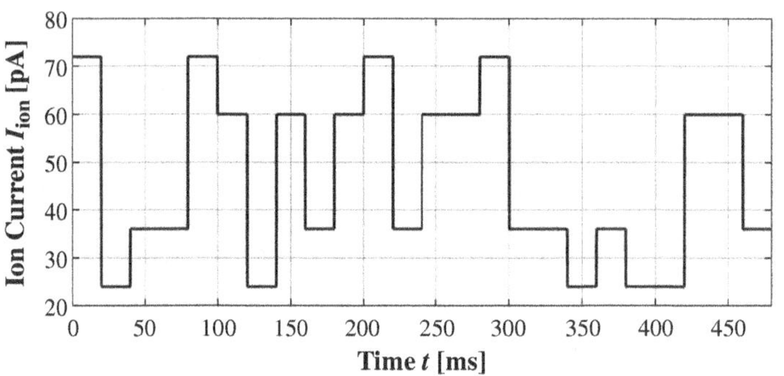

(a) What is the sequence of the first 24 nucleotides of the mRNA?

(b) Based on the results from part (a), what is the sequence of the sense (coding) and antisense (template) strands of the gene which codes for the mRNA sequence? Assume that the promoter sequence of the template strand of the gene is "`ATTAT AATGT CAA`".

(c) For verification, we use Maxam-Gilbert sequencing to sequence the coding strand of the gene which codes for the mRNA. The ssDNA template strands are labeled with radioactive ^{32}P at the 5' end, and four base-specific DNA cleavage reactions are prepared (Table 5-1). Finally, four-lane polyacrylamide-urea gel electrophoresis was carried out. What does the resulting four-lane gel look like after gel electrophoresis is completed? Sketch the four-lane gel with bands showing the first 22 nucleotides.

5-7. We wish to use first-generation DNA sequencing to sequence a dsDNA fragment from a human gene. The sense (coding) strand of the dsDNA fragment has the following sequence:

sense strand = (5') (330 nts) – `AAGAT GAGGA CTGAC ATTAT` (3')

where the sequence of the 330 nucleotides (nts) at the 5' end is unknown.

(a) What is the sequence of the antisense (template) strand of the dsDNA fragment (excluding the sequence of the unknown 330 nts)? For Sanger DNA sequencing, provide the sequences of two different sequencing primers (both 20 nts long) that we could use. Is there a relationship between the two sequencing primers?

(b) The fluorescently labeled variant of Sanger DNA sequencing has been performed to sequence the sense strand of the 350 nts dsDNA fragment from part (a). When exposed to UV light, the bands in the single lane of polyacrylamide-urea gel resulting from electrophoresis fluoresces with four different colors. The fluorescent bands are shown in the figure on the right, which contains the first 24 nucleotides of the sequenced ssDNA (for simplicity, the bands from the remaining nucleotides are not shown). Using the figure on the right to update the sequence provided in part (a), what is the sequence of the sense and antisense strands of the original dsDNA fragment?

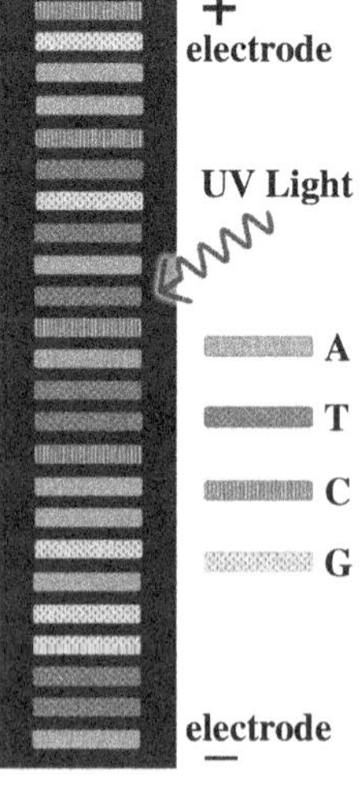

5-8 (Challenging). PCR is a widely used technique for rapid amplification of specific target DNA sequences, where the specificity is achieved by forward and reverse primers. The figure below shows a gene segment containing the specific target DNA sequence to be amplified, along with the primer binding locations. After K full cycles of PCR reaction, the PCR solution is heated to completely dissociate all dsDNA into ssDNA. Because the desired DNA sequence to be amplified is shorter than the gene segment on both ends, some of the ssDNA strands in the resulting PCR solution will be longer than the target DNA sequence.

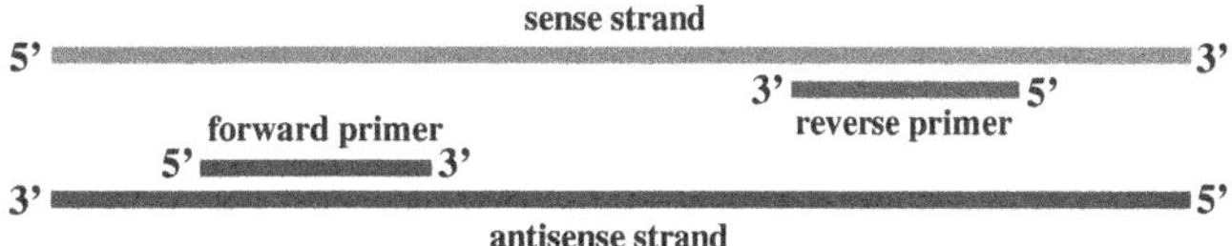

(a) After K full PCR cycles, what is the proportion f_{target} of ssDNA that have the same length as the target DNA sequence? Assume that in the denaturing step of every PCR cycle, the dissociation fraction of the dsDNA product is f_m (a constant between 0 and 1).

(b) It is generally assumed that all of the ssDNA strands resulting from PCR consist of the desired ssDNA target (and its ssDNA complement). The number of ssDNA strands longer than the target strands is considered negligible. From your results in part (a), is this assumption reasonable? If $f_m = 90\%$, what is the minimum number $K_{(min)}$ of PCR cycles required to ensure that $f_{target} \geq 95\%$?

5-9 (Challenging). We have the following eukaryotic mRNA sequence with nucleotides (nts) written from 5' to 3':

CUCGA AACAC GACAC GCCCU GGAAG – (374 nts) – ACUUC GAAUU GCUCU AUUCG – $(A)_N$

where $(A)_N$ is a sequence of A repeated N times, and represents the poly(A) tail of the mRNA. The value of N for each mRNA strand depends on how much the tail has degraded, and it is assumed that $30 \leq N \leq 70$.

We want to sequence the 374 nts in the middle, whose sequence is unknown. First, RT-PCR will be applied to amplify many copies of the cDNA corresponding to this mRNA sequence. During the reverse transcription step of RT-PCR, cDNA strands are successfully reverse transcribed from 85% of the target mRNA strands. During each denaturing step of cDNA amplification, 79% of the cDNA strands dissociate from their ssDNA complements (denoted as $\overline{cDNA}$). Finally, the cDNA will be sequenced to determine the 374 nts of the mRNA sequence.

(a) The first steps of RT-PCR require us to reverse transcribe the initial copies of cDNA from the mRNA template. What (ssDNA) reverse transcription primers could we use? Provide two different options of reverse transcription primers, and give their sequences.

(b) What is the sequence of the cDNA for each of the two options from part (a)?

(c) The latter steps of RT-PCR aim to amplify the cDNA to create enough copies to be sequenced. For cDNA amplification, what combination of forward primer and reverse primer would be compatible with both options of reverse transcription primers and associated cDNA from parts (a) and (b)? Provide the sequences of the forward primer and reverse primer (both 20 nts long).

(d) We require at least 100 million copies of the cDNA for sequencing, and that we start with 4 million copies of the target mRNA. What is the minimum number $K_{(min)}$ of PCR cycles required (excluding the reverse transcription steps), and how many copies of the cDNA will $K_{(min)}$ PCR cycles produce?

(e) As a continuation of part (d), we want to purchase the required primers for $K_{(min)}$ PCR cycles online. For the two options from the previous parts, how many moles and what mass (in picograms) of each primer do we require?

5-10 (Challenging). In Sanger sequencing, the didNTP to dNTP ratio used is critical for the process. The didNTP to dNTP ratio determines the distribution of DNA segments with different lengths in the final product and hence the clarity of the dark bands on the X-ray film (for radioactively labeled didNTP) or the colored bands in UV-illuminated gel (for fluorescently labeled didNTP). If the didNTP to dNTP ratio is too high, the final product will contain only small segments of DNA. Conversely, if the didNTP to dNTP ratio is too low, only a small proportion of the reactions will terminate before the elongation stops when DNA polymerase reaches the 5' end of the ssDNA template. If the ssDNA template is very long, a low didNTP to dNTP ratio will result in a very long reaction time.

We wish to carry out the fluorescently labeled variant of Sanger sequencing with an ssDNA template that is N nucleotides long. In the (sequencing) sample solution, the concentrations of all four types of didNTP is C_{didNTP}, while the concentrations of all four types of dNTP is C_{dNTP}. The didNTP and dNTP molecules are evenly distributed in the sample solution, with a constant ratio of $r = C_{didNTP}/C_{dNTP}$.

(a) Find an expression for the fraction $f(n,r)$ of ssDNA segments with length n (where $1 \leq n \leq N$) that are elongated from the 3' end of the sequencing primers during Sanger sequencing. Since the primers are *never* sequenced, the primers are excluded from the length n.

(b) To verify your results from part (a), show that all of the fractions $f(n,r)$ sum to 1. That is, prove the equation below (left). The sum of a finite geometric series is provided below (right) as a hint.

$$\sum_{n=1}^{N} f(n,r) = 1 \qquad \textbf{Hint:} \; \sum_{k=1}^{K} x^{k-1} = \frac{1-x^K}{1-x} \; \left(\text{for } x \neq 1\right)$$

(c) The signal produced by ssDNA segments with a fraction $f(n,r) \geq F$ can be detected and hence sequenced. For given values of r and F, what is the longest ssDNA segment (with n_0 bases where $n_0 < N$) that we can sequence? That is, find an expression for $n_0(r, F)$, which represents the read length of the Sanger sequencing method. How does n_0 vary with F?

(d) For a constant value of $F = F_{opt}$, find an expression for the optimal value of r (referred to as r_{opt}), which maximizes the length n_0 of the longest ssDNA segment that can be sequenced. Namely, $n_{0(max)} = n_0(r_{opt}, F_{opt})$. In addition, derive an expression for F_{opt}. Express both r_{opt} and F_{opt} as functions of n_0, where $n_0 < N$.

Note: The function $n_0(r)$ has no minima, and only a single maximum.

(e) Calculate r_{opt} and F_{opt} for $n_{0(max)} = 100, 500,$ and 800. To confirm your results, use software to plot the maximum length $n_0(r,F_{opt})$ of ssDNA segments that can be sequenced versus the didNTP to dNTP ratio r for $n_{0(max)} = n_0(r_{opt}, F_{opt}) = 100, 500,$ and 800. Plot all three curves on the same graph, with r on a log scale from 0.0002 to 1, and $n_0(r,F_{opt})$ on a linear scale.

5.10 REFERENCES

[1]   E. W. Sayers, M. Cavanaugh, K. Clark, J. Ostell, K. D. Pruitt, and I. Karsch-Mizrachi, "GenBank," *Nucleic Acids Research*, vol. 48, no. D1, pp. D84–D86, 2020.

[2]   T. van der Straaten, L. Zulianello, A. van Diepen, D. L. Granger, R. Janssen, and J. T. van Dissel, "*Salmonella enterica* Serovar Typhimurium RamA, intracellular oxidative stress response, and bacterial virulence," *Infection and Immunity*, vol. 72, no. 2, pp. 996–1003, 2004.

[3]   "Examining his own body, Stanford geneticist stops diabetes in its tracks," *Science (AAAS Journal)* [Online]. Available: https://www.sciencemag.org/news/2012/03/examining-his-own-body-stanford -geneticist-stops-diabetes-its-tracks, 2012.

[4]   I. Miko, "Gregor Mendel and the principles of inheritance," *Nature Education*, p. 134, 2008 [Online]. Available: https://www.nature.com/scitable/topicpage/gregor-mendel-and-the-principles-of-inheritance-593/

[5]   F. Griffith, "The significance of pneumococcal types," *Journal of Hygiene*, vol. 27, no. 2, pp. 113–159, 1928.

[6]   C. O'Connor, "Isolating hereditary material: Griffith, Avery, Hershey, and Chase," *Nature Education*, p. 105, 2008 [Online]. Available: https://www.nature.com/scitable/topicpage/isolating-hereditary-material -frederick-griffith-oswald-avery-336/

[7]   O. T. Avery, C. M. MacLeod, and M. McCarty, "Studies on the chemical nature of the substance inducing transformation of pneumococcal types induction of transformation by a desoxyribonucleic acid fraction isolated from pneumococcus type III," *Journal of Experimental Medicine*, vol. 79, no. 2, pp. 137–158, 1944.

[8]   A. D. Hershey and M. Chase, "Independent functions of viral protein and nucleic acid in growth of bacteriophage," *Journal of General Physiology*, vol. 36, no. 1, pp. 39–56, 1952.

[9]   D. E. Sadava, D. M. Hillis, H. C. Heller, and M. R. Berenbaum, *Life: The Science of Biology*, 10th ed. Sunderland, MA, USA: Sinauer Associates, Inc., 2014.

[10]   L. A. Pray, "Discovery of DNA structure and function: Watson and Crick," *Nature Education*, p. 100, 2008 [Online]. Available: https://www.nature.com/scitable/topicpage/discovery-of-dna-structure-and-function-watson-397/

[11]   J. Sambrook and D. W. Russell, *Molecular Cloning: A Laboratory Manual*, 3rd ed. Cold Spring Harbor, NY, USA: Cold Spring Harbor Laboratory Press, 2001.

[12]   E. W. Hall and G. W. Faris, "Microdroplet temperature calibration via thermal dissociation of quenched DNA oligomers," *Biomedical Optics Express*, vol. 5, no. 3, pp. 737–751, 2014.

[13]   "Molecular Facts and Figures," Integrated DNA Technologies (IDT) [Online]. Available: https://www.idtdna.com/pages/education/biotech-basics, 2011.

[14]   R. Higuchi, C. Fockler, G. Dollinger, and R. Watson, "Kinetic PCR analysis: real-time monitoring of DNA amplification reactions," *Bio-Technology*, vol. 11, no. 9, pp. 1026–1030, 1993.

[15]   J. J. Kupiec, A. Kay, M. Hayat, R. Ravier, J. Peries, and F. Galibert, "Sequence analysis of the simian foamy virus type 1 genome," *Gene*, vol. 101, no. 2, pp. 185–194, 1991.

[16]   S. A. Bustin, V. Benes, T. Nolan, and M. W. Pfaffl, "Quantitative real-time RT-PCR: a perspective," *Journal of Molecular Endocrinology*, vol. 34, no. 3, pp. 597–601, 2005.

[17]   M. L. Wong and J. F. Medrano, "Real-time PCR for mRNA quantitation," *Biotechniques*, vol. 39, no. 1, pp. 75–85, 2005.

[18]   F. Sanger, S. Nicklen, and A. R. Coulson, "DNA sequencing with chain-terminating inhibitors," *Proceedings of the National Academy of Sciences of the United States of America*, vol. 74, no. 12, pp. 5463–5467, 1977.

[19]   "Human Genome Project Information Archive 1990-2003" [Online]. Available: https://web.ornl.gov/sci/techresources/Human_Genome/index.shtml, 2019.

[20]   L. M. Smith, J. Z. Sanders, R. J. Kaiser, P. Hughes, C. Dodd, C. R. Connell, et al., "Fluorescence detection in automated DNA-sequence analysis," *Nature*, vol. 321, no. 6071, pp. 674–679, 1986.

[21]   A. M. Maxam and W. Gilbert, "A new method for sequencing DNA," *Proceedings of the National Academy of Sciences of the United States of America*, vol. 74, no. 2, pp. 560–564, 1977.

[22]   T. P. Niedringhaus, D. Milanova, M. B. Kerby, M. P. Snyder, and A. E. Barron, "Landscape of next-generation sequencing technologies," *Analytical Chemistry*, vol. 83, no. 12, pp. 4327–4341, 2011.

[23]   D. Branton, D. W. Deamer, A. Marziali, H. Bayley, S. A. Benner, T. Butler, et al., "The potential and challenges of nanopore sequencing," *Nature Biotechnology*, vol. 26, no. 10, pp. 1146–1153, 2008.

[24]   W. Vercoutere, S. Winters-Hilt, H. Olsen, D. Deamer, D. Haussler, and M. Akeson, "Rapid discrimination among individual DNA hairpin molecules at single-nucleotide resolution using an ion channel," *Nature Biotechnology*, vol. 19, no. 3, pp. 248–252, 2001.

[25]   P. J. Russell, *iGenetics: A Molecular Approach*, 3rd ed. San Francisco, CA, USA: Benjamin Cummings, 2010.

[26]   J. Chao, H. Liu, S. Su, L. Wang, W. Huang, and C. Fan, "Structural DNA nanotechnology for intelligent drug delivery," *Small*, vol. 10, no. 22, pp. 4626–4635, 2014.

[27]   V. Kumar, S. Palazzolo, S. Bayda, G. Corona, G. Toffoli, and F. Rizzolio, "DNA nanotechnology for cancer therapy," *Theranostics*, vol. 6, no. 5, p. 710, 2016.

[28]   V. Linko, A. Ora, and M. A. Kostiainen, "DNA nanostructures as smart drug-delivery vehicles and molecular devices," *Trends in Biotechnology*, vol. 33, no. 10, pp. 586–594, 2015.

[29]   P. W. K. Rothemund, "Folding DNA to create nanoscale shapes and patterns," *Nature*, vol. 440, no. 7082, pp. 297–302, 2006.

[30]   C. E. Castro, F. Kilchherr, D.-N. Kim, E. L. Shiao, T. Wauer, P. Wortmann, et al., "A primer to scaffolded DNA origami," *Nature Methods*, vol. 8, no. 3, pp. 221–229, 2011.

[31]   H. Dietz, S. M. Douglas, and W. M. Shih, "Folding DNA into twisted and curved nanoscale shapes," *Science*, vol. 325, no. 5941, pp. 725–730, 2009.

[32]   Y. Ke, L. L. Ong, W. M. Shih, and P. Yin, "Three-dimensional structures self-assembled from DNA bricks," *Science*, vol. 338, no. 6111, pp. 1177–1183, 2012.

[33]   D. Han, S. Pal, Y. Yang, S. Jiang, J. Nangreave, Y. Liu, et al., "DNA gridiron nanostructures based on four-arm junctions," *Science*, vol. 339, no. 6126, pp. 1412–1415, 2013.

[34]   E. Benson, A. Mohammed, J. Gardell, S. Masich, E. Czeizler, P. Orponen, et al., "DNA rendering of polyhedral meshes at the nanoscale," *Nature*, vol. 523, no. 7561, pp. 441–U139, 2015.

[35]   S. Raniolo, G. Vindigni, A. Ottaviani, V. Unida, F. Iacovelli, A. Manetto, et al., "Selective targeting and degradation of doxorubicin-loaded folate-functionalized DNA nanocages," *Nanomedicine: Nanotechnology, Biology and Medicine*, vol. 14, no. 4, pp. 1181–1190, 2018.

[36]   B. Yurke, A. J. Turberfield, A. P. Mills, F. C. Simmel, and J. L. Neumann, "A DNA-fuelled molecular machine made of DNA," *Nature*, vol. 406, no. 6796, pp. 605–608, 2000.

[37]   R. Barrangou, C. Fremaux, H. Deveau, M. Richards, P. Boyaval, S. Moineau, et al., "CRISPR provides acquired resistance against viruses in prokaryotes," *Science*, vol. 315, no. 5819, pp. 1709–1712, 2007.

[38] M. P. Terns and R. M. Terns, "CRISPR-based adaptive immune systems," *Current Opinion in Microbiology*, vol. 14, no. 3, pp. 321–327, 2011.

[39] E. Pennisi, "The CRISPR Craze," *Science*, vol. 341, no. 6148, pp. 833–836, 2013.

[40] W.-J. Dai, L.-Y. Zhu, Z.-Y. Yan, Y. Xu, Q.-L. Wang, and X.-J. Lu, "CRISPR-Cas9 for in vivo gene therapy: promise and hurdles," *Molecular Therapy-Nucleic Acids*, vol. 5, p. e349, 2016.

[41] Z. Chen, F. Liu, Y. Chen, J. Liu, X. Wang, A. T. Chen, et al., "Targeted delivery of CRISPR/Cas9-mediated cancer gene therapy via liposome-templated hydrogel nanoparticles," *Advanced Functional Materials*, vol. 27, no. 46, p. 1703036, 2017.

[42] J. M. Crudele and J. S. Chamberlain, "Cas9 immunity creates challenges for CRISPR gene editing therapies," *Nature Communications*, vol. 9, no. 1, pp. 1–3, 2018.

CHAPTER 6

Lab-on-a-Chip Bionanotechnology and Micro/Nano Fabrication

6.1 OVERVIEW OF LAB-ON-A-CHIP DEVICES

6.1.1 Introduction to Lab-on-a-Chip Devices

Lab-on-a-chip (LOC) is a novel technology invented to replace (or supplement) traditional wet laboratory assays. It is an integrated single-chip device up to a few square centimeters in size that can perform standard laboratory functions. LOC devices are a subset of micro-electro-mechanical systems (MEMS) devices. Since the 1990s, researchers have considered the integration of many functions of conventional wet laboratories on an integrated chip, resulting in the concept of LOC devices. The design and fabrication of LOC devices greatly benefited from the advancement of integrated circuit and MEMS technologies, which have enabled the inexpensive micro/nano fabrication of LOC microchips. Many important processes such as microorganism or biomolecule detection, disease modeling with cell cultures, drug screening, DNA sequencing, enzyme-linked immunosorbent assays (ELISA), molecular separation by chromatography, and even live animal testing—which are completed without relying on microsystems—can also be implemented on LOC systems with a few key advantages. LOC systems enable point-of-care applications owing to their portability, rapid and inexpensive testing, greater automation, and high throughput. Moreover, LOC devices have a wide range of applications which include medical diagnosis, drug and medical device development, disease and toxicological studies, genomic and proteomic studies, smart agriculture, food safety, and environmental monitoring.[1-4]

In resource-limited settings such as rural locations and developing countries where healthcare infrastructure, medical laboratories, and trained medical personnel are highly limited, treatable yet deadly illnesses such as diabetes, cancer, tuberculosis, and malaria often go undiagnosed. Even in high-resource settings such as cities and major towns in developed countries, traditional macroscale assays (for detecting microorganisms or quantifying biomolecules) essential to making accurate diagnosis tend to be time-consuming, labor-intensive, and expensive. As traditional assays need to be performed in specialized medical laboratories by highly trained lab personnel, the time and manpower required for transporting patient samples to the lab and performing the assay will delay the diagnosis and treatment of life-threatening acute illnesses such as sepsis. Moreover, traditional macroscale assays require relatively large amounts (on the order of milligrams to grams) of potentially expensive reagents such as antibodies, enzymes, aptamers, and live cells. Another issue is that traditional drug development and disease studies often involve live animals, which produces imprecise results due to human–animal differences and raises ethical concerns.[1,4]

Well-designed LOC devices have solved the major problems and limitations of traditional macroscale assays. Due to the small size of LOC devices, the amounts of reagents required are reduced by several orders of magnitude (on the order of nanograms to micrograms) compared to macroscale assays, greatly reducing costs and the amounts of hazardous reagents required. Since the reagents can be costly (e.g., ~$200 USD for 50 µg of antibodies), a decrease in the amount used has a significant impact on the overall cost of a process. In addition, LOC systems are highly portable and can be operated by personnel with minimal training, enabling patient bedside testing, clinical point-of-care applications, and eliminating sample transportation time and costs. Owing to their small size, LOC devices offer significantly reduced reactant diffusion distances, increased reaction surface-area-to-volume ratio, and especially greater integration of functions compared with traditional lab assay equipment. Therefore, LOC systems can analyze biosamples much faster than traditional assays, enabling far higher throughput. Furthermore, the throughput of LOC devices can be increased by several orders of magnitude by utilizing parallelization combined with their inherent small size. This is significant for processes which take hours or days to complete. In LOC systems, fluids are typically transported in microchannels using capillary and/or electrokinetic forces rather than manually or by robotic systems. This lends itself better to automation, parallel processing, and integration.[2,5]

The small length scale of the microchannels within a LOC microchip results in a small Reynolds number and therefore highly laminar fluid flow, making fluid mixing much more difficult. Unlike fluid flow within macroscale pipes, pressure-driven flow and flow driven by pumps are far less effective for transporting fluid within the tiny microchannels of LOC devices. Thus, simply shrinking down macroscale systems to create LOC microchips will not work. In general, the design of successful LOC devices requires sophisticated computer simulations combined with extensive experimentation and prototyping.[5]

LOC systems work well with processes that scale well with size. These processes include optical detection (e.g., fluorescence or colorimetric detection) and electrokinetic fluid transport techniques such as electro-osmotic flow (EOF), electrophoretic flow (EPF), and dielectrophoresis (DEP). LOC systems tend not to work well in setups with poorly understood chemistry. For example, the relatively large surface area of high molecular weight proteins makes them difficult to integrate into LOC length scales because proteins and other large molecules can stick to the walls of microchannels. In some other processes, the volume scale cannot be lowered below ~1 µL due to solubility issues. Common LOC devices include:

- *Biosensor Microchips:* LOC biosensor microchips—which are used for medical diagnosis, personal health monitoring, food safety analysis, and environmental monitoring—are especially useful in low-resource environments. These biosensors exploit the portability, high throughput, and ease-of-use of LOC systems to achieve rapid and inexpensive testing in point-of-care applications.[6]

- *Organs-on-Chips:* Organs-on-chips (OOCs) are designed to mimic the behavior of one or more organs *in vitro* (i.e., outside of a living organism). OOCs can be used to study the origins and progression of diseases, the impact of gene expressions, and the role of biomolecules such as proteins or toxins. Additionally, OOCs can be used to screen drug candidates and test medical devices *in vitro*. By replacing macroscale cell cultures and live animal testing, OOC systems promise to accelerate and reduce the cost of drug and medical device development as well as disease studies.[3,4]

- *Array-Type Microchips:* Array-type microchips achieve high throughput via parallel processing. Array-type microchips include protein microarrays, DNA microarrays, DNA hybridization chips, and drug-screening microarrays.[7]

- *Microfluidic Microchips:* Microfluidic microchips rely on electrokinetic (e.g., EOF, EPF, and DEP) as well as mechanical (e.g., capillary forces) methods to drive biosamples such as blood or urine within microchannels. Different functional blocks can be cascaded to achieve the desired functions. Typical examples include micro total analysis systems (µTAS).[8]

Aside from biosensors, other novel LOC applications use live cells or tissues for the inexpensive and rapid screening of drug candidates. As a drug discovery tool, LOC drug-screening microarrays offer dramatically reduced reagent use and costs, as well as high throughput and parallelization.[9] Another recent breakthrough of LOC devices are organs-on-chips, which can potentially replace live animals for toxicity testing as well as drug and vaccine screening. A variation of organ-on-a-chip (OOC) devices, called medical-device-on-a-chip, can also be used for medical-device testing without the need for tests in human subjects.[10,11] Other LOC devices that rely on low costs, parallelization, and high throughput include protein microarrays for probing protein mechanics and DNA microarrays for probing gene expressions.[7] The small scale of LOC microchips also enables exciting novel applications such as single-cell analysis or even the interrogation of individual biomolecules.[12,13]

6.1.2 The Market for Lab-on-a-Chip Devices

Lab-on-a-chip devices have progressed well beyond academic research and hold great market potential as well. Medical diagnosis, cell sorting, drug screening, and organs-on-chips are some of the common biomedical applications of LOC devices. These applications are significant developments for LOC technologies. For instance, organ-on-a-chip (OOC) technology—along with nano-sensors, 2D materials, and autonomous vehicles—was selected as a top emerging technology at the 2016 Davos World Economic Forum.[14] The U.S. Food and Drug Administration (FDA) acknowledged that OOCs could be used to conduct drug toxicity tests, and suggested that drug screening in the United States could use OOCs instead of live animal tests.[11]

According to a report by Yole Développement titled "Status of the Microfluidic Industry (2019 Edition)," the annual global market size for LOC devices (which include microfluidic devices) in 2018 amounts to 8.7 billion USD. The global LOC market size is predicted to reach 17.4 billion USD annually by 2024 with a compound annual growth rate of 11.7% between 2019 and 2024. The Yole Développement report also showed that 15 leading companies occupy more than 75% of the market share for LOC devices. Most low- to medium-income countries lack diagnostic capabilities in community healthcare centers, township healthcare centers, and village clinics. For these countries, LOC technology holds great potential as it can provide much-needed diagnostic capabilities. At present, large multinational manufacturers of LOC devices include Illumina, Abbott Laboratories, bioMérieux, Boehringer Ingelheim, Cepheid, Zoetis, and Hoffmann-La Roche.[15]

6.2 LAB-ON-A-CHIP BIOSENSORS

6.2.1 Design of Lab-on-a-Chip Biosensors

The purpose of LOC biosensors is to detect the presence or quantify the concentration of a target analyte within biological samples such as blood, urine, saliva, swabs, or even environmental air or water. The target analyte can be a type of antigen, virus, toxin, protein, bacteria, metabolite, DNA, or RNA. LOC biosensor systems are comprised of three components: (i) the sample preparation area, (ii) the detection area, and (iii) a signal processing platform comprised of data collection and analysis equipment. The sample preparation (i)

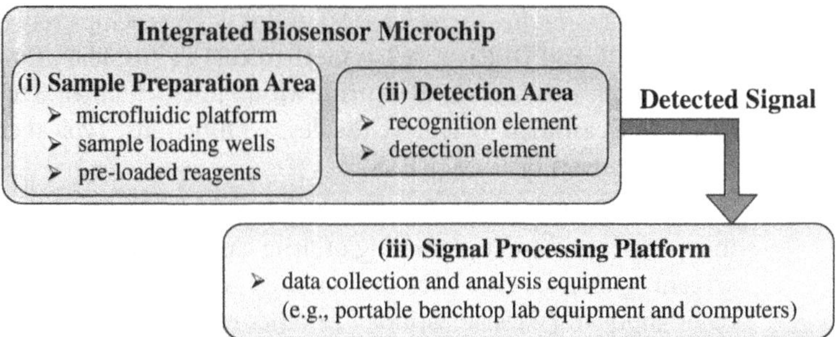

Figure 6-1   The main components of lab-on-a-chip (LOC) biosensor devices.

and detection areas (ii) are located on the integrated biosensor microchip, while the signal processing platform typically includes portable benchtop lab equipment and/or small computers (e.g., tablets). The main components of LOC biosensor systems are illustrated in Figure 6-1.[5]

The sample preparation area (i) can contain wells for loading biofluid samples (e.g., blood, tissue fluids, saliva, urine), pre-loaded reagents, plus a microfluidic platform for carrying out fluid transport, filtration, and preliminary reactions to make the samples easier to detect. The microfluidic platform can contain microchannels for transporting the samples and pre-loaded reagents. The main purpose of the microfluidic platform is to enhance the analyte detection signal-to-noise ratio. This is accomplished by reacting the biofluid samples with pre-loaded reagents to convert the analytes into a form that is easier to detect and/or filter out unwanted molecules and particles that can cause confounding sources of signal to reduce noise. By automatically dispensing the correct volume of biofluid samples into the rest of the microchip, the microfluidic platform greatly simplifies the loading of biosamples. Thus, calibrated micropipettes are not needed to load the biosamples, and a few drops of biosample from a cheap and disposable dropper would be sufficient.[5]

While the microfluidic platform typically employs capillary and electrokinetic (e.g., EOF, EPF, and DEP) forces as the fluid transport methods, other methods including pressure-driven flow, diffusion, and centrifugal forces may also be applied. To carry out fluid transport, mixing, and filtration, microfluidic platforms commonly rely on MEMS components such as micro-pumps, micro-valves, micro-mixers, micro-dispensers, and micro-filters.[6] Instead of employing MEMS components, more recent digital microfluidic platforms use driving microelectrodes—a 2D network of powered and multiplexed microelectrodes—to apply electrokinetic forces. By replacing delicate MEMS structures with powered microelectrodes, digital microfluidic platforms are more durable (less likely to break during transportation), less expensive to fabricate, and more easily reconfigured. However, additional circuitry and software are required to control the driving microelectrodes.[16]

The detection area (ii) and the signal processing platform (iii) vary depending on the detection method employed by the LOC system. In general, the detection area (ii) of LOC biosensors requires a recognition element plus a detection element. The recognition element is an active component which recognizes the target analytes, while the detection element detects and reports the signal generated by the recognition element. The detectable signal can be qualitative or quantitative. For most LOC devices, the recognition element consists of recognition molecules anchored to the detection area surface that have high affinity for the target analyte. Common examples of recognition molecules include antibodies, enzymes, aptamers, proteins, and nucleic acids. In addition to recognition molecules, other suitable recognition elements include live cells (e.g., microorganisms) and tissue. There are three major classes of detection methods for LOC sensors: (1) electrochemical detection, (2) optical detection, and (3) gravimetric detection. More complicated

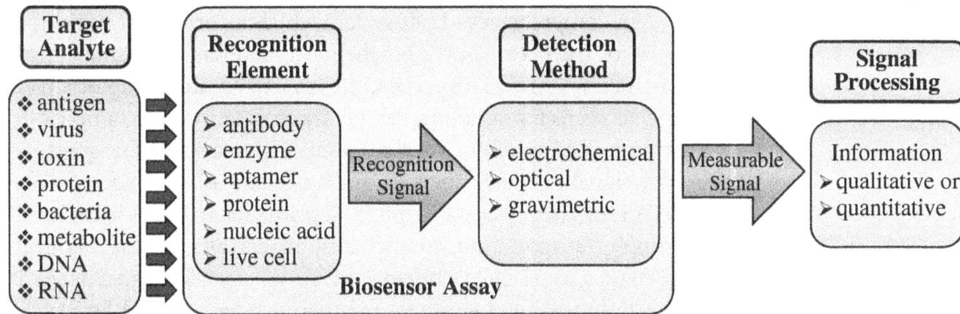

Figure 6-2   The basic principles of lab-on-a-chip (LOC) biosensor devices.

LOC systems can employ a combination of the three methods. An overview of the working principle of LOC biosensor devices is illustrated in Figure 6-2.[5]

(1) *Electrochemical Detection:* For electrochemical LOC sensors, the detection element is comprised of sensing electrodes. The sensing electrodes are commonly configured as 3-electrode systems with working, counter, and reference electrodes. Other sensing electrode configurations include interdigitated electrodes (IDEs), which consist of two interlocking comb-shaped microelectrode arrays. When the target analytes interact with recognition elements in and around the sensing electrodes, there is a change in the potential difference, current, and/or impedance across the sensing electrodes which is measured by equipment such as ammeters, voltmeters, or LCR meters. Electrochemical LOC systems do not require labels and can be simple, highly compact, and require minimal power. Commercial glucose meters for diabetic patients are LOC systems that rely on quantitative electrochemical detection.[6]

(2) *Optical Detection:* In optical LOC sensors, the detection element consists of optical labels which bind to the target analytes. The optical labels can be colored molecules/particles (for colorimetric detection) or fluorophores (for fluorescent detection). Suitable fluorophores include organic fluorescent dyes, fluorescent intercalators, and quantum dots (please refer to Chapter 4 for more details). When the labeled target analytes bind to recognition elements anchored to the detection area, an optical signal is generated that can be measured using absorbance, colorimetry, fluorescence, interferometry, or luminescence. While optical detection can be significantly more accurate and reliable than electrochemical or gravimetric detection, optical LOC systems often require labels as well as potentially bulky optical equipment such as lens systems and light sources. Commercial pregnancy test strips are extremely simple optical LOC biosensors that provide qualitative results.[6]

(3) *Gravimetric Detection:* Gravimetric LOC sensors rely on mechanical deflections and/or oscillation damping for analyte detection. The detection element (upon which the recognition elements are anchored) commonly consist of mass sensing micro/nano-cantilevers, mass sensing nanowires, or oscillating quartz in the form of quartz crystal microbalances. When the target analytes bind to the recognition elements, the mechanical deflections or damped oscillations are detected by specialized data collection equipment. While gravimetric LOC sensors can be highly sensitive and do not require labels, this detection method is highly prone to errors from confounding sources of signal. In addition, the required signal processing platform can be complicated and bulky.[17,18]

A comprehensive LOC system which incorporates and automates all of the steps necessary for the chemical (or biochemical) analysis of a sample is also known as a micro total analysis system (μTAS). Thus, the integrated microchip of a μTAS device includes on-chip mechanisms for sampling, sample transportation, and sample filtration (if necessary), carrying out all required chemical reactions with pre-loaded reagents, as well as generating a detectable signal to enable chemical (or biochemical) analysis with external equipment. Typically, μTAS microchips use microfluidic platforms (MEMS-based or digital) to handle sampling, sample transportation, sample filtration, and all required chemical reactions. The mechanism used on a μTAS microchip to generate a detectable signal depends on the detection method. For instance, on-chip sensor microelectrodes are used for electrochemical detection, while on-chip pre-loaded optical labels (such as fluorophores) are used for optical detection.[19,20]

6.2.2 Lateral Flow Lab-on-a-Chip Biosensors

Lateral flow LOC biosensors consist of either standalone test strips for qualitative detection, or test strips combined with a readout device (typically handheld) for quantitative detection. Lateral flow LOC test strips are made from porous substrates such as cellulose from paper or cloth and cross-linked silica. As such, these test strips rely purely on capillary forces to passively wick a liquid biosample (e.g., blood, urine, saliva, environmental water) from the sample inlet to the detection area. The properties of the porous substrates comprising the test strip can be adjusted by tuning the pore size distribution and the wettability. Most lateral flow LOC sensors employ either optical detection (colorimetric or fluorescent detection in particular) or electrochemical detection.[1,21]

Although quantitative (optical or electrochemical) detection requires a signal processing platform such as a handheld readout device, this is not required for qualitative optical (colorimetric or fluorescent) detection. For instance, commercial home pregnancy test strips rely on qualitative colorimetric optical detection, while most commercial glucose test strips together with glucose meters rely on quantitative electrochemical (amperometric or coulometric) detection.[21,22]

Lateral flow LOC test strips are easy to use, inexpensive, disposable, and require only a few drops of biosample fluid. Hence, lateral flow biosensors are among the earliest commercially successful LOC biosensors, and enjoy widespread use today both at home and in clinical settings. Today, lateral flow LOC biosensors are used to detect a wide range of analytes to test for pregnancy, blood glucose, blood coagulation, heart attack, metabolic disorders, viruses, anthrax, bacteria, antibiotics, illegal drugs, toxins, and even DNA or RNA.[8,21]

(A) Lateral Flow Glucose LOC Biosensors
A famous example of a commercially successful lateral flow LOC biosensor system is the glucose test strip together with glucose meter, which was invented in the 1960s. Many early lateral flow glucose biosensors relied on optical detection using a colorimetric test strip combined with a handheld optical readout device. However, due to issues with reproducibility and accuracy, most modern glucose meters use electrochemical detection instead. An electrochemical glucose test strip contains (i) the sample pad and liquid-attracting layer, (ii) the reagent pad, (iii) a large working electrode, (iv) a counter/reference electrode, and (v) fill-detection electrodes. Figure 6-3 illustrates a lateral flow glucose test strip.[23,24]

To begin the glucose detection process, a drop of blood is loaded onto the sample pad and liquid-attracting layer (i), which draws a reproducible amount of blood onto the reagent pad (ii) via capillary forces. The reagent pad (ii) stores pre-stored *dry* reagents including enzymes (either glucose oxidase or glucose dehydrogenase) and redox mediators such as ferrocenes. Through a series of redox reactions involving glucose within the blood sample, the enzymes, and the redox mediators, electrons are generated at the working electrode (iii). This produces an electric current proportional to the amount of reacted glucose from

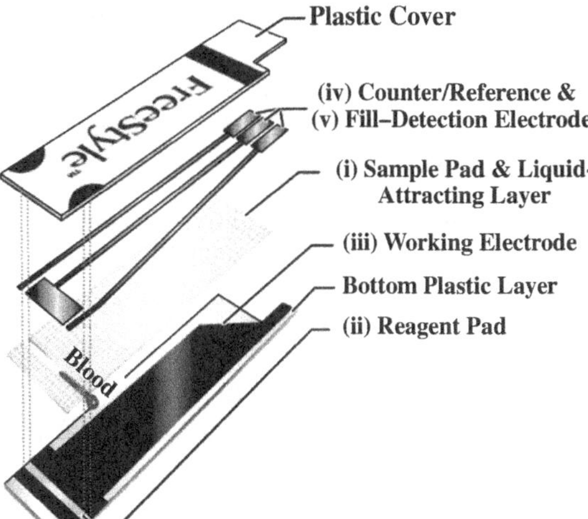

Figure 6-3   An exploded view of a lateral flow glucose test strip. (*The illustration is reprinted with permission from A. Heller and B. Feldman.*[23])

the blood sample, which is used to determine the blood glucose concentration. The redox reactions are listed below.[22,24]

$$(1) \text{ Glucose} + \text{Enzyme} \rightarrow \text{Gluconolactone} + \text{Reduced Enzyme}$$

$$(2) \text{ Reduced Enzyme} + \text{Mediator} \rightarrow \text{Enzyme} + \text{Reduced Mediator}$$

where reaction (2) restores the enzymes, allowing the enzymes to participate in reaction (1) again. At the working electrode (iii), the reaction is

$$(3) \text{ Reduced Mediator} \rightarrow \text{Mediator} + \text{electrons}$$

The counter/reference electrode (iv) completes the conduction path for electrons generated at the working electrode. The electrons generated at the working electrode of the test strip enter the glucose meter and re-enter the test strip via the counter/reference electrode, completing the circuit. To produce reproducible blood glucose detection results, it is important for the test strip to be completely filled with blood when the current detection begins. This is handled by the fill-detection electrodes (v), which sense when the test strip has been entirely filled with blood. Finally, a handheld glucose meter measures the redox electric current to calculate the blood glucose concentration. Electrochemical glucose meters rely on amperometric (i.e., electric current) or coulometric (i.e., electric charge or total electric current) detection.[23]

(B) Optical Lateral Flow LOC Biosensors

Many lateral flow LOC biosensors rely on optical (i.e., colorimetric or fluorescent) detection. The test strip of a typical optical lateral flow biosensor consists of four main components: (i) the sample pad, (ii) the conjugate pad, (iii) the incubation and detection pad, and (iv) the absorbent pad. The sample pad (i) and conjugate pad (ii) together comprise the sample preparation area, while the detection area consists of the incubation and detection pad (iii). Figure 6-4 shows a detailed illustration of an optical lateral flow test strip. The absorbent pad (iv) of the test strip located beyond the incubation and detection pad is designed to control the speed at which the sample fluid is wicked via capillary forces from the sample pad (i) to the incubation and detection pad (iii). Thus, the absorbent pad is made from a highly porous and absorbent material.[8,21]

The optical lateral flow test procedure is as follows. First, a few drops of the fluid biosample is dropped into the sample inlet and onto the sample pad (i). The sample pad (i) wicks

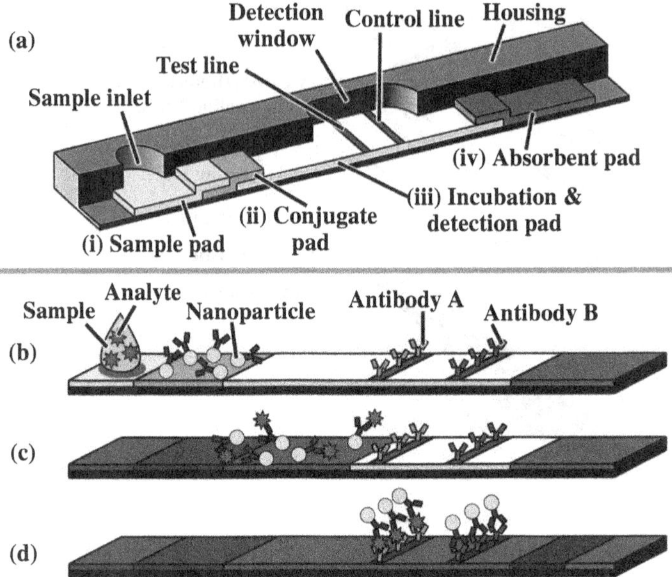

Figure 6-4   (a) An optical lateral flow test strip. (b) Sample fluid containing the target analytes (stars) is loaded into the sample inlet. (c) The target analytes (stars) are conjugated with signal-generating nanoparticles (circles) on the conjugate pad. (d) The analyte-nanoparticle complexes bind to A antibodies on the test line, while the nanoparticles bind to B antibodies on the control line. The detection result is positive. (*The images are reprinted with permission from D. Mark et al.*[8])

desired components of the sample fluid onto the conjugate pad (ii), while simultaneously absorbing (i.e., filtering out) undesirable components to remove confounding sources of signal and reduce noise. The sample pad is typically made from porous cellulose or cross-linked silica substrates, and its filtration properties can be altered by adjusting the substrate. Next, the conjugate pad (ii)—which stores pre-loaded *dry* signal-generating particles in a cross-linked silica substrate—conjugates (i.e., binds) analytes in the sample fluid with signal-generating particles. Then, the resulting fluid is transported into the incubation and detection pad (iii). Upon arriving at the incubation and detection pad (iii), the fluid sample is incubated for a short amount of time (usually seconds to a few minutes), and finally the detection result is read.[21]

For optical detection, the signal-generating particles consist of bioaffinity molecules attached to optical label particles serving as the detection element. These bioaffinity molecules are biomolecules which have high affinity for (i.e., easily bind to) the target analytes. The optical label particles are usually colored molecules/particles (for colorimetric detection), or fluorophores (for fluorescent detection). The incubation and detection pad (iii) contains a test line and a control line visible from the detection window. Different recognition elements are anchored onto the test line and control line. The recognition elements anchored to the control line have high affinity for the signal-generating particles, while the recognition elements anchored to the test line depend on the type of assay used. After incubation, the detection results can be read as a color change of the test and control lines. The readout can be done either by visual observation (for qualitative colorimetric detection), underneath a light source (for qualitative fluorescent detection), or with an optical readout device (for quantitative detection).[21,25]

In general, there are two main types of assays used on the test line of an optical lateral flow test strip: sandwich assays and competition assays (Figure 6-5). Additionally, whether

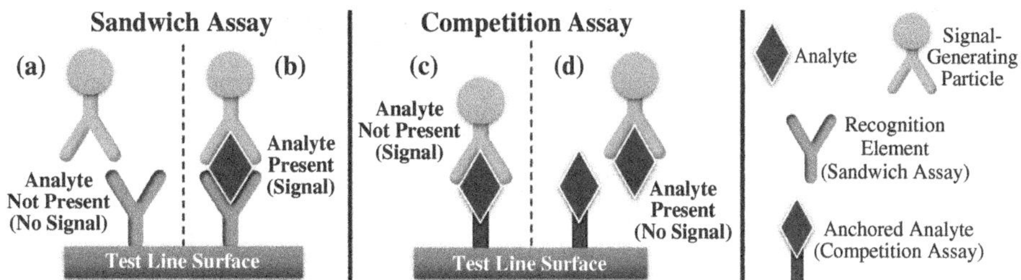

Figure 6-5 Sandwich assay with analyte (a) not present (no signal) and (b) present (signal). Competitive assay with analyte (c) not present (signal) and (d) present (no signal).

the test line surface changes color depends on if the target analytes are present or absent in the sample.[21,25]

- *Target Analytes Are Absent in the Sample:* In this case, the sample fluid will carry signal-generating particles from the conjugate pad to the test line via capillary forces. For sandwich assays, the signal-generating particles cannot bind to the recognition elements on the test line, and thus no signal is produced. For competition assays, the signal-generating particles will bind to the recognition elements on the test line, producing a signal. Usually, sandwich assays are used for the detection of larger analytes with many binding sites (such as proteins).

- *Target Analytes Are Present in the Sample:* If target analytes are present in the sample, (analyte)–(signal-generating particle) complexes formed on the conjugate pad will reach the test line. For sandwich assays, the analyte complexes will bind to recognition elements on the test line, generating a signal. For competition assays, the analyte complexes are not able to bind to the recognition elements on the test line, and no signal is produced. Competition assays are normally used to detect analytes that lack suitable antibody pairs as well as smaller analytes with fewer binding sites (such as some metabolites).

If the control line changes color but the test line remains the same color, the result is negative for sandwich assays and positive for competition assays. If both the control line and the test line change color, the result is positive for sandwich assays and negative for competition assays. A negative result indicates that the concentration of the analyte is below the detection threshold, while a positive result indicates that the concentration of the analyte is above the detection threshold. In all other situations, such as when both lines remain the same color, the test strip is faulty or has been misused and no detection results can be obtained.[21,25]

A well-known example of an optical lateral flow LOC biosensor is the home pregnancy test strip. Since their introduction in the 1970s, over-the-counter home pregnancy test strips have enjoyed global commercial success. These lateral flow pregnancy test strips use qualitative colorimetric detection to detect human chorionic gonadotropin (hCG) in urine using anti-hCG antibodies as the recognition element. Since the concentration of hCG in urine rises quickly and consistently during early pregnancy, hCG is an excellent early pregnancy biomarker. Modern pregnancy test strips can detect early pregnancy 10 days or more following ovulation with accuracies above 90% if used properly. Owing to the large molecular size of hCG, sandwich assays are used on the test lines of home pregnancy test strips.[26]

6.2.3 Non-Faradaic Impedimetric Lab-on-a-Chip Biosensors

Impedimetric LOC biosensors rely on electrochemical detection and often use interdigitated electrodes (IDEs)—which are two interlocking comb-shaped microelectrode arrays

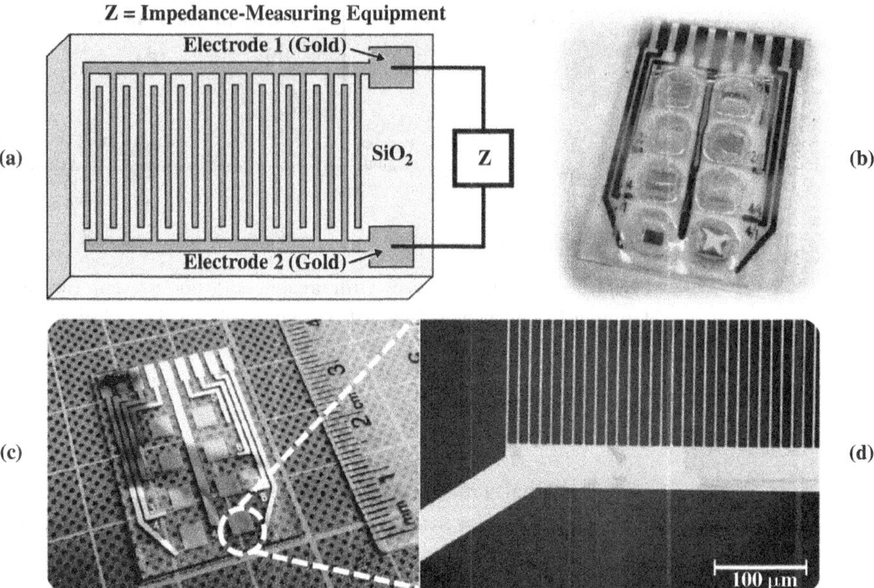

Figure 6-6   (a) Simplified illustration of interdigitated electrodes (IDEs) on a SiO_2 (i.e., glass or quartz) substrate; the microchip of a non-faradaic impedimetric LOC biosensor (b) with eight liquid sample-containing wells and (c) without any samples; (d) optical microscope image of the gold IDEs on the microchip responsible for biosensing. Section 6.5.1 describes the fabrication of this IDE-based LOC biosensor microchip. (*The photographs are provided by Prof. Jie Chen's group.*)

(Figure 6-6)—as the detection element. In particular, the detection technique for impedimetric LOC biosensors is electrochemical impedance spectroscopy (EIS). EIS involves the measurement of impedance (i.e., resistance and reactance) between the two sets of microelectrodes forming the IDEs as a function of AC (i.e., sinusoidal alternating current) excitation frequency. The impedance versus frequency data can be measured with benchtop LCR meters as well as potentiostat/galvanostat impedance analyzers. When the target analytes bind to the recognition elements anchored either on top or in between the IDEs, there is an impedance change across the two sets of microelectrodes comprising the IDEs which is measured. The measured impedance change versus AC frequency spectrum is used to determine the analyte concentration.[6,27]

Compared with other common detection techniques employed on LOC systems, such as optical detection and gravimetric detection, the use of EIS as the detection technique offers unique advantages. Unlike optical-based LOC systems, impedimetric LOC systems do not require labels (e.g., fluorophores) or potentially bulky optical equipment such as lens systems and light sources. Compared to gravimetric-based LOC systems, impedimetric LOC systems are substantially simpler and less prone to error. Thus, impedimetric LOC devices offer a combination of advantages including compactness (high portability), simplicity, and minimal power requirements.[5]

Impedimetric LOC sensors can be classified into two categories: faradaic sensors and non-faradaic sensors. Both faradaic and non-faradaic impedimetric LOC sensors rely on sensing electrodes (such as 3-electrode systems or IDEs) as the detection element and use EIS as the detection technique. The impedance change for faradaic impedimetric sensors is generated by ongoing electrochemical redox reactions at the electrodes. These redox reactions involve both the analytes and redox reagents to generate an electrical current, resulting in the desired impedance change. The impedance change for non-faradaic impedimetric sensors is generated by electrochemical changes on or in between microelectrodes caused by interactions with the analytes. Although faradaic sensors can be more sensitive than non-faradaic sensors, non-faradaic sensors are less complicated and more portable as they do not require redox reagents or redox electrodes.[28,29]

Many early non-faradaic impedimetric LOC biosensor designs before 2005 had poor signal-to-noise ratio and reproducibility issues when quantifying the target analyte concentration. These early LOC designs had high (i.e., poor) detection limits and could only provide qualitative results, whereas traditional lab assays could provide reliable quantitative results. By incorporating metal nanoparticles or magnetic nanobeads as well as an additional recognition element layer in a sandwich assay, later impedimetric LOC biosensor designs offer significantly enhanced signal-to-noise ratio and can accurately quantify analyte concentrations.[30] In a sandwich assay (Figure 6-7), the target analytes are "sandwiched" between two layers of recognition element molecules, with one layer anchored to the detection area surface and the other layer attached to the top of the analytes. For instance, Su et al. (2009) conjugated silver-coated gold nanoparticles with recognition element antibodies and used sandwich assays to detect SpA protein from *Staphylococcus aureus* bacteria, achieving a detection limit of 10 ng/mL.[31] Wang et al. (2018) coated *Escherichia coli* bacteria with silver and gold nanoparticles prior to insertion into the detection area, resulting in an *E. coli* detection limit of 500 cfu/mL.[32] While the detection limits achieved by Su et al. and Wang et al. are still inferior to traditional assays such as ELISA, they are orders of magnitude lower than early designs.

As an example, human immunodeficiency virus (HIV) antigen detection has been shown to demonstrate the potential of non-faradaic impedimetric LOC biosensors. With a traditional macroscale assay, a medical laboratory test such as a western blot or ELISA would need to be performed to detect the concentration of HIV antigens in a patient's blood. Excluding sample transportation time, one such macroscale assay would require many milliliters of blood and at least a full day to complete. For the impedimetric LOC system demonstrated by Shafiee et al. (2013), the highly portable HIV test would require less than 30 min and cost less than $2 USD. The detection procedure for this system is as follows. First, the biofluid sample containing HIV is lysed (i.e., mechanically broken down). Next, the resulting biosample containing lysed HIV is incubated with magnetic nanobeads conjugated with anti-HIV antibodies. Once the lysed HIV has bonded to the nanobead-antibody conjugates, the resulting biofluid is injected onto the surface in between two sensing microelectrodes. Finally, the altered impedance across the two sensing microelectrodes is detected via EIS to quantify the viral concentration. The detection limit of this system is below 10^6 viral copies/mL of biosample, which is sufficient to detect acute HIV infection (10^6 to 10^8 viral copies/mL of blood).[33]

More recent non-faradaic impedimetric LOC designs are able to achieve detection limits comparable to traditional lab assays such as ELISA and PCR-based techniques. Using aptamer-coated magnetic nanobeads, Jin et al. (2017) were able to sense Cry1Ab protein—a

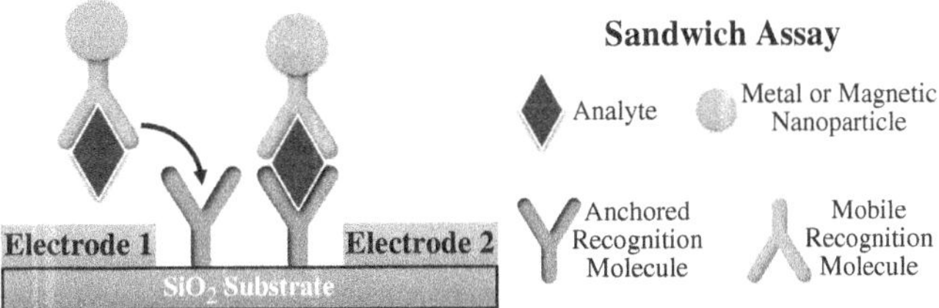

Figure 6-7 Simplified illustration of a sandwich assay applied on the SiO₂ substrate in between two IDE microelectrodes. The metal or magnetic nanoparticles involved in the sandwich assay dramatically enhance the impedance change signal.

common protein insecticide—with a detection limit of 0.96 ng/mL.[34] Prof. Jie Chen's research group has also successfully developed prototype impedimetric LOC biosensors. Using both computer simulations (2015) and prototypes (2017), MacKay et al. demonstrated the feasibility of gold nanoparticle enhanced impedimetric LOC biosensors.[35,36] Based on this work, Abdelrasoul et al. (2018) used antibodies conjugated with gold nanoparticles in a sandwich assay to detect I-FABP proteins, a biomarker for acute mesenteric ischemia. The sandwich assay was created on the SiO_2 substrate surfaces in between the IDEs, achieving an I-FABP protein detection limit of 0.68 ng/mL.[37] In a later work, Abdelrasoul et al. (2020) functionalized the gold surfaces of IDEs with a DNA aptamer having a high affinity for an *E. coli* outer membrane protein, achieving an *E. coli* detection limit of 9 cfu/mL without requiring metal nanoparticles, magnetic nanobeads, or sandwich assays.[38]

In recent years, dramatic advancements in computing power have enabled the use of machine learning algorithms trained on calibrated EIS data for analyzing EIS data.[39] If applied to the EIS data generated by impedimetric LOC sensors, these algorithms could potentially enhance accuracy when determining analyte concentrations. In addition, advancements in signal processing circuitry have enabled complementary metal-oxide-semiconductor (CMOS) LOC sensors. In CMOS non-faradaic impedimetric LOC sensors (Figure 6-8), the IDEs are replaced with a 2D array of sensor microelectrode "pixels" with a CMOS integrated circuit (i.e., network of CMOS transistors) beneath connecting every pixel. Specialized signal processing components and software are able to convert the signals generated by the CMOS integrated circuit into impedance versus frequency (EIS) data. While each set of IDEs only have two terminals, the sensor microelectrode pixels have hundreds to thousands of terminals (with one terminal per pixel). Thus, sensor microelectrode pixels offer vastly improved spatial resolution compared to IDEs, enabling far greater analyte detection accuracy as well as novel applications such as precise cell counting and differentiation. For instance, these CMOS impedance sensors could accurately count tumor cells within a biopsy for early stage cancer detection, which is impossible to achieve with IDEs.[40]

6.2.4 Breakthroughs and Challenges of Lab-on-a-Chip Biosensors

Most LOC biosensor systems have been designed to supplant established macroscale laboratory assays. In recent years, the advancement of LOC systems has enabled many novel applications which are impossible for traditional assays to achieve. Some of these novel applications exploit the portability, rapid diagnostic speed, simplicity of operation, and low cost of LOC biosensors to perform medical diagnostics such as pinprick blood tests in time-critical situations as well as resource-limited settings lacking health infrastructure.[1]

Modern lateral flow LOC sensors have become increasingly sophisticated. For example, modern lateral flow test strips and meters often include automatic internal calibrations and controls to compensate for test strip variations due to batch-to-batch differences, environmental factors, and aging.[8] Lateral flow LOC biosensors can even achieve single-step ELISA, an assay that normally requires five steps in a conventional laboratory.[41] Some recent lateral flow test strips include multiple lanes to achieve greater throughput and parallel screening. Each lane can be designed to test for a different analyte within the same sample, or with all lanes designed to test for the same analyte within different samples.

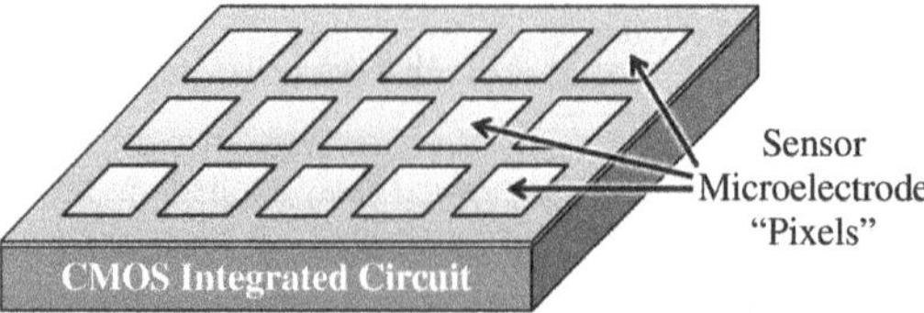

Figure 6-8 Simplified illustration of a CMOS non-faradaic impedimetric LOC sensor. The fabrication of this CMOS LOC sensor microchip is detailed in Section 6.5.3.

However, the accuracy and sensitivity of lateral flow test strips are ultimately limited by the system's ability to achieve precise liquid metering and handling.[21]

Despite the numerous advances made in the field of LOC biosensors during the last two decades, there are still many outstanding challenges before these devices can be adopted for widespread applications in medical diagnostics and environmental monitoring. Depending on the design, the signal-to-noise ratio of LOC biosensors could be inferior to standard macroscale lab assays. Due to the small sizes of the integrated biosensor microchips of LOC systems, the engineering tolerances are very tight and stringent quality control is required to ensure the reproducibility of analyte detection results. Despite being far easier to use than medical lab equipment, LOC systems could still produce inaccurate and irreproducible results when operated by poorly trained personnel. Moreover, the extensive computer simulation, experimentation, and micro/nano fabrication equipment required for prototyping successful LOC biosensors greatly add to the development expense and time. Since LOC biosensor designs in general cannot be easily reconfigured to detect different analytes, a medical laboratory is far more flexible in terms of utility than any LOC biosensor system and commercial development of LOC designs is currently limited in light of the expense and time required.[2]

While the signal processing platform consisting of data collection and analysis equipment of LOC systems can easily be reused, another major unsolved issue is that the integrated microchips of LOC biosensor systems, although cheap to manufacture, are normally single-use for two major reasons. First, once the microfluidic channels within the microchips (e.g., within the sample preparation area) have been used, it is difficult to clean and remove all liquid and bio-contaminants from the microchannels. Second, after the integrated biosensor microchip is used, the analytes are covalently bonded to the recognition elements anchored onto the microchip detection area surface. It is extremely difficult to remove the analytes and replenish the recognition elements without damaging the microchip.[2]

Although the per unit cost of the integrated biosensor microchips of LOC devices tends to be cheap, the microchips normally require specialized micro/nano fabrication equipment to manufacture. The integrated biosensor chips of LOC devices are typically created using standard microelectronic (i.e., integrated circuit and MEMS) micro/nano fabrication techniques. However, micro/nano fabrication equipment can be expensive (>1 million USD) and is operated by trained personnel in the cleanrooms of nanofabrication facilities. Thus, it is a challenge to fabricate LOC microchips in low-resource locations. To help alleviate this issue, 3D printing and laser micromachining techniques have been developed for fabricating LOC microchip components outside of nanofabrication facilities. These developments can greatly reduce the development time of prototype LOC systems and potentially enable the integrated microchips of LOC systems to be created in low-resource environments where portable LOC devices are especially needed.[42]

While any traditional medical or biological laboratory can analyze a very wide range of analytes by altering the biosamples, reagents, and equipment used, this is not the case for LOC systems. A major weakness of nearly all LOC systems is the lack of reconfigurability of the integrated LOC microchip, which significantly increases the time and expense required for LOC development. For instance, an integrated LOC biosensor microchip designed to detect a specific target analyte cannot be easily reconfigured to detect a different analyte without a complete redesign. In other words, the sample preparation and detection areas of each LOC biosensor microchip are designed for sensing specific analytes within a specific type of biofluid sample. For instance, the microfluidic channels of the sample preparation area are designed to transport, filter, and/or carry out reactions utilizing highly precise volumes of a specific type of biosample, and will not work for even a slightly different type of biosample. In addition, the recognition elements anchored to the detection area can bind only to a very specific type of target analyte, and cannot bind to other types of analytes. To overcome this problem, Mark et al. (2010) proposed the idea of modular LOC components.[8] Like modular microelectronic components that can be combined to create integrated circuits for virtually any purpose, modular LOC components can be combined to accomplish an extremely wide range of tasks (e.g., to detect any target analyte or screen any type of drug). Each modular LOC component performs a specific unit operation, such as fluid transport, filtration, fluid metering, fluid mixing, carrying out reactions, or generating impedance changes for detection. In theory, modularity should dramatically decrease LOC development time and expense.

6.3 ORGAN-ON-A-CHIP DEVICES

6.3.1 Introduction to Organ-on-a-Chip Devices

Organ-on-a-chip (OOC) systems, also known as organs-on-chips, are specialized lab-on-a-chip devices designed to mimic the behavior of one or more organs *in vitro*. An OOC device is created by merging a microfluidic chip with live cells and tissues, combining micro/nano fabrication with tissue engineering. OOC systems are 3D lab-on-a-chip devices which use live cells and tissues within a microfluidic chip to mimic organ functions and behavior *in vitro*.

Over the last two decades, OOC devices which mimic most human organs including the skin, blood vessels, heart, brain, lung, intestines, kidney, bone, spleen, and liver have been successfully developed. As illustrated in Figure 6-9, these OOC devices are designed to reproduce the tissue-tissue interactions, tissue micro-architectures, biochemical stimuli (i.e., the biochemical environment), dynamic mechanical cues (i.e., mechanical stresses), and the microvasculature (i.e., blood vessels) within real human organs.[4] By replicating the behavior and functions of human organs *in vitro*, OOC devices can be used in epidemiological studies to elucidate the origins and progression of human diseases, in toxicology studies to determine the toxicity of various toxins, in genomics and epigenomics to study the impact of gene expressions, and in proteomics and metabolomics to examine the role of proteins and metabolites. Additionally, the use of OOC devices can significantly speed up and lower the cost of drug and medical device development by enabling the rapid and

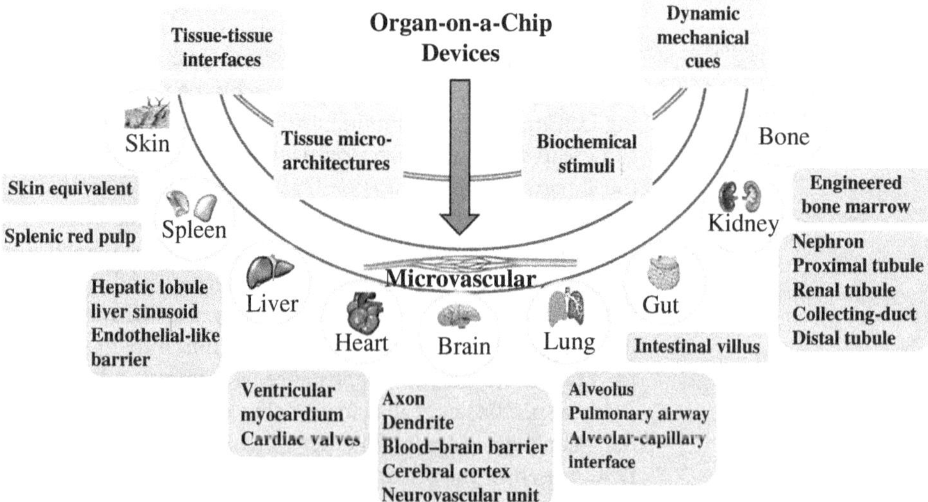

Figure 6-9   Organ-on-chip (OOC) devices are designed to reproduce the tissue-tissue interactions, tissue micro-architectures, biochemical stimuli, dynamic mechanical cues, and the microvasculature within real organs. OOC devices which mimic most human organs have been successfully developed. (*The illustration is reprinted with permission from F. Zheng et al.*[4])

inexpensive screening of drug and drug delivery candidates as well as test medical devices without requiring live animals or humans.[43-45]

The microfluidic chip of an OOC device contains microchambers and microchannels on which living cultured cells and tissues reside. The cells and tissues in an OOC are kept alive through continuous perfusion of a nutrient solution which also carries away their metabolic wastes. Semi-permeable porous membranes can be incorporated to recreate tissue-tissue interfaces such as the blood-brain barrier. The microchannels within an OOC also enable controllable fluid flow, which is essential for modeling fluid circulation within an organ (e.g., organ blood flow). The chip and microfluidic channels of an OOC can be placed under mechanical stresses (i.e., tension and compression) to recreate those in real organs (e.g., air pressure in the lungs).[3,4]

Traditionally, macroscale 2D and 3D cell cultures are used for the *in vitro* modeling of tissues and organs. However, the cells and tissues of real organs are organized in intricate 3D structures on the micrometer scale. Owing to their large size and simplicity in comparison to the 3D structures of real organs, macroscale cell cultures cannot accurately mimic even simple organ functions. Moreover, it is extremely difficult to implement tissue-tissue interfaces, fluid flow, and mechanical stresses in macroscale cell cultures, which all contribute significantly to organ function and behavior. Alternatively, live animal testing can be used to model human organ functions. Unfortunately, such *in vivo* tests are both expensive and potentially unethical, and may not provide accurate results due to the difference between animal and human organs. Well-designed OOCs resolve the major issues associated with both macroscale cell cultures and live animal testing. Such OOCs are inexpensive and can accurately mimic human organ functions *in vitro*.[4,45]

To monitor the cells and tissues within an OOC, optical detection using colorimetric or fluorescent labels under a microscope is commonly employed. To enable optical detection, OOCs are implemented on transparent biocompatible substrates such as glass, quartz, and polymers such as SU-8 (an epoxy-based negative photoresist) and polydimethylsiloxane (PDMS).[46] Despite its name, an OOC is not an artificial recreation of an entire organ. Instead, an OOC is designed to mimic the tissues and tissue-tissue interactions within an organ on a microchip far smaller than any human organs. Thus, an OOC can mimic basic organ functions despite being far simpler than a real organ.[3]

The microchip of an OOC device, which has dimensions on the order of a few centimeters, is typically fabricated using standard and inexpensive MEMS micro/nano fabrication techniques such as photolithography, soft lithography, etching, and 3D micromachining. Compared to macroscale cell cultures, one of the greatest advantages of OOC devices in general is the ease with which their 3D micro-architectures can be altered with modifications to the fabrication process (for instance, changing the photomasks used). The microfabricated 3D microchannels and microchambers of an OOC on which living cells and tissues reside can be designed to closely resemble the 3D micro-architectures and patterns within a real organ.[46]

The small sizes of OOC devices offer a number of advantages compared to macroscale cell cultures. Due to their small size relative to macroscale cell cultures, OOC devices are more portable and easier to transport, and the creation of OOC devices requires far fewer cells. Since human cells can be costly to purchase or cultivate, OOC devices can be significantly cheaper to fabricate than their macroscale cell culture counterparts. OOC devices also offer far greater throughput than macroscale cell cultures for two important reasons. First, the small scale of OOC microchips offers greatly reduced diffusion lengths and increased surface-area-to-volume ratio, which greatly increases the rate of biochemical reactions occurring on the microchip. Second, many OOC microchips can be placed on a single substrate to enable parallel processing.[47] The enhanced throughput of OOC devices is highly useful when screening drug candidates and studying the role of biomolecules such as proteins, toxins, and metabolites.[43]

6.3.2 Working Principles of Organ-on-a-Chip Devices

While early OOC designs had 2D micro-architectures, more recent OOC designs incorporate 3D micro-architectures. 3D OOC designs better model real organs than their 2D counterparts since the intricate microstructures within human organs are inherently 3D. However, 3D OOC microchips are much more difficult to fabricate, and designing successful 3D OOC microchips requires extensive simulation and experimentation. Fortunately, advances in MEMS micro/nano fabrication techniques—namely soft lithography, surface micromachining, bulk micromachining, and 3D printing—have enabled the fabrication of OOC microchips with complex 3D micro-architectures.[48]

The design of a specific OOC device depends on the organ that the OOC is meant to mimic as well as the specific tissues and organ functions that the OOC should model. Most OOCs do not incorporate all of the tissue types in the model organ since OOCs in general are far simpler than the organs they are intended to model.[4] To illustrate the working principles of OOC devices, we will first examine a relatively simple lung-on-a-chip device and then a more sophisticated brain-on-a-chip device.

To begin, we examine a relatively simple human lung-on-a-chip device reported by Huh et al. in 2013, as shown in Figure 6-10. In this OOC device, a microchannel divided into two parts by a porous membrane is placed in between two side chambers. Live lung epithelial

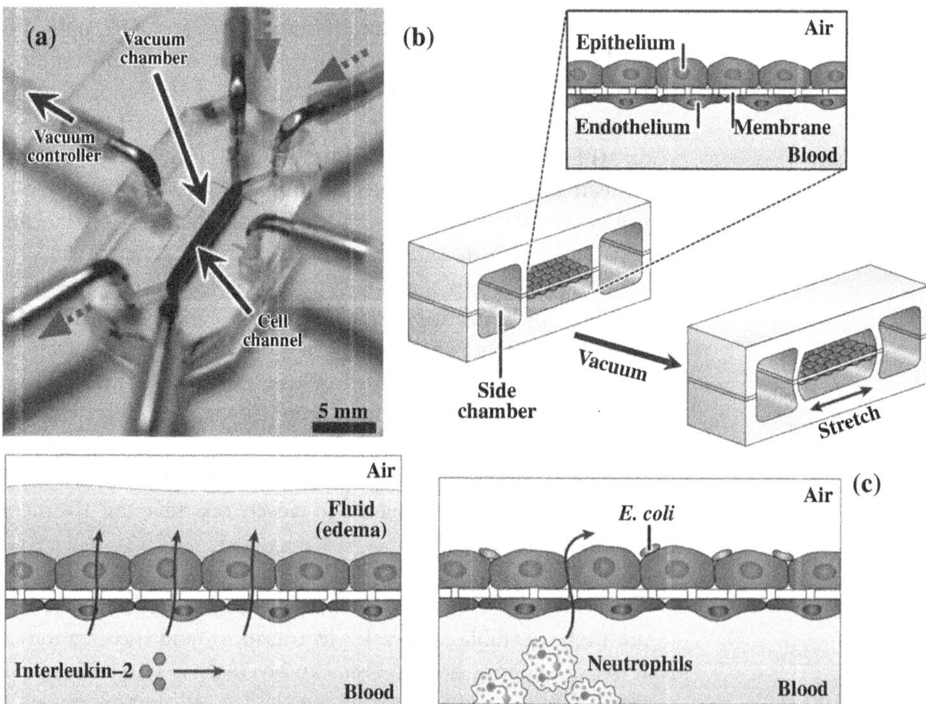

Figure 6-10 (a) Photograph and (b) schematic of a lung-on-a-chip device, which replicates the epithelium, endothelium, alveolar-capillary barrier, air-liquid epithelium interface, and even the mechanical stresses associated with breathing of a real human lung. (c) This lung-on-a-chip device can produce accurate real-time models of (left) pulmonary edema as well as (right) lung inflammation resulting from breathing in bacteria. (*The figures are reprinted with permission from D. Huh et al. and E. W. Esch et al.*[44,46])

cells representing the lung epithelium are placed on the top surface of the membrane, while live lung endothelial cells representing the lung endothelium are placed on the bottom surface of the membrane. The semi-permeable porous membrane represents the alveolar-capillary barrier (i.e., blood-air barrier) of a real lung, while the upper portion of the micro-channel can be filled with air to simulate the air–liquid epithelium interface of a functioning lung. To simulate the mechanical pressures associated with breathing, the air within the two side chambers can be evacuated and re-pressurized with a cycle frequency of 0.25 Hz. When evacuated, a vacuum is created within the two side chambers, which causes the epithelial cells, endothelial cells, and porous membrane in the microchannel to stretch, as would happen during breathing. Inlet and outlet wells are included in this lung-on-a-chip to provide continuous perfusion of a nutrient solution and carry away any metabolic wastes.[46]

In summary, this lung-on-a-chip device models the epithelium, endothelium, alveolar-capillary barrier, air-liquid epithelium interface, and the mechanical stresses associated with breathing of a real human lung. By comparison, a macroscale cell culture would not be able to model the alveolar–capillary barrier, the air–liquid epithelium interface, or the mechanical stresses of breathing. This lung-on-a-chip device has produced accurate real-time models of pulmonary edema as well as lung inflammation resulting from breathing in bacteria or nanoparticles, none of which are possible with conventional cell cultures.[44]

Now we examine a much more sophisticated OOC device: a brain-on-a-chip device reported by Jeong et al. in 2015, as illustrated in Figure 6-11. This OOC device consists of a

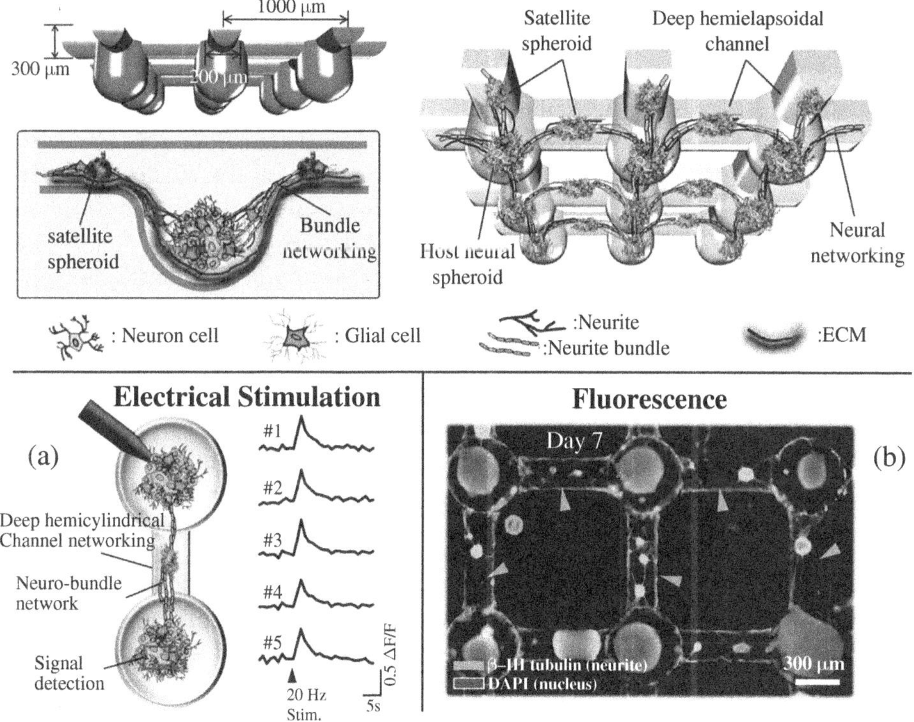

Figure 6-11   A brain-on-a-chip device intended to replicate a neural network within the brain designed using a hemicylindrical channel wall networking system. (Top) Illustration of neuron cells, glial cells, neurites, neurite bundles, and extracellular matrix (ECM) protein membrane within the brain-on-a-chip device. This neural network can be studied in real time by (a) measuring electrical neural signals generated after electrical stimulation via microelectrodes, or (b) using fluorophores combined with appropriate light sources and an optical microscope. (*The figures are from G. S. Jeong et al.*[49])

hemicylindrical channel wall networking system, which is a 2D network of recessed spherical microchambers connected by microchannels. Live neuron cells are cultured in each recessed microchamber along with glial cells which support, feed, and protect the neuron cells. After a few days, a physical neural network is formed between the neuron cells of neighboring microchambers which are connected by neurites and neurite bundles formed in the microchannels. After being successfully cultured, the brain cells secrete a membrane of extracellular matrix proteins (e.g., laminins) between the cells and the OOC substrate. These extracellular matrix proteins both guide and protect the neuron cells and glial cells, and are essential for their survival. There are two options to study the neural network of this brain-on-a-chip device in real time. The first option is to electrically stimulate the neuron cells in one or more of the microchambers using microelectrodes, and then measure the electrical neural signals generated in response in real time. Another option is to label the brain cells with fluorophores, excite the fluorophores with appropriate light sources, and then use an optical microscope to study the neural network in real time.[49]

In macroscale cell cultures of brain cells (i.e., neuron cells and glial cells), the brain cells are clumped together into clusters rather than spread out in a neural network. Hence, most phenomena occurring in the brain cannot be replicated in conventional cell cultures. By mimicking a real neural network within the brain, which is not possible with conventional cell cultures, this brain-on-a-chip device can be used to study the electrical signals generated by the brain as well as the effect of drugs on the brain.[49]

In general, there are two main methods in which the tissues on OOC devices are monitored in real time. One method uses optical detection, which typically involves labeling the tissues on the OOC microchip with stains or fluorophores and then continuously monitoring the tissues under an optical microscope. Another method uses bioelectrical signal detection, in which microelectrodes are used to probe the bioelectrical signals generated by OOC tissues in response to physical or electrochemical cues. For instance, the cue could be electrical excitation from a microelectrode, chemical excitation from introducing a biomolecule, or physical excitation from mechanically bending the OOC microchip. In particular, electrical signal detection is especially useful for brain-on-a-chip, heart-on-a-chip, and muscle-on-a-chip devices in which the tissues generate relatively strong bioelectrical signals.

6.3.3 Applications of Organ-on-a-Chip Devices

(A) Tumor-on-a-Chip Devices

One of the most promising recent developments in OOC systems is the tumor-on-a-chip, an OOC device containing cancer tissue intended to mimic a cancerous tumor. Similar to an organ, a cancerous tumor is comprised of cells and tissues organized in a 3D micro-architecture which act together to create a biochemical and physical microenvironment beneficial to their survival. Cancerous cells and tissues organized in a tumor—as opposed to being disorganized—are far better protected from the immune system as well as anticancer medication and treatments. Because cancer is a genetic disease caused by genetic mutations, animal models of cancer frequency fail due to human–animal genetic differences. On the other hand, macroscale cancer cell cultures cannot recreate the organized 3D microstructures within a tumor, nor the complex biochemical and physical environment created by the interaction between cancer tissues. Therefore, cancer treatments and medications tend to perform far better on macroscale cancer cell cultures than they do in cancer patients. By recreating the 3D micro-architectures along with the biochemical and physical environments resulting from cancerous tissue–tissue interaction in a tumor, a tumor-on-a-chip is a far superior model of a cancerous tumor than a conventional cancer cell culture.[50,51]

The tumor-on-a-chip is used to study the formation and growth of tumors in real time and test the real-world efficacy of cancer medications and treatments *in vitro*. Tumor-on-a-chip devices can also be used to test drug delivery systems intended to treat cancer, which cannot be accomplished with macroscale cancer cell cultures. By incorporating additional microchannels into a tumor-on-a-chip which are intended to replicate the blood vessels entering and exiting a real tumor, cancer metastasis can also be studied in real time. Cancer metastasis is the spread of cancer to other parts of the body at which the cancer becomes deadly and extremely difficult to treat. By studying cancer metastasis, treatments that suppress the spread of cancer and hence significantly improve cancer survival rates can be formulated. Tumor-on-a-chip devices can also be used for personalized cancer treatments. Since cancer is caused by a series of cellular genetic mutations which vary from patient to patient, cancer treatments that work well for one patient may not work at all for another patient, especially if the treatment involves gene therapy or immunotherapy. By culturing cancerous tissue from a specific patient on a tumor-on-a-chip, one can test the efficacy of a personalized cancer treatment prior to treating the patient.[50,51]

A sophisticated tumor-on-a-chip device was reported by Shirure et al. in 2018, as depicted in Figure 6-12.[52] This device utilizes a microfluidic platform incorporating microchambers (to hold live tissues), microchannels (to mimic blood vessels), input/output wells (for continuous perfusion), and microporous walls (i.e., semi-permeable membranes to separate different tissues). This tumor-on-a-chip device is intended to mimic breast cancer

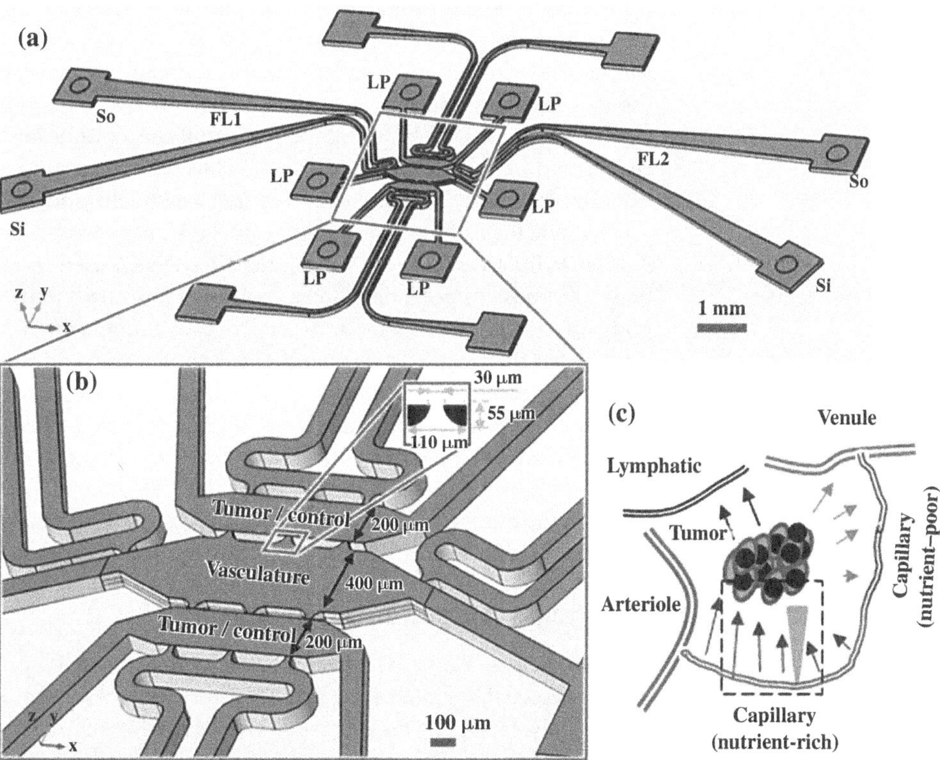

Figure 6-12   (a) Overview and (b) zoomed-in illustration of a sophisticated tumor-on-a-chip device showing microchannels, microchambers, input/output wells, and microporous walls. This tumor-on-a-chip device is intended to model cancerous breast and colorectal tumors, as shown in (c). (*The figures are reprinted with permission from V. S. Shirure et al.*[52])

tumors, and has been used to study the growth and eventual metastasis of breast cancer tumors, in addition to testing the tumor response to anticancer medication. Unlike conventional macroscale cell cultures, this tumor-on-a-chip device can accurately replicate tumor behavior, which is essential to personalized medicine and drug discovery. The establishment of the live cell and tissue cultures (some cancerous) in this tumor-on-a-chip device required less than two weeks, a timeframe that is relevant for personalized cancer treatments.[52]

(B) Multi-Organ Organ-on-a-Chip Systems

Recently, multi-organ OOC systems have been created by integrating multiple OOC devices which model different organs. Complete multi-organ OOC systems called body-on-a-chip systems—which incorporate all major organs in the human body in the form of integrated OOCs—have been developed. In theory, multi-organ OOC systems can mimic the behavior of each organ together with organ–organ interactions. In the human body, different organs interact mainly through blood vessels and the nervous system. Blood vessels and blood cells not only transport oxygen, nutrients, and metabolic wastes throughout the body, but also transport the biomolecules (hormones, metabolites, proteins, etc.) secreted by different bodily organs. These biomolecule secretions are one of main ways in which different organs interact with each other in the human body. In addition, all organs in the human body are connected via the neurons and nerve endings of the peripheral and central nervous system, allowing the work done by different organs to be coordinated by the brain.[3,48]

Although multi-organ OOC systems can easily model the large blood vessels (i.e., arteries and veins) connecting different organs using large microchannels, it is extremely challenging to ensure that the profile of biomolecules secreted by each included organ matches that of a real organ. This issue is especially problematic considering that an OOC device is normally substantially simpler and smaller than a real organ, and typically will not incorporate all of the tissue types found in a real organ. Currently, even the most sophisticated multi-organ OOC systems are not able to mimic the neural connections between different organs via the central and peripheral nervous system. Thus, current multi-organ OOC systems—and by extension body-on-a-chip systems—cannot accurately model organ-organ interactions.[3,48]

Despite their limitations, multi-organ OOC systems still have a number of applications. Skin-intestine-liver-kidney OOC systems have been used to accurately predict the human body's response to potentially toxic molecules absorbed orally or via the skin. In addition, body-on-a-chip systems have been used to study the efficacy of drug delivery systems, revealing whether the drug is delivered into the desired tissues and whether the byproducts of drug delivery bioaccumulate in the body. Also, body-on-a-chip systems have been used to study the side effects of chemotherapy drugs as well as cancer metastasis.[53,54] Figure 6-13 shows a simplified schematic of a lung-heart-bone-kidney-liver-gut multi-organ OOC system. This complex multi-organ OOC system is intended to test the effects of aerosol drugs and oral drugs on the human body, and is capable of simulating drug absorption, metabolism, transport and clearance, and even the immune response to the drug.[47]

6.3.4 Breakthroughs and Challenges of Organ-on-a-Chip Technology

In 2016, the first 3D OOC device created entirely using 3D printing was reported by Lind et al. as depicted in Figure 6-14. The 3D printing process used six different types of biocompatible polymer-based inks to create the microchip of a heart-on-a-chip device, together with embedded strain gage sensors as well as electrical contacts and leads. The strain gages are intended to measure the contractile stresses associated with cardiac tissue contraction, which occurs whenever a real heart beats. Dextran ink was used for the sacrificial layers, while thermoplastic polyurethane (TPU) was used for the structural layers such as load-bearing cantilevers. The wires of embedded strain gage sensors were printed with TPU

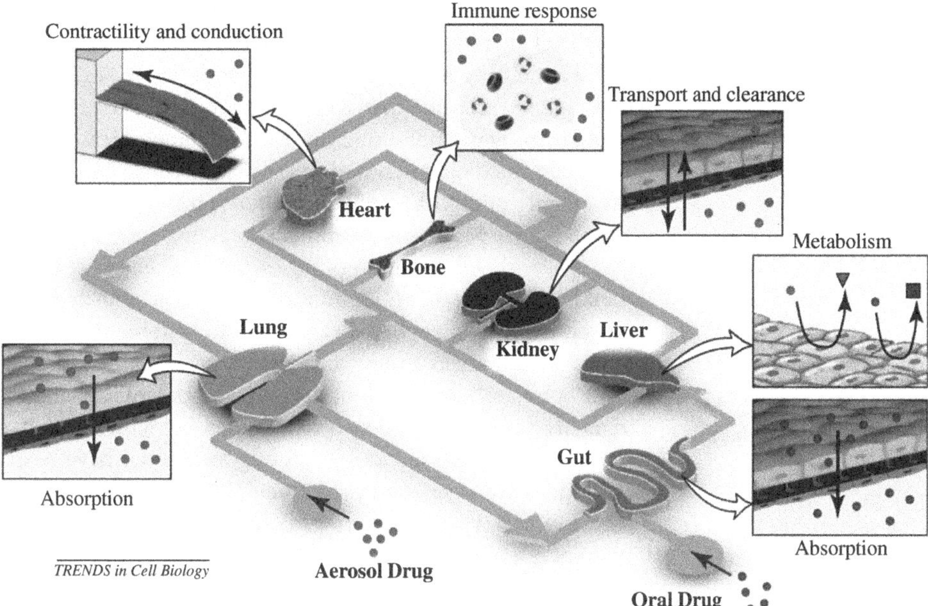

Figure 6-13 A multi-organ organ-on-a-chip (OOC) system which incorporates the functions of the human lung, heart, bone, kidney, liver, and gut. This system can be used to test the effects of aerosol drugs and oral drugs on the human body. (*The illustration is reprinted with permission from D. Huh et al.*[47])

ink strengthened with infused carbon nanoparticles, whereas the electrical contacts and leads were printed using conductive silver particle-infused polyamide ink. Soft portions of the substrate were printed with polydimethylsiloxane (PDMS) ink, but rigid portions were printed with polylactic acid (PLA) or acrylonitrile butadiene styrene (ABS) ink.[55] Compared with other microfabrication techniques, multi ink 3D printing offers greater reproducibility and significantly reduces microfabrication time and expenses in the production of OOC devices. Hence, multi-ink 3D printing can speed up the development and production of complex 3D OOC devices while simultaneously lowering costs.

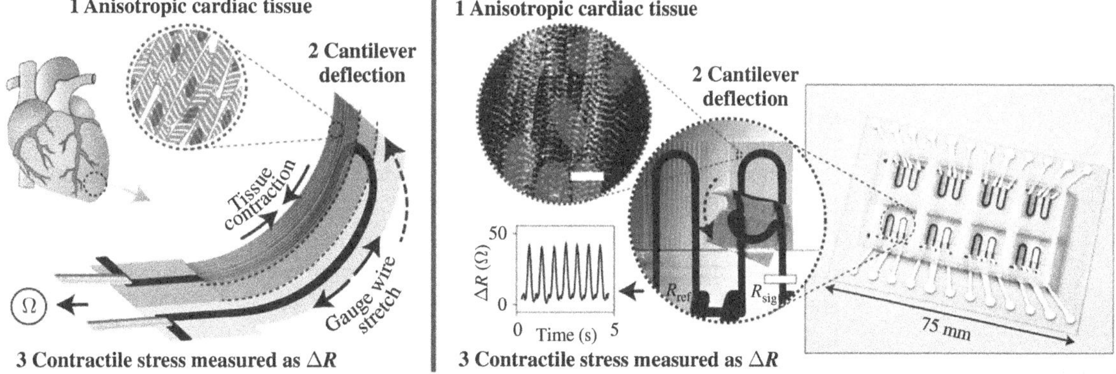

Figure 6-14 A heart-on-a-chip device created entirely using multi-ink 3D printing. In this organ-on-a-chip device, cardiac tissue contractions cause cantilever deflections, which generate a measurable change in electrical resistance ΔR. (*The figures are reprinted with permission from J. U. Lind et al.*[55])

Today, most 3D OOC microchip designs rely on microchambers and microchannels within a 3D microfluidic chip on which living cells and tissues are cultured. The 3D system of microchannels and microchambers can model the 3D micro-architectures within real organs with far greater accuracy than conventional cell cultures. However, the 3D micro-architectures of real organs contain innumerous sub-micrometer features which cannot be reliably replicated using microchannels and microchambers. To overcome this issue, microfluidic scaffolds and microfluidic hydrogels have been proposed. Microfluidic scaffolds are comprised of a biocompatible polymeric elastomer containing networks of nanometer to micrometer-sized pores, where the distribution of pores sizes can be easily tuned during the synthesis of the scaffolds. Although microfluidic scaffolds are not suitable for all organs, liver-on-a-chip and heart-on-a-chip devices have been successfully implemented on microfluidic scaffolds.[56] An alternative solution is to use microfluidic hydrogels. Hydrogels consist of water dispersed in hydrophilic 3D networks of cross-linked polymer chains. Hydrogels are biocompatible and highly permeable to most biomolecules, but tend to be mechanically fragile. Specialized micro/nano fabrication and 3D printing techniques have been developed which can create microfluidic hydrogels with predefined 3D micro-architectures. Due to similarities with the 3D structures in vasculatures (i.e., blood capillaries) and kidneys, vasculature-on-a-chip and kidney-on-a-chip devices have been created using microfluidic hydrogels.[57,58]

Another highly experimental yet promising development in OOC technology is the self-assembly of complex tissue structures. Under the right biochemical conditions, certain cells and tissues will self-assemble into intricate 3D microstructures that closely resemble the micro-architectures within real organs. For example, it has been shown that endothelial cells within a porous substrate can self-assemble into complex microvasculature networks under the influence of biochemical signals such as growth factors. Microvasculature networks are networks of tiny blood capillaries (each 5 to 10 µm in diameter) found in most human tissues. It has also been demonstrated that cultured neuron cells and glial cells can form intricate 3D neural networks under the right biochemical conditions. At present, the self-assembly of tissue microstructures is still a highly experimental topic, since it is a challenge to create the right biochemical environment and stimuli to guide and control the self-assembly.[59,60]

As with all microfluidic and LOC devices, a major issue currently facing OOC devices is the lack of standardized components, which greatly increases the time and expense required to develop novel OOC devices. In the fabrication of microelectronic devices and integrated circuits, standardized components (e.g., resistors, capacitors, transistors, and operational amplifiers) are readily available which can be assembled into circuits for virtually any application. Replicating or troubleshooting an integrated circuit design is fairly straightforward since the components used in the integrated circuit are all standardized. However, this is not the case with OOC devices. Since there are currently no standardized components that can be integrated together to design an OOC device, prototype OOC devices can be difficult to replicate or troubleshoot.[61]

Another major issue with all OOC devices is the lack of standard validation protocols at present. The main purpose of any OOC device is to replicate organ functions *in vitro*. However, there are no standard validation protocols to assess how well any OOC device replicates intended organ functions. Currently, different groups rely on totally different statistical measures and algorithms to assess how well their OOC devices perform. The lack of standard validation protocols makes it extremely difficult to compare the real-world performance of different OOC designs. Since most current OOC devices are designed to be used in healthcare for drug screening and disease (e.g., cancer) studies, the absence of standard validation protocols is likely a major barrier to the widespread adoption and commercialization of OOC devices.[61]

Most OOC devices today rely on optical detection to monitor the artificial "organs" in real time. In particular, the tissues on the OOC microchip are stained with fluorophores, excited with appropriate light sources, and then monitored under an optical microscope. In this situation, water-soluble QD (quantum dot) fluorophores are highly desirable since they have exceptional photostability, brightness, a relatively long fluorescence lifetime, and very large Stokes shift. Due to their photostability, water-soluble QDs will last far longer than organic fluorescent dyes under continuous optical excitation required for real-time monitoring. While organic fluorescent dyes require a different light source for each dye, water-soluble QDs designed to emit different colors can all be excited with a single (usually UV or blue) light source due to the large effective Stokes shift, greatly simplifying the optics involved. Moreover, water-soluble QDs are far brighter than organic fluorescent dyes under the same illumination conditions, and the longer fluorescence lifetime of QDs enable their emission signal to be more easily distinguished from background autofluorescence, which can be problematic since OOC microchips commonly incorporate polymers.

To non-invasively monitor the tissues in an OOC device in real time, a conventional optical microscope is usually used. However, conventional optical microscopes have limited resolution due to the diffraction limit of light, and limited total focused area due to the optics and the depth of field. The advent of non-invasive next-generation optical microscopy techniques promise to resolve both limitations of conventional optical microscopes. By combining specialized light sources with advanced optics and computer algorithms, next-generation super-resolution optical microscopes offer superior resolution while simultaneously observing a larger focused area or volume. In particular, deep tissue super-resolution imaging can image labeled tissues in 3D, which is especially useful for monitoring 3D OOC devices. Another promising technique for real-time OOC imaging is the next-generation *ex vivo* optical microscopy, which can image tissues in 3D without requiring labels, freezing, or fixing.[62,63]

On a final note, the two main methods in which the tissues on OOC devices are monitored in real time—optical detection and bioelectrical signal detection—generate video and bioelectrical signal data which can be difficult and time-consuming for a human to interpret. This could be potentially resolved with the use of machine learning techniques.

6.4 MICRO/NANO FABRICATION TECHNIQUES

6.4.1 Substrates and Overview of Micro/Nano Fabrication

A significant portion of this book has been dedicated to microfluidic and lab-on-a-chip (LOC) systems, whose functions are made possible by integrated chips at the heart of such systems. These integrated chips are usually 1 to 10 cm in length and width, and 0.5 to 5 mm in thickness. We will cover how these integrated chips are fabricated. LOC and microfluidic chips are created using MEMS (micro-electro-mechanical system) micro/nano fabrication techniques. MEMS fabrication techniques include standard techniques used for integrated circuit fabrication such as lithography, doping, thin film deposition/growth, and etching. More specialized MEMS fabrication techniques such as soft lithography, 3D micromachining, surface modification, and bonding are also commonly employed in the fabrication of microfluidic/LOC chips. Microfluidic and LOC device designers must be familiar with MEMS fabrication techniques because such devices can be complex and there are numerous fabrication choices that affect device performance and cost.[6]

Substrate Selection   An important consideration in the design of any microfluidic or LOC system is the substrate of the integrated chip at the core of the system. The integrated chip is normally fabricated on silicon (Si), glass (amorphous solid comprised mainly of SiO_2), quartz (crystalline SiO_2), PDMS (polydimethylsiloxane, a type of silicone polymer), SU-8 (an epoxy-based negative photoresist), or thermoplastic substrates. The choice of substrate material depends mainly on which detection method will be employed (if applicable), whether the integrated chip is disposable, the ease of fabrication and any desired surface modifications, as well as biocompatibility and mechanical strength considerations.[1]

If optical detection is to be employed—such as for OOCs that rely on optical microscope observation of labeled tissues and for optical LOC sensors—transparent substrates such as glass, quartz, and transparent polymers (e.g., PDMS and SU-8) are preferred. For the disposable parts of microfluidic and LOC devices (e.g., lateral flow LOC test strips), cheaper substrates such as paper, wax, and cloth are also used for easy disposal of biohazardous samples. These destructible substrate LOC devices use capillary forces to passively wick biofluid samples, and often rely on colorimetric optical detection.[1] In this case, the substrate does not need to be transparent because the detection method relies on color changes displayed on the substrate.

By far the most common substrate used for the integrated chips of microfluidic and LOC devices is silicon, which offers ease of fabrication together with favorable mechanical properties. In particular, single-crystal silicon substrates are used since silicon wafers are well characterized from use in the semiconductor and MEMS industries, and many micro/nano fabrication techniques have been established for silicon substrates. Polycrystalline silicon (also known as polysilicon) is comprised of many crystalline silicon grains with different sizes and orientations. Unlike polycrystalline silicon, the crystal lattice of single-crystal silicon is continuous throughout the entire wafer without any grain boundaries. Single-crystal silicon wafers are heavily used in the semiconductor and MEMS industries because the local electronic and physical properties are virtually identical throughout the entirety of each wafer. In addition, silicon has excellent mechanical properties: compared to steel, crystalline silicon has far higher strength-to-weight ratio, higher thermal conductivity, greater hardness, and far better machinability.

However, silicon substrates have a drawback: single-crystal and polycrystalline silicon surfaces are difficult to chemically modify. Surface modification involves the covalent attachment of functional groups (e.g., $-COOH$) and/or more complex molecules (e.g., antibodies) onto the surface of an integrated chip. Recognition elements can be anchored onto the sensing surface of a LOC biosensor via surface modification. A popular workaround for the issue of surface modification is to use SiO_2-coated silicon wafers, which can be purchased directly or created through the thermal oxidation of silicon wafers. Unlike silicon surfaces, SiO_2 surfaces are much more amenable to chemical modification.

Material biocompatibility is another consideration in the design of integrated chips that will be exposed to biofluids (e.g., saliva, urine, sweat, and blood) and/or live cells. Silicon, glass, quartz, PDMS, and SU-8 are all biocompatible materials. Most metals, however, are not biocompatible since they can oxidize or react with biological samples. As a noble metal with low reactivity, gold is a suitable biocompatible metal. In integrated chips where metal electrodes/interconnects are exposed to biological samples, gold is the preferred electrode/interconnect material.

Fabrication Process Overview   Once a suitable substrate has been selected, the next step is to design the micro/nano fabrication process for the integrated chip of the microfluidic/LOC system (Figure 6-15). In general, each integrated chip is constructed layer by layer from the bottom up starting with the substrate. Each subsequent layer is applied onto the layer beneath using a thin film deposition or growth technique. Popular thin film deposition/growth techniques include physical vapor deposition (PVD), chemical vapor deposition (CVD), electrochemical deposition (ECD), and thermal oxidation. If the applied layer

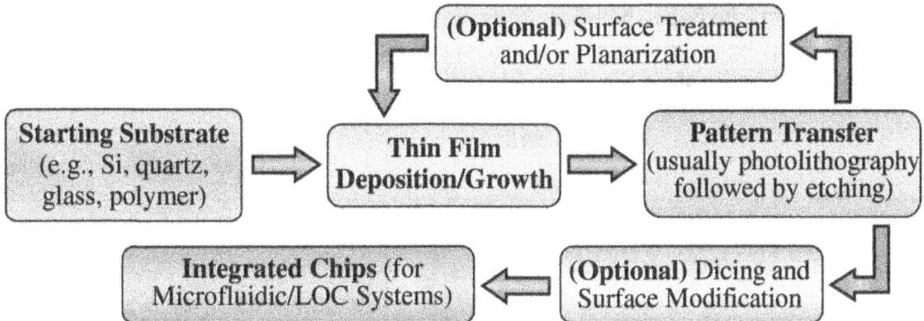

Figure 6-15 An overview of the micro/nano fabrication process for creating the integrated chips of microfluidic and LOC systems.

needs to be patterned, pattern transfer techniques are employed. Pattern transfer techniques include lithography, etching, and lift-off patterning. The most common pattern transfer method involves photolithography followed by etching. In situations where the surface topography of the top layer is uneven, surface planarization is often applied prior to the application of the next layer to prevent fabrication problems. To modify the electrical, structural, and optical properties of a semiconductor, impurities can be introduced into the semiconductor crystal lattice via doping, a type of surface treatment. Together, these fabrication techniques are sufficient for making integrated circuits, but are often not enough for creating the integrated chips of microfluidic/LOC systems.

In combination with the aforementioned integrated circuit fabrication techniques, the creation of integrated chips for microfluidic/LOC devices often requires specialized MEMS fabrication techniques. Prominent examples of such techniques include soft lithography, surface modification, 3D printing, 3D micromachining (i.e., bulk or surface micromachining), and bonding. If required, surface modification and dicing are carried out during the final step of integrated chip fabrication. Surface modification—such as anchoring recognition elements onto the sensing surface of an LOC biosensor—enhances the surface chemistry of the integrated chip. To reduce costs (per chip), multiple identical integrated chips are frequently created on a single substrate (e.g., wafer), and physically separated by dicing.

6.4.2 Thin Film Deposition and Growth

Similar to integrated circuits and MEMS devices, integrated chips for microfluidic/LOC devices are built up layer by layer from the bottom up. Each layer is formed through a thin film deposition or growth technique. The thickness of deposited film material is usually between 5 nm and 10 μm. The most prominent categories of thin film deposition/growth techniques include physical vapor deposition (PVD), chemical vapor deposition (CVD), electrochemical deposition (ECD), and thermal oxidation. An overall summary of common thin film deposition/growth techniques is shown in Table 6-1.

Thin Film Quality Different deposition/growth techniques produce thin films of different quality. Here, "quality" is an umbrella term which refers to the uniformity, density, and coverage of the thin film. Higher quality thin films have greater uniformity, higher density, and better coverage. Uniform thin films have consistent thicknesses and physical (e.g., mechanical, electrical, and optical) properties throughout the substrate surface on which they are deposited. Due to the presence of voids and defects, deposited/grown thin films always have lower densities than the corresponding bulk solid material. High-density thin films have lower concentrations of voids and defects, thereby achieving densities closer to the bulk material. Coverage refers to the thickness uniformity of a thin film on non-flat topography—a surface with microscale/nanoscale trenches. Thin films with

TABLE 6-1   A Summary of Common Thin Film Deposition/Growth Techniques

Deposition/Growth Technique	Suitable Thin Film Materials	Advantages	Disadvantages
Evaporation (PVD)	Elemental metals and semiconductors	No noxious gases	Slow deposition rates; high vacuum required
Sputtering (PVD)	Alloys, metals, semiconductors, and compounds	High-quality thin films; low substrate temperatures; no noxious gases	
Atmospheric-Pressure CVD (APCVD)	Solids that can be formed through vapor phase chemical reactions (most commonly Si, SiO_2, Si_3N_4, W, and WSi_x) *Note:* CVD reactors are often limited to just one material/process	Very high maximum deposition rates; vacuum not required	High substrate temperatures; noxious gases; wastage of reactant gases
Low-Pressure CVD (LPCVD)		Improved thin film uniformity and coverage	High substrate temperatures; noxious gases; vacuum required
Plasma-Enhanced CVD (PECVD)		High maximum deposition rates; reduced substrate temperatures	Noxious gases; vacuum required
Epitaxial CVD	Single-crystal materials (usually Si or GaAs)	Deposits single-crystal thin films	Especially high substrate temperatures; noxious gases; slow deposition rates
Electrochemical Deposition (ECD)	Conductive metals (most commonly Cu and Ni)	Superb coverage; very low substrate temperatures; vacuum not required	Substrate surface must be conductive
Thermal Oxidation	Amorphous SiO_2 on underlying Si surface	Very high-quality thin films; excellent adhesion and superb SiO_2–Si interface	Very high substrate temperatures; slow deposition rates; consumes underlying Si

good coverage have consistent thicknesses across the bottom, sidewalls, and surrounding flat topography of microscale/nanoscale trenches. Deposition/growth techniques with excellent coverage can completely fill microscale/nanoscale trenches without leaving behind air pockets or numerous voids.

Process Substrate Temperature   The temperature of the substrate during thin film deposition/growth is extremely important. Low substrate temperature is highly desirable because it reduces unwanted diffusion, thermal stresses, and (if present) the softening/degradation of amorphous materials such as polymers and glass. To avoid these issues, thin film deposition/growth methods with high substrate temperatures should be carried out close to the beginning of any fabrication process and before temperature-vulnerable thin film materials have been deposited. After that, only deposition/growth methods with low substrate temperatures can be used.

- *Unwanted Diffusion:* The concentrations of dopant atoms are essential to the function of transistors, diodes, and other microelectronic components. Unwanted diffusion can cause integrated circuits and microelectronic devices to fail. Additionally, unwanted diffusion can damage integrated chips at the nanoscale, potentially resulting in non-functional devices.

- *Thermal Stresses:* Thermal stresses are caused by differences in thermal expansion coefficients between different materials. When a substrate coated with a thin film is cooled from a high temperature, thermal stresses can cause the thin film to delaminate, crack, or otherwise fail. If the thin film is sufficiently thick, the substrate may even bend at high thermal stresses. Thermal stresses are especially problematic for substrates that are coated with multiple layers of patterned thin films, each comprising a different material. Fortunately, thermal stresses can be alleviated through annealing, which allows thin films to expand or contract to relieve stress. During the annealing process, the thin film coated substrate is heated to a moderately high temperature (depending on the thin film and substrate materials), then remains at that temperature, and finally slowly cools down.

- *Softening/Degradation of Amorphous Materials:* In general, the softening/degradation of any present amorphous materials will likely destroy any integrated chip. Amorphous materials are non-crystalline solids that lack a regular crystalline structure. Unlike crystalline materials (both single-crystal and polycrystalline), the atoms of amorphous materials are arranged in a disorderly fashion. For instance, glass is mainly comprised of amorphous SiO_2, while quartz is comprised of crystalline SiO_2. Because of their disorderly structure, amorphous materials begin to soften at their glass transition temperature, which is usually far lower than their melting point. In contrast, crystalline materials do not significantly soften until the temperature is close to their melting point. Although glass will not melt until temperatures well over 1000°C are achieved, glass begins to soften above 400°C. Polymers are also amorphous materials, and are often used as dielectrics (i.e., thermal and electrical insulators) since polymers are easy to shape, usually biocompatible, and sometimes transparent. In general, polymers have relatively low melting points (usually between 100°C and 300°C), and even lower glass transition temperatures (usually <100°C) at which they begin to soften. When heated to above their melting points, polymers will often thermally degrade.

(A) Physical Vapor Deposition (PVD)

During physical vapor deposition (PVD), the desired thin film material is deposited onto the substrate as a vapor, forming a solid thin film through condensation at the substrate surface. In general, PVD suffers from slow deposition rates, and is thus limited to the creation of thin films less than about 500 nm thick. Moreover, PVD is carried out under high vacuum, and requires a vacuum chamber that can achieve pressures below 10^{-3} Pa. There are two main PVD techniques: evaporation and sputtering. At present, some of the most common materials deposited by the evaporation technique are Al, Ag, Au, C, Cr, Cu, Pb, Pt, Si, Ta, Ti, and W. The most common materials deposited by sputtering include Al, Ag, Au, Cr, Pt, TiN (diffusion barrier and hardness coating), TiW (diffusion barrier), metal alloys, oxides, and nitrides.

Evaporation (PVD)   The evaporation technique involves the evaporation of a solid source material (called the "charge") in a vacuum chamber followed by deposition onto the substrate surface, condensing as a solid thin film. In order to evaporate the solid source material (i.e., convert the source material from solid to vapor phase), the source material is heated with either a large electrical current, a directed electron beam, or (less commonly) a laser beam. The entire evaporation process is conducted under high vacuum background pressures ($<10^{-3}$ Pa) to ensure a high deposition rate and to reduce impurities in the resulting thin film. The deposition rate by evaporation is increased under vacuum for two main reasons. First, most solid materials (at standard temperature and pressure) have relative low vapor pressures, and evaporate substantially faster under vacuum. Second, vacuum pressures prevent the desired vapor phase atoms from colliding with background gas molecules before reaching and condensing at the substrate. Under vacuum, the concentrations of background gas molecules are reduced by many orders of magnitude, thereby preventing their incorporation into the resulting thin film and reducing impurities.

Although the evaporation technique used to be popular due to its simplicity, it has many limitations. Evaporation is usually (but not always) limited to elemental metals and semiconductors since it is difficult to deposit compounds or alloys with evaporation, especially if the deposited thin film must have a specific stoichiometry. Also, the uncooled substrate temperature can rise to 200 to 500°C during evaporation due to heat transfer from the heated source material, limiting the applications of evaporation. Additionally, thin films produced by evaporation tend to have lower quality and uniformity than those produced by sputtering. Finally, evaporation offers much less control over the resulting thin films than sputtering, resulting in less repeatability and lower chip yields.

Sputtering (PVD) Currently, sputtering is the predominant and most popular PVD process.[64] During sputtering, a solid source material (called the "target") is bombarded by energetic ions, dislodging (i.e., "sputtering") the source material in atomic form. Atoms of the source material are then deposited onto the substrate forming a solid thin film. By far the most common ions used are noble gas ions with bombarding energies of 100 to 1000 eV per ion since noble gases are inert and will not chemically react with the target. In particular, Ar^+ ions are frequently used since argon is inexpensive and has sufficiently high atomic mass to be effective at sputtering solid targets. The bombarding ions are created in a low-pressure plasma glow discharge through electron impact ionizations, and are accelerated toward the target by a strong electric field generated by powered electrodes. The electrodes can be powered by DC, radio frequency AC, or pulsed-DC potentials. The entire sputtering process is conducted in a vacuum chamber because the low-pressure plasma glow discharge cannot be sustained under atmospheric pressure. Moreover, vacuum pressures enhance the sputter deposition rate and efficiency by reducing collisions between unwanted background gas molecules and desired atoms (i.e., the sputtered atoms and bombarding ions). As with evaporation, vacuum pressures significantly reduce impurities in the thin film deposited by sputtering.

The most popular sputtering method is magnetron sputtering, which offers far greater deposition rate and efficiency compared to the older diode sputtering method. In magnetron sputtering, magnets are used to confine electrons in the plasma glow discharge close to the target. Since the bombarding ions are created by electron impact ionizations, confining electrons near the target greatly increases ionization efficiency, thereby improving sputter deposition rates by several-fold.

A major advantage of sputtering compared to evaporation is that the substrates are kept at relatively low temperatures during sputtering (often <150°C). Generally, sputtering produces much higher quality thin films with better coverage than evaporation, while offering more control over the process, greater repeatability, and higher chip yields. Unlike evaporation, sputtering can be used to deposit alloys and compounds in addition to elemental metals and semiconductors. Compounds are often sputtered reactively, where gases (usually oxygen or nitrogen) are intentionally introduced. The introduced gases chemically react with the target material atoms to form compounds that are then deposited onto the substrate. Such reactions can take place at the target surface and/or the substrate surface. For instance, to sputter alumina (Al_2O_3), one can use a solid Al target in combination with introduced oxygen gas.

(B) Chemical Vapor Deposition (CVD)

In chemical vapor deposition (CVD), vapor phase reactants react at the substrate surface to form the desired solid thin film. Unlike PVD, the deposition rate of CVD can be adjusted over a very wide range. Compared to PVD, CVD usually offers a much larger maximum deposition rate, and thus CVD is suitable for depositing thin films thicker than 500 nm, as well as thin films thinner than 500 nm. However, PVD is much safer to carry out than CVD because the reactant and waste byproduct gases of CVD are often noxious (i.e., toxic, corrosive, flammable, and/or explosive). While sputtering can be carried out at relatively low temperatures (often <150°C), CVD usually requires substrate temperatures well above 300°C. Due to the gases and chemical reactions involved, CVD processes are much more vulnerable to cross-contamination than PVD. Hence, CVD reactors are often limited to just one material and one process, while a PVD system can deposit multiple materials.

During CVD, care must be taken to prevent chemical reactions from occurring outside of the substrate surface, or else solid particles will form that can contaminate the deposited thin film. CVD is a multi-step process where the deposition rate is determined by the slowest step. First, the reactant gas molecules diffuse and then adsorb onto the substrate surface. Second, the reactants chemically react with each other at the substrate surface, forming a solid product that is incorporated into the desired thin film. Finally, gaseous waste byproducts desorb and then diffuse away from the substrate surface. During CVD, the substrate is heated to high temperatures (300°C to over 1000°C) to activate the chemical reaction occurring at the substrate surface and speed up the diffusion of gas molecules to and from the substrate. Carrier gases (e.g., $N_{2(g)}$ or $H_{2(g)}$) that do not participate in reactions are often added to control the flow rate of reactant gases and the CVD reactor pressure.

Common variants of CVD include, but are not limited to, atmospheric-pressure CVD, low-pressure CVD, plasma-enhanced CVD, and epitaxial CVD.

Atmospheric-Pressure CVD   Atmospheric-pressure CVD (APCVD), the simplest variant of CVD, is performed under atmospheric pressure with a high flow rate of carrier gases to ensure that the CVD process proceeds at an acceptable rate. Although APCVD offers very high maximum deposition rates, it is inefficient because the majority of reactant gases used are wasted during APCVD.[65]

Low-Pressure CVD   Low-pressure CVD (LPCVD) is carried out in a vacuum chamber at pressures of 1 to 100 Pa, where carrier gases are not used at all. Compared to APCVD, LPCVD is much more efficient in the use of reactant gases. Because the diffusion coefficient of any gas is inversely related to pressure, low-pressure CVD greatly increases the rate of diffusion to and from the substrate surface, significantly improving gas transport uniformity. As a result, thin films deposited by LPCVD are much more uniform with better coverage than those deposited by APCVD. Due to the lower pressures, LPCVD processes tend to have lower maximum deposition rates.

Plasma-Enhanced CVD   Plasma-enhanced CVD (PECVD) is intended to lower the required substrate temperature, which is achieved by activating chemical reactions occurring at the substrate surface with a low-pressure plasma glow discharge instead of with high substrate temperatures. To sustain the plasma, PECVD is conducted in a vacuum chamber with plasma pressures of around 10 to 700 Pa. Compared to other CVD methods, PECVD reduces the required substrate temperature by hundreds of degrees (°C or K) to between 200°C and 400°C. Compared to LPCVD, PECVD offers much higher maximum deposition rates, but the thin films produced tend to be of lower quality.

Epitaxial CVD   Epitaxial CVD is the only CVD method that can deposit single-crystal thin films. In other words, the thin films deposited by other CVD methods are polycrystalline.

During epitaxial CVD, the single-crystal thin film is (relatively) slowly "grown" on a substrate heated to high temperatures through the reaction of reactant gases. For epitaxial CVD to work, the top surface of the substrate must be single-crystalline, must have similar lattice spacings as the thin film to be grown, and must be clean with low defect densities. The single-crystal thin film grown by epitaxial CVD has the same crystallographic orientation as the surface of the underlying substrate. Epitaxial CVD is mainly used in the semiconductor industry for the creation of silicon-on-insulator wafers, bipolar junction transistors, and GaAs semiconductor devices. Depending on the exact process, epitaxial CVD may be carried out under atmospheric pressure or in a vacuum.

CVD Materials and Examples   CVD can deposit most solid materials that could be formed through vapor phase chemical reactions. In particular, CVD can deposit a much wider range of compound materials than sputtering. In practice, CVD is usually used to deposit thin films that are difficult or too thick to be deposited by other means (e.g., sputtering). Common thin film materials deposited by CVD include—but are not limited to—silicon (single-crystal or polycrystalline), silicon dioxide (etch mask, electrical/thermal insulator, and passivation material), silicon nitride (etch mask, diffusion/oxidation barrier, and passivation material), tungsten (electrical interconnection material), and tungsten silicide (electrical contact material on silicon). Due to the ubiquity of sputtering, tungsten is the only significant metal that is commonly deposited by CVD.

The most common CVD reaction for depositing polycrystalline or single-crystal silicon (Si) is

$$SiH_{4(g)} \rightarrow Si_{(s)} + 2H_{2(g)} \quad \left(300 \text{ to } 1200°C, \text{ depending on CVD technique}\right) \tag{6.1}$$

To introduce n-type (e.g., phosphorus or arsenic) or p-type (e.g., boron) dopants into the resulting silicon (polycrystalline or single-crystal) thin film, gases such as phosphine ($PH_{3(g)}$), diborane ($B_2H_{6(g)}$), or arsine ($AsH_{3(g)}$) can be added in situ during the CVD deposition of silicon. In practice, doping (if required) is usually done after CVD deposition of silicon.

There are many CVD reactions that are suitable for producing silicon dioxide (SiO_2) or silicon nitride (Si_3N_4) thin films. Two of the most common reactions are shown below. To prevent the incorporation of hydrogen (H) in the Si_3N_4 thin film, nitrogen (N_2) gas is often added during PECVD.

$$SiH_{4(g)} + O_{2(g)} \rightarrow SiO_{2(s)} + 2H_{2(g)} \quad \left(\sim 400°C\right) \tag{6.2}$$

$$3SiH_{4(g)} + 4NH_{3(g)} \rightarrow Si_3N_{4(s)} + 12H_{2(g)} \quad \left(300 \text{ to } 900°C, \text{ depending on CVD technique}\right) \tag{6.3}$$

Tungsten (W) thin films can be deposited using the following CVD reactions. Note that reaction [Equation (6.5)] also produces tungsten silicide ($WSi_{x(s)}$)

$$WF_{6(g)} + 3H_{2(g)} \rightarrow W_{(s)} + 6HF_{(g)} \quad \left(\sim 400°C\right) \tag{6.4}$$

$$2WF_{6(g)} + 3SiH_{4(g)} \rightarrow 2W_{(s)} + 3SiF_{4(g)} + 6H_{?(g)} \quad \left(\sim 400°C\right) \tag{6.5}$$

(C) Electrochemical Deposition (ECD)

In the semiconductor industry, by far the most prevalent type of electrochemical deposition (ECD) used is electroplating, where electrolysis is used to deposit a metal thin film on a conductive substrate surface. ECD is most often used to deposit copper (Cu) and nickel (Ni). Compared with other inexpensive conductors (e.g., aluminum), copper offers substantially higher electrical conductivity and excellent electromigration resistance. Electromigration is the unwanted movement of metal atoms from the momentum transferred by electrons in an electrical current, especially if the current density is high. Over time, electromigration can result in short and/or open circuits, potentially causing device failure.

ECD offers two main advantages: superb coverage and very low substrate temperatures (normally below 60°C). In the microelectronics/MEMS industry, the most common application of ECD is the creation of copper electrical interconnects, especially vias. Vias are vertical electrical connections that link different planes/layers of integrated circuits or other devices. During ECD, the very low substrate temperatures allow copper electrical interconnects to be created without damaging the underlying integrated circuits or other microelectronic components. Furthermore, the excellent coverage of ECD allows microscale/nanoscale trenches to be completely filled with copper to create vias, even if the trenches are relatively narrow and deep. Filling such trenches with PVD or CVD can result in numerous voids and/or air pockets due to the poorer coverage, producing low-quality vias that may easily fail.

ECD Procedure (Copper)   To deposit copper (Cu) through ECD, a conductive substrate surface is immersed in copper sulfate ($CuSO_4$) solution, with a block of solid copper acting as the anode and the conductive substrate surface acting as the cathode. Various chemical additives such as sulfuric acid (H_2SO_4, to control pH), brighteners, carriers, and levelers could be added into the $CuSO_4$ solution to adjust the ECD process and modify the properties of deposited copper. A DC voltage applied between the cathode and anode supplies an electrical current through the $CuSO_4$ solution, which deposits solid copper onto the substrate surface (i.e., the cathode) while consuming the copper anode. The overall electrochemical reaction is

$$Cu^{2+}_{(aq)} + 2e^- \rightarrow Cu_{(s)} \ (20 \text{ to } 50°C) \tag{6.6}$$

ECD Procedure (Nickel)   The ECD process for depositing nickel (Ni) is similar to that of copper. A conductive substrate serves as a cathode in a solution containing nickel sulfate ($NiSO_4$) and nickel chloride ($NiCl_2$), while a solid block of nickel acts as the anode. Electrical current in the solution supplied by a DC voltage applied between the cathode and anode deposits solid nickel on the conductive substrate surface (i.e., cathode) while consuming the nickel anode. Chemical additives such as boric acid (H_3BO_3, to adjust pH), brighteners, carriers, and levelers can be added into the solution to adjust the process and alter the properties of deposited nickel. For depositing nickel (Ni), the overall electrochemical reaction is

$$Ni^{2+}_{(aq)} + 2e^- \rightarrow Ni_{(s)} \ (40 \text{ to } 65°C) \tag{6.7}$$

(D) Thermal Oxidation

In the semiconductor/MEMS industry, thermal oxidation is a very high temperature process used to grow amorphous (i.e., non-crystalline) silicon dioxide (SiO_2) on a silicon surface. The SiO_2 thin film grown by thermal oxidation is of extremely high quality, with excellent adhesion to the underlying silicon surface and superb SiO_2–Si interface. Thermal oxidation is typically used to create high-quality dielectric thin films for electrical and thermal insulation, as structural layers, as masks to protect patterned regions from diffusion or etching, or as gate oxides for metal-oxide semiconductor field-effect transistors (MOSFETs). Although thermal oxidation produces better quality SiO_2 thin films than PVD or CVD, the very high temperatures required (800 to 1200°C) limits the use of thermal oxidation to the first few steps of a fabrication process, before the creation of any layers sensitive to high temperatures. Another disadvantage of thermal oxidation is the slow oxide (i.e.,

SiO$_2$) growth rate, which usually limits the thickness of oxide grown by thermal oxidation to under 1 μm. Unlike PVD or CVD, thermal oxidation consumes the underlying silicon to form the resulting oxide. To protect patterned regions of a surface from thermal oxidation, a sufficiently thick patterned silicon nitride (Si$_3$N$_4$) mask is used.

There are three main variants of thermal oxidation: dry oxidation, non-pyrogenic wet oxidation, and pyrogenic wet oxidation. During thermal oxidation, the silicon surface is exposed to either oxygen gas (dry oxidation), water vapor (non-pyrogenic wet oxidation), or water vapor formed by the reaction of hydrogen and oxygen gases (pyrogenic wet oxidation). At the same temperatures, dry oxidation grows oxide (i.e., SiO$_2$) significantly more slowly than the two forms of wet oxidation, but produces slightly better quality thin films. In general, higher thermal oxidation temperatures grow oxide at faster rates. For single-crystal silicon surfaces, the rate of oxide growth by thermal oxidation also depends on the crystallographic orientation. Unfortunately, metal ions which can damage microelectronic components can easily become dissolved in the water vapor used during non-pyrogenic wet oxidation. Compared to non-pyrogenic wet oxidation, pyrogenic wet oxidation greatly reduces metal ion contamination due to the use of clean water vapor formed through the chemical reaction of hydrogen and oxygen gases.[66] The overall chemical reactions for dry and wet thermal oxidation are listed below.

$$\text{Dry Oxidation: } Si_{(s)} + O_{2(g)} \rightarrow SiO_{2(s)} \left(800 \text{ to } 1200°C\right) \tag{6.8}$$

$$\text{Wet Oxidation: } Si_{(s)} + 2H_2O_{(g)} \rightarrow SiO_{2(s)} + 2H_{2(g)} \left(800 \text{ to } 1200°C\right) \tag{6.9}$$

In non-pyrogenic wet oxidation, water vapor is added directly. In pyrogenic wet oxidation, water vapor is introduced through the following reaction:

$$2H_{2(g)} + O_{2(g)} \rightarrow 2H_2O_{(g)} \left(\text{Pyrogenic Wet Oxidation Only}\right) \tag{6.10}$$

Silicon wafers that are already coated with a surface layer of SiO$_2$ (called "thermal oxide") can be readily purchased. If we want to apply thermal oxidation on an entire blank silicon wafer, it may be easier and less expensive to instead purchase silicon wafers coated with thermal oxide.

6.4.3 Pattern Transfer

Pattern transfer techniques are intended to transfer a desired pattern to either the top layer of the substrate or the substrate surface itself. Unlike a flat surface, the surface of a patterned layer contains topographical features such as trenches and mesas. Commonly used pattern transfer methods include lithography, etching, and lift-off patterning. Lithography is an additive pattern transfer technique which transfers the desired pattern to a layer of deposited resist, a cured polymeric material that is usually 1 to 5 μm in thickness. Etching is a subtractive pattern transfer technique that etches (i.e., removes) unprotected regions of the substrate surface to create the desired surface topography. In fact, the patterned surface layer of resist created by lithography is commonly used as an etch mask or protective barrier. Etch masks are meant to protect desired regions of the substrate surface from being etched during etching, while protective barriers prevent certain regions of the substrate surface from being treated during surface treatments. Finally, lift-off patterning is used to create a patterned layer of thin film without etching. Lift-off patterning is used for materials that are difficult to etch, since the quality of patterned thin film obtained by lift-off patterning is generally inferior to that obtained by etching. The common pattern transfer techniques used in micro/nano fabrication are summarized in Table 6-2.

TABLE 6-2   A Summary of Common Pattern Transfer Techniques

Pattern Transfer Technique	Purpose	Advantages	Disadvantages
Photolithography	Transfers pattern from a photomask onto a layer of photoresist	Highly cost effective; high throughput	Requires a patterned photomask; works only on planar surfaces
Direct-Write Lithography	Transfers pattern directly onto a layer of resist; commonly used to create photomasks	No mask required; works on non-planar surfaces	Extremely low throughput; expensive
Isotropic Wet Etching	Uses a liquid etchant to remove patterned regions of a surface which are not protected by an etch mask; may require a mask to protect the backside of the substrate	Suitable for etching deep structures (fast etch rates); simple and inexpensive	Cannot etch small features; undercutting; challenging to control; noxious etchant solutions
(Alkaline) Anisotropic Wet Etching of Silicon		Directional etch of {100} Si; nearly vertical etch of {100} Si; simple and inexpensive	Depends on silicon crystal lattice structure; noxious etchant solutions
Physical Dry Etching	Uses ion bombardment to physically remove patterned regions of a surface which are not protected by an etch mask	Directional etch; can etch any solid material; safe	No/poor selectivity (~1); very slow etch rates; etch artifacts
Chemical Dry Etching	Uses reactive gases to chemically remove patterned regions of a surface which are not protected by an etch mask	Good selectivity; adjustable etch rates; safe	Cannot etch small features; undercutting; can only etch materials with suitable chemical reactions
Reactive Ion Etching (RIE)	(Physical-Chemical Dry Etching) Uses a combination of ion bombardment and reactive gases to remove patterned regions of a surface which are not protected by an etch mask	Can etch small features; adjustable etch rates; vertical etching; good selectivity; safe	Etch artifacts; cannot etch deep features with high aspect ratios; complicated
Deep Reactive Ion Etching (DRIE)		Can etch small features and deep structures with high aspect ratios; safe; vertical etching; adjustable and very fast etch rates; excellent selectivity;	Complicated and expensive; etch artifacts
Lift-Off Patterning	Creates patterned thin film(s) in an additive process without using etching	Can pattern alloys/mixed materials/multi-material stacks	Patterning accuracy and reliability issues

Etching methods can be classified as either wet etching or dry etching. Wet etching uses a liquid solution (i.e., a liquid etchant) to chemically remove regions of the substrate surface which are not protected by a mask. In contrast, dry etching uses energetic ions and/ or electrically neutral reactive gas molecules to remove unprotected regions of the substrate surface. Overall, wet etching methods are much simpler and less expensive to carry out than dry etching methods. However, dry etching methods can etch smaller features more accurately than wet etching methods, and are more flexible and safer to carry out than wet etching methods.

In wet etching, the substrate is submerged in a wet etchant solution, and all sides of the substrate are exposed to the etchant solution. A problem arises if the top and bottom surfaces of the substrate can both be significantly etched by the wet etchant (for instance, both surfaces are comprised of the same material), which is generally undesirable. Therefore, depositing an unpatterned mask on the bottom side of the substrate is sometimes necessary prior to wet etching to protect the entire bottom side from being etched. During wet etching, unwanted etching can also occur on the sides and edges of the substrate. Fortunately, most substrates used in micro/nano fabrication are thin enough (≤1 mm) that unwanted etching of sides/edges is rarely an issue, especially if dicing is performed which will cut away the edges of the substrate. Instead of masking the backside of a wafer, one can also use a liquid-tight and etchant-resistant wafer chuck to protect the wafer backside.

Compared to wet etching, one major advantage of dry etching is that dry etchants (i.e., energetic ions and/or electrically neutral reactive gas molecules) do not etch the backside of the substrate. Hence, there is no need to deposit a mask on the backside of the substrate prior to dry etching, and liquid-tight wafer chucks are not required.

Etching methods can also be categorized as either isotropic, partially anisotropic (directional), or completely anisotropic (vertical), as shown in Figure 6-16. Isotropic etching involves etching in all directions, while completely anisotropic (vertical) etching involves etching purely in the vertical direction. Partially anisotropic (directional) etching is in between isotropic and completely anisotropic (vertical) etching. For pattern transfer (etching in particular), three important parameters are the aspect ratio, etch rate, and (etch mask) selectivity which are defined in Equations (6.11), (6.12), and (6.13), respectively.

Aspect Ratio   The aspect ratio of any pattern transfer technique is defined as follows:

$$\text{Aspect Ratio} = \frac{\text{Depth (or Height) of Feature}}{\text{Width of Feature}} \tag{6.11}$$

For example, the aspect ratio of an etched trench is the depth of the trench divided by the trench width. In general, pattern transfer techniques that can achieve high aspect ratios are highly desirable.

Etch Rate   The etch rate of any etching technique is

$$\text{Etch Rate} = \frac{\text{Depth of Etched Feature}}{\text{Etch Time}} \tag{6.12}$$

The etch rate is same in all directions for isotropic etching. For partially anisotropic (directional) etching and completely anisotropic (vertical) etching, the etch rate is significantly faster in the vertical direction than the horizontal direction. If the etch rate is high, much deeper structures can be feasibly etched, but it is more difficult to control the etched structure.

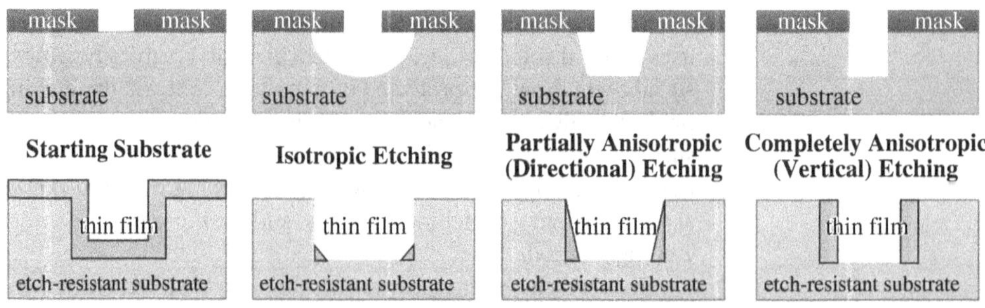

Figure 6-16   Isotropic etching, partially anisotropic (directional) etching, and completely anisotropic (vertical) etching. (Top) Etching a substrate covered with a patterned and protective etch mask. (Bottom) Etching a coating of unprotected thin film deposited on an etch-resistant substrate.

(Etch Mask) Selectivity   When choosing a suitable etch mask, the (etch mask) selectivity is an important parameter to consider. It is defined as follows:

$$(\text{Etch Mask}) \text{ Selectivity} = \frac{\text{Etch Rate of Material (To Be Etched)}}{\text{Etch Rate of (Etch) Mask}} \quad (6.13)$$

The thickness of etch mask required depends on both the etch mask selectivity and the desired etch depth. For an etch mask material, we want the selectivity to be high, which enables the use of a thin etch mask. If the selectivity is equal to one—which is generally undesirable—the material to be etched and the mask material are etched at the same rate.

(A) Lithography

Lithography is a process used to transfer a desired pattern to a layer of resist. The patterned resist can then be used as an etch mask or protective barrier (i.e., to protect desired regions of the substrate surface from being etched during etching, or from being treated during surface treatments). The two most common lithography techniques are photolithography and direct-write lithography. Photolithography requires a patterned photomask, while direct-write lithography does not require any kind of mask. Furthermore, photolithography offers far greater throughput and is more cost effective than direct-write lithography. Thus, direct-write lithography is mainly used to create patterned photomasks and low-volume/ prototype chips.

Photolithography   Photolithography uses UV (ultraviolet) light to transfer the pattern on a photomask to a layer of photoresist with the help of a developer. The most critical components of photolithography are the UV light source, photomask, photoresist, and developer.

- *UV Light Source:* The UV light source used has a wavelength between 10 nm and 440 nm, from extreme UV to violet light. Typically, less expensive photolithography equipment uses filtered broadband UV light from high-pressure mercury-vapor lamps (436 nm/405 nm/365 nm for the G/H/I-lines). However, the production of cutting-edge integrated circuits such as computer processors require short-wavelength monochromatic UV light. These light sources include deep UV light from KrF lasers (248 nm) or ArF lasers (193 nm), as well as extreme UV (~13.5 nm) generated by laser-driven plasma.

- *Photomask:* A photomask consists of an opaque layer of patterned thin film deposited on a transparent substrate. Here, opaque and transparent are defined with respect to the wavelength(s) of the UV light source used. For UV wavelengths above 200 nm, the photomask is typically a glass substrate (soda lime, crown, or fused silica glass) coated with a patterned ~100-nm-thick layer of chromium (Cr). More exotic and far more expensive photomasks are required for UV wavelengths below 200 nm.

- *Photoresist (PR):* Photoresists are polymers dissolved in a solvent along with additives such as photosensitive cross-linking agents. Photoresists can be classified as positive or negative. Positive photoresists become soluble in the developer after exposure to UV light, while negative photoresists become insoluble in the developer after exposure to UV light. One of the most popular photoresists for the fabrication of microfluidic/LOC integrated chips is SU-8, a negative epoxy-based photoresist that is both biocompatible and transparent.

- *Developer:* A developer is a solvent that dissolves cured positive photoresists exposed to UV light, or cured negative photoresists not exposed to UV light. Developers are critical to the creation of patterned layers of photoresist, and different photoresist formulations require different developers.

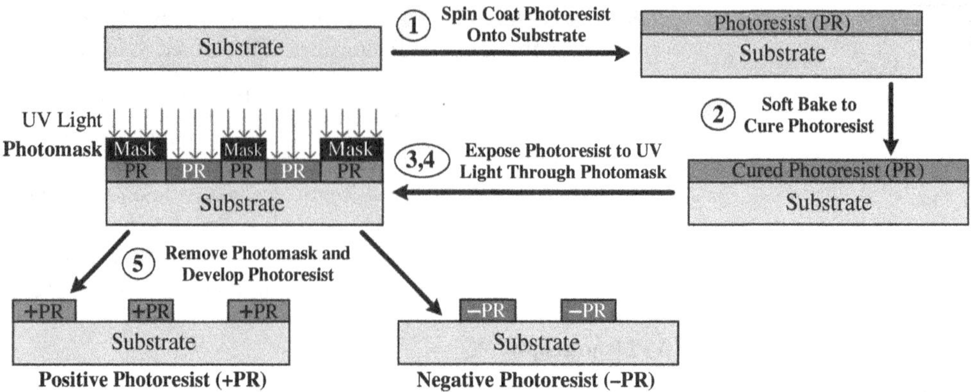

Figure 6-17   The overall process for photolithography, which deposits and patterns a layer of photoresist.

Photolithography Procedure   The overall procedure for photolithography, as illustrated in Figure 6-17, is as follows.

(1)   Spin coat photoresist onto the substrate surface using a spin coater capable of reaching thousands of RPM (revolutions per minute). The substrate surface must be planar (i.e., flat).

(2)   Use a hotplate to "soft bake" the photoresist coating dry (usually ≤100°C) by driving off any remaining solvents in the photoresist solution. The cured (i.e., dry) photoresist coating is usually 1 to 5 μm thick, depending on the photoresist formulation and the spin speed during spin coating.

(3)   Use a mask aligner to align the photomask onto and above the cured photoresist surface.

(4)   Use the UV light source to expose the cured photoresist layer through the photomask. The exposure typically lasts a few seconds to a minute. The ideal UV exposure dose/time depends on the type of photoresist used, the thickness of the photoresist, and the UV reflectivity of the material right underneath the photoresist.

(5)   Remove the photomask and then develop the photoresist by immersing the exposed photoresist coating in a suitable developer solution.

(6)   *(Optional)* Use a hotplate to "hard bake" the photoresist coating (at about 120 to 180°C) to further cure the photoresist coating, improve photoresist adhesion to the substrate below, and completely remove any remaining solvents. This step is optional, but is helpful if the cured photoresist will be used as a structural layer, etch mask, or protective barrier.

(Planar) Resolution of Photolithography   There are many factors limiting the (planar) resolution of photolithography, which is the dimension of the smallest feature that can be reliably transferred to the cured and patterned photoresist coating. The (planar) resolution of photolithography r_{min} is limited by optical diffraction (which depends on the wavelength of light λ), the gap g between the photomask and the photoresist surface, and the thickness t of the cured photoresist as follows.[65]

$$r_{min} = \frac{3}{2}\left[\lambda\left(g + \frac{1}{2}t\right)\right]^{1/2}$$

$$(6.14)$$

Here, λ is the (vacuum or air) peak wavelength of the monochromatic UV light source. If the UV light source has multiple peaks, such as UV light filtered from a high-pressure mercury-vapor lamp, λ is the peak wavelength of the longest-wavelength peak (usually 436 nm or 405 nm).

In contact photolithography, there is physical contact between the photomask and photoresist surface (i.e., $g \cong 0$), which minimizes the resolution r_{min}. In proximity photolithography, there is a gap between the photomask and photoresist surface (i.e., $g > 0$), limiting the achievable resolution r_{min}. Compared to proximity photolithography, contact photolithography can transfer smaller features to the cured and patterned photoresist coating, but is more likely to degrade the photomask used. The cleanliness of the photoresist coating and photomask is especially important during contact lithography, since micrometer-sized dust particles trapped between the photoresist coating and photomask (i.e., $g > 1\,\mu m$) will result in significantly poorer resolution r_{min}. In addition, reducing the thickness t of the cured photoresist will also improve the achievable resolution r_{min}. Equation (6.14) does *not* apply to projection photolithography systems, where lenses are used to focus UV light onto the photomask, and then focus the UV light transmitted through the photomask onto the cured photoresist surface.

Using contact photolithography ($g \cong 0$) with less expensive equipment where $\lambda = 405$ nm (the H-line of mercury-vapor lamps), and with a cured photoresist thickness of $t = 1\,\mu m$, a resolution of

$$r_{min} \cong \frac{3}{2}\left[(405\ \text{nm})\left(\frac{1}{2}\cdot 1\,\mu m\right)\right]^{1/2} = 675\ \text{nm}$$

can be achieved. By filtering light from mercury-vapor lamps leaving behind only the 365 nm I-line, and reducing the cured photoresist thickness to $t = 500$ nm, the resolution can be improved to

$$r_{min} \cong \frac{3}{2}\left[(365\ \text{nm})\left(\frac{1}{2}\cdot 500\ \text{nm}\right)\right]^{1/2} = 453\ \text{nm}$$

For contact photolithography, filtering the light source and reducing the cured photoresist thickness are the simplest and least inexpensive methods for obtaining better (planar) resolution. A (planar) resolution of less than 500 nm is more than sufficient for the fabrication of most microfluidic/LOC integrated chips. Nevertheless, the fabrication of more sophisticated complementary metal-oxide-semiconductor (CMOS) LOC devices can require (planar) resolutions of as low as 150 nm.

To attain even lower (planar) resolutions in the semiconductor industry, projection photolithography combined with a deep UV laser (248 nm KrF laser or 193 nm ArF laser) is often used. A (planar) resolution of about 100 to 150 nm—which is sufficient for virtually all microfluidic/LOC integrated chips—can be feasibly attained with a deep UV laser in combination with projection photolithography. To obtain even better (planar) resolutions, techniques requiring extremely expensive equipment (>10 million USD) such as immersion projection photolithography or extreme UV projection photolithography are used in the semiconductor industry.

Direct-Write Lithography   Aside from photolithography, another popular lithography technique is direct-write lithography, which scans (i.e., rasters) a focused beam line by line across a resist-covered surface to transfer the desired pattern to the layer of resist. Compared to photolithography, the most important advantage of direct-write lithography is that no masks (e.g., photomasks) are required. Another advantage is that direct-write lithography can create patterned resist on non-planar surfaces, while photolithography is limited to the creation of patterned photoresist on planar surfaces. Owing to the long time required for rastering, direct-write lithography is extremely slow, often requiring more than 10 min for a single 100 mm wafer compared to less than 30 s for photolithography. While the focused beam of direct-write lithography can only process a single wafer at a time, the UV light source used in photolithography can process an entire batch of wafers simultaneously. Moreover, direct-write lithography proceeds more slowly for larger wafers and for finer (planar) resolutions, since more/longer lines must be rastered. Taken altogether, direct-write lithography is very time-consuming, yielding far lower throughput than photolithography. As such, direct-write lithography is used to create photomasks for photolithography, low-volume chips, and prototype chips for research and development. Note that once a single photomask has been created with direct-write lithography, additional photomasks of the same design can be more quickly and economically created with photolithography.

The focused beam used for rastering during direct-write lithography is typically either a UV laser beam (with a peak wavelength between 150 nm and 450 nm), or an electron beam (e-beam). For (UV) laser direct-write lithography, the same photoresists and developers suitable for photolithography are used. On the other hand, electron beam direct-write lithography requires e-beam resists and their corresponding developers. Like photoresists, e-beam resists can also be positive (i.e., become soluble in the developer after e-beam exposure) or negative (i.e., become insoluble in the developer after e-beam exposure). Similar to photoresists, e-beam resists are usually comprised of polymers dissolved in a solvent with additives.

With laser direct-write lithography, a (planar) resolution of about 300 to 500 nm can be feasibly achieved. Electron beam direct-write lithography can achieve (planar) resolutions below 50 nm, but requires far more expensive equipment than laser direct-write lithography. However, rastering a complex pattern with fine (planar) resolution can require many hours for an e-beam direct-write lithography system.

Direct-Write Lithography Procedure   The procedure for direct-write lithography is as follows.

(1) Spin coat resist (photoresist or e-beam resist) onto the substrate surface using a spin coater capable of reach thousands of revolutions per minute (RPM).

(2) Use a hotplate to "soft bake" the resist coating dry by driving off any remaining solvents in the resist solution.

(3) Raster the focused UV laser beam or electron beam across the 2D resist surface.

(4) Develop the exposed resist by immersion in a suitable developer solution.

(5) **(Optional)** Use a hotplate to "hard bake" the resist coating to further cure the coating and improve coating adhesion to the substrate below. Again, this optional step can be helpful if the cured resist will be used as a structural layer, etch mask, or protective barrier.

Resist Removal   A final concern in the application of both photolithography and direct-write lithography is the removal of resist. A cured and patterned layer of resist created through lithography is typically used as a temporary etch mask or protective barrier. As such, the cured and patterned layer of resist at the substrate surface often needs to be removed (i.e., stripped) before the next layer of thin film can be deposited/grown on the substrate surface. Most resists can be removed with specialized solvents. For instance, immersion in acetone solvent followed by rinsing with isopropyl alcohol (IPA) is a common method for

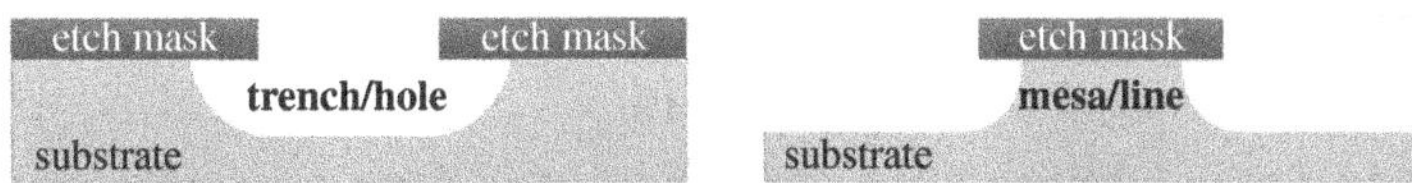

Figure 6-18 Isotropic etching etches in all directions, which results in undercutting. Undercutting is the over-etching of (left) trenches/holes and (right) mesas/lines.

removing cured resist. However, resists that are difficult to remove with solvents will need to be removed with plasma dry etching.

(B) Isotropic Wet Etching

During isotropic wet etching, a liquid etchant solution chemically removes regions of the substrate surface which are not protected by an etch mask. The etch is isotropic if the desired material is etched away equally in all directions that are exposed to the etchant. Isotropic wet etching can be used to etch silicon (single-crystal or polycrystalline), silicon dioxide (e.g., quartz), silicon nitride, glass, many metals (e.g., Al, Au, Pt, Ti, Ta, and Cr), and many compounds (e.g., TiN, TaN).

In general, the etch rate of isotropic wet etching is very high. The high etch rate is advantageous if relatively deep features (> 5 µm) must be etched, but it makes the etching process difficult to control. Another issue with isotropic wet etching is undercutting (Figure 6-18)—the over-etching of topographical features such as trenches, holes, mesas, and lines. It is challenging to accurately etch small features (<5 µm in width, length, or depth) with isotropic wet etching due to the high etch rate combined with undercutting. To compensate for undercutting, the etch mask can be designed such that trench/hole openings are made narrower, while masked regions covering mesas/lines are made wider. An additional disadvantage of isotropic wet etching is the extensive use of noxious etchant solutions which commonly contain highly corrosive and toxic acids. In situations where the wet etchant can significantly etch both the front and back sides of the substrate, the backside needs to be protected either by an unpatterned mask deposited prior to wet etching or with a liquid-tight wafer chuck that is resistant to the etchant solution used.

HNA Wet Etching of Silicon   HNA is a mixture of hydrofluoric acid (HF), nitric acid (HNO_3), and acetic acid (CH_3COOH). The isotropic wet etching of silicon utilizes HNA, and does *not* depend on the crystallographic orientation of silicon. HNA etching of silicon proceeds in the same way regardless of the crystallographic orientation, and regardless of whether the silicon is single-crystal or polycrystalline. Because HNA will aggressively attack most resists as well as SiO_2, Si_3N_4 or gold etch masks are used for HNA etching. The HNA etching of silicon involves the following chemical reactions:

(1) Nitric acid (HNO_3) is a strong acid and can oxidize the surface silicon (Si), converting silicon to silicon dioxide. The chemical reaction is as follows:

$$3Si_{(s)} + 4HNO_{3(aq)} \rightarrow 3SiO_{2(s)} + 4NO_{(g)} + 2H_2O_{(l)} \tag{6.15A}$$

(2) Hydrofluoric acid (HF) can further oxidize silicon dioxide (SiO_2), producing water-soluble hexafluorosilicic acid (H_2SiF_6). The chemical reaction is as follows:

$$3SiO_{2(s)} + 18HF_{(aq)} \rightarrow 3H_2SiF_{6(aq)} + 6H_2O_{(l)} \tag{6.15B}$$

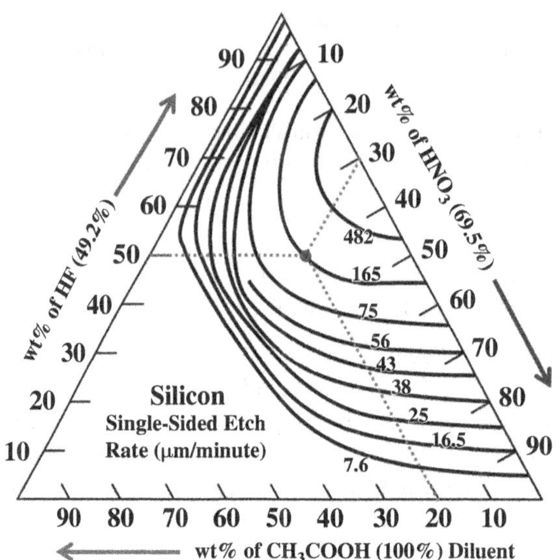

Figure 6-19 The isotropic etch rate of silicon attainable through HNA etching. (*The figure is redrawn with permission using data from H. Robbins and B. Schwartz.*[67])

The overall reaction for HNA wet etching of silicon is

$$3Si_{(s)} + 4HNO_{3(aq)} + 18HF_{(aq)} \rightarrow 4NO_{(g)} + 8H_2O_{(l)} + 3H_2SiF_{6(aq)} \tag{6.16}$$

Nitric acid is a strong oxidizing agent that is reduced in chemical reactions. Acetic acid helps prevent the dissociation of nitric acid and maintains the oxidizing ability of nitric acid. Isotropic etching is very fast, and the etch rate depends on the concentration of hydrofluoric acid, nitric acid, and acetic acid. The etch rate also depends on the dopant concentration of the silicon substrate. Although water can be used, acetic acid is more commonly used because it can prevent the dissociation and evaporation of nitric acid.

The etch rate can be predicted using the plot in Figure 6-19, where the left axis is the weight ratio of 49.2% HF, the right axis is the weight ratio of 69.5% HNO₃, and the bottom axis is the weight ratio of 100% CH₃COOH. If we want to obtain a single-sided silicon etch rate of 165 μm/min, we can select a point (e.g., the red dot) in the plot. We then draw three lines parallel to the three sides of the triangle (e.g., the three blue dashed lines) to obtain an HNA mixture consisting of (50 parts of 49.2% HF), (30 parts of 69.5% HNO₃) and (20 parts of 100% CH₃COOH diluent).

It is difficult to etch a controllable structure with HNA wet etching of silicon due to the extremely high etch rate. Therefore, HNA wet etching of silicon is normally used for polishing uneven silicon surfaces or for making the silicon substrate thinner by etching from the backside of the silicon wafer.

BOE Wet Etching of SiO₂ or Glass   To etch SiO₂ (e.g., quartz) or glass (amorphous solid comprised mainly of SiO₂) with isotropic wet etching, a solution of hydrofluoric acid (HF) plus ammonium fluoride (NH₄F) as an acidity buffer is used. To allow small features to be more accurately etched, a surfactant is often added into the etchant solution for reducing surface tension during etching. This etchant solution is called a buffered oxide etchant (BOE) or buffered HF (BHF) etchant. By using the NH₄F acidity buffer, a constant (instead of steadily decreasing) SiO₂/glass etch rate of ~100 nm/min can be maintained.

For BOE etching, Si₃N₄, silicon (single-crystal or polycrystalline), or gold masks are preferred as they offer very high selectivity. However, gold is expensive and does not adhere well to glass or SiO₂ (e.g., quartz), requiring an adhesion layer of chromium. Although resists can be used as etch masks for BOE etching, BOE solution can both attack resists and cause resists to peel off. The chemical reaction for BOE etching of SiO_2 is

$$SiO_{2(s)} + 6HF_{(aq)} \rightarrow H_2SiF_{6(aq)} + 2H_2O_{(l)} \qquad (6.17A)$$

The above reaction is identical to reaction (2) of HNA etching of silicon. The difference here is that the NH_4F acidity buffer maintains a constant concentration of HF through the following reaction:

$$NH_4F_{(aq)} \rightarrow NH_{3(aq)} + HF_{(aq)} \qquad (6.17B)$$

Wet Etching of Silicon Nitride   The isotropic wet etching of silicon nitride (Si_3N_4) is performed using concentrated phosphoric acid (H_3PO_4) heated to 140 to 180°C in a reflux system. In this acid vapor reflux system, H_3PO_4 is continually evaporated and then condensed on the substrate surface to be etched. This reflux system ensures that the condensed H_3PO_4 remains highly concentrated, providing a relatively constant Si_3N_4 etch rate. Unlike other isotropic wet etch chemistries, wet etching of Si_3N_4 is generally very slow (~10 nm/min). Suitable masks for this process include Si (selectivity of ~30) and SiO_2 (selectivity of ~10). Due to the relatively high temperatures involved, resists (and polymeric materials in general) are not suitable masks for this process.[68]

Wet Etching of Metals   The isotropic wet etching of metals can be done with acidic solutions containing a combination of acids/oxidizers (e.g., HF, HCl, HNO_3, and H_3PO_4) together with diluents (e.g., water or acetic acid) and aqueous additives such as pH buffers. For metal wet etching, photoresist etch masks made through photolithography are most commonly used. Depending on the etch solution, more expensive etch masks comprised of Si, SiO_2, Si_3N_4, or even e-beam resists can also be used.

(C) Anisotropic Wet Etching of Silicon

Anisotropic wet etching of silicon involves etching along a particular direction (i.e., along an angle) into a single-crystal silicon substrate with a liquid etchant solution. Anisotropic wet etching utilizes alkaline etchant solutions, since the relative alkaline etch rate of single-crystal silicon depends on the crystallographic orientation. Anisotropic wet etching only works on single-crystal silicon, the predominant substrate used in the semiconductor industry. Depending on the crystallographic orientation of the single-crystal silicon surface to be etched, alkaline wet etchants can achieve either partially anisotropic (directional) or completely anisotropic (vertical) etching. If alkaline wet etchants are used to etch polycrystalline silicon, they would act instead as isotropic wet etchants. For anisotropic wet etching where both the front and back sides of the substrate are comprised of silicon, the backside needs to be protected either by an unpatterned mask deposited prior to wet etching or with a liquid-tight wafer chuck that is resistant to alkaline solutions.

Unlike isotropic wet etching which uses acidic solutions to etch single-crystal or polycrystalline silicon, anisotropic wet etching uses alkaline solutions to etch single-crystal silicon. Alkaline wet etching solutions include inorganic solvents such as potassium hydroxide (KOH), sodium hydroxide (NaOH), or cesium hydroxide (CsOH), as well as organic solvents such as ethylenediamine pyrocatechol (EDP) or tetramethylammonium hydroxide (TMAH). The anisotropic alkaline etching mechanism for single-crystal silicon can be explained by two commonly accepted models: the Seidel model and the Elwenspoek model. The Seidel model is outlined as follows.[69]

$$Si_{(s)} + 2OH^-_{(aq)} \rightarrow Si(OH)^{2+}_{2(aq)} + 4e^- \qquad (6.18A)$$

$$4H_2O_{(l)} + 4e^- \rightarrow 4OH^-_{(aq)} + 2H_{2(g)} \tag{6.18B}$$

$$Si(OH)^{2+}_{2(aq)} + 4OH^-_{(aq)} \rightarrow SiO_2(OH)^{2-}_{2(aq)} + 2H_2O_{(l)} \tag{6.18C}$$

The overall reaction for anisotropic alkaline etching of silicon is

$$Si_{(s)} + 2OH^-_{(aq)} + 2H_2O_{(l)} \rightarrow SiO_2(OH)^{2-}_{2(aq)} + 2H_{2(g)} \tag{6.19}$$

On the other hand, the Elwenspoek model explains why the alkaline wet etching of single-crystal silicon is anisotropic.[70] However, a detailed description of the Elwenspoek model is beyond the scope of this book.

Miller indices describe specific directions or planes within a crystal lattice, which can be used to better understand the anisotropic wet etching of silicon. Using Miller indices, crystallographic directions (i.e., directions in a crystal lattice) can be denoted with $[hk\ell]$, which represents the vector $h\hat{x} + k\hat{y} + \ell\hat{z}$ for cubic crystal lattices such as that of single-crystal silicon. For Miller indices, negative values are written with a bar (e.g., $[0\bar{1}0]$). A family of crystallographically equivalent directions is represented with $\langle hk\ell \rangle$. For example, $\langle 100 \rangle$ represents the family of directions that include $[100]$, $[010]$, $[001]$, $[\bar{1}00]$, $[0\bar{1}0]$, and $[00\bar{1}]$. Likewise, $\langle 110 \rangle$ represents the family of directions that include $[110]$, $[101]$, $[011]$, $[\bar{1}10]$, $[1\bar{1}0]$, $[\bar{1}\bar{1}0]$, $[\bar{1}01]$, $[10\bar{1}]$, $[\bar{1}0\bar{1}]$, $[0\bar{1}1]$, $[01\bar{1}]$, and $[0\bar{1}\bar{1}]$. Similarly, $\langle 111 \rangle$ represents the family of directions that include $[111]$, $[\bar{1}11]$, $[1\bar{1}1]$, $[11\bar{1}]$, $[\bar{1}\bar{1}1]$, $[1\bar{1}\bar{1}]$, $[\bar{1}1\bar{1}]$, and $[\bar{1}\bar{1}\bar{1}]$.

Crystallographic planes (i.e., planes in a crystal lattice) can also be represented with Miller indices (Figure 6-20). $(hk\ell)$ represents a plane that is normal (i.e., perpendicular) to the direction $[hk\ell]$, while $\{hk\ell\}$ represents a crystallographically equivalent family of symmetric planes that are normal to $\langle hk\ell \rangle$. The three most common surface crystallographic orientations of single-crystal silicon wafers are $\langle 100 \rangle$, $\langle 111 \rangle$, and $\langle 110 \rangle$. Here, the surface crystallographic orientation refers to the crystallographic direction normal (i.e., perpendicular) to the wafer surface. For any single-crystal silicon wafer, the surface crystallographic orientation is stated as a family of crystallographically equivalent directions $\langle hk\ell \rangle$, since it is meaningless to distinguish between crystallographic directions that belong to the same family. Silicon wafers with surface orientations of $\langle 100 \rangle$ are the most common, with surfaces represented by $\{100\}$ crystallographic planes. Silicon wafers with surface orientations of $\langle 111 \rangle$ and $\langle 110 \rangle$ are less common, with surfaces represented respectively by $\{111\}$ and $\{110\}$ crystallographic planes. Crystallographic planes that belong to the same family $\{hk\ell\}$ are equivalent, so there is no need to distinguish between them.

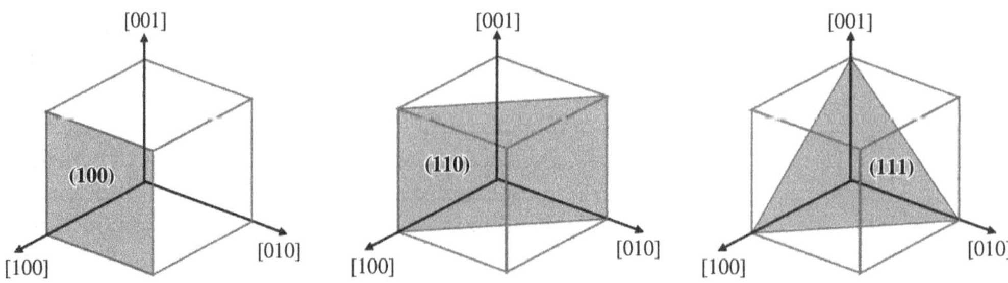

Figure 6-20   Crystallographic planes with Miller indices of (100), (110), and (111).

Using the figure on the right, we can derive the angle θ_{Si} as follows. Because single-crystal silicon has a cubic crystal lattice, we can let the lattice spacing be a. The length of line AD is $L_{AD} = \sqrt{a^2 + a^2} = \sqrt{2}\,a$, while the length of line AB is $L_{AB} = \sqrt{2}\,a/2$. Since the length of line AC is $L_{AC} = a$, we have

$$\theta_{Si} = \arctan\left(\frac{L_{AC}}{L_{AB}}\right) = \arctan\left(\frac{a}{\sqrt{2}\,a/2}\right) \quad (6.20)$$
$$= 54.74°$$

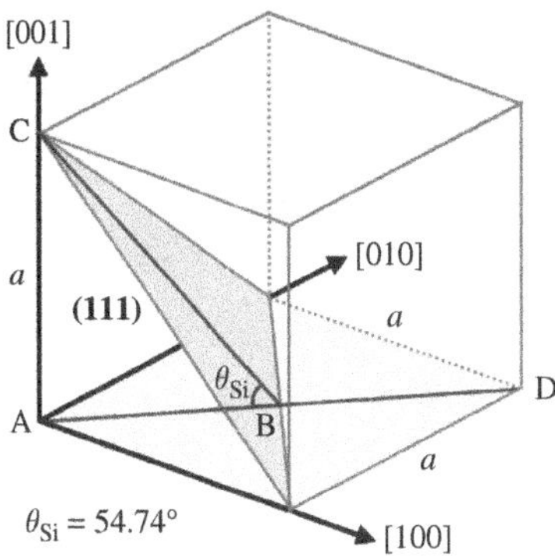

For single-crystal silicon, the {100} and {111} planes (i.e., families of planes) intersect each other at angles of either $\theta_{Si} = 54.74°$ or $90° - \theta_{Si} = 35.26°$. The {110} and {111} planes intersect each other at angles of either $90°$, $90° - \theta_{Si} = 35.26°$, or $90° + \theta_{Si} = 144.74°$.

The alkaline etch rate of single-crystal silicon depends mainly on the crystal lattice structure, temperature, concentration of the alkaline solution, and dopant concentration in the silicon. Aside from the crystal lattice structure, many other factors can impact the alkaline etch rate of silicon. As the temperature increases, the rate of alkaline etching increases exponentially.

Let us first examine the relationship between etch rate and the silicon crystal lattice structure. The alkaline etch rate of silicon varies significantly along different crystallographic directions, and is considerably faster along the $\langle 110 \rangle$ and $\langle 100 \rangle$ directions, and slower along the $\langle 111 \rangle$ direction. The relative inorganic alkaline etch rates for silicon are $\langle 110 \rangle : \langle 100 \rangle : \langle 111 \rangle = 600:400:1$.[71] Therefore, we can assume that etching along the $\langle 111 \rangle$ direction is insignificant, and that etching stops once it touches the {111} surface/plane. Consequently, {111} surfaces determine the resulting etched structure. Let us use common {100} silicon to illustrate anisotropic etching (Figure 6-21). In an open window delineated by "UXYV," the resulting etched structure (highlighted by the black lines) depends on the contacted {111} surfaces. Here we need to note that etching stops when four {111} surfaces ("UVW", "XYZ", "UXZW", and "VYZW") meet. In general, alkaline etching of silicon occurs parallel to the {111} surfaces but virtually stops in the direction perpendicular to {111} surfaces.

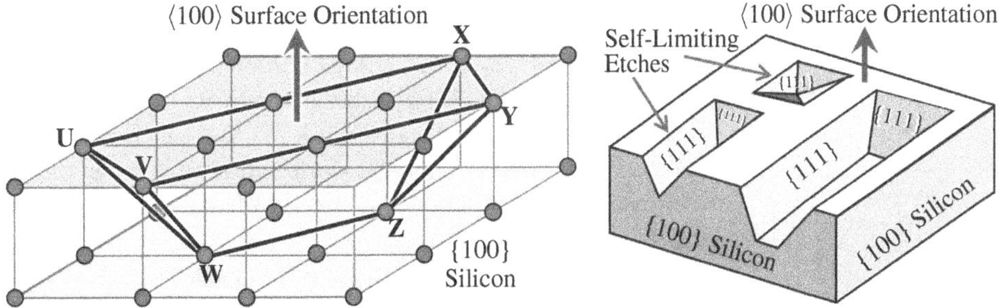

Figure 6-21   Alkaline anisotropic wet etching of {100} single-crystal silicon, with each etched structure determined by {111} surfaces and the size of the open window.

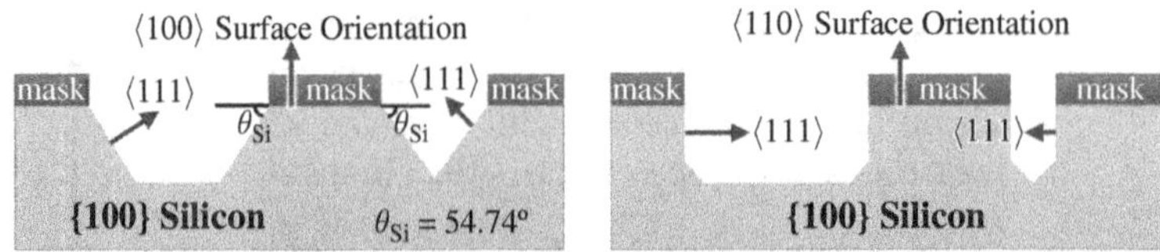

Figure 6-22   Akaline anistropic wet etching is (left) partially anistropic (directional) for {100} single-crystal silicon, and (right) almost completely anisotropic (almost vertical) for {110} single-crystal silicon.

{100} Silicon: We have shown that the angle between the {100} and {111} planes in silicon is $\theta_{Si} = 54.74°$ (or $90° - \theta_{Si} = 35.26°$). That is, etching occurs along a slope of $\theta_{Si} = 54.74°$ in a {100} silicon substrate, as shown in Figure 6-22 (left). This angle is determined by the silicon crystal lattice structure and cannot be varied. Thus, the alkaline wet etching of {100} silicon is partially anisotropic (directional). If the window is large enough, etching along the slope of $\theta_{Si} = 54.74°$ continues. A hole will form once the etch depth equals the wafer thickness.

{110} Silicon: Recall that the {110} and {111} planes in silicon intersect each other at angles of either $90°$, $90° - \theta_{Si} = 35.26°$, or $90° + \theta_{Si} = 144.74°$. Hence, the alkaline wet etching of {110} silicon is *almost* vertical (i.e., *almost* completely anisotropic), as shown in Figure 6-22 (right). Compared to {100} silicon, the alkaline wet etching of {110} silicon can achieve far greater aspect ratios.

{111} Silicon: Due to the extremely slow rate of alkaline etching along the {111} direction of silicon, alkaline etching is *never* used on {111} single-crystal silicon wafers.

Etch Masks (Alkaline Wet Etching)   Both Si_3N_4 and SiO_2 masks are used for alkaline wet etching. Si_3N_4 is the primary mask used, because it has much better (i.e., higher) selectivity than SiO_2 for the alkaline etching of silicon. Typically, the patterned Si_3N_4 or SiO_2 etch mask is applied using CVD followed by photolithography and etching. Since strong bases easily dissolve organic materials, photoresist and e-beam resist masks cannot be used. Resists cannot withstand the strong alkaline etchants used in this process and could contaminate the wet etch solution.

Alkaline Wet Etchants   The most popular etchant for the alkaline wet etching of silicon is KOH, since KOH is inexpensive, less toxic than other alkaline etchants (i.e., NaOH, EDP, and TMAH), and produces smooth etched surfaces. The optimal temperature for KOH etching is 80°C and the optimal concentration of KOH is about 30% by weight. The reaction needs mechanical or ultrasonic stirring. Under optimal conditions, the KOH etch rate of silicon along the ⟨100⟩ direction is 1.4 μm/min. The ideal mask for KOH etching is Si_3N_4, which can almost completely resist etching by KOH. SiO_2 is generally not a good mask for KOH etching due to its poor (i.e., low) selectivity. A thick layer of SiO_2 is needed to serve as a mask for KOH etching, which is not desirable. Another vital consideration is that metal hydroxides can damage the metal interconnects/wires of microelectronic components, so metal hydroxide etching is generally not compatible with integrated circuits.[72]

In addition to inorganic alkaline etchants, organic etchants such as tetramethylammonium hydroxide (TMAH) are also used. As a commonly used alkaline silicon etchant, TMAH has the following etching conditions: concentration at 22% by weight and temperature at 80°C to 90°C. The silicon etch rate of TMAH is 0.5 to 1 μm/min along the ⟨100⟩

direction, slower than that of KOH. The relative etch rates of $\langle100\rangle$:$\langle111\rangle$ silicon surfaces are reduced from 400:1 for inorganic alkaline etchants to within the range of [10:1 to 35:1] for TMAH. Consequently, the greatly increased etch rate along the {111} surface cannot be ignored. Either SiO_2 (etch rate of 1 nm/min) or Si_3N_4 (etch rate of 0.05–0.25 nm/min) can be used as a mask, with Si_3N_4 being the better mask. Because TMAH does not contain any metal ions (e.g., Li^+, Na^+, or K^+), it will not damage the metal interconnects of any integrated circuits. Furthermore, the etching of aluminum wire by TMAH is very slow. As a result, TMAH is the second most widely used alkaline silicon etchant.[73,74]

Another organic alkaline etchant is the earlier developed ethylenediamine pyrocatechol (EDP). It has an etching temperature of 115°C, with a silicon etch rate of 0.75 μm/min along the $\langle100\rangle$ direction, and relative etch rates of $\langle100\rangle$:$\langle111\rangle$ = 35:1. The etch mask can be either SiO_2 (1 to 80 nm/min) or Si_3N_4. The advantages of EDP are that its etching process is stable, repeatable, controllable, and produces highly smooth etched surfaces. However, EDP is carcinogenic and highly corrosive and thus is seldomly used.[71,75]

Control Methods (Alkaline Wet Etching)   While alkaline solvents can be used to anisotropically etch single-crystal silicon, the issue is how to control or stop etching at a desired silicon etch depth.

- *Time Control Method:* The easiest method is using the time control method to stop etching after a specified period. After measuring the etching thickness, we calculate the etch rate by dividing the etched thickness by elapsed time. We then estimate how far it is from the desired target thickness and calculate the remaining time. This method is straightforward but not very accurate. We need to increase the measuring frequency as the etch approaches the targeted depth to avoid over-etching.

- *Pattern Control Method:* The second method is the pattern control method (Figure 6-23), where etching stops when multiple {111} surfaces meet. Based on the desired etch depth, we can calculate beforehand the size of the open window required and then apply etching. This method is more accurate than the time control method but requires more chip area.

- *Doping Control Method:* The third and most accurate method is the doping control method, by which we dope (i.e., add impurities to) the silicon substrate to stop etching (Figure 6-24). The alkaline etch rate will decrease at least 40-fold when encountering single-crystal silicon that is heavily doped with boron (i.e., with boron concentrations of [B] > 10^{20} atoms/cm³ of silicon). We can dope a high concentration of boron on part of the silicon substrate prior to alkaline etching to ensure that etching (virtually) stops upon reaching the highly doped silicon. The side effect is that the resistivity of silicon drastically decreases after being highly doped, which is not desirable in integrated circuits. Furthermore, doping can damage the

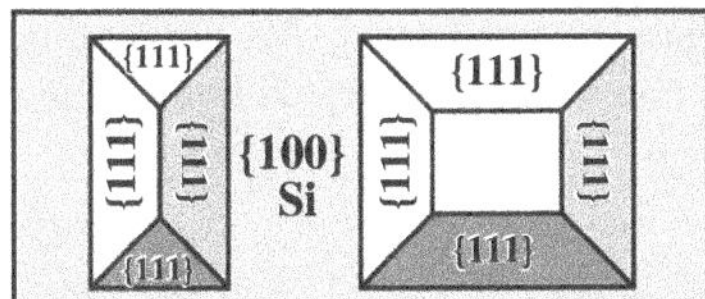

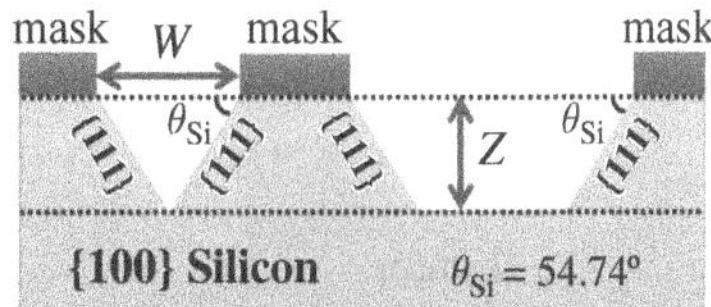

Figure 6-23   Pattern control method for the alkaline wet etching of silicon (Si). The left rectangular pattern formed by four {111} surfaces is used as a reference to time and control the etch depth of the right square pattern. For a desired etch depth Z, we can calculate the required width W of the open widow.

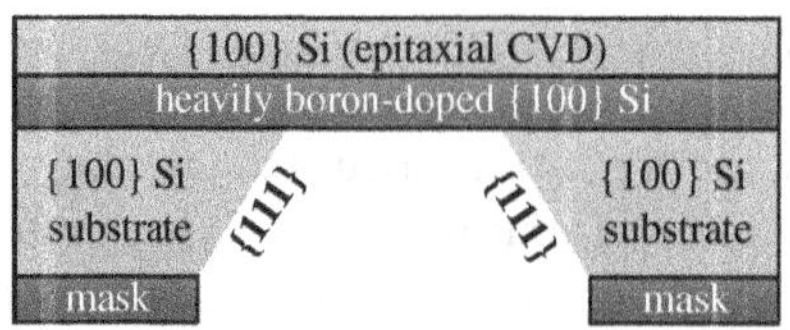

Figure 6-24 Doping control method for the alkaline anisotropic wet etching of single-crystal silicon (Si).

surrounding silicon crystal lattice structure, resulting in electrical and mechanical defects. To overcome this shortfall, we can deposit a thick single-crystal silicon layer on top of the doped area with epitaxial CVD.[71]

EXAMPLE 6-1 You wish to etch a {100} single-crystal silicon chip to produce the microstructure shown on the right. The silicon chip already has integrated circuits (ICs) on it, which are all located outside of the areas to be etched. You have access to the following wet etchants: BOE (i.e., BHF), EDP, HNA, H_3PO_4 (with reflux system), KOH, NaOH, and TMAH.

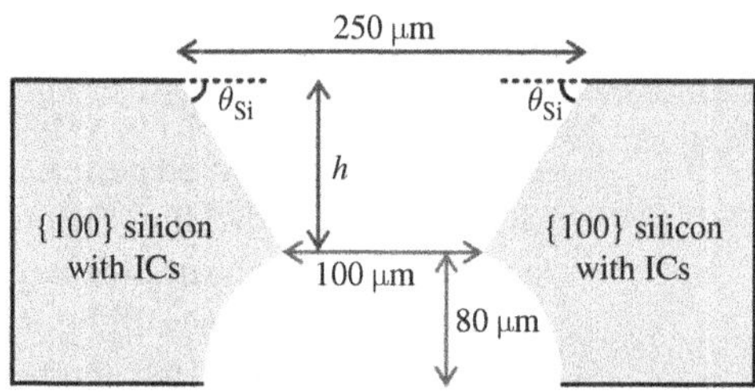

(a) Which etchant should be used to etch the trapezoidal top part, and which etchant should be used to etch the ellipsoidal bottom part of the microstructure? Assume that etchant cost is not an issue.

(b) What is the length of h? For (i) etching the trapezoidal top part and (ii) etching the semi-elliptical bottom part, what etch mask material is ideal and how thick should the mask be? Assume that the etch mask material has a selectivity of 500 against alkaline etching and 200 against BOE or HNA etching.

(c) The alkaline etchant you selected has an etch rate of 0.75 µm/min along the $\langle 100 \rangle$ direction of silicon, and relative silicon etch rates of $\langle 100 \rangle : \langle 111 \rangle = 20{:}1$. The isotropic wet etchant you chose has a single-sided silicon etch rate of 16.5 µm/min. Excluding the time required for depositing and patterning the etch masks, how long does it take to etch the entire microstructure? For the anisotropic etching step, is the undesired etching along the {111} silicon surface less than 10 µm?

(d) Propose a process flow for etching the entire microstructure starting with a silicon chip which contains ICs, including the steps required to deposit and remove the etch masks. Assume that the etch masks are patterned with photolithography followed by anisotropic dry etching (no explanation is needed). Sketch figures showing the intermediate structure at key steps of the process.

Solution

(a) To etch the trapezoidal top part, TMAH is the ideal anisotropic alkaline wet etchant. Unlike NaOH and KOH, TMAH does not contain metal ions and will not damage the existing ICs on the silicon chip. Unlike EDP, TMAH is not highly carcinogenic.

To etch the semi-elliptical bottom part, HNA is the ideal isotropic wet etchant. BOE (i.e., BHF) is intended to etch SiO_2 (e.g., quartz) or glass, and is not suitable for etching silicon. Likewise, H_3PO_4 (with reflux system) is designed to etch Si_3N_4 and should not be used to etch silicon.

(b) The length of h is calculated as follows using $\theta_{Si} = 54.74°$:

$$\frac{h}{(250\ \mu m - 100\ \mu m)\ /\ 2} = \tan\theta_{Si} = \tan 54.74° \;\Rightarrow\; h = (75\ \mu m)(\tan 54.74°) = 106\ \mu m$$

(i) Since the trapezoidal top part should be etched with anisotropic alkaline wet etching, the ideal etch mask material is silicon nitride (Si_3N_4), which offers the best (i.e., highest) selectivity. Photoresist masks are not suitable as they cannot withstand strong alkaline etchants. Assuming a selectivity of 500, the minimum thickness required for the etch mask is

$$\text{Mask Thickness (Alkaline Etching)} \geq \frac{\text{Etch Depth}}{\text{Selectivity}} = \frac{h}{500} = \frac{106\ \mu m}{500} = 212\ nm$$

(ii) Because the semi-elliptical bottom part should be etched with HNA isotropic wet etching, Si_3N_4 is the ideal mask material. Gold is also a suitable mask material, but does not adhere well to silicon. We cannot use photoresist masks, which will be aggressively attacked by the HNA etchant. With a selectivity of 200, the minimum thickness required for the etch mask is

$$\text{Mask Thickness (HNA Etching)} \geq \frac{\text{Etch Depth}}{\text{Selectivity}} = \frac{80\ \mu m}{200} = 400\ nm$$

To withstand both TMAH alkaline etching and HNA etching, the etch mask should be at least $212\ nm + 400\ nm = 612\ nm$ thick.

(c) The time required for etching the trapezoidal top part with anisotropic alkaline etching is

$$t_{anisotropic} = \frac{106\ \mu m}{0.75\ \mu m/min} = 141\ min$$

Likewise, the time required for etching the semi-elliptical bottom part with isotropic wet etching is

$$t_{isotropic} = \frac{80\ \mu m}{16.5\ \mu m/min} = 4.85\ min$$

The time required to etch the entire structure is $141\ min + 4.85\ min = 146\ min$.

We estimate the maximum length $L_{\{111\}\ max}$ of undesired etching along the $\{111\}$ silicon surface. With the anisotropic etching time of $t_{anisotropic} = 141\ min$, silicon etch rate of $0.75\ \mu m/min$ along the $\langle 100 \rangle$ direction, and relative silicon etch rates of $\langle 100 \rangle : \langle 111 \rangle = 20:1$, we have

$$L_{\{111\}\ max} = (141\ min)\left(\frac{0.75\ \mu m/min}{20}\right) = 5.3\ \mu m < 10\ \mu m$$

Thus, the undesired etching along the $\{111\}$ silicon surface is much less than $10\ \mu m$.

(d) As shown in the figure below, we can etch the desired shape as follows.

(1) Deposit a layer of Si_3N_4 on *both sides* of the silicon chip that is at least $612\ nm$ thick with plasma-enhanced CVD (PECVD) to protect against both alkaline and HNA wet etching. For wet etching, the bottom side of the silicon substrate needs to be protected. PECVD is carried out at relatively low substrate temperatures, which avoids damaging the integrated circuits on the silicon chip. Since the Si_3N_4 layer is relatively thick, sputtering may take a long time.

(2) Apply photolithography to obtain a patterned layer of photoresist (PR) above the Si_3N_4 surface on one side of the silicon chip.

(3) Etch away regions of Si_3N_4 not protected by photoresist with anisotropic dry etching to create the patterned Si_3N_4 etch mask. Then, strip all photoresist to avoid reactions with HNA etchant.

(4) Using HNA (an isotropic wet etchant), etch the semi-elliptical structure into the silicon chip through the patterned Si_3N_4 etch mask. Etch for a duration of $t_{isotropic} = 4.85$ min.

(5) Flip the silicon chip, and apply photolithography to obtain a patterned layer of photoresist above the Si_3N_4 surface on the other side of the chip.

(6) Use anisotropic dry etching to etch and pattern the second Si_3N_4 etch mask. Next, strip all photoresist to avoid reactions with alkaline etchant.

(7) Place the silicon chip in a liquid-tight chuck that is resistant to alkaline solutions to protect the backside. Then, use TMAH (an anisotropic alkaline wet etchant) to etch the trapezoidal structure into the silicon chip through the second Si_3N_4 etch mask. To stop etching at the desired silicon etch depth of 106 μm, use the time control method by waiting for $t_{anisotropic} = 141$ min.

(8) Remove all Si_3N_4 mask layers with isotropic wet etching. Place the etched silicon chip in a reflux system with concentrated H_3PO_4 heated to 140 to 180°C. With a selectivity of ~30, silicon will not be significantly etched by the heated H_3PO_4.

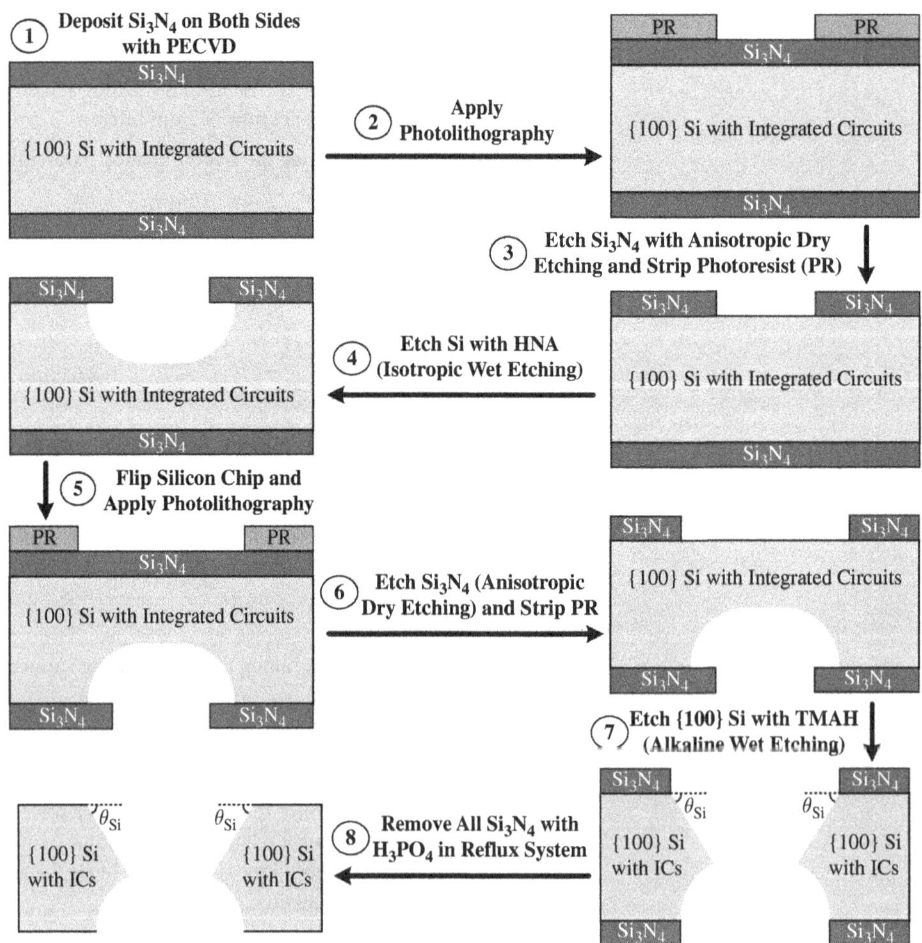

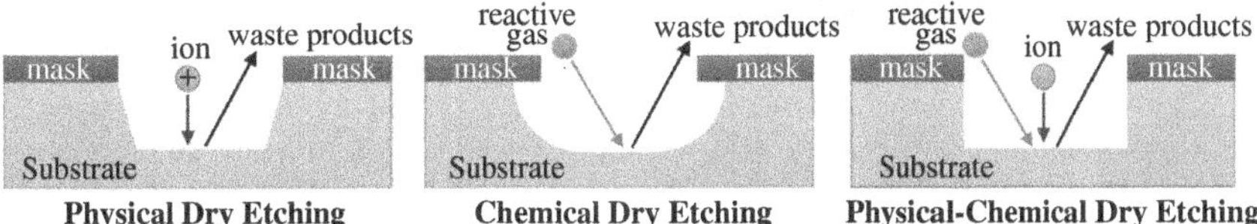

Figure 6-25 The three main categories of dry etching methods are physical dry etching (partially anisotropic), chemical dry etching (isotropic), and physical-chemical dry etching (completely anisotropic).

(D) Dry Etching

Dry etching utilizes energetic ions and/or electrically neutral reactive gas molecules to etch away areas of the substrate surface that are not protected by an etch mask. Compared to wet etching, which is carried out in open air with noxious liquid etchants, dry etching is instead performed in a sealed chamber and is safer to carry out. In contrast to wet etching, the backside of the substrate is never etched during dry etching and does not need any protection. In recent years, dry etching techniques have become more popular than the wet etching techniques discussed in Sections 6.4.3(B) and 6.4.3(C). Although more complicated and expensive than wet etching methods, dry etching methods can etch smaller features more accurately and offer better control. Unlike isotropic wet etching, anisotropic dry etching is capable of accurately etching small features (<5 μm in width, length, or depth), as well as high aspect ratio features (e.g., deep vertical structures). In addition, dry etching is far more suitable than wet etching for fabricating 3D microscale/nanoscale structures. Thus, dry etching has been used to fabricate 3D integrated circuits as well as 3D integrated chips for microfluidic/LOC devices. In general, dry etching can be classified as physical dry etching, chemical dry etching, or physical-chemical dry etching (Figure 6-25).

Physical Dry Etching   In physical dry etching, energetic ions are accelerated to bombard and physically remove (i.e., sputter away) unprotected regions of the substrate surface. Atoms in exposed regions of the substrate surface are dislodged and etched away by energetic ions through momentum transfer. The mechanism for physical dry etching is similar to that of sputtering, where the target is sputtered away by energetic non-reactive ions. For physical dry etching, Ar^+ ions are most frequently used, since argon is chemically inert, inexpensive, and has sufficiently high atomic mass to be effective at etching via momentum transfer. The bombarding ions are created by electron impact ionizations in a low-pressure plasma glow discharge, and are accelerated toward the substrate surface with large electric fields produced by electrodes powered either by DC or radio frequency AC potentials. To sustain the low-pressure plasma glow discharge and reduce collisions between unwanted background gas molecules and the bombarding ions which would significantly decrease the etch rate, physical dry etching is carried out in a vacuum chamber.

The two most common variants of physical dry etching are sputter etching and ion milling. Sputter etching uses a two-electrode (i.e., diode) setup, where the substrate is placed on the cathode with the substrate surface facing the bombarding ions, while the anode is sometimes grounded. Alternatively, ion milling uses a three-electrode (i.e., triode) setup, where two electrodes are used to generate and sustain the plasma, while the third electrode accelerates the ions to bombard the substrate surface. By decoupling the plasma sustainment process from the ion acceleration process, ion milling offers more control, higher ion energies, and substantially faster maximum etch rates than sputter etching.

The etch profile created by physical dry etching is partially anisotropic (directional) because the flux of bombarding ions is highly directional. Here, flux refers to the number of

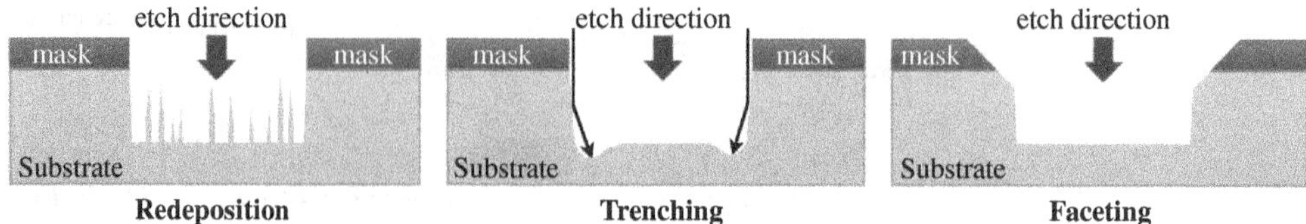

Figure 6-26 Physical dry etching and physical-chemical dry etching both suffer from etch artifacts which include redeposition, trenching, and faceting. In this figure, the three etch artifacts are exaggerated for illustrative purposes. To minimize etch artifacts, the etch process parameters may need to be tuned.

incident ions per unit area per unit time. Since the flux of bombarding ions is reduced near the bottom corners of trenches, the etch profile is not entirely anisotropic (i.e., not vertical). In physical dry etching, no chemical reactions are involved. Therefore, physical dry etching can be used to etch virtually any solid material and has no selectivity for the targeted material or the etch mask. In other words, the selectivity of physical dry etching is ~1 and both the targeted material and the mask are etched away at the same rate. Due to its very slow etch rate, physical dry etching is usually only used to etch materials that are difficult to etch by other methods, especially when a directional etch is desired.

Three potential issues with physical dry etching are redeposition, trenching, and faceting—as shown in Figure 6-26—which reduce the quality of etched features. Unwanted grass-like structures are formed by the redeposition of dislodged material (from both the material to be etched and the mask) back onto the substrate surface. Trenching refers to the formation of unwanted pits at the bottom corners of trenches and mesas due to ions reflecting off sidewalls at glancing incidence. Finally, faceting is the over-etching of the top corners of the etch mask which are more easily dislodged than the rest of the mask by bombarding ions. If the faceting is severe enough, undercutting of the etched features may result.[76]

A relatively thick patterned layer of photoresist can be cheaply and easily created through photolithography. Due to the poor selectivity and the relatively low substrate temperatures involved, photoresists are most commonly used as etch masks for physical dry etching. Alternatively, more expensive mask materials such as SiO_2, Si_3N_4, and e-beam resists are also suitable, but a relatively thick mask may be required due to the poor selectivity of physical dry etching.

Chemical Dry Etching   Chemical dry etching utilizes electrically neutral reactive gas molecules to etch away unprotected areas of the substrate surface. The neutral reactive gas molecules can be neutral radicals generated in a plasma (most common), or neutral non-radical gas molecules that do not require a plasma (less common). Neutral radicals are electrically neutral gas molecules or atoms that are highly reactive because they have unpaired valence electrons. Due to their highly reactive nature and short lifespan, neutral radicals are generated in a plasma relatively close to the substrate within a vacuum chamber. Neutral non radical gas molecules are relatively stable and electrically neutral molecules having valence electrons that are all paired.

An example of a neutral non-radical gas molecule used for chemical dry etching is xenon difluoride (XeF_2), which is used to etch silicon (single-crystal or polycrystalline) in the fabrication of MEMS devices through the following chemical reaction [77]:

$$Si_{(s)} + 2XeF_{2(g)} \rightarrow SiF_{4(g)} + 2Xe_{(g)} \tag{6.21}$$

Alternatively, the most popular neutral radicals used for chemical dry etching rely on fluorine-based and/or chlorine-based chemistries. For instance, the non-radical gas carbon tetrafluoride ($CF_{4(g)}$) can be converted into $CF^*_{x(g)}$ and $F^*_{(g)}$ radicals by colliding with energetic electrons in a plasma as follows: [78]

$$CF_{4(g)} \xrightarrow{\text{electron impact}} CF^*_{x(g)} + (4-x)F^*_{(g)} \quad \text{where } x = 1,\ 2,\ \text{or } 3 \qquad (6.22)$$

and where the asterisk ($*$) indicates that a molecule is a neutral radical.

The resulting $F^*_{(g)}$ radicals can etch silicon (single-crystal or polycrystalline), silicon dioxide (SiO_2), and silicon nitride (Si_3N_4) through the following reactions: [78]

$$Si_{(s)} + 4F^*_{(g)} \rightarrow SiF_{4(g)} \qquad (6.23)$$

$$SiO_{2(s)} + 4F^*_{(g)} \rightarrow SiF_{4(g)} + O_{2(g)} \qquad (6.24)$$

$$Si_3N_{4(s)} + 12F^*_{(g)} \rightarrow 3SiF_{4(g)} + 2N_{2(g)} \qquad (6.25)$$

Silicon can also be etched using chlorine-based chemistries with chemical dry etching. For example, chlorine radicals $Cl^*_{(g)}$ can be created from non-radical chlorine gas $Cl_{2(g)}$ through energetic electron impacts in a plasma as follows:

$$Cl_{2(g)} \xrightarrow{\text{electron impact}} 2Cl^*_{(g)} \qquad (6.26)$$

The chlorine radicals can be used to chemically etch silicon (single-crystal or polycrystalline) as follows:

$$Si_{(s)} + 4Cl^*_{(g)} \rightarrow SiCl_{4(g)} \qquad (6.27)$$

While physical dry etching can etch almost any solid material, chemical dry etching can only etch solid materials that have suitable chemical reactions for vapor-phase etching. In practice, chemical dry etching is used for etching silicon (single-crystal or polycrystalline), SiO_2 (e.g., quartz), Si_3N_4, many metals (e.g., Al, Au, Cr, W, and Mo), and many compounds (e.g., GaAs, TiW, some organic solids and polymers, and some silicides).

Like isotropic wet etching, chemical dry etching also results in isotropic etch profiles with poor directionality and undercutting issues (please refer to Figure 6-18), because the chemical etchant gases etch exposed materials equally in all directions. It is difficult to accurately etch small features (<5 μm in width, length, or depth) with chemical dry etching due to undercutting. Unlike physical dry etching, chemical dry etching generally offers good (i.e., high) selectivity, and can selectively etch away targeted materials instead of the mask. Furthermore, redeposition and trenching do not occur during chemical dry etching. In contrast with physical dry etching, the etch rates of chemical dry etching can be easily adjusted (e.g., by increasing the process temperature), offering substantially higher maximum etch rates.

The choice of suitable etch mask materials for chemical dry etching depends on the etch chemistry and substrate temperature during etching. Typically, substrate temperatures during chemical dry etching are sufficiently low ($<150°C$) that photoresist etch masks can be used. While the selectivity of photoresist masks during chemical dry etching is not high (~ 1 to 10), an adequately thick layer of patterned photoresist can be created easily and inexpensively via photolithography. Generally, SiO_2 and Si_3N_4 masks offer much better (i.e., significantly higher) selectivity than photoresists. For instance, SiO_2 masks are suitable when etching silicon or Si_3N_4 using $CF_{4(g)}/O_{2(g)}$ plasma.

Physical-Chemical Dry Etching   Physical-chemical dry etching combines both physical dry etching (energetic ions) and chemical dry etching (neutral reactive gas molecules). This combination overcomes the weaknesses of both physical dry etching and chemical dry etching.

Reactive Ion Etching (RIE)   The predominant physical-chemical dry etching method is reactive ion etching (RIE). RIE combines the best aspects of both physical dry etching and chemical dry etching. RIE can achieve completely anisotropic (vertical) etching with etch rates higher than physical or chemical dry etching, while simultaneously offering good selectivity. Moreover, RIE offers far more control over the etching process than either physical dry etching or chemical dry etching. The other significant advantage of RIE is that crystal lattice structures—such as $\{111\}$ silicon surfaces—do not impact the etch rate, since RIE etching occurs independently of the crystal lattice structure.

In the simplest form of RIE, energetic ions and neutral reactive gas molecules are generated in the same plasma with a two-electrode (i.e., diode) setup. Let us consider the reactive ion etching of silicon, SiO_2, or Si_3N_4 with $CF_{4(g)}$. In a plasma, $CF_{4(g)}$ can be converted into both $F^*_{(g)}$ neutral radicals and $CF^+_{3(g)}$ ions through energetic electron impacts as follows:

$$CF_{4(g)} \xrightarrow{\text{electron impact}} CF^+_{3(g)} + F^*_{(g)} + e^- \tag{6.28}$$

Just like $Ar^+_{(g)}$ ions, $CF^+_{3(g)}$ ions are accelerated toward the substrate to bombard and physically etch the substrate surface. Meanwhile, the $F^*_{(g)}$ neutral radicals chemically etch the substrate surface.

As another example, let us consider the reactive ion etching of silicon (single-crystal or polycrystalline) with $Ar^+_{(g)}$ ions combined with $XeF_{2(g)}$ (a neutral non-radical gas). Both $Ar^+_{(g)}$ physical dry etching and $XeF_{2(g)}$ chemical dry etching can etch silicon at a rate of about 0.5 nm/min. By contrast, the physical-chemical dry etching of silicon with $Ar^+_{(g)}$ plus $XeF_{2(g)}$ can achieve an etch rate of 6 nm/min, which is six times faster than the combined etch rates of physical dry etching and chemical dry etching.

The fast etch rates of physical-chemical dry etching can be attributed to the synergistic effects of combining physical and chemical dry etching. The bombardment of energetic ions breaks chemical bonds at the substrate surface, increasing the reactivity of the neutral reactive gas molecules. Additionally, the ion bombardment physically removes waste products generated by chemical reactions, allowing reactive gas molecules to react with newly exposed areas of the substrate surface. The physical removal of waste products is especially prominent when the waste products are solids, which can be difficult to remove by other means. Furthermore, the combination of energetic ion bombardment and reactive gas molecules dramatically increases the formation of volatile byproducts, speeding up the etching process.

More complicated RIE setups use plasmas to create both Ar^+ ions as well as neutral radicals. The Ar^+ ions are accelerated to bombard the substrate surface, whereas the neutral radicals chemically etch away the substrate surface. As an example, let us consider the reactive ion etching of aluminum (Al) with $Ar^+_{(g)}/Cl_{2(g)}$ plasma. Some of the $Cl_{2(g)}$ gas is converted to $Cl^*_{(g)}$ radicals through energetic electron impacts in a plasma. Unlike $Cl_{2(g)}$, the $Cl^*_{(g)}$ radicals readily react with (Al) to form the solid byproduct aluminum chloride ($AlCl_{3(s)}$). The reactions are as follows:

$$Cl_{2(g)} \xrightarrow{\text{electron impact}} 2Cl^*_{(g)} \qquad\qquad Al_{(s)} + 3Cl^*_{(g)} \rightarrow AlCl_{3(s)} \qquad (6.29)$$

Here, the $Ar^+_{(g)}$ ions bombarding the substrate surface are extremely helpful as they physically remove (dislodge) the solid byproduct $AlCl_{3(s)}$, thereby dramatically increasing the etch rate.

The foremost advantage of RIE is the completely anisotropic etch profile (i.e., vertical and without any undercutting) that can be achieved with proper tuning of the process parameters. The vertical etch profile of RIE is mainly due to the highly directional flux of bombarding ions that initiate and promote etching, combining with the neutral reactive gas molecules that etch away exposed regions of the substrate, especially the bottom corners of trenches where the ion flux is reduced. Since many RIE formulations include carbon (for instance, in the form of CF_4 gas), a passivation layer of etch-resistant polymer will often form on the surfaces where the ion flux is small—in particular the sidewalls of trenches, mesas, and lines. In regions where the ion flux is large, such as the bottoms of trenches, ion bombardment quickly removes any passivation layers. The passivation layers that form on sidewall surfaces, which are not always polymeric, further increases the anisotropy of RIE. Thus, passivation gases such as halocarbons (e.g., CF_4, CCl_4, CHF_3, and CF_2Cl_2) and some inorganic gases (e.g., BCl_3 and SF_6) can be introduced during RIE to improve anisotropy. Note that many passivation gases can also act as sources of neutral radical etchants in a plasma.

RIE can etch a wider range of materials than chemical dry etching, especially materials whose vapor phase chemical reactions create solid byproducts. RIE can be used to etch silicon (single-crystal or polycrystalline), SiO_2 (e.g., quartz), Si_3N_4, glass, most metals (e.g., Al, Au, Cr, W, and Mo), and many compounds (e.g., GaAs, TiW, some organic solids and polymers, and some silicides). Also, RIE is more suitable and effective than chemical dry etching for etching glass or quartz, because energetic ion bombardment weakens the strong oxide bonds holding together glass/quartz.

The selectivity of RIE is comparable to that of chemical dry etching, but is substantially better (i.e., much higher) than that of physical dry etching. Like physical dry etching and chemical dry etching, substrate temperatures during RIE are also sufficiently low ($<150°C$) that photoresist etch masks can be used. Generally, the etch mask selectivity of RIE is similar to that of chemical dry etching: the selectivity of photoresist masks in RIE is not high (only ~1 to 10). While SiO_2 and Si_3N_4 masks have better selectivity (on the order of ~30) during RIE, the thickness of the etch mask required can be problematic when etching deep features with RIE.

The main weaknesses of RIE are the very long time required to etch deep features (>20 µm in depth), and the inability to accurately etch deep features (>10 µm in depth) that have high aspect ratios. For RIE, etch rates on the order of 20 to 200 nm/min can be reliably obtained. Even though the maximum etch rate is higher than that of chemical dry etching or physical dry etching, etching features that are tens of micrometers deep would take many hours for RIE. Another issue is that the selectivity of RIE, while good, is not high enough for the etching of deep features—particularly with respect to photoresist etch masks. For example, etching a 50-µm-deep feature with RIE would typically require a layer of cured photoresist mask that is at least 10 µm thick, which is challenging to obtain with photolithography. Generally, etching features deeper than about 50 µm with RIE would require an etch mask (e.g., SiO_2 or Si_3N_4) that is at least a few micrometers thick, which can be time-consuming and potentially expensive to deposit/grow and pattern. Like physical dry etching, RIE is also susceptible to trenching, redeposition, and faceting (please refer to Figure 6-26). Careful control and tuning of the process parameters may be required to minimize these etch artifacts.[76]

Deep Reactive Ion Etching (DRIE)   Deep reactive ion etching (DRIE) is a completely anisotropic (vertical) etch technique designed to etch deep features (>10 μm in depth), especially for those requiring high aspect ratios. Like RIE, DRIE etching is unaffected by the crystal lattice structure. DRIE offers a combination of very high maximum etch rates, excellent (i.e., very high) selectivity, and the ability to etch deep features with high aspect ratios. Thus, DRIE overcomes the main limitations of RIE. The DRIE process is popular in semiconductor processing and integrated circuit fabrication as it allows many etching characteristics including etch profile, selectivity, reproducibility, and uniformity to be controlled.[79]

ICP-RIE (DRIE Setup)   In physical-chemical dry etching processes, the etchants are ions together with neutral reactive gas molecules (usually neutral radicals), which are often both generated in the same low-pressure plasma. Crucially, the concentrations of ions and neutral radicals are proportional to the density of the plasma. The predominant DRIE setup is called inductively coupled plasma–reactive ion etching (ICP-RIE). There is an alternative DRIE setup called electron cyclotron resonance–reactive ion etching (ECR-RIE), which is not commonly used due to issues with control and scalability. When discussing DRIE, we will focus exclusively on the ICP-RIE setup.

In ICP-RIE, the mechanism for sustaining the plasma is decoupled from the mechanism for accelerating the bombarding ions. In particular, the plasma density is increased about 10- to 100-fold by utilizing electromagnetic induction, which sustains the conductive plasma with electric currents generated by alternating magnetic fields. Electromagnetic induction of the plasma is maintained with an inductive coil powered by a radio frequency AC potential. Meanwhile, a second power source handles ion acceleration to bombard unmasked regions of the substrate surface, with the substrate usually located away from the plasma. With the denser plasma, ICP-RIE can achieve a maximum etch rate that is 10 to 100 times higher than regular RIE, with typical etch rates of about 0.5 to 50 μm/min.[80]

When DRIE (ICP-RIE setup) is used to etch deep features with low aspect ratios (≤ 2), passivation techniques may not be required at all. For example, silicon carbide (SiC)—a promising MEMS material for replacing silicon in applications with hot and/or corrosive environments—can be etched using ICP-RIE without any passivation technique. Since SiC is chemically inert, etching of SiC is induced/promoted by ion bombardment, thereby greatly reducing sidewall etching and enhancing anisotropy. With an Ni or Al etch mask, SiC can be etched at a rate of ~300 nm/min with ICP-RIE.[81]

Passivation techniques are intended to prevent the etching of sidewall surfaces, which is crucial for the vertical etching of deep and high aspect ratio (> 2) features. There are three main DRIE techniques that include passivation: DRIE with passivation gases, the Bosch process (DRIE), and cryogenic DRIE. The Bosch process (DRIE) is used to etch silicon and polymers, whereas cryogenic DRIE is generally used to etch silicon. Similar to regular RIE, DRIE processes are also susceptible to trenching, redeposition, and faceting (please refer to Figure 6-26), which can all be minimized by tuning process parameters.

DRIE with Passivation Gases   The simplest passivation technique is the addition of passivation gases during ICP-RIE, which allows the etching of deep and high aspect ratio features. The most common passivation gases are halocarbons (e.g., CF_4, CCl_4, CHF_3, and CF_2Cl_2), and some inorganic gases (e.g., BCl_3 and SF_6). In a plasma, many passivation gases

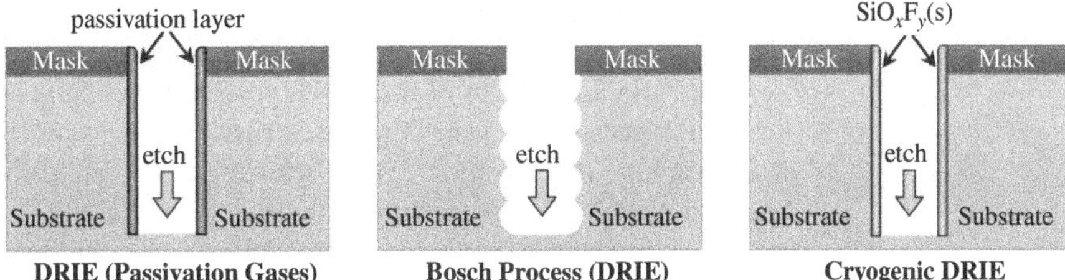

Figure 6-27   The three main deep reactive ion etching (DRIE) techniques include (left) DRIE with passivation gases, (center) the Bosch DRIE process, and (right) cryogenic DRIE.

can also act as sources of neutral radical etchants. As shown in Figure 6-27 (left), passivation gases enhance anisotropy by forming an etch resistant passivation layer (e.g., a polymeric layer) on the sidewall surfaces of etched features where the incident ion flux is low. On the other hand, surfaces where etching is desired (e.g., trench bottoms) receive high ion flux, which quickly sputters away any passivation layers that form. DRIE with passivation gases is used to etch silicon, SiO$_2$ (e.g., quartz), Si$_3$N$_4$, glass, many metals (most commonly Al, Au, Cu, Cr, and Pt), and many compound semiconductors (e.g., GaAs, AlGaAs, GaN, and InP). This DRIE method offers substantially higher etch rates (on the order of 0.1 to 1 μm/min) than regular RIE. Unfortunately, the selectivity of this DRIE method is not high (i.e., comparable to regular RIE), and is only ~4 for photoresist masks and ~30 for SiO$_2$ or Si$_3$N$_4$ masks.[65]

The Bosch Process (DRIE)   The Bosch process (DRIE) is currently the most popular DRIE technique for etching silicon (single-crystal or polycrystalline), and is carried out using an ICP-RIE setup. As illustrated in Figure 6-28, the Bosch process is cyclical and alternates between (1) a passivation step and (2) a fast isotropic etching step.[82]

Let us consider the etching of silicon with the Bosch process. (1) During the passivation step, C$_x$F$_{y(g)}$ (usually either C$_4$F$_{8(g)}$ or C$_3$F$_{6(g)}$) is introduced, forming chemically inert polytetrafluoroethylene (PTFE, also known as Teflon®) through plasma polymerization. The PTFE is then deposited on all exposed surfaces, especially on the sidewalls. (2) During the fast isotropic etching step, both ions (e.g., SF$_{x(g)}^+$) and neutral radicals (e.g., F$_{(g)}^*$) are generated in SF$_{6(g)}$ plasma. The ions remove any PTFE on trench bottoms through ion

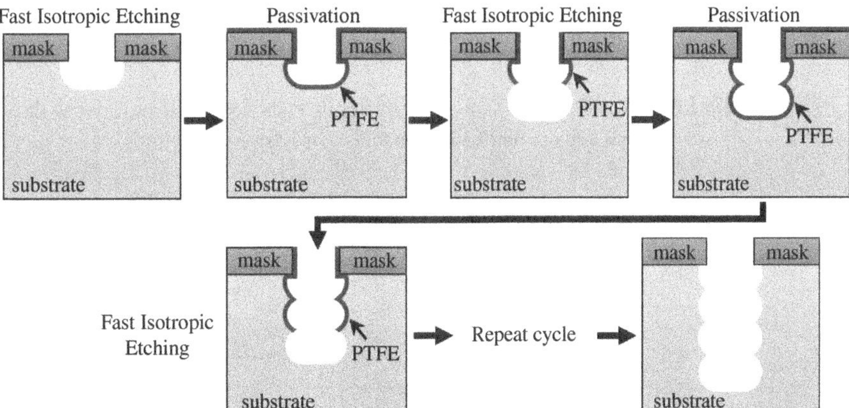

Figure 6-28   The Bosch DRIE process is cyclical, alternating between a fast isotropic etching step and a passivation step. The etched structure exhibits sidewall scalloping due to the isotropic etching steps.

bombardment, while the neutral radicals etch deeper into trenches. This etch step is both fast and isotropic, resulting in sidewall scalloping (Figure 6-27, center).[80,82]

The main advantages of the Bosch process for etching silicon are the extremely high etch rate, excellent (i.e., very high) selectivity, and the capability of easily etching deep features with high aspect ratios. The Bosch process can etch silicon with an etch rate of 2 to 50 μm/min, which is significantly faster than any other DRIE or dry etching process. By far the most popular etch mask for etching silicon with the Bosch process is photoresist patterned through photolithography (selectivity of ~40 to 140). Alternatively, SiO_2 masks can also be used (selectivity of ~100 to 300). [80,82]

Aside from etching silicon, the Bosch process is less commonly used to etch polymers such as polymethyl methacrylate (i.e., acrylic), SU-8, and polyimide (e.g., Kapton). The method used to etch polymers is almost the same as that for etching silicon; the only differences are that $O_{2(g)}$ plasma is used instead of $SF_{6(g)}$ plasma in step (2), and that $CF_{4(g)}$ or $SF_{6(g)}$ is sometimes added to increase the etch rate. A polymer etch rate of about 0.15 to 1.5 μm/min can be attained with the Bosch process. Suitable masks for etching polymers with the Bosch process include silicon (polycrystalline is the cheapest), oxides (especially SiO_2), and some metals. Because resists are usually polymeric materials, resist etch masks offer very poor selectivity (~1) in this process.[80]

Cryogenic DRIE   Cryogenic DRIE is carried out using an ICP-RIE setup with the substrate cooled by liquid nitrogen, achieving typical substrate temperatures between −110°C and −90°C. At these low temperatures, isotropic etching processes are significantly slowed down, virtually stopping the etching of sidewalls. The preservation of sidewalls allows cryogenic DRIE to etch deep and high aspect ratio features. Even though cryogenic DRIE is normally used to etch silicon, cryogenic temperatures in combination with passivation gases may also improve the etching of some metals and compounds. Most resist masks are not suitable for cryogenic DRIE due to their tendency to shatter or crack at the cold temperatures used. Instead, mask materials such as SiO_2, Al, Al_2O_3, Cr, and specialized resists are used, which generally offer exceptional selectivity (>100) at cryogenic temperatures.[82]

The etching of silicon (single-crystal or polycrystalline) by cryogenic DRIE is carried out with $SF_{6(g)}/O_{2(g)}$ plasma. At low cryogenic temperatures, a passivating (i.e., etch resistant) layer of silicon oxyfluoride $SiO_xF_{y(s)}$ is formed on the sidewalls, while silicon oxyfluoride that forms elsewhere is rapidly removed by ion bombardment (Figure 6-27, right). Although slower than the Bosch process, cryogenic DRIE does not suffer from scalloping, and can etch silicon at a rate of ~3 μm/min.[83,84]

EXAMPLE 6-2   Consider the "step" microstructure etched in a silicon wafer as shown on the right. The silicon wafer has a diameter of 100 mm and a thickness of 525 μm.

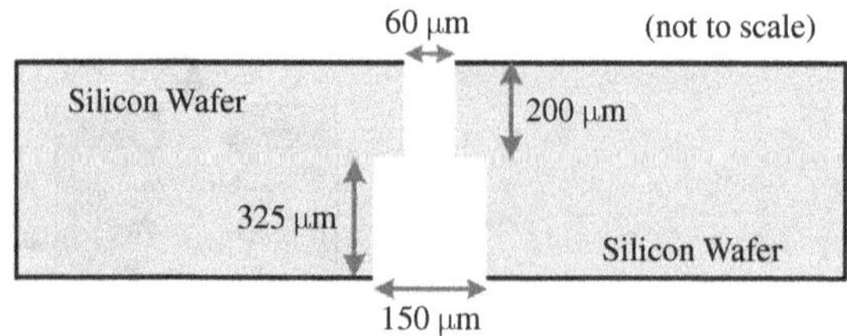

(a) If a very high degree of anisotropy is required, what etching methods are appropriate? Take into consideration the depth and aspect ratio of etched features. For each of the suitable etching methods, what etch mask material should be used and how thick should the etch mask be? Assume that the etch mask material has a selectivity of ~100.

(b) How should the etch mask be deposited and patterned? Sketch figures depicting the process for creating the patterned etch mask.

(c) Propose a process flow for fabricating the "step" microstructure. Sketch figures illustrating the intermediate structure at key steps of the process.

Solution

(a) The aspect ratio of the "step" microstructure is greater than 2, since

$$\text{Aspect Ratio (top hole)} = \frac{200 \ \mu m}{60 \ \mu m} = 3.33 \qquad \text{Aspect Ratio (bottom hole)} = \frac{325 \ \mu m}{150 \ \mu m} = 2.10$$

Considering the relatively high aspect ratio (>2) required, and the very deep features that need to be etched (200 μm for the top hole, and 325 μm for the bottom hole), there are only two suitable etching methods: the Bosch process (DRIE) and cryogenic DRIE. DRIE with passivation gases is not suitable because of its subpar selectivity, which would require an extremely thick SiO_2 or Si_3N_4 mask. For both the Bosch process and cryogenic DRIE, SiO_2 is the most suitable mask material given the very deep features that need to be etched. With an etch mask selectivity of ~100, the SiO_2 etch masks need to be at least 2.00 μm thick (top surface), and at least 3.25 μm thick (bottom surface). That is,

$$\text{Mask Thickness} \geq \frac{\text{Etch Depth}}{\text{Selectivity}} = \frac{200 \ \mu m \ (\text{top}) \text{ or } 325 \ \mu m \ (\text{bottom})}{100} = \begin{cases} 2.00 \ \mu m \ (\text{top}) \\ 3.25 \ \mu m \ (\text{bottom}) \end{cases}$$

(b) Given the required thickness (at least 2.00 μm or 3.25 μm) of SiO_2 etch mask on each side of the wafer, PVD and thermal oxidation processes are not suitable for depositing the thick SiO_2 masks due to their low deposition rates. CVD processes (including APCVD, LPCVD, and PECVD) are suitable for depositing the SiO_2 etch masks on each side of the wafer.

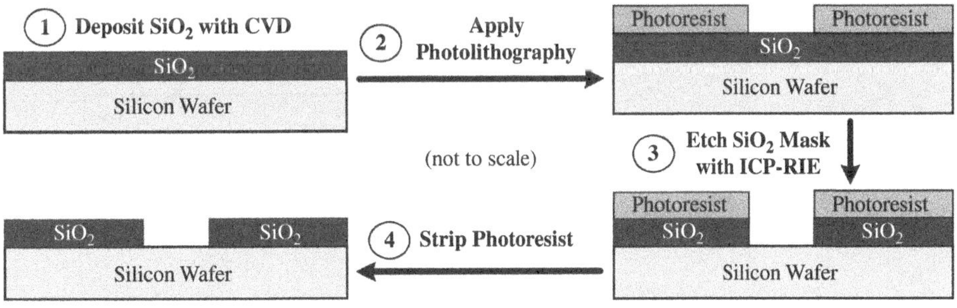

As shown in the figure above, the fabrication process for each SiO_2 mask is as follows.

(1) Deposit the SiO_2 mask using CVD.

(2) Apply photolithography to deposit a patterned layer of photoresist above the SiO_2 mask.

(3) Use any ICP-RIE technique to pattern the SiO_2 mask (i.e., etch regions of the SiO_2 mask that are not protected by photoresist). Isotropic wet etching is not suitable due to under-cutting, and regular RIE may take a long time to etch the thick SiO_2 mask. ICP-RIE offers vertical etching, and passivation is not required here since the aspect ratio of the patterned mask is extremely low (i.e., $\ll 2$). Assuming a SiO_2 mask thickness of ~5 μm on each side of the wafer, we have

$$\text{Aspect Ratio} \left(SiO_2 \text{ mask} \right) = \frac{5 \ \mu m}{60 \ \mu m \ (\text{top}) \text{ or } 150 \ \mu m \ (\text{bottom})} < 0.1$$

(**4**) Finally, strip the layer of photoresist.

(**c**) We start with a silicon wafer with a diameter of 100 mm and thickness of 525 μm. As illustrated in the figure below, we can fabricate the "step" microstructure in the silicon wafer as follows.

(**1**) Create a patterned SiO_2 etch mask (at least 3.25 μm thick) on the bottom wafer surface using the procedure outlined in part (b).

(**2**) Use DRIE to etch the larger hole (325 μm deep and 150 μm wide) into the silicon substrate.

(**3**) Flip the silicon wafer, and create a patterned SiO_2 mask (at least 2.00 μm thick) on the top wafer surface again using the procedure from part (b).

(**4**) Use DRIE to etch the smaller hole (200 μm deep and 60 μm wide) by etching all the way through the silicon wafer.

(**5**) Strip the patterned SiO_2 masks on both sides of the wafer simultaneously by submerging the wafer in buffered oxide etchant (BOE), also known as buffered HF (BHF). Since BOE (an isotropic wet etchant) etches SiO_2 far faster than silicon, undesired BOE etching of the silicon wafer should not be an issue.

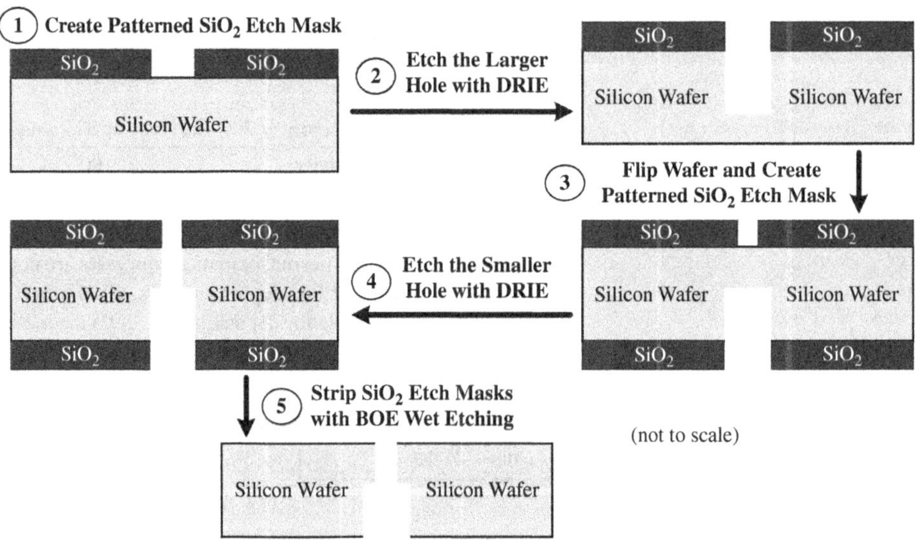

(E) Lift-Off Patterning

The lift-off patterning technique is designed to pattern any deposited thin film without using etching. Compared to etching (especially anisotropic dry etching), lift-off patterning is generally less reliable and less accurately patterns thin films. Consequently, lift-off patterning is used in situations where etching is not suitable, such as for thin films comprised of alloys or a mixture of materials, or a multi-material stack of thin films. Unlike etching, which is a subtractive pattern transfer technique, lift-off patterning is an additive pattern transfer technique.

In theory, lift-off patterning can be accomplished in a few steps just using photolithography and thin film deposition. However, this simplistic lift-off patterning method is seldom used because it produces patterned thin films of very low quality. Instead, lift-off patterning is typically performed with a more sophisticated approach. In particular, a special kind of resist called lift-off resist (LOR) is employed. Like photoresists and e-beam resists, lift-off resists are also polymers dissolved in a solvent. Lift-off resists are neither

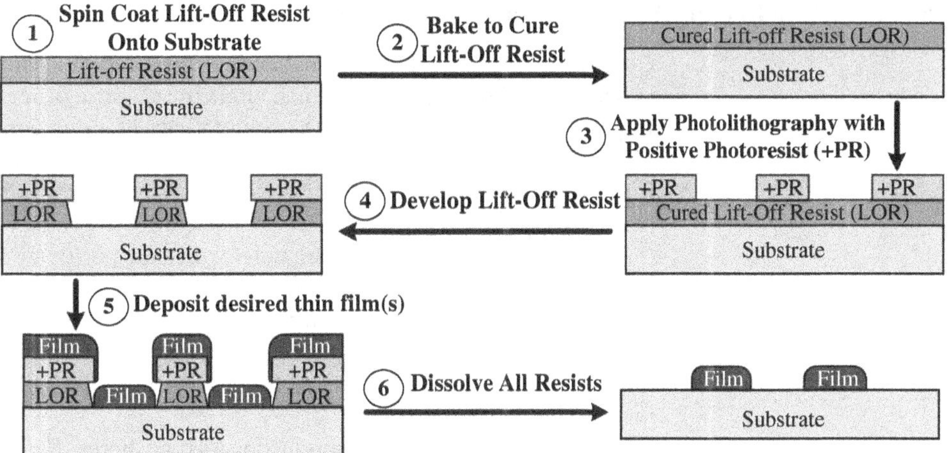

Figure 6-29   The procedure for lift-off patterning, which patterns any deposited thin film without etching.

photosensitive (unlike photoresists), nor electron beam sensitive (unlike e-beam resists). The procedure for lift-off patterning, as illustrated in Figure 6-29, is as follows.

(1)   Starting with a substrate that does *not* contain the thin film(s) to be patterned, spin coat lift-off resist onto the substrate surface using a spin coater.

(2)   Use a hotplate to bake the lift-off resist coating dry (usually 150 to 200°C) by driving off any remaining solvents in the lift-off resist solution.

(3)   Apply photolithography to deposit a patterned layer of *positive* photoresist above the lift-off resist coating. Positive photoresists are used here for compatibility.

(4)   Develop the lift-off resist by immersing the lift-off resist coating in its unique developer solution, which removes patterned regions of the lift-off resist that are not protected by photoresist. Unlike photoresists, lift-off resists are designed to develop isotropically, resulting in intentional undercutting which assists the lift-off process and prevents retention.

(5)   Deposit the desired thin film which needs to be patterned. If multiple layers of thin films need to be patterned together, they can be deposited one after another in this step. To prevent the softening and degradation of the cured photoresist and lift-off resist, only thin film deposition methods with relatively low substrate temperatures (<200°C) can be used. These low temperature deposition techniques include sputtering, evaporation (with substrate cooling), and plasma-enhanced CVD.

(6)   Finally, dissolve (i.e., remove) all photoresist and lift-off resist by immersing the substrate surface in a solvent that will not damage the desired thin film(s) to be patterned. Thin film(s) with resist underneath will "lift-off" and be removed, while the remaining patterned regions of thin film(s) will remain. Undercutting of the lift-off resist in step (4) ensures that the thin film(s) will lift-off cleanly.

The main issues with lift-off patterning are retention and redeposition. Retention occurs when the thin film(s) do not lift-off cleanly. This can result in unwanted parts of the thin film(s) remaining stuck to the substrate instead of lifting-off. These unwanted parts can be pillar-like structures from thin film material deposited on the sidewalls of the patterned resists, which can fall over and damage the patterned thin film(s). On the other hand, redeposition occurs when particles of the thin film(s) that have been lifted-off fall back and become attached to the substrate surface.

6.4.4 Surface Treatments, Modification, and Planarization

Doping   Doping involves the deliberate incorporation of impurity atoms into the crystal lattice of a semiconductor, which alters the physical properties of the semiconductor. In particular, doping increases the conductivity of a semiconductor material by several orders of magnitude. There are two types of dopants: p (positive)-type dopants and n (negative)-type dopants. In n-type (i.e., n-doped) semiconductors, the primary (electric) charge carriers are electrons. Conversely, the primary charge carriers in p-type (i.e., p-doped) semiconductors are holes which are positively charged electron vacancies. Combinations of p-doped and n-doped semiconductor material are essential to the operation of microelectronic components such as transistors, diodes, op-amps, and integrated circuit components. For example, light-emitting diodes (LEDs), photodiodes, field-effect transistors (FETs), and bipolar junction transistors (BJTs) all rely on doped semiconductor materials to function.

For silicon, the most common dopants are boron (B, p-type dopant), phosphorus (P, n-type dopant), and arsenic (As, n-type dopant). Pre-doped p-type or n-type silicon wafers can be readily purchased. If we want to dope the entire surface of a blank silicon wafer, it is likely easier and cheaper to purchase a pre-doped (p-type or n-type) silicon wafer. Aside from silicon, other semiconductor materials (e.g., GaAs, GaP, and GaN) can also be doped. However, the p-type and n-type dopants for these other semiconductor materials are different than that of silicon.

There are two common surface treatments for doping desired regions of a semiconductor surface: diffusion and ion implantation. Even though both diffusion and ion implantation can be applied to dope other semiconductor materials, we will focus exclusively on the doping of silicon which is by far the most popular semiconductor material.

Diffusion (Doping)   Diffusion (doping) is a very high temperature surface treatment process for doping unprotected regions of a semiconductor surface. The procedure for diffusion (doping), which can require up to a few hours to complete, is as follows.

(1)   First, a patterned mask needs to be deposited on the silicon surface to protect regions where doping is undesired. SiO_2 masks created through CVD or thermal oxidation and patterned by etching are the most appropriate. Resist masks are completely unsuitable as polymeric materials will degrade at the high temperatures required for diffusion.

(2)   (**Pre-deposition**) Expose the silicon surface to gases (e.g., AsH_3, PH_3, or B_2H_6) containing the desired dopant atoms at high temperatures (900 to 1200°C). These highly noxious gases can either be directly introduced (potentially dangerous), or created by heating liquid or solid sources in a sealed chamber (safer). At the high temperatures, the gases will react with the silicon surface to form a silicate glass with a high concentration of the dopant atoms.

(3)   (**Drive-in**) Finally, the silicon surface is maintained at high temperatures (again 900 to 1200°C) for an extended period of time to allow dopant atoms from the silicate glass to diffuse into areas of the silicon surface that are not protected by the mask, resulting in a more uniform distribution of dopants over a larger volume of silicon.

Ion Implantation (Doping)   Ion implantation, sometimes abbreviated as I^2, dopes unprotected areas of a semiconductor surface with ion bombardment (i.e., "implantation"). Compared to diffusion (doping), ion implantation offers better controllability, greater repeatability, substantially lower substrate temperatures, and greatly reduced process time. Industrially, ion implantation is the most popular doping technique. In research settings, diffusion is still preferred since ion implantation is conducted under high vacuum with very expensive equipment (>1 million USD). The procedure for ion implantation is as follows.

(1) First, deposit a patterned mask on the silicon surface to protect regions where doping is unwanted. Although many mask materials are suitable for ion implantation, SiO_2, Si_3N_4, and photoresist masks are most commonly used. Photoresist masks can be used, but are not ideal since they can polymerize from ion bombardment or flow if the substrate temperature is too high.

(2) Bombard exposed silicon surfaces with highly energetic ions (5 to 200 keV) that contain the desired dopant atoms. These ions are typically created in a plasma arc discharge and accelerated by strong electric fields. Implantation requires much higher ion energies than sputtering or physical etching.

(3) **(Annealing/Diffusion)** The final step is to anneal the silicon surface to repair crystal lattice damages caused by ion implantation, and diffuse the implanted ions further and more evenly into the silicon surface. Annealing/diffusion are carried out together by heating the silicon surface (~500 to 600°C) and maintaining the temperature for about an hour. A shorter and higher temperature anneal may also be required to "activate" the dopants.

Surface Planarization   The surface topography of the top layer of a substrate can be uneven, especially following etching or thin film deposition/growth. To prevent fabrication problems, the surface of the top layer of the substrate is often planarized (i.e., made flat/planar) prior to the application of the next layer. For instance, the substrate surface should be planar prior to the application of photolithography. Surface planarization is also used to planarize layers of electrical interconnects, passivation layers, and much more.

The standard method of surface planarization is chemical-mechanical polishing (CMP). In CMP, the substrate (usually a wafer) is pressed against a porous polishing pad saturated with an abrasive slurry. Both the substrate and polishing pad are rotated, allowing the highly abrasive slurry to planarize the substrate surface. The abrasive slurry consists of nanoscale particles (for mechanical polishing) immersed in a buffered acid or base (for chemical polishing). The nanoscale particles are usually comprised of hard materials such as silica (SiO_2), alumina (Al_2O_3), and ceria (CeO_2).

Piranha Surface Treatment   Piranha solution is a 3:1 (by volume) mixture of concentrated ($\geq$ 95% by weight) sulfuric acid to 30% (by weight) hydrogen peroxide. Piranha solution is extremely corrosive and dangerous if mishandled. To prevent violent boiling and potential explosion, hydrogen peroxide must be added into sulfuric acid when preparing piranha solution. ***Never*** add sulfuric acid into hydrogen peroxide, because a 1:1 mixture of concentrated sulfuric acid and 30% hydrogen peroxide can explode.

Piranha solution is most often used to clean the surfaces of silicon, quartz, and glass substrates by removing (i.e., dissolving) all organic and metal contaminants. Though less common, piranha solution can also be used to clean other semiconductor (e.g., GaAs) surfaces. In particular, piranha solution is highly effective at removing resist (e.g., photoresist) residues. Note that piranha solution is incompatible with substrates that contain organic compounds, polymers, and/or metals (unless we want to remove them).

Piranha solution also alters the surface chemistry of SiO_2 (e.g., quartz) and glass surfaces, temporarily making these surfaces highly hydrophilic through the creation of silanol (Si−O−H) functional groups. The silanol functional groups are produced through the hydroxylation of the SiO_2. Highly hydrophilic SiO_2 (e.g., quartz) and glass surfaces greatly enhance the adhesion and uniformity of any deposited metal (e.g., Cr). Thus, metals are sometimes deposited on SiO_2 (e.g., quartz) and glass surfaces within a few hours of piranha surface treatment.

Surface Modification   Surface modification intentionally alters the surface chemistry of a substrate. Due to their complexity and small size, the integrated chips in microfluidic/LOC devices have relatively high surface-area-to-volume ratio, making surface modification especially impactful. Surface modification can be used to alter many surface properties of a substrate such as biocompatibility, wettability, reactivity, adhesion, adsorption, and hydrophilicity/hydrophobicity. For instance, surface modification can render surfaces biocompatible by reducing the chemical reactivity of the surface with biofluids.[85]

To exemplify the importance of surface modification, let us consider materials with naturally hydrophobic surfaces such as SiO_2 (e.g., quartz), glass, and many polymers. Microchannel (e.g., capillary) walls comprised of these materials can easily become constricted or clogged because cells and many biomolecules (e.g., proteins) easily adsorb onto hydrophobic surfaces. After applying surface modification to make hydrophobic microchannel wall surfaces hydrophilic, unwanted adsorption of biomolecules and cells will be significantly reduced.

Surface modification can be classified as either dynamic or static. Generally, silicon (single-crystal or polycrystalline) surfaces are difficult to modify, while SiO_2 (e.g., quartz), glass, and polymeric surfaces are much easier to modify. For dynamic surface modification, surface-active agents (i.e., surfactants) are added into the buffer solution flowing through microchannels. The surface-active agents adsorb onto the microchannel walls, forming a dynamic (and temporary) coating. Dynamic surface modification is both simple and quick to carry out, and is most suitable for disposable integrated chips. Conversely, static surface modification is more complicated and time consuming to carry out, and is more appropriate for reusable integrated chips where permanent surface modification is desired.

During static (i.e., permanent) surface modification, functional groups (e.g., −COOH) and/or more complex molecules (e.g., antibodies) are covalently attached onto the substrate surface. For example, static surface modification can be used to form a self-assembled monolayer on the substrate surface to tune the surface chemistry. For SiO_2 (e.g., quartz), glass, and polymeric surfaces, the first step of static surface modification is often the creation of hydroxyl (−OH) functional groups on the substrate surface, which makes the surface hydrophilic. Hydroxyl functional groups can be temporarily created by exposing the substrate surface to a low-pressure oxygen plasma, or with piranha surface treatment. Oxygen plasma treatment is usually more suitable because piranha surface treatment is incompatible with substrates that contain layers of polymers and/or metals. Once hydroxyl functional groups have been created, the substrate surface can be further and permanently modified through a series of chemical reactions. For example, recognition elements (e.g., antibodies) can be covalently anchored onto the sensing surface of a LOC biosensor via surface modification.

EXAMPLE 6-3   Propose a process flow for fabricating the silicon membrane nozzle shown on the right, which has dimensions of 25 mm (length) × 23 mm (width) × 525 μm (thickness). At each key step of the process, sketch the cross-sectional view of the intermediate structure. Note that p^{++} Si refers to heavily doped p-type silicon, and the p^{++} silicon membrane is ~5 μm thick. This silicon membrane nozzle design is by I. Brodie and J. J. Muray.[86]

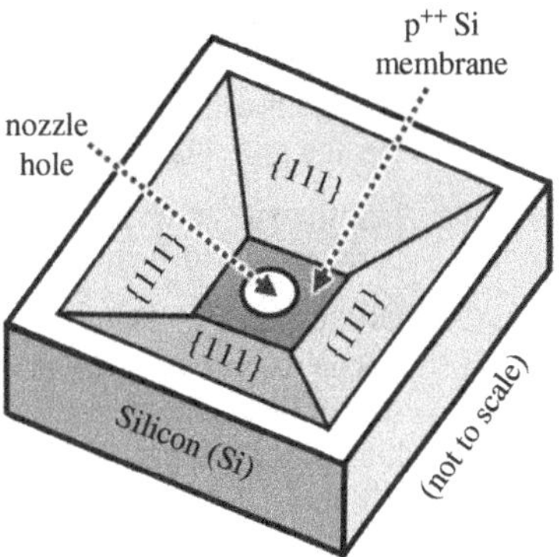

Solution   We start with a {100} single-crystal silicon (Si) substrate that is 525 µm thick, and etch the structure with alkaline anisotropic wet etching utilizing the doping control method. Because directional etch is required, {110} and {111} single-crystal silicon substrates are not suitable.

As shown in the figure below, the process for fabricating the silicon membrane nozzle is as follows.

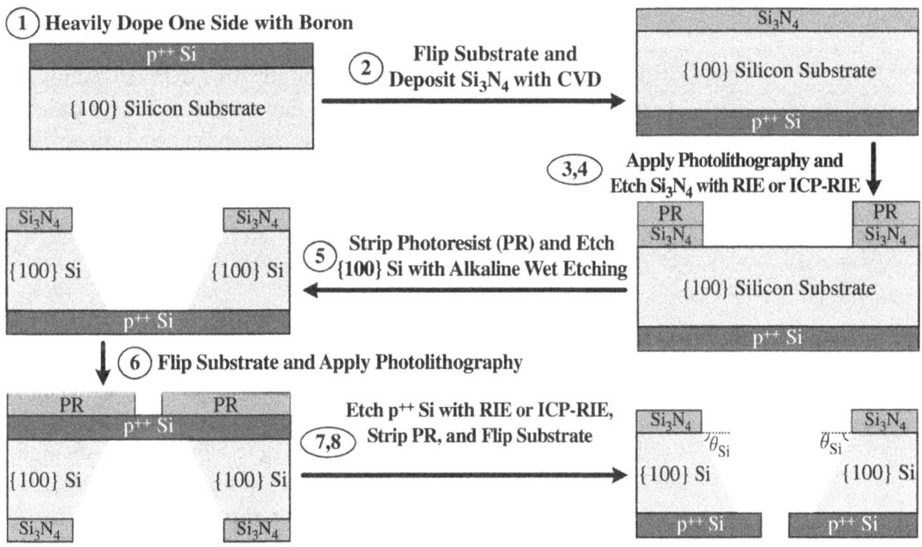

(1) First, heavily dope one side of the {100} silicon substrate with boron (B) to create a surface layer of p^{++} silicon that is ~5 µm thick. Because we are doping a blank silicon substrate, we can either use diffusion or ion implantation to dope the silicon with boron (B).

(2) Flip the silicon substrate, and then deposit a layer of silicon nitride (Si_3N_4) on the other side with CVD (APCVD, LPCVD, or PECVD). This Si_3N_4 layer will serve as an etch mask, which has to be relatively thick because we have to etch deep (~520 µm) into the silicon substrate. Thus, CVD is most suitable.

(3) Apply photolithography to obtain a layer of patterned photoresist (PR) with a rectangular opening above the Si_3N_4 layer.

(4) Etch away the large rectangular region of Si_3N_4 not protected by photoresist to create the patterned Si_3N_4 etch mask. To avoid undercutting, which will change the shape of the rectangular opening, use RIE or ICP-RIE anisotropic dry etching.

(5) Strip all photoresist to avoid reactions with alkaline etchants, and then apply alkaline wet etching using the patterned Si_3N_4 layer as an etch mask. Etch all the way through the silicon substrate to obtain the desired pyramidal hole structure. Since there are no microelectronic components, both KOH and TMAH are suitable alkaline etchants. The doping control method is used here, and alkaline wet etching will virtually stop when the etchant encounters the p^{++} silicon, forming the p^{++} silicon membrane.

(6) Flip the substrate and then apply photolithography to obtain a patterned layer of cured photoresist with a circular opening above the p^{++} silicon layer.

(7) Use ICP-RIE (anisotropic dry etching) to etch away the exposed circular region of p^{++} silicon not protected by photoresist to create the nozzle hole. Isotropic etching techniques should be avoided because undercutting will enlarge and change the shape of the nozzle hole. Since the p^{++} silicon membrane layer is ~5 μm thick, etching the hole with regular RIE may take a long time.

(8) Strip all photoresist and flip the substrate.

(9) Finally, dice the silicon substrate to cut out the rectangular silicon membrane nozzle. ▲

6.5 MICRO/NANO FABRICATION OF MICROFLUIDIC AND LAB-ON-A-CHIP DEVICES

In Section 6.4, we covered a wide range of micro/nano fabrication techniques which can be used to create integrated circuits, MEMS devices, and integrated chips for microfluidic and LOC devices. To demonstrate the use of micro/nano fabrication for creating bionanotechnological devices, we will go through three detailed examples. The first example is a simplistic LOC biosensor microchip that utilizes IDEs for detection and does not include any microfluidic components. To show the fabrication processes for microfluidic platforms, the second example is a microfluidic platform-based microchip designed to selectively capture single cells. The third and final example is a complementary metal-oxide-semiconductor (CMOS) LOC sensor microchip, which is used to illustrate the fabrication of sophisticated microchips for CMOS LOC devices.

6.5.1 Fabricating Interdigitated Electrode Biosensor Microchips

In Section 6.2.3, we discussed the working principles of non-faradaic impedimetric LOC biosensors, which detect target analyte concentrations via impedance changes following the addition of biosample fluids. To detect impedance changes, non-faradaic impedimetric LOC biosensors typically rely on sets of interdigitated electrodes (IDEs) together with recognition elements anchored either on top or in between the IDEs. Each set of IDEs consists of two interlocking comb-shaped microelectrode arrays.

The simplest non-faradaic impedimetric LOC biosensor design consists of multiple sets of IDEs on a microchip, plus one liquid sample loading well on top of each set of IDEs (Figure 6-30). This simple IDE-based LOC biosensor is inexpensive and straightforward to fabricate. Although simple, the signal-to-noise ratio, sensitivity, and detection limit of this simplistic IDE-based LOC biosensor tends to be inferior to traditional lab assays. Its signal-to-noise ratio and sensitivity are relatively low, and the detection limit is relatively high. Also, biosample fluids have to be loaded into the sample loading wells manually with a micropipette. Loading the correct amount of biosample is key to assuring reproducible detection results.

Sample Loading Wells   The sample loading wells can be made from PDMS, a type of silicone polymer. PDMS is preferred because one can temporarily bond a smooth piece of PDMS to a flat substrate without needing an adhesive. The PDMS wells can also be reused after cleaning with acetone and isopropyl alcohol (IPA). Furthermore, PDMS is an electrically insulating material which will not interfere with the impedance signal. PDMS is also inexpensive,

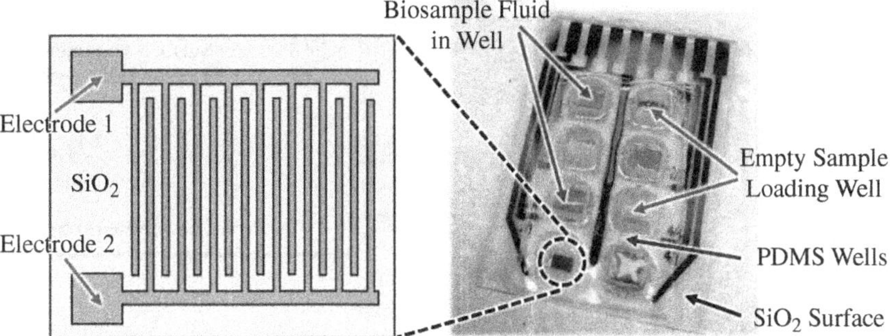

Figure 6-30 A simple IDE-based LOC biosensor, which consists of eight sets of IDEs on a microchip covered with eight PDMS liquid sample loading wells. (*The photograph on the right is provided by Prof. Jie Chen's group.*)

non-toxic, biocompatible, and transparent. Although highly detailed PDMS designs are traditionally fabricated using PDMS micromolding, the advancement of 3D printing technology has allowed cheaper fabrication of less detailed PDMS designs without requiring microfabrication equipment or cleanrooms. To fabricate PDMS sample loading wells, one can pour liquid PDMS base mixed with a curing agent into a high-resolution 3D printed mold, place the mold containing the PDMS mixture in a vacuum desiccator to remove air bubbles, and finally solidify the PDMS in an oven set at about 90°C for an hour.[87,88]

Fabrication of Microelectrodes Interdigitated electrodes (IDEs) or other similar microelectrodes can be fabricated starting with a flat SiO_2-coated substrate such as SiO_2-coated silicon, glass (mainly amorphous SiO_2), or quartz (crystalline SiO_2). It is important to have a SiO_2 surface, which can be activated with silanol (Si–O–H) groups through surface treatment. The activated SiO_2 surface greatly improves the adhesion and uniformity of any deposited metal, and enables further surface modification to chemically anchor recognition elements onto the surface. Therefore, if starting from a silicon substrate lacking a SiO_2 surface, the first step is to create a SiO_2 surface.

(**Silicon Substrates Only**) Apply thermal oxidation (~1000°C) to obtain the SiO_2 top layer (~500 nm). Compared to CVD, thermal oxidation results in a higher quality insulating SiO_2 top layer and higher quality Si–SiO_2 interface which will be less likely to interfere with the impedance signal. If starting from a glass, quartz, or SiO_2-coated silicon substrate, this step is unnecessary.

The procedure for fabricating IDE-based LOC biosensor microchips is as follows (Figure 6-31).

(1) Start with a flat glass, quartz, or SiO_2-coated silicon substrate. Immerse the substrate in piranha solution (please refer to Section 6.4.4) to clean the substrate and activate the SiO_2 surface with silanol (Si–O–H) groups, which allows chromium to adhere more strongly and with better uniformity.

(2) Use sputtering (PVD) to deposit an adhesion layer of chromium (~10 nm Cr) onto the activated SiO_2 surface, followed by a layer of gold (~100 nm Au) for the IDEs. Gold is highly biocompatible (i.e., less likely to oxidize or react with biological samples), but does not adhere well to SiO_2 surfaces. On the other hand, chromium is not biocompatible but acts as an adhesion layer between the gold and SiO_2. Compared to evaporation, sputtering offers better control, repeatability, and coverage which are all important for biosensors.

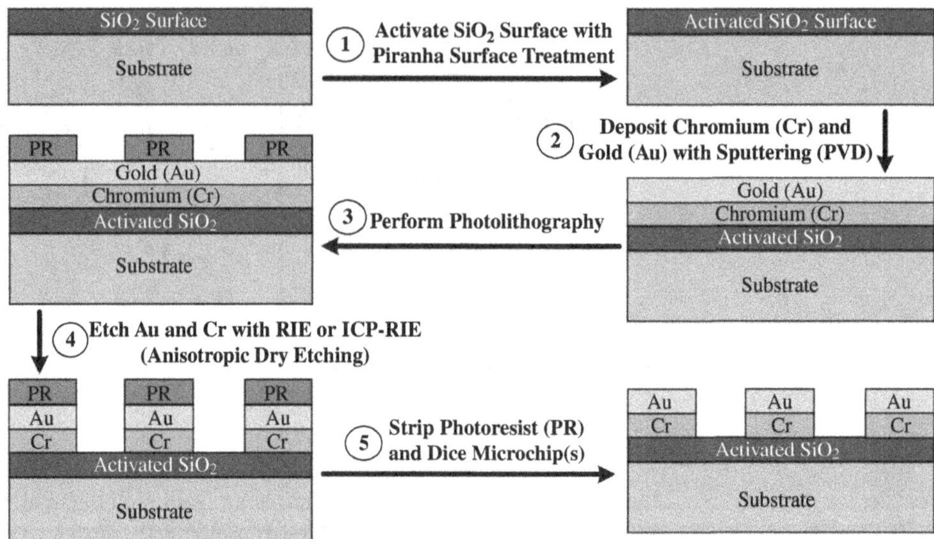

Figure 6-31   Procedure for fabricating microelectrodes such as interdigitated electrodes (IDEs). Suitable substrates include glass, quartz, or SiO$_2$-coated silicon. If starting from a silicon substrate lacking a SiO$_2$ surface, thermal oxidation can grow a high-quality SiO$_2$ surface layer.

(3)   Apply photolithography to create a patterned layer of photoresist (PR) above the gold surface, which will serve as an etch mask for etching the Au/Cr layers.

(4)   Etch the patterned regions of gold and chrome which are not protected by photoresist to define the IDEs. Use RIE or ICP-RIE anisotropic dry etching to prevent open-circuit issues resulting from undercutting. Wet etching methods should be avoided because they are fast, difficult to control, and prone to undercutting.

(5)   Strip the photoresist etch mask. If multiple microchips are fabricated on the same substrate, perform dicing to physically separate the microchips.

Surface Modification   Before the IDE-based LOC biosensor can be used for analyte detection, either the gold (Au) surfaces of the IDEs or the SiO$_2$ surfaces between the IDEs must be modified by anchoring recognition elements onto the surface (Figure 6-32). The exact surface modification procedure varies depending on the type of recognition element to be anchored.

To anchor aptamers (i.e., short strands of DNA, RNA, or peptide) onto the gold surfaces (Figure 5), one can (i) coat the gold IDE surfaces with carboxy aliphatic thiol compounds to create carboxylic (–COOH) groups on the gold surfaces. Next, (ii) introduce the aptamers onto the surface to anchor aptamer recognition elements onto the gold electrode surfaces of the IDEs. Aptamer recognition elements can be used to detect peptides, proteins, toxins, bacteria, carbohydrates, and some small biomolecules.[38]

Alternatively, one can functionalize the SiO$_2$ surfaces between the IDEs. To achieve this, (i) first apply oxygen plasma treatment to activate the SiO$_2$ surfaces with silanol (Si–O–H) groups. The silanol groups allow organic molecules to attach to the SiO$_2$ surface via covalent bonding. Piranha solution cannot be used for the activation, since it easily dissolves the gold and chromium of the microelectrodes. The following step depends on the type of recognition element used. If antibody recognition elements are used, (ii) the silanol-activated SiO$_2$ surface could be coated with 3-aminopropyltriethoxysilane (APTES) followed by glutaraldehyde and then the antibody recognition elements. This will anchor the antibody recognition elements onto the SiO$_2$ surfaces between the IDEs, which is suitable for detecting proteins, antigens, viruses, and bacteria.[89]

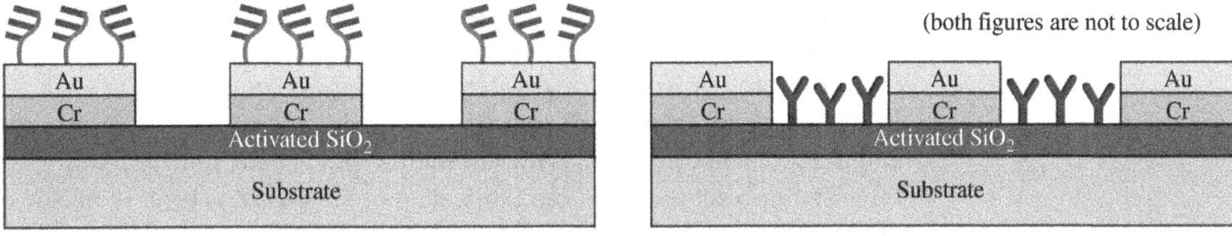

Figure 6-32 Recognition elements for biosensing can be chemically anchored (left) on the gold (Au) surfaces of the IDEs, or alternatively (right) on the SiO$_2$ surfaces between the IDEs.

Analyte Detection   The overall procedure for using an IDE-based LOC biosensor microchip for analyte detection is as follows.

(1) First, attach the two electrodes of each set of IDEs to portable impedance sensing equipment such as an LCR meter or a potentiostat/galvanostat impedance analyzer.

(2) Next, place the piece of PDMS containing all of the sample loading wells on the microchip. The PDMS piece will temporarily adhere to the microchip surface without requiring an adhesive.

(3) Then, load biosample fluid into each sample loading well, which changes the impedance spectra.

(4) Wait and then wash out the biosample fluids from the sample loading wells, so that only bound analytes can contribute to impedance change.

(5) With calibrated computer software, the measured impedance change versus AC excitation frequency spectra can be used to obtain the analyte concentration in the biosample fluid loaded into each well.

6.5.2 Fabricating Microfluidic Platforms

As discussed in Section 2.1, a microfluidic platform is comprised of a combination of microfluidic components, where each component is responsible for carrying out a fluidic unit operation. Common microfluidic components include microchannels, microchambers, inlets, outlets, micro-valves, micro-mixers, micro-dispensers, micro-filters, micro-pumps, and fluid-handling microelectrodes (some of which are shown in Figure 6-33). Microfluidic platforms are integral parts of many LOC, OOC, cell capture and sorting, and microchip electrophoresis devices. Furthermore, microfluidic platforms have a wide range of applications ranging from improving biomedical assays to assisting drug delivery.

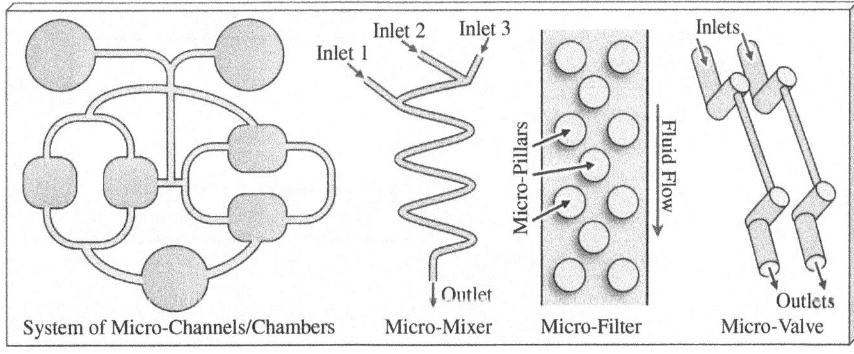

Figure 6-33 Examples of common microfluidic components found on microfluidic platforms.

(A) Fabricating Systems of Microchannels and Microchambers

Two of the most common techniques for fabricating systems of microchannels and micro-chambers are (1) isotropic wet etching of glass or quartz and (2) soft lithography with PDMS. Both techniques are capable of creating a transparent system of microchannels and microchambers, which is important for optical detection. Soft lithography with PDMS offers better resolution and can fabricate more intricate features than isotropic wet etching of glass/quartz which suffers from undercutting and controllability issues. Unfortunately, both techniques are not suitable for fabricating more complex microfluidic components. 3D printing techniques cannot be used to fabricate systems of micro-channels/chambers because of the small features sizes (on the order of a few micrometers) involved.

Isotropic Wet Etching of Glass/Quartz   One common way of creating systems of micro-channels and microchambers in a glass or quartz substrate is with BOE (buffered oxide etchant) isotropic wet etching. Glass and quartz substrates are biocompatible, usually optically transparent, and have surfaces that are relatively easy to modify. Due to undercutting issues and the high etch rate, BOE isotropic wet etching is only suitable for etching micro-channels/chambers that are wider and deeper than about 5 μm, and is generally not suitable for creating more complicated microfluidic components. The main advantage of isotropic etching is that it produces micro-channels/chambers with smooth edges by uniformly etch-ing in all directions. Conversely, anisotropic etching creates micro-channels/chambers with sharp edges that can lead to turbulent flow.

The procedure for fabricating a system of microchannels and microchambers in a flat glass or quartz substrate is as follows (Figure 6-34).

(1)   Start with a flat and clean glass or quartz substrate. Deposit a layer of mask mate-rial resistant to BOE on *both sides* of the substrate to mask the top surface and pre-vent the bottom side of the substrate from being etched. Suitable mask materials

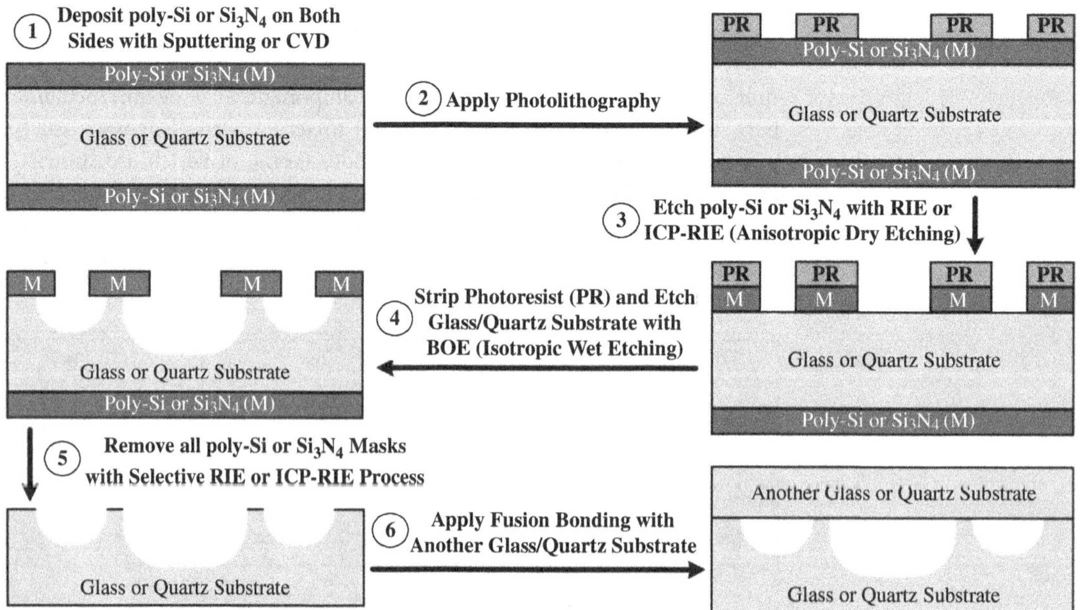

Figure 6-34   Process for fabricating a system of microchannels and microchambers with isotropic wet etching of a glass or quartz substrate.

include polycrystalline silicon (poly-Si) or silicon nitride (Si_3N_4) deposited by CVD or sputtering. Due to the higher deposition rates, CVD is preferred if a thick mask is required (i.e., the micro-channels/chambers are relatively deep).

Note: Gold (Au) is also a suitable mask material that is highly resistant to BOE. We will not use gold here since it is costly and does not adhere well to glass/quartz, requiring an adhesion layer of chromium (Cr).

(2) Next, apply photolithography to obtain a patterned layer of photoresist (PR) above the top mask material layer (i.e., poly-Si or Si_3N_4). To compensate for undercutting during BOE isotropic wet etching, the openings for the micro-channels/chambers should be intentionally made narrower when designing the photomask for this photolithography step.

(3) Use RIE or ICP-RIE anisotropic dry etching to etch away regions of the top mask material layer that are not protected by photoresist, creating the etch mask for BOE wet etching. Here, isotropic etching should be avoided because undercutting in this step will change the shapes of the micro-channels/chambers.

(4) Strip the photoresist layer. Then, submerge the substrate in BOE to etch unprotected regions of the glass/quartz substrate through isotropic wet etching, creating the system of microchannels and microchambers.

(5) Remove the mask material layers (i.e., poly-Si or Si_3N_4) from both sides of the substrate with a selective RIE or ICP-RIE anisotropic dry etching process. Glass/quartz is highly resistant to RIE etching. For example, we can use $CF_{4(g)}$ plasma with added $O_{2(g)}$ during RIE etching, which easily etches both poly-Si and Si_3N_4 but not SiO_2 (the main constituent of glass/quartz).

(6) Finally, use fusion bonding to bond the glass/quartz substrate containing the micro-channels/chambers to another flat glass/quartz substrate. Bonding seals the top surfaces of the micro-channels/chambers and will protect liquids in the microfluidic system from contamination and evaporative losses. Do not use adhesives for bonding since adhesives can damage the micro-channels/chambers and reduce the optical transparency of glass or quartz, making optical detection more difficult. The procedure for fusion bonding is as follows.[90]

(i) Immerse the glass/quartz substrate containing the micro-channels/chambers together with another clean and flat glass/quartz substrate in piranha solution (Section 6.4.4). The piranha solution will remove organic and metallic contaminants on both glass/quartz substrates and activate the SiO_2 surfaces with silanol (Si–O–H) groups.

(ii) Press the two glass/quartz substrates against each other. Due to the hydrophilic silanol groups on the surfaces of both substrates, van der Waals forces temporarily bond the two substrates. To achieve a permanent bond, the two substrates are placed in an oven and heated to between 400°C and 600°C for a few hours. To prevent thermal stresses, the substrates should be heated and cooled slowly.

Soft Lithography (with PDMS) The soft lithography technique is also commonly used to fabricate systems of microchannels and microchambers. Soft lithography creates a system of microchannels and microchambers in a patterned piece of PDMS that is sealed against a flat SiO_2 surface such as glass, quartz, or SiO_2-coated silicon. PDMS is used due to its low cost, non-toxicity, transparency, biocompatibility, elasticity (easy to remove from molds for

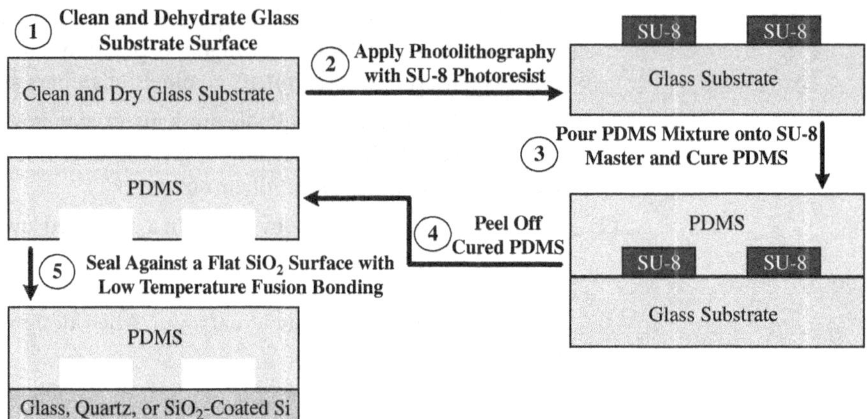

Figure 6-35   Overall process for soft lithography (with PDMS), which can be used to fabricate systems of microchannels and microchambers.

feature replication), and ability to easily bond to glass, quartz, plastic, and other flat surfaces without requiring any adhesives. Additionally, PDMS is inherently hydrophobic, but exposure to oxygen plasma can make PDMS temporarily hydrophilic.

The major advantage of soft lithography is that etching is not required, so the micro-channels are much cheaper and simpler to fabricate, and the fabrication does not involve strong acids or strong bases. Soft lithography is especially well suited for creating deep micro-channels/chambers (i.e., >100 µm deep), which takes a long time to etch even with DRIE processes. While isotropic wet etching can only achieve a resolution of ~5 µm due to undercutting and the high etch rates, soft lithography can achieve a resolution of ~1 µm which is sufficient for most micro-channels/chambers. Thus, soft lithography is able to create narrower and shallower micro-channels/chambers than isotropic wet etching. Overall, soft lithography is superior to isotropic wet etching for creating systems of microchannels and microchambers.

The procedure for fabricating a system of microchannels and microchambers with soft lithography is as follows (Figure 6-35).

(1) Immerse a flat glass substrate in piranha solution (Section 6.4.4) to clean the glass surface, and then dehydrate the glass surface for improving the adhesion of SU-8. Although silicon wafer substrates can also be used, glass substrates are cheaper and less prone to fracturing when peeling off PDMS.

(2) Apply photolithography to obtain a patterned layer of SU-8 photoresist "master" on the glass substrate surface. SU-8 is an epoxy-based negative photoresist with many advantages. With most other photoresists, we can obtain a dry thickness of about 1 to 4 µm with spin coating followed by soft baking. With SU-8, spin coating and soft baking can be repeated multiple times to obtain a very thick dry layer up to about 2 mm, which is extremely useful for deep micro-channels/chambers. The cured SU-8 surface is also very flat compared to other photoresists, allowing one to obtain microchannels and microchambers of uniform depth. Vertical sidewalls can also be produced with cured SU-8, which is helpful for specialized high aspect ratio microchannels.[91]

(3) Place the substrate with SU-8 master in a suitable container. Next, mix liquid PDMS base with a curing agent and pour the mixture onto the SU-8 master in the container. Put the container holding the substrate and PDMS mixture in a vacuum

desiccator to remove air bubbles, and then cure the PDMS by baking in an oven set at about 90°C for an hour.[88]

(4) Gently peel the cured and patterned PDMS from the SU-8 master. As PDMS is elastic, it can be easily removed from the SU-8 master for feature replication. If required, the patterned and cured piece of PDMS can be cut into the desired shape(s) with a scalpel or razor blade.[92]

(5) Finally, permanently bond the patterned PDMS to a flat SiO_2 surface such as glass, quartz, or SiO_2-coated silicon to seal the system of microchannels and microchambers. Because cured PDMS can only withstand temperatures up to about 350°C, high temperature bonding processes cannot be used. The procedure for low temperature plasma-activated fusion bonding is as follows.[93]

    (i) Use low-pressure oxygen plasma treatment to activate the SiO_2 surface of the substrate as well as the PDMS surface with silanol (Si–O–H) groups, making both surfaces hydrophilic and allowing them to adhere to each other.

    (ii) Press the patterned PDMS and flat SiO_2 surface together at room temperature to permanently seal the system of microchannels and microchambers.

(B) Fabricating MEMS Components

Aside from microchannels and microchambers, microfluidic platforms often incorporate MEMS microfluidic components such as micro-valves, micro-mixers, micro-pumps, micro-dispensers, and micro-filters. In both LOC and microfluidic devices, these MEMS components enable on-chip preparation and staging of the sample. For instance, MEMS microfluidic components on a biosensor microchip can be used to greatly enhance the signal and reduce noise, thereby improving the sensitivity and detection limit of the biosensor.

Fluid-Handling Microelectrodes   Before fabricating MEMS microfluidic components, it is highly worthwhile to consider whether they are necessary. Digital microfluidics in the form of fluid-handling microelectrodes powered by electric potentials can carry out the functions of some MEMS microfluidic components such as micro-valves, micro-dispensers, and micro-mixers. Fluid-handling microelectrodes use electrokinetic forces to direct fluid transport, dispensing, mixing, and other fluidic operations (Figure 6-36). The electrokinetic forces used primarily include electro-osmosis (EOF), electrophoresis (EPF), and dielectrophoresis (DEP) as detailed in Chapters 2 and 3. To fabricate fluid-handling microelectrodes, one can follow the procedure for fabricating microelectrodes given in Section 6.5.1.[16,95]

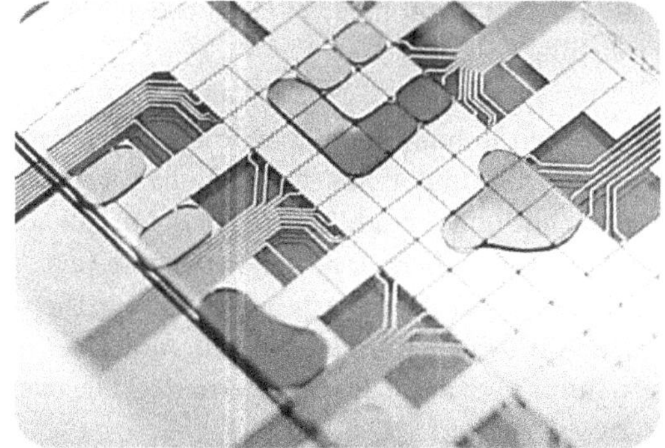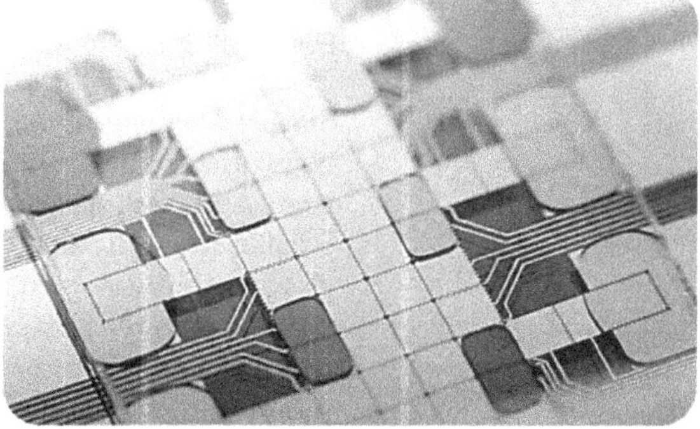

Figure 6-36   In digital microfluidics, fluid-handling microelectrodes use electrokinetic forces to carry out microfluidic functions. (*The photographs are reprinted with permission from A. Wheeler and D. Rackus [University of Toronto/ NSERC].*[94])

Fluid-handling microelectrodes can be a major improvement over the MEMS microfluidic structures they replace, as the electrodes are more durable than delicate MEMS structures and are far less likely to break during transportation and handling. Compared to complex MEMS microfluidic components, fluid-handling microelectrodes can be easier and less expensive to fabricate, and are more easily reconfigured since the external software controlling the fluid-handling microelectrodes can easily be changed.

The main drawback of fluid-handling microelectrodes is the external equipment (e.g., a function generator controlled by computer software) required to power and control them. Adding fluid-handling microelectrodes to a chip increases the number of electrical terminals on the chip that need to be connected to external equipment, which may necessitate the inclusion of a CMOS integrated circuit on the chip (please refer to Section 6.5.3 for more details).

3D Micromachining   MEMS components are frequently created using 3D micromachining processes which include bulk micromachining and surface micromachining. 3D micromachining can be used to fabricate systems of microchannels and microchambers, as well as MEMS microfluidic components. The two micromachining techniques can either be used individually, or combined to create highly complex MEMS components. For fabricating simpler MEMS components, bulk micromachining is preferred since it is simpler, faster, less expensive, and requires fewer steps than surface micromachining. Moreover, bulk micromachining can be used to create relatively deep MEMS structures (>100 μm in depth), which is difficult to accomplish with surface micromachining. Nevertheless, surface micromachining is still required for many complex MEMS structures, especially structures with overhangs such as cantilevers.[96]

Bulk Micromachining   Bulk micromachining involves the application of a patterned etch mask, followed by anisotropic etching of exposed areas of the substrate. Bulk micromachining is usually performed using either DRIE anisotropic dry etching or alkaline anisotropic wet etching. In particular, DRIE is used for the microfabrication of MEMS structures which can be relatively large (up to hundreds of micrometers deep), where a high etch rate is required for process efficiency. Regular RIE is not suitable due to the slow etch rate, since it would take many hours or even a few days to etch a deep MEMS structure. While DRIE is compatible with silicon, glass, quartz, and polymer substrates, alkaline anisotropic wet etching is only compatible with $\{100\}$ and $\{110\}$ single-crystal silicon substrates. Unlike alkaline anisotropic wet etching, DRIE etches anisotropic structures independent of crystallographic orientations. Please refer to Sections 6.4.3(C) and 6.4.3(D) for more details about anisotropic wet and dry etching.

Surface Micromachining   In addition to bulk micromachining, surface micromachining is also used for the fabrication of MEMS components. Unlike bulk micromachining (a substrative process), surface micromachining is an additive process. Surface micromachining requires the application of a patterned sacrificial layer on a substrate (e.g., silicon, quartz, glass, or polymer). Next, a patterned structural layer is applied above the sacrificial layer. Finally, the sacrificial layer is etched away which "frees" the structural layer, allowing for the creation of complex MEMS structures such as those with overhangs. The overall process for surface micromachining is as follows (Figure 6-37).

(1)   First, deposit a sacrificial layer on the substrate surface. Sputtering (PVD) can be used to deposit thinner films (≤ 500 nm thick), while much faster CVD (e.g., APCVD, LPCVD, and PECVD) can be used to deposit thicker films (>500 nm thick).

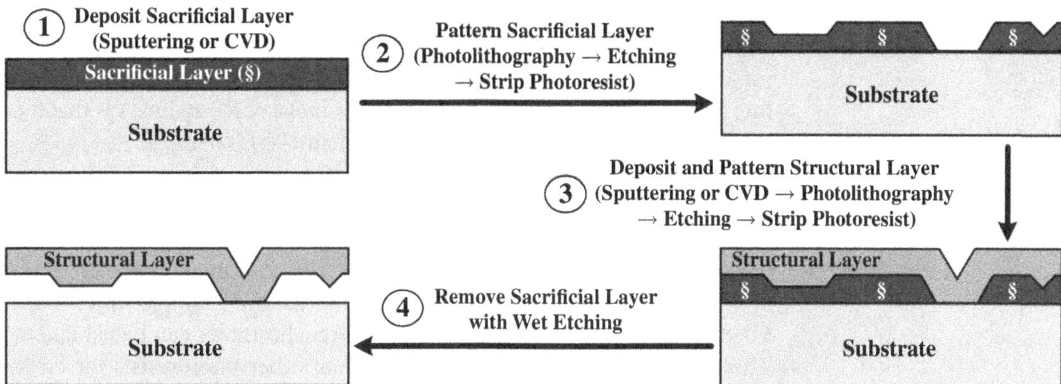

Figure 6-37   Overall process for surface micromachining, which is used to fabricate MEMS components.

(2) Pattern the sacrificial layer by using photolithography followed by etching and photoresist stripping. Any etching process or combination of etching processes can be used to pattern the sacrificial layer. For high resolution (i.e., highly detailed) features to be created with the sacrificial layer, anisotropic etching techniques are preferred.

(3) Deposit a structural layer above the sacrificial layer, and use photolithography followed by etching and photoresist stripping to pattern the structural layer. Depending on its thickness, sputtering or CVD is used to deposit the structural layer. Any single or combination of etching processes can be used for etching the structural layer.

(4) Finally, remove the sacrificial layer using a wet etching technique with an etchant highly selective to the sacrificial layer but not to the substrate or structural layer.

For surface micromachining, the sacrificial layer material must be different from the substrate material, or else the substrate will be etched when removing the sacrificial layer. Furthermore, the substrate material must be resistant against the etchant used to remove the sacrificial layer. Silicon dioxide (SiO_2) deposited by CVD or grown using thermal oxidation is commonly used for the sacrificial layer. However, SiO_2 sacrificial layers are incompatible with quartz and glass substrates as they are mostly comprised of SiO_2. To remove the SiO_2 sacrificial layer, BOE is effective and highly selective to SiO_2 compared to silicon and Si_3N_4. Other suitable sacrificial layer materials include polycrystalline silicon (for non-silicon substrates) and metals (e.g., Al).

The choice of structural layer material for surface micromachining depends on the required physical properties as well as adhesion to the underlying substrate. Polycrystalline silicon deposited by CVD is frequently used for the structural layer due to the excellent mechanical properties of silicon. Other common structural layer materials include Si_3N_4, polymers (e.g., cured photoresists), and metals. For example, metals such as tungsten or titanium may be used in specialized applications as they have increased fracture toughness, higher durability, and better biocompatibility than silicon.

UV LIGA (with SU-8)   LIGA (a German acronym for lithography, electroplating, and molding) is a MEMS fabrication technique capable of creating complex microstructures. There are two variants of LIGA: UV LIGA and X-ray LIGA. X-ray LIGA is an extremely expensive process, because it requires an X-ray lithography step that can only be carried out with a powerful collimated X-ray source such as that from a synchrotron particle accelerator. UV LIGA is performed with standard UV photolithography equipment and is relatively inexpensive to carry out. The primary advantage of X-ray LIGA is that it can produce more detailed and higher aspect ratio features than UV LIGA.[91,97]

Here, we focus exclusively on UV LIGA because it is affordable and can be carried out in standard micro/nano fabrication facilities. UV LIGA relies on the use of SU-8, an epoxy-based negative photoresist which can offer many benefits. SU-8 is transparent and biocompatible. Unlike most other photoresists, we can achieve a dry layer of SU-8 as thick as 2 mm by repeating spin coating and soft baking multiple times. Furthermore, the dry SU-8 surface is very flat and cured SU-8 trenches/holes can have highly vertical sidewalls. This makes SU-8 much more suitable than other photoresists for creating complex and higher aspect ratio microstructures.

Starting with a flat and conductive nickel (Ni) substrate, the overall procedure for UV LIGA (with SU-8) is as follows (Figure 6-38).

(1) First, apply photolithography to create a patterned layer of cured SU-8 on a flat and conductive nickel substrate. If a thick layer of SU-8 is required, spin coating and soft baking of the SU-8 can be repeated many times prior to UV exposure to obtain a thick layer up to ~2 mm. The UV exposure duration needs to be increased if the SU-8 layer is thick.

(2) Use electrochemical deposition (ECD) of nickel to completely fill all of the trenches/holes of the patterned SU-8 starting at the exposed conductive surfaces of the underlying nickel substrate. Please refer to Section 6.4.2(C) for more details about ECD.

(3) Apply chemical-mechanical polishing (CMP) to planarize the nickel/SU-8 surface. For more details about surface planarization, please refer to Section 6.4.4.

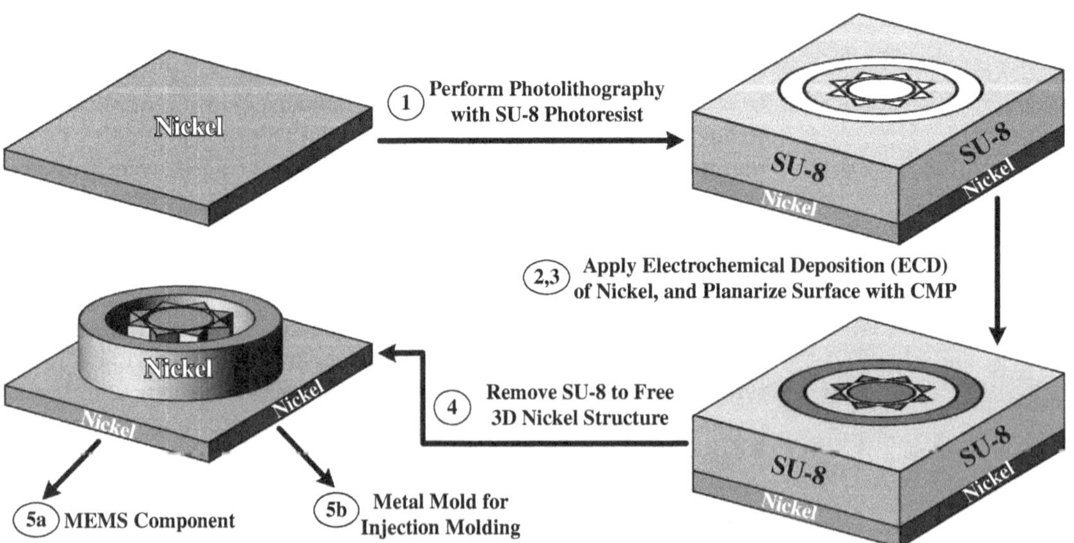

Figure 6-38 Process for UV LIGA (with SU-8 photoresist), which is capable of creating complex 3D MEMS microstructures. The result 3D nickel structure can be used directly as a MEMS component, or as a metal mold for the injection molding of glass, polymer, and ceramic MEMS components.

(4) Remove all of the SU-8 to free the 3D nickel structure. Unlike most photoresists, cured SU-8 contains cross-linked epoxy and thus cannot be removed with organic solvents such as acetone. Although piranha solution can remove cured SU-8, it will also dissolve the nickel. A suitable technique for removing cured SU-8 without damaging nickel is downstream chemical etching (DCE), which is carried out with oxygen plasma plus added $CF_{4(g)}$ in a vacuum chamber at substrate temperatures of ~225°C. During DCE, highly reactive oxygen radicals are blown "downstream" onto the SU-8, which etches away the cured SU-8 at a rate of 7 to 10 μm/min.[98]

(5) Finally, the freed and patterned 3D nickel structure can serve as a metal mold for injection molding, which can be used to create glass, polymer/plastic, and ceramic MEMS components. Alternatively, the patterned 3D nickel structure can be used directly as a MEMS component.

Note: Injection molding involves the injection of heated and molten material into a mold, which then solidifies with the desired shape and is subsequently removed from the mold. With a melting point of 1455°C, nickel molds can be used for the injection molding of a wide variety of non-metallic materials. In general, metal molds cannot be used for the injection molding of other metals due to the formation of metallic alloys which bonds the injected and solidified metal to the mold.

(C) Fabricating a Microfluidic Platform for Selective Single-Cell Capture

Here, the fabrication of a microchip designed to selectively capture single cells is used to illustrate the fabrication of an entire microfluidic platform. An overhead view of the microfluidic microchip is shown in Figure 6-39. The working principles of this microchip is as follows. After the biosample fluid enters the microchip via input wells A and B, DEP powered by IDEs is used to either capture (pDEP = positive DEP) or reject (nDEP = negative DEP) cells. The desired cells are transported into recessed microwells for single-cell capture via pDEP, while unwanted cells are transported into waste wells A and B via nDEP. Any excess fluids carried with the captured cells are transported into the output well. Please refer to Section 3.5.2 for more details about cell capture and separation by DEP.

The microfluidic-platform-based microchip is comprised of three main layers (Figure 6-40): the bottom glass substrate with IDEs and recessed microwells, the middle SU-8 layer with microchannels and wells, and the top PDMS cover with holes for wells and electrodes. The main design choices for this microfluidic platform-based microchip are as follows.

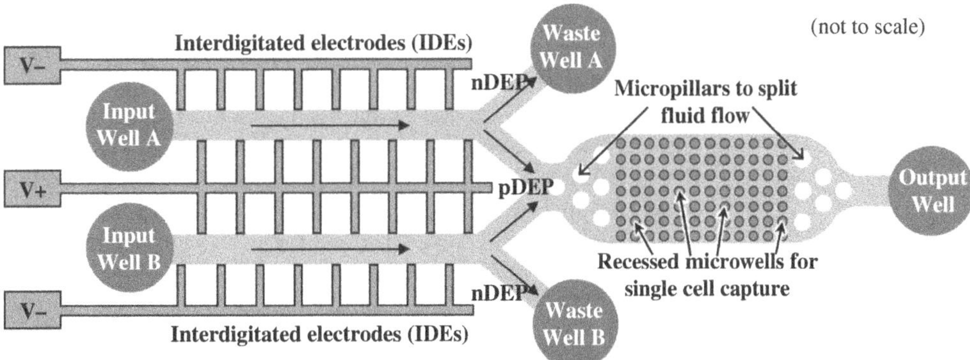

Figure 6-39 A microfluidic platform-based microchip designed to selectively capture single cells using dielectrophoresis (DEP) powered by interdigitated electrodes (IDEs).

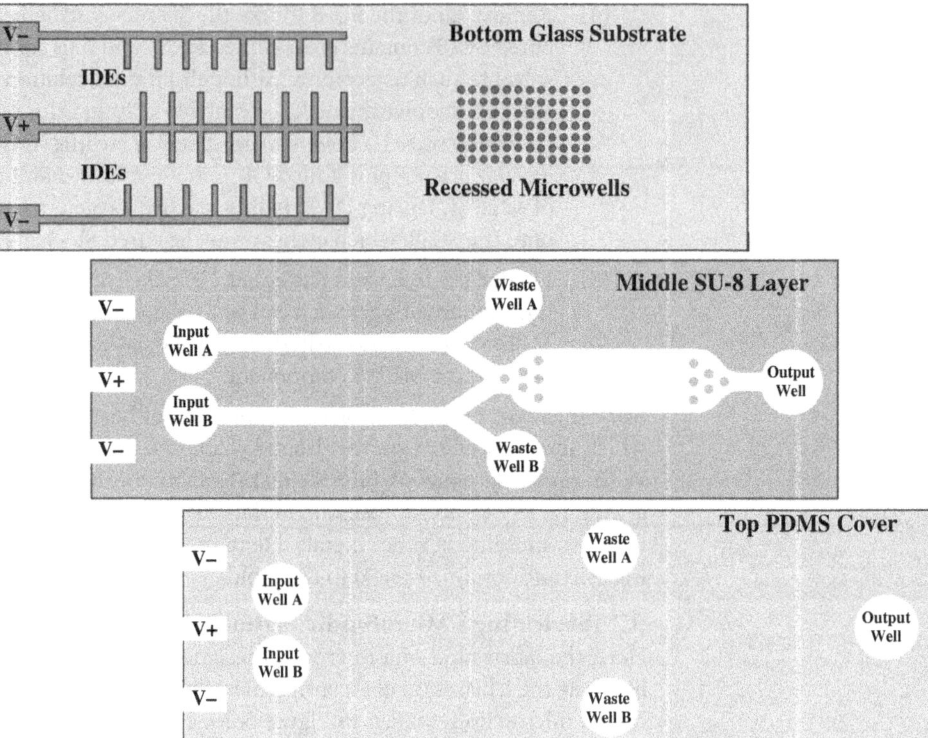

Figure 6-40 The three main layers comprising the microfluidic-platform–based microchip for selective single-cell capture.

Material Choices   The microchip substrate material is glass, which is optically transparent, inexpensive, and biocompatible. The recessed microwells for single-cell capture are etched into the glass substrate. A PDMS cover with holes for the wells and electrodes is used, since PDMS is optically transparent, chemically inert, cheap, and easy to mold into the desired geometry. Optical transparency is important as it allows us to visualize the cell capture process by eye or using an optical microscope, and is crucial if colorimetric or fluorescent dyes are used to stain the cells. The microchannels are created in a ~50 μm thick layer of cured SU-8 photoresist via photolithography. SU-8 is optically transparent, biocompatible, and is capable of producing high-quality and relatively deep microchannels.

Electrode Structures   This microchip utilizes two sets of IDEs, which are connected to three electrodes with AC voltages of V_-, V_+, and V_-. The required amplitude and frequency of the AC voltages depend on the sample biofluid and what cell type we want to capture. The electrodes are composed of gold above an adhesion layer of chromium since gold does not stick well to glass. Gold is unlikely to react with biological samples and cannot be easily oxidized, which ensures none or negligible interfere with cell capture. There are three holes on the left side of the SU-8 layer and the PDMS cover, allowing for the connection of the three electrodes to external equipment (e.g., a function generator) via pogo pins or micro-alligator clips.

Microfluidic Channels   The SU-8 layer contains recessed microfluidic channels, along with cylindrical holes for the five wells and rectangular holes for the three electrodes. Microfluidic tubing can easily be inserted into the SU-8 layer containing the microchannels through the PDMS cover, which also has cylindrical holes for the wells. This design allows the five wells to be connected to external parts. Syringe pumps can be used to pump sample fluids into the microfluidic tubing connected to the two input wells A and B. The pressure provided by the syringe pumps (along with any capillary and DEP forces) helps the sample fluid move through the microchannels and into the output and waste wells.

Single-Cell Capture   The tiny round recessed microwells are designed for single cell capture. The recessed microwells are etched into the glass substrate, and are therefore at greater depths than the microchannels, allowing the desired cells to be individually captured inside each microwell (i.e., one cell per microwell). The cylindrical micropillars are designed to split incoming fluid flow to help prevent cell clusters, instead of single cells, from being captured.

Dimensions   The overall size of the microchip is 20 mm (length) $\times$ 10 mm (width). The input, waste, and output wells have diameters of ~2 mm, which would allow microfluidic tubing to be inserted. The size of the three electrodes is about 3 mm (length) $\times$ 2 mm (width), which enables external electrical connections with pogo pins or micro-alligator clips. The dimensions of the recessed microwells etched into the glass substrate depend on the type of cell we wish to capture. If we want to capture human white blood cells (~15 µm in diameter), we can set the recessed microwells to be about 20 µm (diameter) $\times$ 18 µm (depth).

The overall procedure for fabricating the microfluidic-platform-based microchip for selective capture of single cells is as follows.

(1) Start with a flat and transparent glass substrate that is sufficiently durable (i.e., 0.5 mm or thicker). Clean the glass substrate by immersing it in piranha solution (please refer to Section 6.4.4).

(2) Apply photolithography to obtain a patterned mask layer of cured photoresist on the glass substrate surface with small round openings for the recessed microwells. To ensure that the cured photoresist can be easily removed, epoxy-based photoresists (e.g., SU-8) cannot be used here.

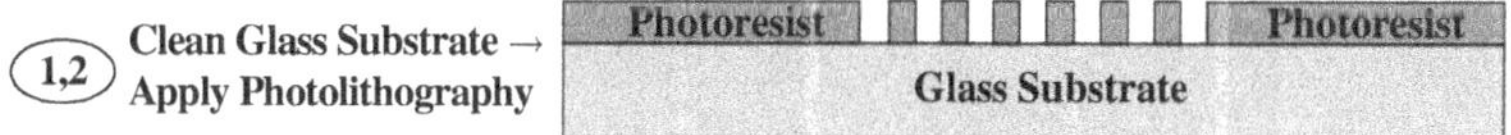

(3) Use ICP-RIE anisotropic dry etching to etch the recessed microwells (which should have uniform dimensions) into the glass through the photoresist etch mask. To avoid undercutting which will alter the shapes of the microwells, isotropic etch processes cannot be used here. Due to the depth of the microwells (e.g., ~18 µm for white blood cells), regular RIE may take a long time. In this step, passivation is not required during ICP-RIE due the low aspect ratio (~1) of each microwell.

(4) Strip the cured photoresist etch mask. Next, immerse the substrate in piranha solution to clean the substrate and activate the glass surface with silanol (Si–O–H) groups to allow chromium to adhere more strongly and with better uniformity in the next step.

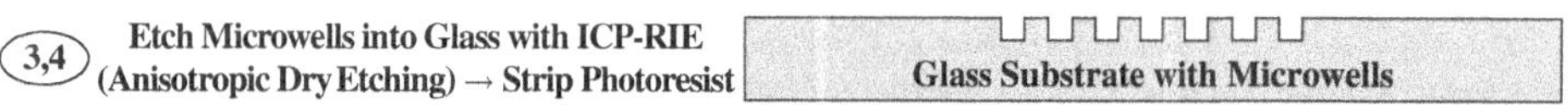

(5) Use sputtering (PVD) to coat the glass substrate surface with a ~10 nm-thick adhesion layer of chromium (Cr), followed by a ~100 nm-thick layer of gold (Au). Sputtering is more suitable than evaporation since it offers better control, repeatability, and coverage.

(6) Apply photolithography to obtain a patterned layer of cured photoresist above the gold layer, which will serve as an etch mask for creating the IDEs and metal interconnects. Because we want to remove the cured photoresist later, epoxy-based photoresists (e.g., SU-8) cannot be used here.

(5,6) Deposit Chrome (Cr) and Gold (Au) with Sputtering (PVD) → Apply Photolithography

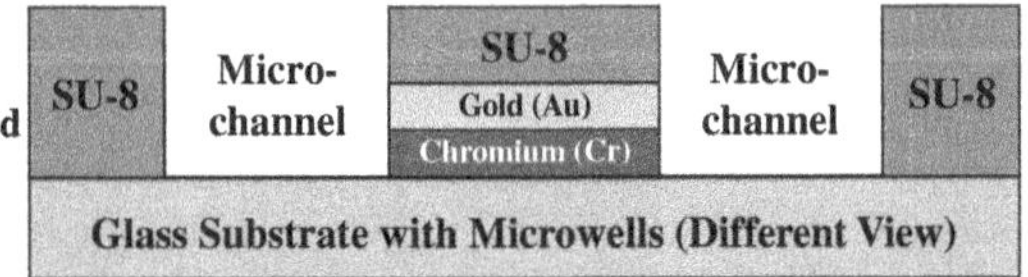

(7) Use RIE or ICP-RIE anisotropic dry etching to etch away the regions of gold and chromium not protected by cured photoresist, forming the IDEs and all metal interconnects. Compared to isotropic wet etching, RIE or ICP-RIE offers far greater anisotropy as well as better control, repeatability, and higher yield. The IDE "fingers" have widths of ~20 μm, and opposing IDE "fingers" are spaced ~20 μm apart, which are large enough to be relatively easy to fabricate.

(8) Remove the cured photoresist etch mask, and then dehydrate the Au/Cr coated glass substrate surface to improve adhesion of SU-8 in the next step.

(7,8) Etch Au and Cr with RIE or ICP-RIE (Anisotropic Dry Etching) → Strip Photoresist and Dehydrate Surface

(9) Apply photolithography to obtain a ~50 μm-thick (or slightly thicker) patterned layer of cured SU-8 photoresist on the glass and gold substrate surfaces with holes for the microchannels, five wells, and three electrodes. Spin coating and soft baking of the SU-8 can be repeated many times prior to UV exposure to obtain a thick layer up to ~2 mm. The UV exposure duration will need to be adjusted accordingly.

(10) Dice the microchip(s) out of the glass substrate with a dicing saw. To reduce costs per chip, multiple microchips can be created simultaneously on a single substrate.

(9,10) Perform Photolithography to Get Patterned SU-8 Photoresist → Dice Microchip(s)

(11) For each microchip, create a PDMS cover (~4 mm thick) with holes for the five wells and three electrodes using a high-resolution 3D printed mold. There is no need to use more advanced techniques to create the PDMS cover because of the relatively large dimensions of the wells and electrodes (i.e., 2 mm or greater). Finally, press the PDMS cover against the SU-8 microchip surface to temporarily seal the microchannels. To allow for the retrieval of cells captured in the microwells, the PDMS cover should not be permanently bonded to the microchip surface.

(11) Create PDMS Cover to Temporarily Seal Microchannels

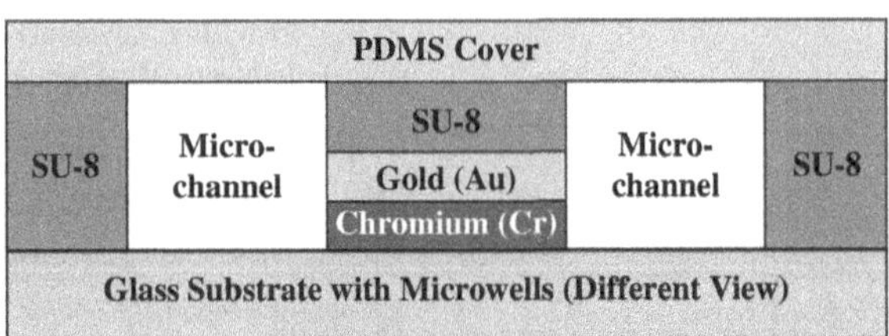

6.5.3 Fabricating CMOS Lab-on-a-Chip Devices

The integrated chips of sophisticated LOC devices often contain many electrical terminals (i.e., tens of terminals or more). With so many terminals on a small chip, it becomes infeasible to connect every terminal to external signal processing equipment. Instead, the terminals can be internally connected to complementary metal-oxide-semiconductor (CMOS) integrated circuits built into the chip. The internal integrated circuits process the signals from the terminals, and produce outputs that can be relayed to external signal processing equipment via a small number of (i.e., far fewer) terminals. For CMOS LOC devices that incorporate microfluidic platforms, fluid-handling microelectrodes can be connected to CMOS integrated circuits on the same microchip to be more easily controlled and powered by external equipment. By handling some of the signal processing and control internally, the use of CMOS LOC microchips can also reduce the required complexity of external control and signal processing circuitry. CMOS integrated circuits are used in particular because they are small enough to easily fit on a microchip, and because the technology for fabricating them is well-established.[2,40]

In Section 6.2.3, we discussed the working principles of CMOS non-faradaic impedimetric LOC sensors (Figure 6-41), which uses a 2D array of sensor microelectrode "pixels" with a network of CMOS transistors (i.e., a CMOS integrated circuit) underneath connecting every pixel. The signals generated by the CMOS integrated circuit are converted into impedance versus frequency data by external equipment, which allows the analyte concentration to be quantified with high spatial resolution. This CMOS LOC sensor can also incorporate an on-chip microfluidic platform to improve the analyte detection signal-to-noise ratio. Moreover, the fluid-handling microelectrodes in the microfluidic platform can be easily controlled and powered by external equipment through the on-chip CMOS integrated circuit. To illustrate the fabrication of CMOS LOC devices, we now cover the fabrication process of this CMOS LOC sensor.

The first step to fabricate the chip of the CMOS LOC device is to create the on-chip CMOS integrated circuit which is comprised of a network of CMOS transistors. Each CMOS transistor consists of an n-type metal-oxide-semiconductor field-effect transistor (MOSFET) and a p-type MOSFET. MOSFETs are four-terminal transistor devices each containing a gate, source, drain, and body. For CMOS LOC devices, the MOSFETs are nanofabricated using 150 to 500 nm CMOS fabrication processes. Therefore, the minimum features size (e.g., gate length) of the MOSFETs is between 150 nm and 500 nm, and there are at least thousands of MOSFET transistors within the CMOS integrated circuit. Due to the very low CMOS transistor densities and relatively large transistor sizes, the network of CMOS transistors is relatively inexpensive to fabricate with standard CMOS microelectronic fabrication processes.

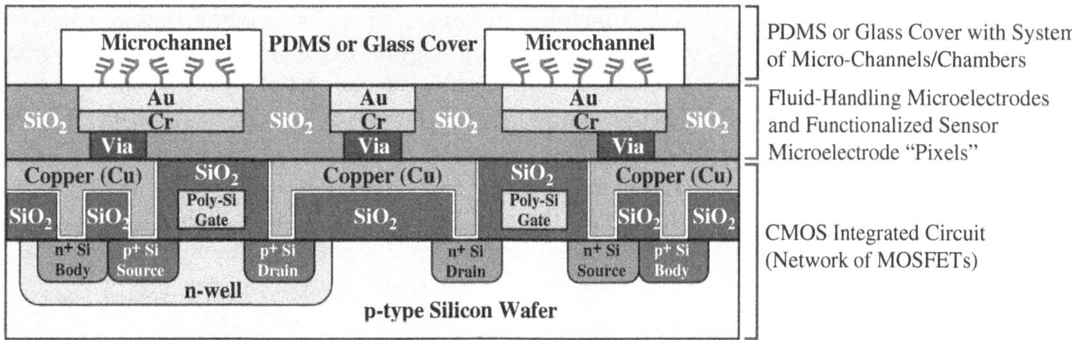

Figure 6-41   A side view of the CMOS non-faradaic impedimetric LOC sensor discussed in Section 6.2.3.

Due to the small dimensions of CMOS transistors, RIE and DRIE (anisotropic dry etching) are the two predominant etching processes used in CMOS integrated circuit fabrication. RIE and DRIE allow many important etching characteristics such as etch profile, selectivity, reproducibility, and uniformity to be controlled. It is challenging to accurately etch small features (<5 μm in width, length, or depth) with isotropic etching processes due to undercutting and controllability issues. The fabrication process for creating the on-chip CMOS integrated circuit is as follows.

(1) Start with a p-type single-crystal silicon wafer substrate. Unlike glass, quartz, and polymer substrates, silicon wafers are compatible with well-established CMOS fabrication processes. The p-type silicon substrate will serve as p-wells for separating the source and drain of every n-type MOSFET. First, apply thermal oxidation (~1000°C) to grow a mask layer of SiO_2 on the silicon substrate surface.

(2) Perform photolithography to create a patterned layer of cured photoresist above the SiO_2 mask layer. Then, etch the SiO_2 mask layer with RIE or DRIE through the cured photoresist.

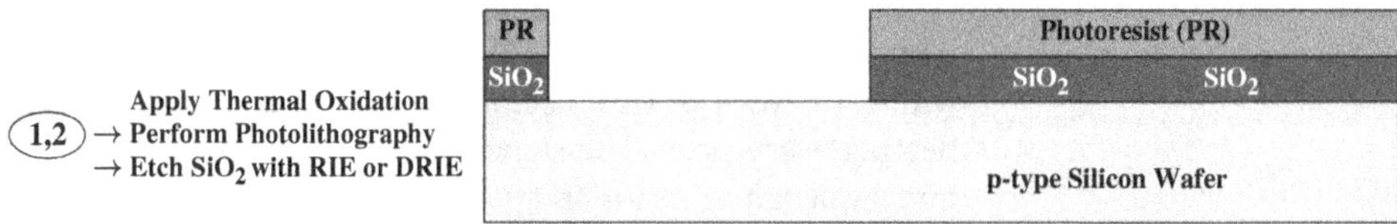

(3) Strip the photoresist layer to prevent its thermal decomposition during diffusion. Then, use diffusion (a high temperature doping technique) of phosphorus (P) dopant to create the n-wells for separating the source and drain of every p-type MOSFET.

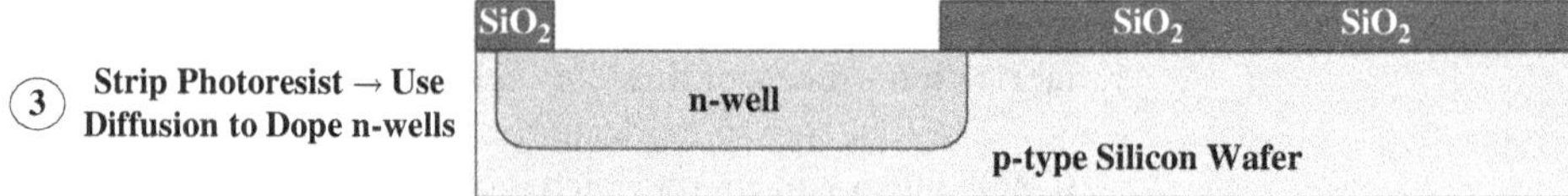

(4) Completely remove the SiO_2 mask layer with a selective dry etching process (e.g., RIE) that will significantly etch SiO_2 but not silicon.

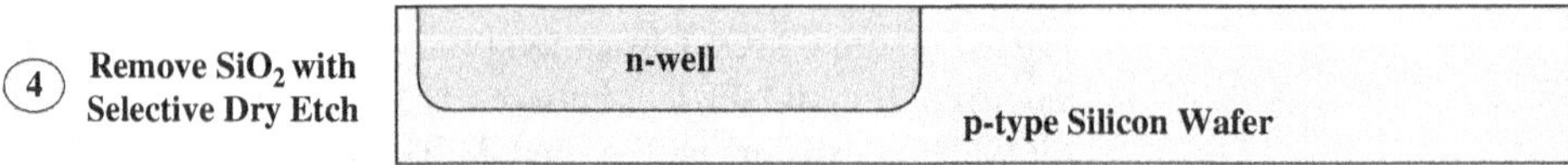

(5) Apply thermal oxidation (~1000°C) again to grow an electrically insulating layer of SiO_2 on the silicon substrate surface for the MOSFET gates. Compared to PVD and CVD, thermal oxidation produces a higher quality layer of SiO_2 and an excellent Si–SiO_2 interface. Pyrogenic wet oxidation is preferred since wet oxidation is much faster than dry oxidation at the same temperatures, and unlike non-pyrogenic wet oxidation does not result in contamination by metal ions such as Na^+.

(6) Use low-pressure CVD (LPCVD) to deposit a high-quality layer of heavily doped polycrystalline silicon (poly-Si, also called polysilicon). It is important for the polysilicon to be a good conductor (i.e., heavily doped) since it will serve as electrical contacts for the MOSFET gates. Due to its higher melting point, polysilicon is used instead of metals such as copper and aluminum.

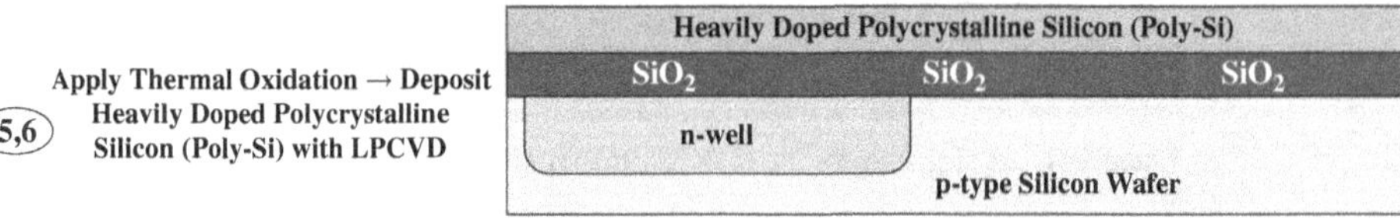

(7) Perform photolithography followed by RIE or DRIE to pattern both the heavily-doped polycrystalline silicon (Poly-Si) and SiO$_2$ layers, creating the MOSFET gates. Next, strip the cured photoresist layer.

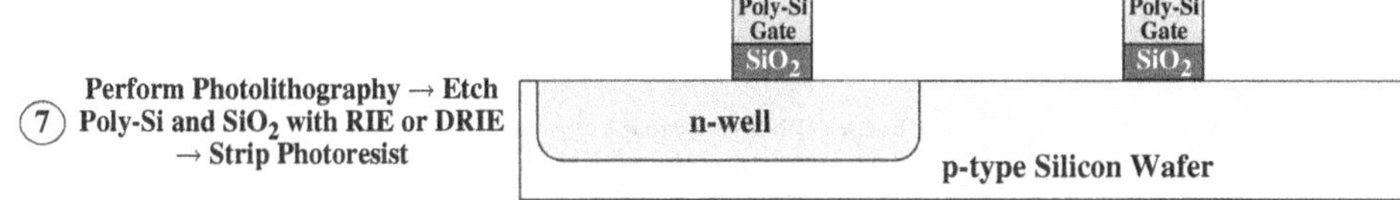

(8) Create a patterned mask layer of SiO$_2$ with plasma-enhanced CVD (PECVD), followed by SiO$_2$ etching with RIE or DRIE, and then photoresist stripping. PECVD is suitable as it involves lower substrate temperatures (200 to 400°C) than other CVD processes. From this point onward, high substrate temperatures can cause the MOSFETs to fail from unwanted diffusion and thermal stresses.

(9) Perform ion implantation of boron (B, p-type) through the SiO$_2$ mask to form the p$^+$ (heavily doped p-type silicon) source, drain, and body wells of every MOSFET. Compared to diffusion, ion implantation occurs at much lower substrate temperatures which reduces unwanted diffusion.

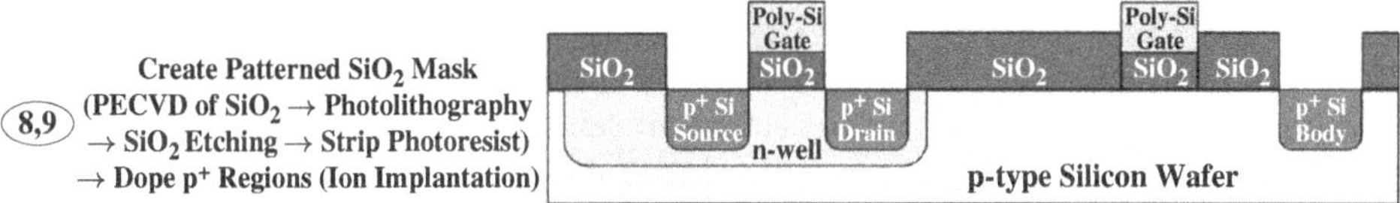

(10) Remove the SiO$_2$ mask layer with a selective dry etching process. Next, create a different patterned mask layer of SiO$_2$ using the same procedure as in step (8). Then, perform ion implantation of phosphorus (P, n-type) with the SiO$_2$ mask to form the n$^+$ (heavily doped n-type silicon) source, drain, and body wells of every MOSFET.

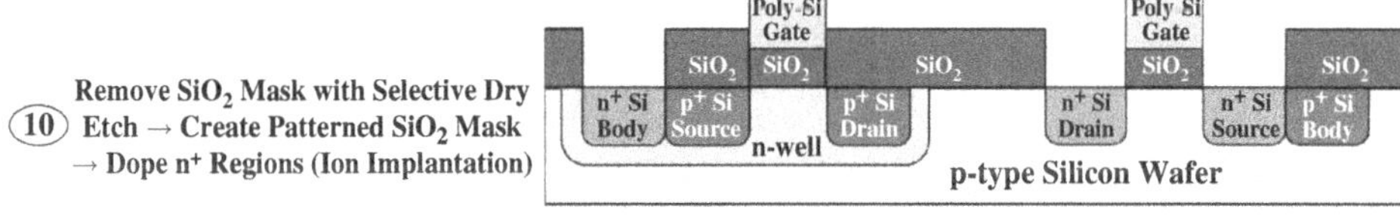

(11) Strip the SiO$_2$ mask layer with a selective dry etching process.

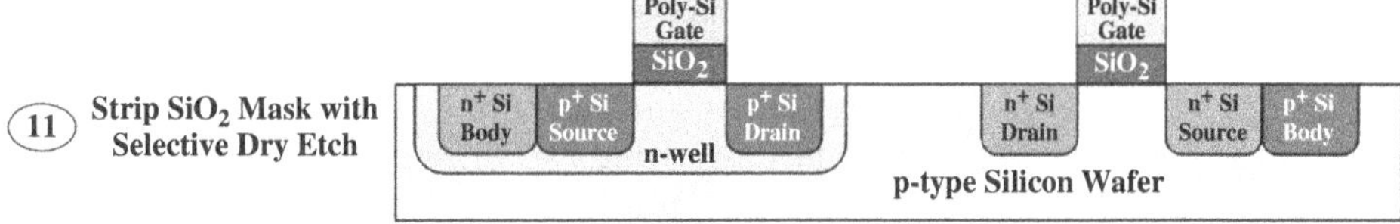

(12) Deposit a blanket layer of SiO$_2$ with plasma-enhanced CVD (PECVD) for electrical insulation and to serve as a diffusion barrier. Again, the low substrate temperatures involved during PECVD help prevent the MOSFETs from failing.

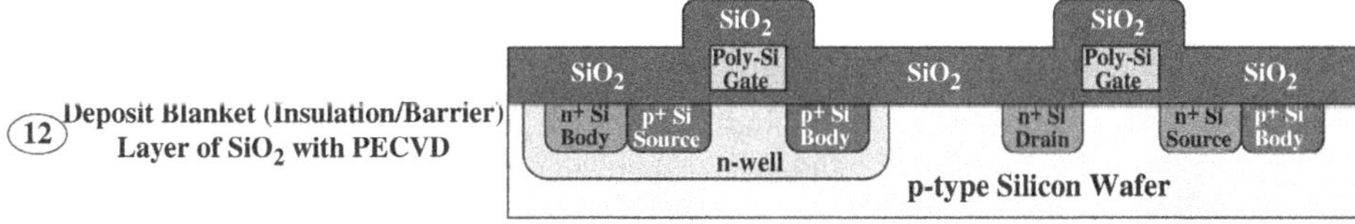

(13) Perform photolithography followed by SiO_2 etching with RIE or DRIE to pattern the SiO_2 blanket layer, creating openings for the electrical interconnects. Then, strip the cured photoresist layer.

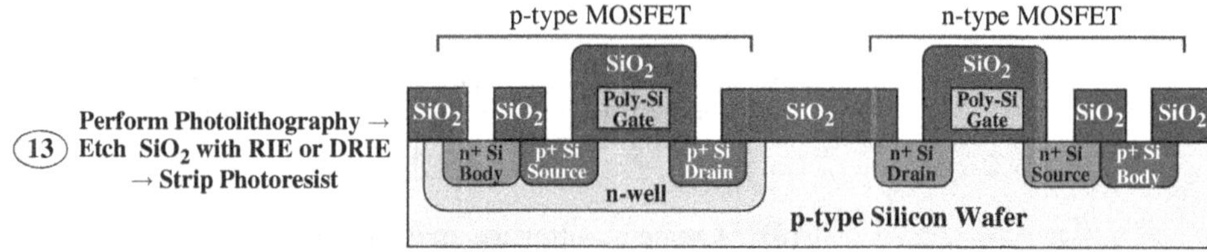

(14) Finally, connect the terminals (i.e., source, drain, gate, and body) of the MOS-FETs to form a CMOS integrated circuit. At present, dual damascene is the most popular microelectronic fabrication process for creating electrical interconnections. The procedure for dual damascene, which simultaneously creates copper (Cu) horizontal interconnects and vias (i.e., vertical interconnects), is as follows.

   (i) First, a diffusion barrier layer (usually Ta, TaN, TiN, or TiW) is deposited on the substrate surface by sputtering. This barrier layer prevents the diffusion of copper into the substrate below as well as any diffusion from the substrate into the copper.[99]

   (ii) Deposit a thin seed layer of copper on the barrier layer with sputtering to make the substrate surface highly conductive. Next, deposit copper with electrochemical deposition (ECD) to completely fill all of the trenches/holes of the patterned integrated circuit to create the vias. Continue the ECD process to create a horizontal surface layer of copper, forming the horizontal interconnects. Please refer to Section 6.4.2(C) for more details about ECD.

   (iii) Apply chemical-mechanical polishing (CMP) to planarize the copper surface. For more details about surface planarization, please refer to Section 6.4.4.

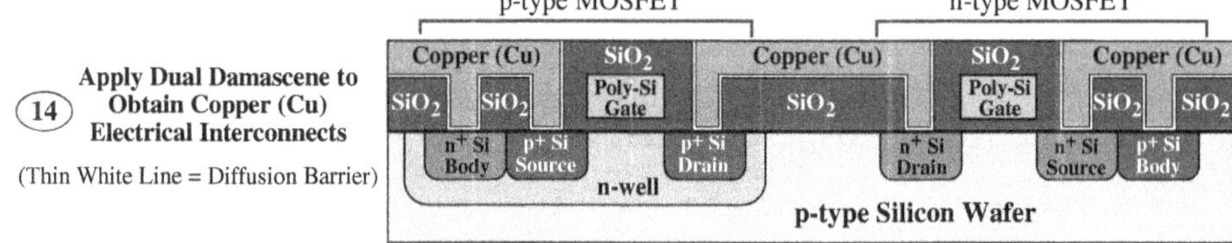

Note: The dual damascene process creates copper interconnects without etching. Copper vias and interconnects are desirable since they can be deposited simultaneously, and have low resistivity and good electromigration resistance. Unlike aluminum, copper will not form brittle or low conductivity intermetallic compounds with gold.

After the underlying CMOS integrated circuit has been fabricated, the next step is to fabricate the rest of the CMOS LOC microchip. The fabrication processes for any included microfluidic platform have already been discussed in Section 6.5.2. However, the fabrication procedure for the 2D array of sensor microelectrode "pixels" as well as any fluid-handling microelectrodes is different due to the network of CMOS transistors underneath. A process sequence for fabricating the 2D array of sensor microelectrode "pixels" together with fluid-handling microelectrodes is as follows.

   (1) Start with a silicon substrate which already contains a CMOS integrated circuit, including the CMOS transistor network and all required interconnects. Perform plasma-enhanced CVD (PECVD) to deposit a layer of SiO_2 (~1 μm) for electrical isolation between the substrate and surface. The low substrate temperatures during PECVD (200 to 400°C) avoids damaging the on-chip CMOS integrated circuit.

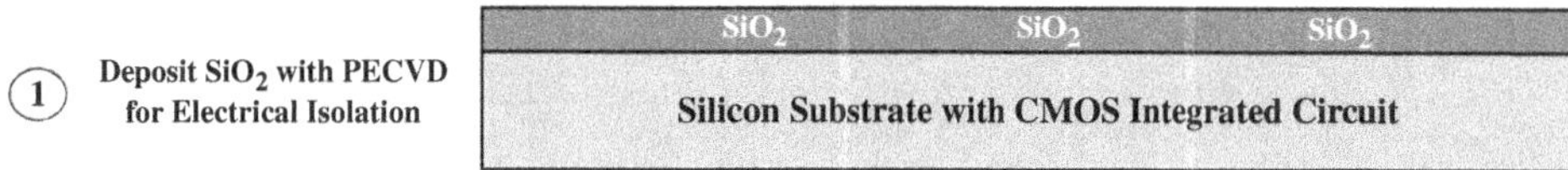

(2) Pattern the SiO_2 layer using photolithography followed by RIE or ICP-RIE anisotropic dry etching for a vertical etch. To prevent damaging the on-chip integrated circuit and avoid undercutting, wet etching processes cannot be used. Next, strip the cured layer of photoresist created during photolithography.

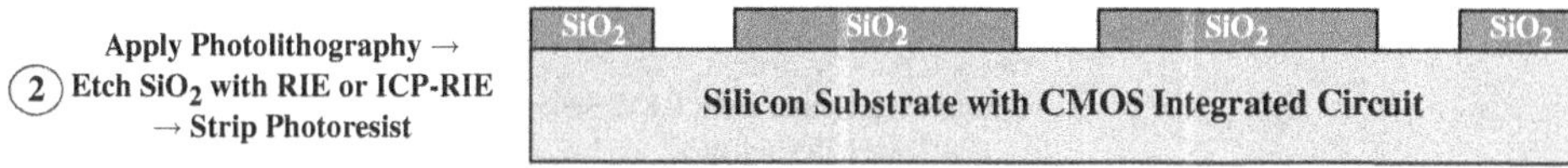

(3) Create the vertical electrical interconnects (i.e., vias) between the underlying CMOS integrated circuit and the microelectrode layer which contains the sensor microelectrode "pixels" and fluid-handling microelectrodes. This can be accomplished in two different ways.

> **(Option 1)** We can deposit a thin diffusion barrier layer (usually Ta, TaN, TiN, or TiW), followed by tungsten (W) for filling the trenches/holes of the patterned surface to create the vias. For depositing the barrier layer and the tungsten vias, we can use either sputtering (PVD) or PECVD since both techniques involve relatively low substrate temperatures. Finally, we planarize the resulting surface with CMP.
>
> **(Option 2)** Alternatively, we can use dual damascene to simultaneously create copper (Cu) vias and any required horizontal interconnects.

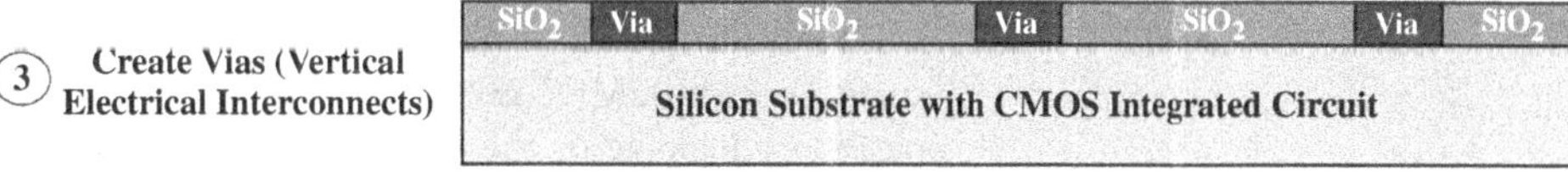

(4) Use sputtering to deposit a ~50 nm adhesion/barrier layer of chromium (Cr), followed by a ~150 nm layer of gold (Au). Gold has excellent biocompatibility, but requires an adhesion layer of chromium underneath to stick to SiO_2. The chromium layer also acts as a diffusion barrier between the gold layer and the layer underneath (i.e., SiO_2 and the via material). Sputtering is used because it offers better control, repeatability, and coverage compared to evaporation (another PVD process).

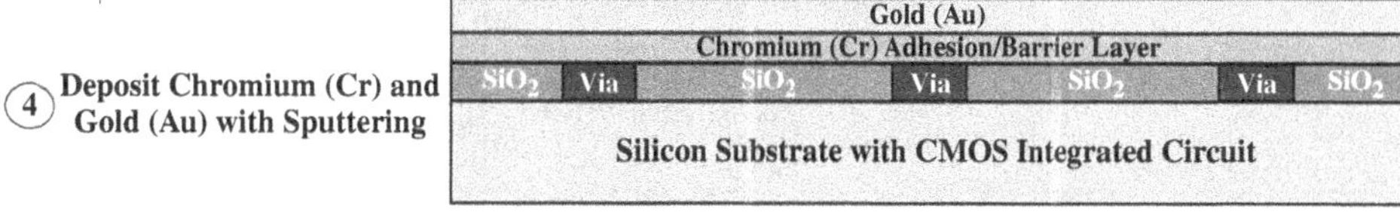

(5) Perform photolithography followed by RIE or ICP-RIE anisotropic dry etching to define the required openings for the 2D array of sensor microelectrode pixels plus the fluid-handling microelectrodes. The gold microelectrode surfaces will be exposed to biological samples. In order to accurately etch the microelectrodes, isotropic etching processes should be avoided.

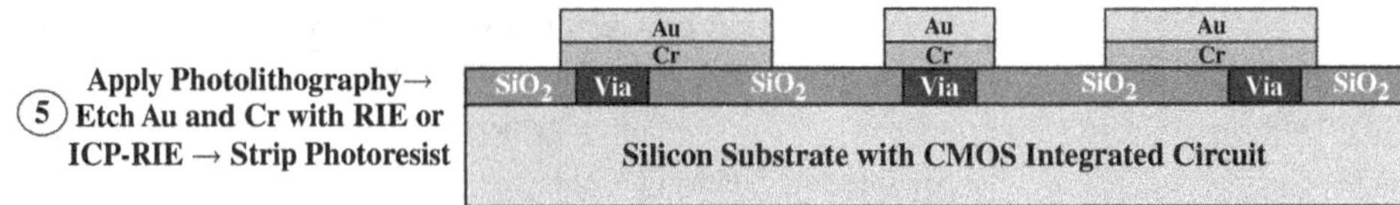

(6) Deposit SiO_2 with PECVD to completely fill the spaces between the Au/Cr microelectrodes, and then planarize the surface with CMP (please refer to Section 6.4.4). If necessary, dice the CMOS LOC microchip(s) out of the silicon substrate with a dicing saw. Recall that we can create multiple microchips simultaneously on a single substrate to reduce costs per chip.

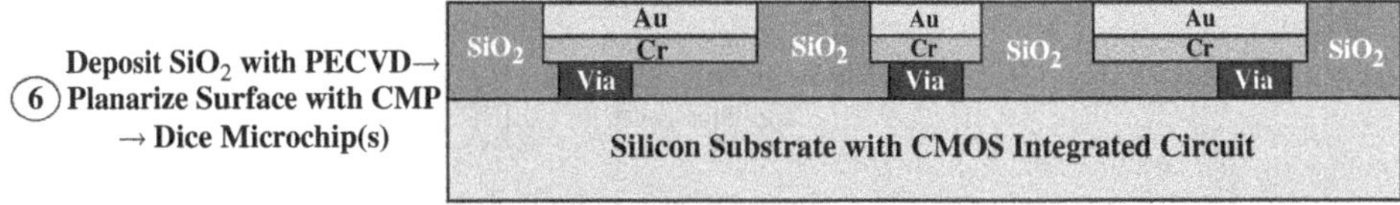

(7) To be capable of analyte detection, the gold (Au) surfaces of the 2D array of sensor microelectrode pixels need to be functionalized by anchoring recognition elements onto them. For the detection of multiple types of analytes, multiple types of recognition elements may need to be anchored.

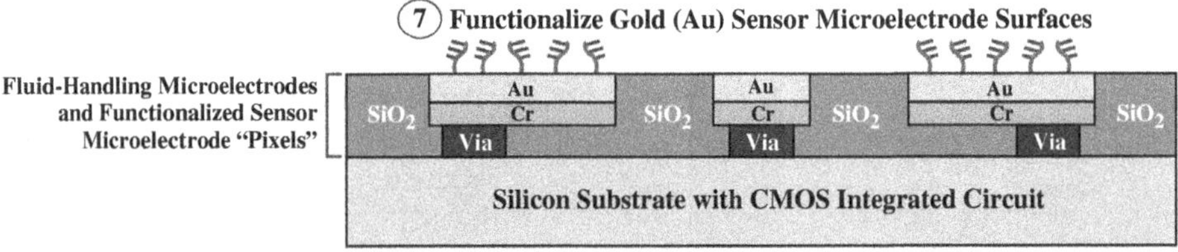

(8) To enable the transport of biosample fluids to and from the sensor microelectrode pixel surfaces, we can bond a cover piece of PDMS or glass that contains a system of microchannels and microchambers onto the gold (Au) and SiO_2 surfaces of the CMOS LOC microchip. The cover piece helps prevent contamination or leakage of the biological samples, while the fluid-handling microelectrodes carry out on-chip fluidic operations with electrokinetic forces. For a permanent bond with a glass or PDMS cover piece, use low temperature plasma-activated fusion bonding as discussed in Section 6.5.2(A). Alternatively, we can press a PDMS cover piece against the microchip surface for a temporary bond.

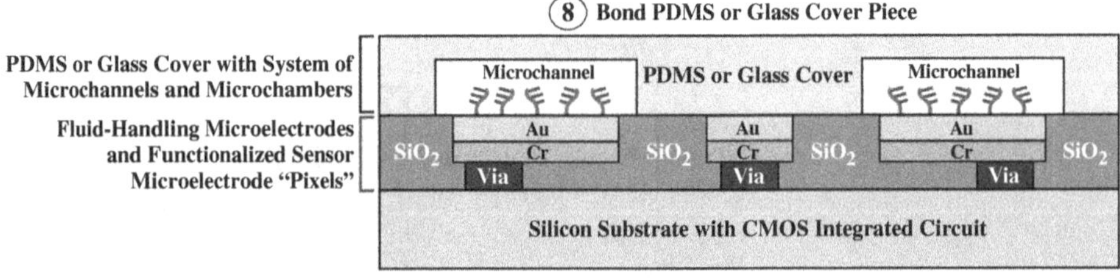

6.6 REFERENCES

[1] E. K. Sackmann, A. L. Fulton, and D. J. Beebe, "The present and future role of microfluidics in biomedical research," *Nature*, vol. 507, no. 7491, pp. 181–189, 2014.

[2] Y. H. Ghallab and W. Badawy, *Lab-on-a-Chip: Techniques, Circuits, and Biomedical Applications*. Norwood, MA, USA: Artech House, 2010.

[3] S. N. Bhatia and D. E. Ingber, "Microfluidic organs-on-chips," *Nature Biotechnology*, vol. 32, no. 8, pp. 760–772, 2014.

[4] F. Zheng, F. Fu, Y. Cheng, C. Wang, Y. Zhao, and Z. Gu, "Organ-on-a-chip systems: microengineering to biomimic living systems," *Small*, vol. 12, no. 17, pp. 2253–2282, 2016.

[5] J. Castillo-León and W. E. Svendsen, Eds., *Lab-on-a-Chip Devices and Micro-Total Analysis Systems: A Practical Guide*, 1st ed. Cham, Switzerland: Springer International Publishing, 2015.

[6] E. Iannone, *Labs on Chip: Principles, Design, and Technology*. Boca Raton, FL, USA: CRC Press, Taylor & Francis Group, 2015.

[7] M. Otten, W. Ott, M. A. Jobst, L. F. Milles, T. Verdorfer, D. A. Pippig, et al., "From genes to protein mechanics on a chip," *Nature Methods*, vol. 11, no. 11, pp. 1127–1130, 2014.

[8] D. Mark, S. Haeberle, G. Roth, F. von Stetten, and R. Zengerle, "Microfluidic lab-on-a-chip platforms: requirements, characteristics and applications," *Chemical Society Reviews*, vol. 39, no. 3, pp. 1153–1182, 2010.

[9] P. S. Dittrich and A. Manz, "Lab-on-a-chip: microfluidics in drug discovery," *Nature Reviews Drug Discovery*, vol. 5, no. 3, pp. 210-218, 2006.

[10] A. Guan, P. Hamilton, Y. Wang, M. Gorbet, Z. Y. Li, and K. S. Phillips, "Medical devices on chips," *Nature Biomedical Engineering*, vol. 1, no. 3, article 0045, 2017.

[11] "Organs-on-Chips Technology," U.S. Food and Drug Administration (FDA) [Online]. Available: https://www.fda.gov/media/104288/download, 2017.

[12] H. Craighead, "Future lab-on-a-chip technologies for interrogating individual molecules," *Nature*, vol. 442, no. 7101, pp. 387–393, 2006.

[13] M. R. Bennett and J. Hasty, "Microfluidic devices for measuring gene network dynamics in single cells," *Nature Reviews Genetics*, vol. 10, no. 9, pp. 628–638, 2009.

[14] "These are the top 10 emerging technologies of 2016," World Economic Forum [Online]. Available: https://www.weforum.org/agenda/2016/06/top-10-emerging-technologies-2016/, 2016.

[15] "Status of the Microfluidics Industry (2019)," Yole Développement [Online]. Available: http://www.yole.fr/iso_upload/News/2019/PR_STATUS_MICROFLUIDIC_INDUSTRY_MarketStatus_YOLE_September2019.pdf, 2019.

[16] L. Malic, D. Brassard, T. Veres, and M. Tabrizian, "Integration and detection of biochemical assays in digital microfluidic LOC devices," *Lab on a Chip*, vol. 10, no. 4, pp. 418–431, 2010.

[17] K. M. Hansen and T. Thundat, "Microcantilever biosensors," *Methods*, vol. 37, no. 1, pp. 57–64, 2005.

[18] C. Yao, T. Zhu, Y. Qi, Y. Zhao, H. Xia, and W. Fu, "Development of a quartz crystal microbalance biosensor with aptamers as bio-recognition element," *Sensors*, vol. 10, no. 6, pp. 5859–5871, 2010.

[19] M. L. Kovarik, D. M. Ornoff, A. T. Melvin, N. C. Dobes, Y. Wang, A. J. Dickinson, et al., "Micro total analysis systems: fundamental advances and applications in the laboratory, clinic, and field," *Analytical Chemistry*, vol. 85, no. 2, pp. 451–472, 2013.

[20] C. T. Culbertson, T. G. Mickleburgh, S. A. Stewart-James, K. A. Sellens, and M. Pressnall, "Micro Total Analysis Systems: fundamental Advances and Biological Applications," *Analytical Chemistry*, vol. 86, no. 1, pp. 95–118, 2014.

[21] G. A. Posthuma-Trumpie, J. Korf, and A. van Amerongen, "Lateral flow (immuno) assay: its strengths, weaknesses, opportunities and threats. A literature survey," *Analytical and Bioanalytical Chemistry*, vol. 393, no. 2, pp. 569–582, 2009.

[22] J. D. Newman and A. P. F. Turner, "Home blood glucose biosensors: a commercial perspective," *Biosensors & Bioelectronics*, vol. 20, no. 12, pp. 2435–2453, 2005.

[23] A. Heller and B. Feldman, "Electrochemical glucose sensors and their applications in diabetes management," *Chemical Reviews*, vol. 108, no. 7, pp. 2482–2505, 2008.

[24] E. H. Yoo and S. Y. Lee, "Glucose biosensors: an overview of use in clinical practice," *Sensors*, vol. 10, no. 5, pp. 4558–4576, 2010.

[25] K. M. Koczula and A. Gallotta, "Lateral flow assays," *Essays in Biochemistry*, vol. 60, no. 1, pp. 111–120, 2016.

[26] C. Gnoth and S. Johnson, "Strips of hope: accuracy of home pregnancy tests and new developments," *Geburtshilfe Und Frauenheilkunde*, vol. 74, no. 7, pp. 661–669, 2014.

[27] J. G. Guan, Y. Q. Miao, and Q. J. Zhang, "Impedimetric biosensors," *Journal of Bioscience and Bioengineering*, vol. 97, no. 4, pp. 219–226, 2004.

[28] R. A. Dorledo de Faria, L. G. Dias Heneine, T. Matencio, and Y. Messaddeq, "Faradaic and non-faradaic electrochemical impedance spectroscopy as transduction techniques for sensing applications," *International Journal of Biosensors & Bioelectronics*, vol. 5, no. 1, pp. 29–31, 2019.

[29] J. S. Park, H. J. Kim, J. H. Lee, J. H. Park, J. Kim, K. S. Hwang, et al., "Amyloid beta detection by Faradaic electrochemical impedance spectroscopy using interdigitated microelectrodes," *Sensors*, vol. 18, no. 2, p. 11, 2018.

[30] E. B. Bahadir and M. K. Sezginturk, "A review on impedimetric biosensors," *Artificial Cells Nanomedicine and Biotechnology*, vol. 44, no. 1, pp. 248–262, 2016.

[31] K.-L. Su, H.-H. Huang, T. C. Chang, H.-P. Lin, Y.-C. Lin, and W.-T. Chen, "An immunoassay using an electro-microchip, nanogold probe and silver enhancement," *Microfluidics and Nanofluidics*, vol. 6, no. 1, pp. 93–98, 2009.

[32] R. Wang, Y. Xu, T. Sors, J. Irudayaraj, W. Ren, and R. Wang, "Impedimetric detection of bacteria by using a microfluidic chip and silver nanoparticle based signal enhancement," *Microchimica Acta*, vol. 185, no. 3, article 184, 2018.

[33] H. Shafiee, M. Jahangir, F. Inci, S. Wang, R. B. M. Willenbrecht, F. F. Giguel, et al., "Acute on-chip HIV detection through label-free electrical sensing of viral nano-lysate," *Small*, vol. 9, no. 15, pp. 2553–2563, 2013.

[34] S. R. Jin, Z. Z. Ye, Y. X. Wang, and Y. B. Ying, "A novel impedimetric microfluidic analysis system for transgenic protein Cry1Ab detection," *Scientific Reports*, vol. 7, article 43175, 2017.

[35] S. MacKay, G. N. Abdelrasoul, M. Tamura, D. H. Lin, Z. M. Yan, and J. Chen, "Using impedance measurements to characterize surface modified with gold nanoparticles," *Sensors*, vol. 17, no. 9, article 2141, 2017.

[36] S. MacKay, P. Hermansen, D. Wishart, and J. Chen, "Simulations of interdigitated electrode interactions with gold nanoparticles for impedance-based biosensing applications," *Sensors*, vol. 15, no. 9, pp. 22192–22208, 2015.

[37] G. N. Abdelrasoul, S. MacKay, S. Y. Salim, K. P. Ismond, M. Tamura, C. Khalifa, et al., "Non-invasive point-of-care device to diagnose acute mesenteric lschemia," *ACS Sensors*, vol. 3, no. 11, pp. 2296–2302, 2018.

[38] G. N. Abdelrasoul, A. Anwar, S. MacKay, M. Tamura, M. A. Shah, D. P. Khasa, et al., "DNA aptamer-based non-Faradaic impedance biosensor for detecting *E. coli*," *Analytica Chimica Acta*, vol. 1107, pp. 135–144, 2020.

[39] S. Buteau and J. R. Dahn, "Analysis of thousands of electrochemical impedance spectra of lithium-ion cells through a machine learning inverse model," *Journal of the Electrochemical Society*, vol. 166, no. 8, pp. A1611–A1622, 2019.

[40] H. Yu, M. Yan, and X. Huang, *CMOS Integrated Lab-on-a-Chip System for Personalized Biomedical Diagnosis*. Hoboken, NJ, USA: John Wiley & Sons, Ltd., 2018.

[41] A. Apilux, Y. Ukita, M. Chikae, O. Chailapakul, and Y. Takamura, "Development of automated paper-based devices for sequential multistep sandwich enzyme-linked immunosorbent assays using inkjet printing," *Lab on a Chip*, vol. 13, no. 1, pp. 126–135, 2013.

[42] A. A. Yazdi, A. Popma, W. Wong, N. Tammy, Y. Pan, and J. Xu, "3D printing: an emerging tool for novel microfluidics and lab-on-a-chip applications," *Microfluidics and Nanofluidics*, vol. 20, no. 3, article 50, 2016.

[43] A. Skardal, T. Shupe, and A. Atala, "Organoid-on-a-chip and body-on-a-chip systems for drug screening and disease modeling," *Drug Discovery Today*, vol. 21, no. 9, pp. 1399–1411, 2016.

[44] E. W. Esch, A. Bahinski, and D. Huh, "Organs-on-chips at the frontiers of drug discovery," *Nature Reviews Drug Discovery*, vol. 14, no. 4, pp. 248–260, 2015.

[45] D. Huh, Y.-s. Torisawa, G. A. Hamilton, H. J. Kim, and D. E. Ingber, "Microengineered physiological biomimicry: organs-on-Chips," *Lab on a Chip*, vol. 12, no. 12, pp. 2156–2164, 2012.

[46] D. Huh, H. J. Kim, J. P. Fraser, D. E. Shea, M. Khan, A. Bahinski, et al., "Microfabrication of human organs-on-chips," *Nature Protocols*, vol. 8, no. 11, pp. 2135–2157, 2013.

[47] D. Huh, G. A. Hamilton, and D. E. Ingber, "From 3D cell culture to organs-on-chips," *Trends in Cell Biology*, vol. 21, no. 12, pp. 745–754, 2011.

[48] B. Zhang, A. Korolj, B. F. L. Lai, and M. Radisic, "Advances in organ-on-a-chip engineering," *Nature Reviews Materials*, vol. 3, no. 8, pp. 257–278, 2018.

[49] G. S. Jeong, J. Y. Chang, J. S. Park, S.-A. Lee, D. Park, J. Woo, et al., "Networked neural spheroid by neuro-bundle mimicking nervous system created by topology effect," *Molecular Brain*, vol. 8, article 17, 2015.

[50] J. J. F. Sleeboom, H. E. Amirabadi, P. Nair, C. M. Sahlgren, and J. M. J. den Toonder, "Metastasis in context: modeling the tumor microenvironment with cancer-on-a-chip approaches," *Disease Models & Mechanisms*, vol. 11, no. 3, article 033100, 2018.

[51] H.-F. Tsai, A. Trubelja, A. Q. Shen, and G. Bao, "Tumour-on-a-chip: microfluidic models of tumour morphology, growth and microenvironment," *Journal of the Royal Society Interface*, vol. 14, no. 131, article 20170137, 2017.

[52] V. S. Shirure, Y. Bi, M. B. Curtis, A. Lezia, M. M. Goedegebuure, S. P. Goedegebuure, et al., "Tumor-on-a-chip platform to investigate progression and drug sensitivity in cell lines and patient-derived organoids," *Lab on a Chip*, vol. 18, no. 23, pp. 3687–3702, 2018.

[53]   I. Maschmeyer, A. K. Lorenz, K. Schimek, T. Hasenberg, A. P. Ramme, J. Huebner, et al., "A four-organ-chip for interconnected long-term co-culture of human intestine, liver, skin and kidney equivalents," *Lab on a Chip*, vol. 15, no. 12, pp. 2688–2699, 2015.

[54]   C. Oleaga, C. Bernabini, A. S. T. Smith, B. Srinivasan, M. Jackson, W. McLamb, et al., "Multi-Organ toxicity demonstration in a functional human in vitro system composed of four organs," *Scientific Reports*, vol. 6, article 20030, 2016.

[55]   J. U. Lind, T. A. Busbee, A. D. Valentine, F. S. Pasqualini, H. Yuan, M. Yadid, et al., "Instrumented cardiac microphysiological devices via multimaterial three-dimensional printing," *Nature Materials*, vol. 16, no. 3, pp. 303–308, 2017.

[56]   B. Zhang, M. Montgomery, M. D. Chamberlain, S. Ogawa, A. Korolj, A. Pahnke, et al., "Biodegradable scaffold with built-in vasculature for organ-on-a-chip engineering and direct surgical anastomosis," *Nature Materials*, vol. 15, no. 6, pp. 669–678, 2016.

[57]   K. A. Homan, D. B. Kolesky, M. A. Skylar-Scott, J. Herrmann, H. Obuobi, A. Moisan, et al., "Bioprinting of 3D Convoluted Renal Proximal Tubules on Perfusable Chips," *Scientific Reports*, vol. 6, article 34845, 2016.

[58]   G. Ligresti, R. J. Nagao, J. Xue, Y. J. Choi, J. Xu, S. Ren, et al., "A novel three-dimensional human peritubular microvascular system," *Journal of the American Society of Nephrology*, vol. 27, no. 8, pp. 2370–2381, 2016.

[59]   X. Wang, D. T. T. Phan, A. Sobrino, S. C. George, C. C. W. Hughes, and A. P. Lee, "Engineering anastomosis between living capillary networks and endothelial cell-lined microfluidic channels," *Lab on a Chip*, vol. 16, no. 2, pp. 282–290, 2016.

[60]   J. H. Yeon, H. R. Ryu, M. Chung, Q. P. Hu, and N. L. Jeon, "In vitro formation and characterization of a perfusable three-dimensional tubular capillary network in microfluidic devices," *Lab on a Chip*, vol. 12, no. 16, pp. 2815–2822, 2012.

[61]   V. Allwardt, A. J. Ainscough, P. Viswanathan, S. D. Sherrod, J. A. McLean, M. Haddrick, et al., "Translational Roadmap for the organs-on-a-chip industry toward broad adoption," *Bioengineering*, vol. 7, no. 3, article 112, 2020.

[62]   L. P. Hariri, "Next-generation microscopy optical imaging for in vivo and ex vivo microscopy in pathology," *Archives of Pathology & Laboratory Medicine*, vol. 143, no. 3, p. 287, 2019.

[63]   R. Roy, "Next-generation optical microscopy," *Current Science*, vol. 105, no. 11, pp. 1524–1536, 2013.

[64]   A. Baptista, F. Silva, J. Porteiro, J. Miguez, and G. Pinto, "Sputtering physical vapour deposition (PVD) coatings: a critical review on process improvement and market trend demands," *Coatings*, vol. 8, no. 11, article 402, 2018.

[65]   M. J. Madou, *Fundamentals of Microfabrication and Nanotechnology Volume II: Manufacturing Techniques for Microfabrication and Nanotechnology*, 3rd ed. Boca Raton, FL, USA: CRC Press, 2012.

[66]   W. Lerch, G. Roters, P. Munzinger, R. Mader, and R. Ostermeir, "Wet rapid thermal oxidation of silicon with a pyrogenic system," *Materials Science and Engineering B: Advanced Functional Solid-State Materials*, vol. 54, no. 3, pp. 153–160, 1998.

[67]   H. Robbins and B. Schwartz, "Chemical Etching of Silicon: II. The System HF, HNO_3, H_2O, and $HC_2H_3O_2$," *Journal of the Electrochemical Society*, vol. 107, no. 2, pp. 108–111, 1960.

[68]   W. Vangelder and V. E. Hauser, "The Etching of silicon nitride in phosphoric acid with silicon dioxide as a mask," *Journal of the Electrochemical Society*, vol. 114, no. 8, pp. 869–872, 1967.

[69]   H. Seidel, L. Csepregi, A. Heuberger, and H. Baumgartel, "Anisotropic etching of crystalline silicon in alkaline solutions: I. Orientation dependence and behavior of passivation layers," *Journal of the Electrochemical Society*, vol. 137, no. 11, pp. 3612–3626, 1990.

[70]   M. Elwenspoek, "On the mechanism of anisotropic etching of silicon," *Journal of the Electrochemical Society*, vol. 140, no. 7, pp. 2075–2080, 1993.

[71]   G. T. A. Kovacs, N. I. Maluf, and K. E. Petersen, "Bulk micromachining of silicon," *Proceedings of the IEEE*, vol. 86, no. 8, pp. 1536–1551, 1998.

[72]   K. R. Williams and R. S. Muller, "Etch rates for micromachining processing," *Journal of Microelectromechanical Systems*, vol. 5, no. 4, pp. 256–269, 1996.

[73]   O. Tabata, R. Asahi, H. Funabashi, K. Shimaoka, and S. Sugiyama, "Anisotropic etching of silicon in TMAH solutions," *Sensors and Actuators A: Physical*, vol. 34, no. 1, pp. 51–57, 1992.

[74]   M. Shikida, K. Sato, K. Tokoro, and D. Uchikawa, "Differences in anisotropic etching properties of KOH and TMAH solutions," *Sensors and Actuators A: Physical*, vol. 80, no. 2, pp. 179–188, 2000.

[75]   S. Dutta, M. Imran, P. Kumar, R. Pal, P. Datta, and R. Chatterjee, "Comparison of etch characteristics of KOH, TMAH and EDP for bulk micromachining of silicon (110)," *Microsystem Technologies*, vol. 17, no. 10-11, pp. 1621–1628, 2011.

[76]   S. Franssila and L. Sainiemi, "Reactive ion etching (RIE)," in *Encyclopedia of Microfluidics and Nanofluidics*, D. Li, Ed., 2nd ed. New York, NY, USA: Springer, 2015, pp. 2911–2921.

[77]   J. D. Brazzle, M. R. Dokmeci, and C. H. Mastrangelo, "Modeling and characterization of sacrificial polysilicon etching using vapor-phase xenon difluoride," in *17th IEEE International Conference on Micro Electro Mechanical Systems*, 2004, pp. 737–740.

[78]   I. Brodie and J. J. Muray, *The Physics of Microfabrication*, 1st ed. New York, USA: Plenum Press, 1982.

[79]   K. S. Chen, A. A. Ayon, X. Zhang, and S. M. Spearing, "Effect of process parameters on the surface morphology and mechanical performance of silicon structures after deep reactive ion etching (DRIE)," *Journal of Microelectromechanical Systems*, vol. 11, no. 3, pp. 264–275, 2002.

[80]   F. Laermer, S. Franssila, L. Sainiemi, and K. Kolari, "Chapter 21: Deep reactive ion etching," in *Handbook of Silicon Based MEMS Materials and Technologies*, M. Tilli, T. Motooka, V.-M. Airaksinen, S. Franssila, M. Paulasto-Kröckel, and V. Lindroos, Eds., 2nd ed. London, UK: Elsevier Inc., 2015, pp. 444–469.

[81]   G. M. Beheim, "Chapter 21: Deep reactive ion etching for bulk micromachining of silicon carbide," in *The MEMS Handbook*, M. Gad-el-Hak, Ed., 1st ed. Boca Raton, FL, USA: CRC Press, 2002.

[82]   M. J. Walker, "Comparison of Bosch and cryogenic processes for patterning high aspect ratio features in silicon," in *Conference on MEMS Design, Fabrication, Characterization, and Packaging (Proceedings of SPIE)*, 2001, pp. 89–99.

[83]   X. Mellhaoui, R. Dussart, T. Tillocher, P. Lefaucheux, P. Ranson, M. Boufnichel, et al., "SiOxFy passivation layer in silicon cryoetching," *Journal of Applied Physics*, vol. 98, no. 10, article 104901, 2005.

[84]   H. Jansen, M. de Boer, H. Wensink, B. Kloeck, and M. Elwenspoek, "The black silicon method. VIII. A study of the performance of etching silicon using SF6/O2-based chemistry with cryogenical wafer cooling and a high density ICP source," *Microelectronics Journal*, vol. 32, no. 9, pp. 769–777, 2001.

[85]   S. K. Mitra and A. A. Saha, "Surface modification, methods," in *Encyclopedia of Microfluidics and Nanofluidics*, D. Li, Ed., 2nd ed. New York, NY, USA: Springer, 2015, pp. 3115–3123.

[86]   I. Brodie and J. J. Muray, *The Physics of Micro/Nano-Fabrication*, Revised ed. New York, NY, USA: Springer, 1992.

[87]   N. Bhattacharjee, A. Urrios, S. Kanga, and A. Folch, "The upcoming 3D-printing revolution in microfluidics," *Lab on a Chip*, vol. 16, no. 10, pp. 1720–1742, 2016.

[88]   S. A. MacKay, "Design of an impedance-based, gold nanoparticle enhanced biosensor system," Ph.D. dissertation, Department of Electrical and Computer Engineering, University of Alberta, Edmonton, AB, Canada, 2017.

[89]   G. N. Abdelrasoul, S. MacKay, S. Y. Salim, K. P. Ismond, M. Tamura, C. Khalifa, et al., "Supporting Information: Non-invasive Point-of-Care Device To Diagnose Acute Mesenteric Ischemia," *ACS Sensors*, vol. 3, no. 11, pp. 2296–2302, 2018.

[90]   T. Mayer, A. N. Marianov, and D. W. Inglis, "Comparing fusion bonding methods for glass substrates," *Materials Research Express*, vol. 5, no. 8, article 085201, 2018.

[91]   E. H. Conradie and D. F. Moore, "SU-8 thick photoresist processing as a functional material for MEMS applications," *Journal of Micromechanics and Microengineering*, vol. 12, no. 4, pp. 368–374, 2002.

[92]   D. Qin, Y. Xia, and G. M. Whitesides, "Soft lithography for micro- and nanoscale patterning," *Nature Protocols*, vol. 5, no. 3, pp. 491–502, 2010.

[93]   S. Bhattacharya, A. Datta, J. M. Berg, and S. Gangopadhyay, "Studies on surface wettability of poly(dimethyl) siloxane (PDMS) and glass under oxygen-plasma treatment and correlation with bond strength," *Journal of Microelectromechanical Systems*, vol. 14, no. 3, pp. 590–597, 2005.

[94]   A. Wheeler. "Shrinking the Lab - Darius Rackus - University of Toronto," Wheeler Microfluidics Laboratory (University of Toronto) [Online]. Available: https://microfluidics.utoronto.ca/ or https://www.youtube.com/watch?v=NAVrYQqpwMQ, 2016.

[95]   E. Samiei, M. Tabrizian, and M. Hoorfar, "A review of digital microfluidics as portable platforms for lab-on a-chip applications," *Lab on a Chip*, vol. 16, no. 13, pp. 2376–2396, 2016.

[96]   V. R. Mamilla and K. S. Chakradhar, "Micro machining for micro electro mechanical systems (MEMS)," *Procedia Materials Science*, vol. 6, pp. 1170–1177, 2014.

[97]   V. Saile, U. Wallrabe, O. Tabata, and J. G. Korvink, Eds., *Advanced Micro & Nanosystems Volume 7: LIGA and Its Applications*, 1st ed. Weinheim, Germany: WILEY-VCH Verlag GmbH & Co. KGaA, 2009.

[98]   P. M. Dentinger, W. M. Clift, and S. H. Goods, "Removal of SU-8 photoresist for thick film applications," *Microelectronic Engineering*, vol. 61-2, pp. 993–1000, 2002.

[99]   T. Hara and K. Sakata, "Stress in copper seed layer employing in the copper interconnection," *Electrochemical and Solid State Letters*, vol. 4, no. 10, pp. G77–G79, 2001.

CHAPTER 7

Applications of Bionanotechnology

Bionanotechnology can be used for diagnosing medical problems as well as monitoring and treating diseases such as cancer, diabetes, and bacterial infections. In the previous chapters, we discussed microfluidic and lab-on-a-chip (LOC) devices which can be used for inexpensive and portable biosensing, capturing and sorting cells, screening drug candidates and testing medical devices *in vitro*, and studying diseases. We have also discussed the importance of enhancing cell and tissue imaging with quantum dot probes for monitoring diseases. In this chapter, we will present examples of other important applications of bionanotechnology including microreactors for carrying out polymerase chain reaction (PCR), continuous glucose monitoring (CGM) for diabetes, targeted and potentially personalized therapies for treating cancer and antibiotic-resistant bacterial infections, targeted drug delivery for treating cancer and obesity, neural implants for alleviating hearing loss and neuropsychiatric disorders, and nanomaterial-based fertilizers and pesticides for use in agriculture. The main applications of bionanotechnology that are discussed in this book are shown in Figure 7-1.

7.1 EQUIVALENT CIRCUIT MODELS FOR MECHANICAL, FLUIDIC, AND THERMAL SYSTEMS

7.1.1 Equivalent Parameters

An integral part of applying bionanotechnology is the design of microsystems such as microreactors, microfluidic systems, lab-on-a-chip devices, and other micro-electro-mechanical systems (MEMS). When designing microsystems, it is usually necessary to model the desired microsystems to ensure that they will function as intended. Microsystem modeling can be accomplished with equivalent circuits, where we transform mechanical, fluidic, and thermal parameters into their equivalent counterparts in electrical circuits, as shown in Table 7-1. By doing so, we can model the properties and components of a mechanical, fluidic, or thermal system as an equivalent circuit—a combination of voltage and current sources plus resistive, capacitive, and inductive elements. Such an equivalent circuit representation enables the use of standard electrical circuit solving techniques to analyze a mechanical, fluidic, or thermal system.[1-3]

Table 7-2 lists the equations governing equivalent parameters for electrical circuits, mechanical translations, incompressible fluid flows, and thermal systems. While Equations (7.1) to (7.3) apply to all four types of systems (i.e., electrical circuits, mechanical translations, incompressible fluid flows, and thermal systems), Equations (7.4) to (7.9)

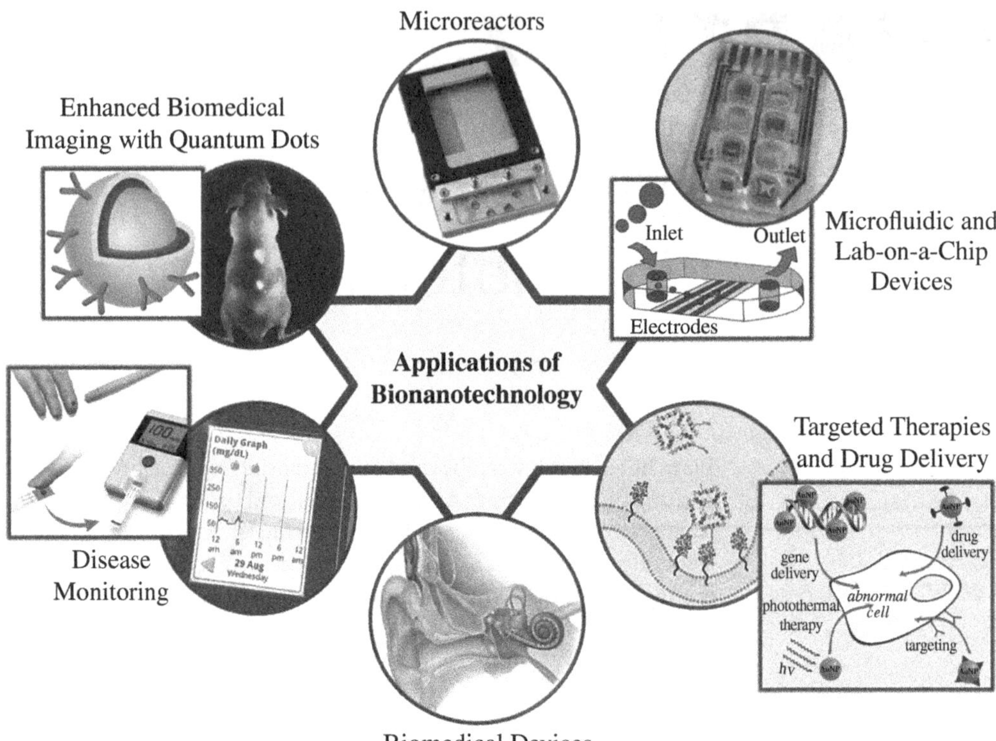

Figure 7-1 The main applications of bionanotechnology discussed in this book include microfluidic and lab-on-a-chip devices (Chapters 2, 3, and 6), enhanced biomedical imaging with quantum dots (Chapter 4), microreactors (Chapter 7), disease monitoring (Chapter 7), targeted therapies and drug delivery (Chapter 7), and nanomaterial-based biomedical devices (Chapter 7).

TABLE 7-1 Modeling Mechanical, Fluidic, and Thermal Parameters as Electrical Circuit Parameters[1-3]

Parameter [unit]	Electrical Circuit	Mechanical Translation*	Incompressible Fluid Flow	Thermal System
Potential	Voltage V or ΔV [V]	Velocity v [m/s]	Pressure P or ΔP [Pa]	Temperature T or ΔT [K]
Flow	Current I [A]	Force F [N]	Volumetric Flow Rate Q_f [m³/s]	Heat Flow Rate q_t [W]
Accumulated Flow	Charge q_e [C]	Momentum p or Impulse Δp [N·s]	Fluid Volume V_f or ΔV_f [m³]	Thermal Energy Q_t [J]
Generalized Resistance	Resistance R_e [Ω]	Inverse Damping Coefficient b^{-1} [s/kg]	Fluid Resistance in Vessel R_f [kg/(s·m⁴)]	Thermal Resistance R_t [K/W]
Generalized Capacitance	Capacitance C_e [F]	Mass m [kg]	Fluid Vessel Compliance C_f [s²·m⁴/kg]	Heat Capacity C_t [J/K]
Generalized Inductance	Inductance L_e [H]	Inverse Spring Constant k^{-1} [s²/kg]	Fluid Vessel Inertance L_f [kg/m⁴]	N/A†

*Some sources prefer to use force F as the potential parameter and velocity v as the flow parameter. However, such a representation makes it more cumbersome to generate equivalent circuit models.[3]

†Although thermal inductance can theoretically exist, it is uncommon and hence usually excluded from thermal equivalent circuit models.[4]

TABLE 7-2   Equations Governing Equivalent Circuit Parameters[1,2]

$$\text{Flow} = \frac{d(\text{Accumulated Flow})}{dt} \quad (7.1) \qquad\qquad \text{Resistance} = \frac{\text{Potential}}{\text{Flow}} \quad (7.2)$$

$$\text{Flow} = \text{Capacitance} \cdot \frac{d(\text{Potential})}{dt} \quad\Leftrightarrow\quad \text{Capacitance} = \frac{d(\text{Accumulated Flow})}{d(\text{Potential})} \quad (7.3)$$

$$\text{Potential} = \text{Inductance} \cdot \frac{d(\text{Flow})}{dt} \quad\Leftrightarrow\quad \text{Inductance} = \text{Potential} \cdot \left[\frac{d(\text{Flow})}{dt}\right]^{-1} \quad (7.4)$$

$$\text{Power} = \frac{d(\text{Work})}{dt} = \text{Potential} \cdot \text{Flow} \quad\Rightarrow\quad \begin{cases} \text{Electric Power} = \Delta V \cdot I \\ \text{Mechanical Power} = \boldsymbol{F} \cdot \boldsymbol{v} \quad (7.5) \\ \text{Fluid Power} = \Delta P \cdot Q_f \end{cases}$$

$$\text{If the potential is constant over time: Work} = \text{Potential} \cdot (\text{Accumulated Flow}) \quad (7.6)$$

$$\text{Power} = \text{Resistance} \cdot (\text{Flow})^2 = \frac{(\text{Potential})^2}{\text{Resistance}} \quad (7.7)$$

$$\text{Energy} = \frac{1}{2}\text{Capacitance} \cdot (\text{Potential})^2 \quad (7.8) \qquad\qquad \text{Energy} = \frac{1}{2}\text{Inductance} \cdot (\text{Flow})^2 \quad (7.9)$$

do *not* apply to thermal systems, but do apply to electrical circuits, mechanical translations, and incompressible fluid flows. Equations (7.7) to (7.9) assume that the generalized resistance, capacitance and inductance are constant over time. Using Equations (7.1) to (7.6), we can obtain the formulas in Table 7-3.[1,2]

TABLE 7-3   Formulas Governing Electrical, Mechanical, Fluidic, and Thermal Systems*

System Domain	Electrical Circuit	Mechanical Translation	Incompressible Fluid Flow	Thermal System
Equation (7.1)	$I = \dfrac{dq_e}{dt}$	$\boldsymbol{F} = \dfrac{d\boldsymbol{p}}{dt} = \dfrac{d(m\boldsymbol{v})}{dt} = m\boldsymbol{a}$	$Q_f = \dfrac{dV_f}{dt}$	$q_t = \dfrac{dQ_t}{dt}$
Equation (7.2)	$R_e = \dfrac{\Delta V}{I}$	$b^{-1} = \dfrac{|\boldsymbol{v}|}{|\boldsymbol{F}|} \Leftrightarrow |\boldsymbol{F}| = b|\boldsymbol{v}|$	$R_f = \dfrac{\Delta P}{Q_f}$	$R_t = \dfrac{\Delta T}{q_t}$
Equation (7.3)	$I = C_e \dfrac{dV}{dt}$	$\boldsymbol{F} = m\dfrac{d\boldsymbol{v}}{dt} = m\boldsymbol{a}$	$Q_f = C_f \dfrac{dP}{dt}$	$q_t = C_t \dfrac{dT}{dt}$
Equation (7.4)	$\Delta V = L_e \dfrac{dI}{dt}$	$\boldsymbol{v} = k^{-1}\dfrac{d\boldsymbol{F}}{dt} \Leftrightarrow \boldsymbol{F} = k\boldsymbol{x}$	$\Delta P = L_f \dfrac{dQ_f}{dt}$	N/A
Equation (7.5)	$\dfrac{dW}{dt} = \Delta V \cdot I$	$\dfrac{dW}{dt} = \boldsymbol{F} \cdot \boldsymbol{v}$	$\dfrac{dW}{dt} = \Delta P \cdot Q_f$	N/A
Equation (7.6)	$W = \Delta V \cdot q_e$	$W = \boldsymbol{v} \cdot \Delta \boldsymbol{p}$	$W = P \cdot \Delta V_f$	N/A

*For Equation (7.6), it is assumed that the potential (ΔV, $\boldsymbol{v}$, or P) is constant over time. W represents work done, dW/dt represents instantaneous power, and $\boldsymbol{a}$ represents acceleration.

For mechanical translations, it is assumed that the force F, velocity v, and position x are vectors all parallel to each other. In classical mechanics, Equations (7.1) and (7.3) are equivalent to Newton's second law. Moreover, Equation (7.2) represents the linear damping force $|F|$, which is proportional to the speed $|v|$. We can show that Equation (7.4) is Hooke's law as follows:

$$v = \frac{dx}{dt} = k^{-1}\frac{dF}{dt} \quad \Rightarrow \quad dF = k\, dx \quad \Rightarrow \quad F = kx$$

Applying Equation (7.9) to mechanical translations, we have

$$\text{Energy} = \frac{1}{2}k^{-1}\left|F\right|^2 = \frac{1}{2}k^{-1}\left|kx\right|^2 = \frac{1}{2}k\left|x\right|^2$$

Therefore, Equation (7.8) represents kinetic energy and Equation (7.9) represents elastic potential energy for mechanical translations. That is,

$$(\text{Kinetic})\ \text{Energy} = \frac{1}{2}m\left|v\right|^2 \qquad (\text{Elastic Potential})\ \text{Energy} = \frac{1}{2}k\left|x\right|^2 \qquad (7.10)$$

For thermal systems, we can use Equation (7.3, right) to obtain

$$\text{heat capacity} = C_t = \frac{dQ_t}{dT} = \text{mass} \times \text{specific heat capacity} \qquad (7.11)$$

If the temperature gradient ΔT across the thermal "capacitor" (i.e., a component that can store thermal energy) is constant, the energy stored by the thermal "capacitor" is given by

$$C_t = \frac{\Delta Q_t}{\Delta T} \quad \Leftrightarrow \quad \text{Energy Stored} = \Delta Q_t = C_t \cdot \Delta T \qquad (7.12)$$

EXAMPLE 7-1

(a) Show that the two definitions of generalized capacitance in Equation (7.3) are equivalent and that the two definitions of generalized inductance in Equation (7.4) are equivalent.

(b) Derive Equations (7.6) to (7.9) using Equations (7.1) to (7.5).

(c) Prove that Equation (7.5) applies to electrical circuits, mechanical translations and incompressible fluid flows using the following line integral, where F represents force. That is, use Equation (7.13) to prove the equations for electric power, mechanical power, and fluid power in Equation (7.5).

$$\text{Work} = \int_{\text{Line}} F \cdot dx \qquad (7.13)$$

Solution

(a) We can derive Equation (7.3, right) using Equations (7.1) and (7.3, left) as follows:

$$\text{Flow} = \frac{d(\text{Accumulated Flow})}{dt} = \text{Capacitance} \cdot \frac{d(\text{Potential})}{dt}$$

$$d(\text{Accumulated Flow}) = \text{Capacitance} \cdot d(\text{Potential}) \quad \Rightarrow \quad \text{Capacitance} = \frac{d(\text{Accumulated Flow})}{d(\text{Potential})}$$

Starting with Equation (7.4, left), we can easily derive Equation (7.4, right):

$$\text{Potential} = \text{Inductance} \cdot \frac{d(\text{Flow})}{dt} \quad \Rightarrow \quad \text{Inductance} = \text{Potential} \cdot \left[\frac{d(\text{Flow})}{dt}\right]^{-1}$$

(b) We can derive Equation (7.6) using Equations (7.1) and (7.5):

$$\text{Power} = \text{Potential} \cdot \text{Flow} \quad \Rightarrow \quad \text{Power } dt = \text{Potential} \cdot \text{Flow } dt$$

$$\text{Work} = \int \text{Power } dt = \int \text{Potential} \cdot \text{Flow } dt = \text{Potential} \cdot \int \text{Flow } dt$$

where we assumed that the potential is constant over time. In addition, we have

$$\int \text{Flow } dt = \int \frac{d(\text{Accumulated Flow})}{dt} \, dt = \int d(\text{Accumulated Flow}) = \text{Accumulated Flow}$$

Finally, we obtain Equation (7.6):

$$\text{Work} = \text{Potential} \cdot \int \text{Flow } dt = \text{Potential} \cdot (\text{Accumulated Flow})$$

With Equations (7.2) and (7.5), we can derive Equation (7.7) as follows:

$$\text{Resistance} = \frac{\text{Potential}}{\text{Flow}} \quad \Rightarrow \quad \text{Potential} = \text{Resistance} \cdot \text{Flow} \quad \Rightarrow \quad \text{Flow} = \frac{\text{Potential}}{\text{Resistance}}$$

$$\text{Power} = \text{Potential} \cdot \text{Flow} = (\text{Resistance} \cdot \text{Flow}) \cdot \text{Flow} = \text{Resistance} \cdot (\text{Flow})^2$$

$$\text{Power} = \text{Potential} \cdot \text{Flow} = \text{Potential} \cdot \left(\frac{\text{Potential}}{\text{Resistance}}\right) = \frac{(\text{Potential})^2}{\text{Resistance}}$$

To derive Equation (7.8), we use Equations (7.3, left) and (7.5) as follows:

$$\text{Power} = \text{Potential} \cdot \text{Flow} = \text{Potential} \cdot \left[\text{Capacitance} \cdot \frac{d(\text{Potential})}{dt}\right]$$

Using $d(\text{Potential}^2) = 2 \cdot \text{Potential} \cdot d(\text{Potential})$, we have

$$\text{Power } dt = \text{Capacitance} \cdot \text{Potential} \cdot d(\text{Potential}) = \text{Capacitance} \cdot \frac{1}{2} d(\text{Potential}^2)$$

Integrating both sides and assuming that the capacitance is constant, we obtain

$$\int \text{Power } dt = \frac{1}{2} \int \text{Capacitance} \cdot d(\text{Potential}^2) = \frac{1}{2} \text{Capacitance} \cdot \int d(\text{Potential}^2)$$

$$\text{Energy} = \frac{1}{2} \text{Capacitance} \cdot (\text{Potential})^2$$

Assuming that the inductance is constant, Equation (7.9) can be derived in a similar fashion using Equations (7.4, left) and (7.5) as follows:

$$\text{Power} = \text{Potential} \cdot \text{Flow} = \left[\text{Inductance} \cdot \frac{d(\text{Flow})}{dt}\right] \cdot \text{Flow}$$

$$\text{Power } dt = \text{Inductance} \cdot \text{Flow} \cdot d(\text{Flow}) = \text{Inductance} \cdot \frac{1}{2} d(\text{Flow}^2)$$

$$\int \text{Power } dt = \frac{1}{2}\text{Inductance} \cdot \int d(\text{Flow}^2) \quad \Rightarrow \quad \text{Energy} = \frac{1}{2}\text{Inductance} \cdot (\text{Flow})^2$$

(c) For electrical circuits, we will use the following definitions for the 1D electric field E and electric force F_{electric}. In addition, we note that $d\boldsymbol{x} = \hat{\boldsymbol{x}}\, dx$. Using Equation (7.13), we have

$$E = -\boldsymbol{\nabla} V = -\frac{dV}{dx}\,\hat{\boldsymbol{x}} \qquad F_{\text{electric}} = q_e E = -q_e \frac{dV}{dx}\,\hat{\boldsymbol{x}}$$

$$\text{Work} = \int_{\text{Line}} F_{\text{electric}} \cdot d\boldsymbol{x} = \int -q_e \frac{dV}{dx}\,\hat{\boldsymbol{x}} \cdot \hat{\boldsymbol{x}}\, dx = q_e \int (-dV)\,\hat{\boldsymbol{x}} \cdot \hat{\boldsymbol{x}}\,\frac{dx}{dx} = q_e \int (-dV) = q_e \cdot \Delta V$$

Assuming that the electric potential difference $\Delta V = \int(-dV)$ is constant over time t, we have

$$\text{Electric Power} = \frac{d(\text{Work})}{dt} = \frac{d}{dt}\big(q_e \cdot \Delta V\big) = \Delta V \cdot \frac{dq_e}{dt} = \Delta V \cdot I$$

For mechanical translations, we use Equation (7.13) as well as $\boldsymbol{v} = d\boldsymbol{x}/dt$ to obtain

$$\text{Work} = \int_{\text{Line}} F \cdot d\boldsymbol{x} = \int F \cdot \boldsymbol{v}\, dt = \int \text{Power} \cdot dt \quad \Rightarrow \quad \text{Mechanical Power} = F \cdot \boldsymbol{v}$$

For incompressible fluid flow, we use Equation (7.13) and the fact that the force F and position $\boldsymbol{x}$ vectors are parallel to obtain

$$\text{Power} = \frac{d(\text{Work})}{dt} = \frac{d}{dt}\int_{\text{Line}} F \cdot d\boldsymbol{x} = \frac{d}{dt}\int F \cdot dx = \frac{d}{dt}\int \frac{F}{\text{Area}} \cdot (\text{Area} \cdot dx)$$

where Area represents the cross-sectional area perpendicular to the position vector $\boldsymbol{x}$. Using the equations $d(\text{Volume}) = \text{Area} \cdot dx$ and $Q_f = dV_f/dt$, we get

$$\text{Power} = \frac{d}{dt}\int \text{Pressure} \cdot d(\text{Volume}) = \frac{d}{dt}\int P \cdot dV_f = \int dP \cdot \frac{dV_f}{dt} = \int dP \cdot Q_f = Q_f \int dP = Q_f \cdot \Delta P$$

$$\Rightarrow \quad \text{Fluid Power} = \Delta P \cdot Q_f \quad \blacktriangle$$

7.1.2 Equivalent Circuit Components

In terms of equivalent circuit components, voltage sources generate potential while current sources generate flow. Generalized resistance, capacitance, and inductance each have an associated impedance and are represented respectively as resistors, capacitors, and inductors. Table 7-4 lists equivalent circuit components and their associated parameters for electrical, mechanical, fluidic, and thermal systems.

In general, impedance in the s-domain (i.e., Laplace domain) $Z(s)$ is defined as follows:

$$\text{Impedance} = Z(s) = \frac{\text{Potential}(s)}{\text{Flow}(s)} \qquad \text{where} \begin{cases} s = \sigma + j\omega \\ \omega = 2\pi f \end{cases} \tag{7.14}$$

$$\text{Potential}(s) = \mathcal{L}\{\text{Potential}(t)\} \quad \text{and} \quad \text{Flow}(s) = \mathcal{L}\{\text{Flow}(t)\} \tag{7.15}$$

TABLE 7-4   Circuit Representation of Mechanical, Fluidic, and Thermal Properties and Components

Circuit Element (Parameter)	Electrical Circuit	Mechanical Translation	Incompressible Fluid Flow	Thermal System
Voltage Source (Potential)	ΔV [V]	v [m/s]	ΔP [Pa]	ΔT [K]
Current Source (Flow)	I [A]	F [N]	Q_f [m³/s]	q_t [W]
Resistor (Resistive Impedance)	R_e [Ω]	b^{-1} [s/kg]	R_f [kg/(s · m⁴)]	R_t [K/W]
Capacitor (Capacitive Impedance)*	$\dfrac{1}{s \cdot C_e}$ [Ω]	$\dfrac{1}{s \cdot m}$ [s/kg]	$\dfrac{1}{s \cdot C_f}$ [kg/(s·m⁴)]	$\dfrac{1}{s \cdot C_t}$ [K/W]
Inductor (Inductive Impedance)*	$s \cdot L_e$ [Ω]	$s \cdot k^{-1}$ [s/kg]	$s \cdot L_f$ [kg/(s · m⁴)]	N/A

*Here, we assume that there is no energy initially stored in the capacitor or inductor.

where s [rad/s] is the complex frequency, σ [rad/s] is a measure of attenuation, $\omega = 2\pi f$ [rad/s] is the (real) angular frequency, f [Hz] is the (real) frequency, $\mathcal{L}$ is the Laplace transform, and $j = \sqrt{-1}$ is the imaginary unit (for a review of complex numbers, please refer to Appendix F). In the time (t) domain, Potential(t) and Flow(t) are given by

$$\text{Potential}(t) = P_0 \exp(\sigma t)\cos(\omega t + \theta) = \text{Re}\left\{P_0 e^{j\theta} e^{st}\right\} \tag{7.16}$$

$$\text{Flow}(t) = F_0 \exp(\sigma t)\cos(\omega t + \phi) = \text{Re}\left\{F_0 e^{j\phi} e^{st}\right\} \tag{7.17}$$

By modeling mechanical, fluidic, and thermal systems as equivalent circuits, we can apply standard electrical circuit analysis techniques to analyze other systems. These circuit analysis techniques include—but are not limited to—Kirchhoff's current law, Kirchhoff's voltage law, and equivalent impedances resulting from series and parallel impedance elements. Kirchhoff's voltage law arises from the conservation of energy and states that the algebraic sum of the voltages around any closed path (i.e., any closed loop) is zero. Kirchhoff's current law is an expression of the conservation of charge and states that the algebraic sum of the currents entering any node (i.e., any junction) is zero; that is, the total current entering a junction is equal to the total current leaving that same junction. By generalizing voltage as potential and current as flow, we can generalize Kirchhoff's laws as follows:[1]

$$\overset{\text{Closed Path}}{\sum_{n}} \left(\text{Potential}\right)_n = 0 \qquad (7.18) \qquad \overset{\text{Into Node}}{\sum_{n}} \left(\text{Flow}\right)_n = 0 \qquad (7.19)$$

Similar to electrical circuit elements, the equivalent impedance of series and parallel generalized impedance elements can be expressed as follows:

$$\left(Z_{\text{equivalent}}\right)_{\text{series}} = \sum_{n=1}^{N} Z_n = Z_1 + Z_2 + Z_3 + \cdots + Z_N \tag{7.20}$$

$$\left(Z_{\text{equivalent}}\right)_{\text{parallel}}^{-1} = \sum_{n=1}^{N} Z_n^{-1} = Z_1^{-1} + Z_2^{-1} + Z_3^{-1} + \cdots + Z_N^{-1} \tag{7.21}$$

If there are only two parallel generalized impedance elements Z_1 and Z_2, it can be shown that

$$Z_{\text{equivalent}} = Z_1 \parallel Z_2 = \frac{Z_1 Z_2}{Z_1 + Z_2} \tag{7.22}$$

EXAMPLE 7-2

(a) Show that if $Y(t) = Y_0 \exp(\sigma t)\cos(\omega t + \varphi)$, then $Y(t) = \mathrm{Re}\{Y_0 e^{j\varphi} e^{st}\}$. This will prove Equations (7.16) and (7.17).

(b) Show that $Z(s) = R$ for a generalized resistor R with constant resistance, $Z(s) = 1/(s \cdot C)$ for a generalized capacitor with constant capacitance C, and that $Z(s) = s \cdot L$ for a generalized inductor with constant inductance L. Assume that there is no energy initially stored in the capacitor or inductor.

Hint: Use $\mathcal{L}\{df/dt\} = sF(s) - f(t = 0)$, which can be found in standard Laplace transform tables.

Solution

(a) Using Euler's formula $\exp(j\Phi) = \cos\Phi + j\sin\Phi$, we have $\cos\Phi = \mathrm{Re}\{\exp(j\Phi)\}$ and hence

$$\cos(\omega t + \varphi) = \mathrm{Re}\left\{\exp\left[j(\omega t + \varphi)\right]\right\}$$

$$Y(t) = Y_0 \exp(\sigma t)\cos(\omega t + \varphi) = Y_0 \exp(\sigma t) \cdot \mathrm{Re}\left\{\exp\left[j(\omega t + \varphi)\right]\right\}$$

Since $Y_0 \exp(\sigma t)$ is a purely real quantity, we have

$$Y(t) = \mathrm{Re}\left\{Y_0 \exp(\sigma t)\exp\left[j(\omega t + \varphi)\right]\right\} = \mathrm{Re}\left\{Y_0 \exp\left[\sigma t + j(\omega t + \varphi)\right]\right\}$$

$$Y(t) = \mathrm{Re}\left\{Y_0 \exp\left[(\sigma + j\omega)t + j\varphi\right]\right\} = \mathrm{Re}\left\{Y_0 \exp(st)\exp(j\varphi)\right\} \quad \Rightarrow \quad Y(t) = \mathrm{Re}\left\{Y_0 e^{j\varphi} e^{st}\right\}$$

We can prove Equation (7.16) by letting $Y(t) = \mathrm{Potential}(t)$, $Y_0 = P_0$, and $\varphi = \theta$. Similarly, we can prove Equation (7.17) by letting $Y(t) = \mathrm{Flow}(t)$, $Y_0 = F_0$, and $\varphi = \phi$.

(b) Using the definition of generalized resistance R in Equation (7.2), and assuming that the resistance R is constant, we obtain

$$R = \mathrm{Potential}(t)/\mathrm{Flow}(t) \quad \Rightarrow \quad \mathcal{L}\{\mathrm{Potential}(t)\} = \mathcal{L}\{R \cdot \mathrm{Flow}(t)\} = R \cdot \mathcal{L}\{\mathrm{Flow}(t)\}$$

$$\mathrm{Potential}(s) = R \cdot \mathrm{Flow}(s) \quad \Rightarrow \quad Z_{\mathrm{resistor}}(s) = \mathrm{Potential}(s)/\mathrm{Flow}(s) = R$$

Starting with the definition of generalized capacitance C in Equation (7.3, left), and assuming that the capacitance C is constant, we have

$$\mathrm{Flow}(t) = C \cdot \frac{d\left[\mathrm{Potential}(t)\right]}{dt} \quad \Rightarrow \quad \mathcal{L}\{\mathrm{Flow}(t)\} = \mathcal{L}\left\{C \cdot \frac{d\left[\mathrm{Potential}(t)\right]}{dt}\right\} = C \cdot \mathcal{L}\left\{\frac{d\left[\mathrm{Potential}(t)\right]}{dt}\right\}$$

$$\mathrm{Flow}(s) = C \cdot [s \cdot \mathrm{Potential}(s) - \mathrm{Potential}(t = 0)]$$

Since there is no energy initially stored in the capacitor, the potential across the capacitor at time $t = 0$ is zero: $\mathrm{Potential}(t = 0) = 0$. Thus,

$$\mathrm{Flow}(s) = C \cdot s \cdot \mathrm{Potential}(s) \quad \Rightarrow \quad Z_{\mathrm{capacitor}}(s) = \frac{\mathrm{Potential}(s)}{\mathrm{Flow}(s)} = \frac{1}{s \cdot C}$$

For the generalized inductance L, we start with the definition in Equation (7.4, left) and assume the inductance L is constant. Therefore,

$$\mathrm{Potential}(t) = L \cdot \frac{d\left[\mathrm{Flow}(t)\right]}{dt} \quad \Rightarrow \quad \mathcal{L}\{\mathrm{Potential}(t)\} = L \cdot \mathcal{L}\left\{\frac{d\left[\mathrm{Flow}(t)\right]}{dt}\right\}$$

$$\mathrm{Potential}(s) = L \cdot [s \cdot \mathrm{Flow}(s) - \mathrm{Flow}(t = 0)]$$

Since there is no energy initially stored in the inductor, the flow through the inductor at time $t = 0$ is zero: Flow$(t = 0) = 0$. Thus,

$$\text{Potential}(s) = L \cdot s \cdot \text{Flow}(s) \quad \Rightarrow \quad Z_{\text{inductor}}(s) = \text{Potential}(s)/\text{Flow}(s) = s \cdot L \quad \blacktriangle$$

7.1.3 Applying Equivalent Circuits for Modeling Microsystems

We will use three different examples to demonstrate the application of equivalent circuit models for modeling microsystems. The first example—a MEMS (micro-electro-mechanical-system) sensor—is a mechanical microsystem. The second example is a microfluidic system (i.e., an incompressible fluidic microsystem), which is similar to the ones found on microfluidic and lab-on-a-chip devices. The third example is a thermal microsystem similar to heated microsystems such as microreactors.

(A) Modeling a MEMS Sensor

We use a MEMS sensor as an example to illustrate the modeling of mechanical microsystems with equivalent circuits. As shown in Figure 7-2, the MEMS sensor is designed to measure single-axis forces and accelerations. Depending on the configuration of the MEMS sensor, it can be used as a microbalance to measure weight at the microscale, as a vehicle accelerometer to determine when airbags should be deployed, or as a smart phone or tablet accelerometer to determine device orientation.

In this MEMS sensor, the external force F_{ext} (or equivalently acceleration a_{ext}) causes a solid block with mass (m_B) to move. The motion of the solid block (m_B) is damped with two dampers in series (having damping coefficients of b_2 and b_3) and transferred to electrode A, which is mobile with mass m. This damping is crucial as it allows the MEMS sensor to measure much larger forces, since the force experienced by the durable solid block (m_B) is greatly attenuated before reaching the potentially fragile electrode A (m). Electrode A (m) is connected to a fixed enclosure with two springs having spring constants of k_1 and k_2, which allows the position of electrode A to be restored (i.e., resets the sensor) when the external force is zero. One of the springs (k_1) is non-ideal and also has an associated damping coefficient of b_1. Electrode A (m) is electrically connected to two smaller fixed electrodes B and C, and there is a capacitance sensor (not shown) which senses the capacitance $C_{\text{electrodes}}(t)$ in real time between electrode A and electrodes B and C. The capacitance $C_{\text{electrodes}}(t)$, which is a function of time t, is

$$C_{\text{electrodes}}(t) = \epsilon_m \frac{A_{\text{effective}}}{d(t)} \quad \text{where} \quad d(t) = d_0 + \int_0^t v(t)\, dt \tag{7.23}$$

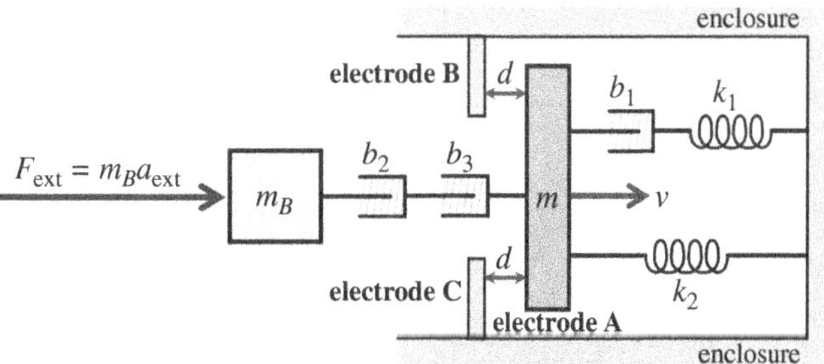

Figure 7-2 An example of a MEMS sensor for measuring single-axis forces and accelerations.

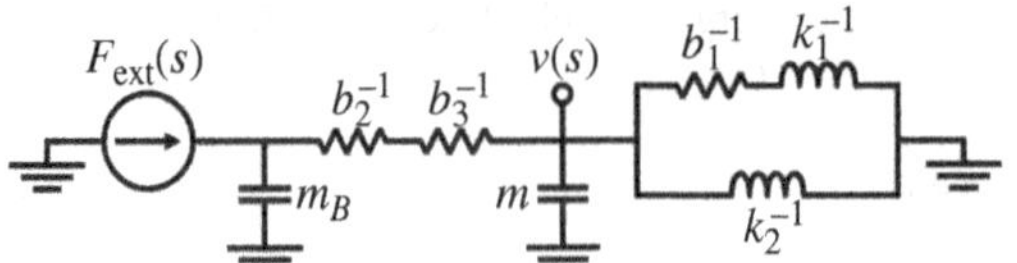

Figure 7-3 The MEMS sensor represented by an equivalent circuit model.

where $A_{\text{effective}}$ is the effective surface area of the three-electrode system, ϵ_m is the permittivity of the medium, $d(t)$ is the distance between the surface of electrode A and the surfaces of electrodes B and C, d_0 is the value of d when the external force is zero (i.e., $F_{\text{ext}} = 0$) and electrode A is stationary, and $v(t)$ is the velocity of electrode A. Note that the sign of $F_{\text{ext}} = m_B a_{\text{ext}}$ or v can be positive or negative, depending on the direction (i.e., to the left or to the right).

Because ϵ_m is known and $A_{\text{effective}}$ can be obtained empirically by calibrating the capacitance sensor, $d(t)$ can be calculated from the measured real-time capacitance $C_{\text{electrodes}}(t)$. Therefore, in order to use the MEMS sensor to measure forces F_{ext} (or equivalently acceleration a_{ext}) in real time, we require an expression for $F_{\text{ext}}(s)$ in terms of $d(s)$ and the provided constants (i.e., the transfer function of the MEMS sensor), which relates the external force F_{ext} to the gap distance d of the capacitance sensor in the Laplace domain. With this transfer function, we can compute the external force $F_{\text{ext}}(t)$ in real time using $C_{\text{electrodes}}(t)$ obtained from the real-time capacitance sensor.

The equivalent circuit of the MEMS sensor is shown in Figure 7-3 (please refer to Table 7-3 for an overview of equivalent circuit elements for mechanical translation). Similar to the electrical ground of an electrical circuit, the mechanical ground of this equivalent circuit occurs at the locations where the (relative) potential is zero. Since the potential is the (relative) velocity v in mechanical systems, the ground is comprised of locations where $v = 0$. Thus, the fixed enclosure (where $v = 0$) is considered to be a mechanical ground. The two masses m_B (solid block) and m (electrode A) are represented by capacitors with mechanical capacitances of m_B and m. Because the motion (i.e., potential or velocity v) of the two masses m_B and m is considered relative to the enclosure, both masses must also be connected to the ground at one end. The external force F_{ext} is represented as a current source connected to ground on the left end, since F_{ext} is also considered relative to the fixed enclosure. The three dampers with damping coefficients of b_1, b_2, and b_3 are respectively represented by resistors with resistances of b_1^{-1}, b_2^{-1}, and b_3^{-1}. Finally, the two springs with spring constants of k_1 and k_2 are respectively represented as inductors with inductances of k_1^{-1} and k_2^{-1}.

To obtain the transfer function relating $F_{\text{ext}}(s)$ to $d(s)$, we first find an expression for $v(s)$ in terms of $F_{\text{ext}}(s)$, which is represented as the potential (i.e., velocity) of electrode A (mass m) relative to the mechanical ground (i.e., the enclosure). In Figure 7-4, the mechanical

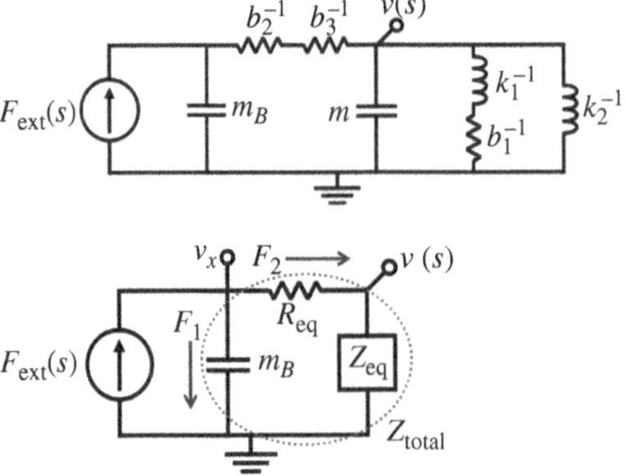

Figure 7-4 Two entirely equivalent mechanical circuit models of the MEMS sensor, where

$$R_{\text{eq}} = b_2^{-1} + b_3^{-1}$$

$$Z_{\text{eq}} = m \,\|\, (k_1^{-1} + b_1^{-1}) \,\|\, k_2^{-1}$$

$$Z_{\text{eq}}(s) = \left(\frac{1}{s \cdot m}\right) \,\|\, (s \cdot k_1^{-1} + b_1^{-1}) \,\|\, (s \cdot k_2^{-1})$$

equivalent circuit of the MEMS sensor is simplified and redrawn. In terms of $F_{ext}(s)$, $v(s)$ can be expressed as

$$v(s) = Z_{eq} \cdot F_2(s) = Z_{eq} \cdot \frac{v_x(s)}{R_{eq} + Z_{eq}} = \frac{Z_{eq} \cdot Z_{total}}{R_{eq} + Z_{eq}} \cdot F_{ext}(s) \quad \text{with} \quad \begin{cases} v_x(s) = Z_{total} \cdot F_{ext}(s) \\ R_{eq} = b_2^{-1} + b_3^{-1} \end{cases}$$

Using Equation (7.22) for two parallel impedances, we can find Z_{total} as

$$Z_{total} = \left(\frac{1}{s \cdot m_B}\right) \| \left(R_{eq} + Z_{eq}\right) = \frac{\left(\dfrac{1}{s \cdot m_B}\right)\left(R_{eq} + Z_{eq}\right)}{\left(\dfrac{1}{s \cdot m_B}\right) + \left(R_{eq} + Z_{eq}\right)} = \frac{R_{eq} + Z_{eq}}{s \cdot m_B\left(R_{eq} + Z_{eq}\right) + 1}$$

Next, we use Equation (7.21) to combine the three parallel impedances to obtain Z_{eq} as

$$Z_{eq}(s) = \left(\frac{1}{s \cdot m}\right) \| \left(s \cdot k_1^{-1} + b_1^{-1}\right) \| \left(s \cdot k_2^{-1}\right) \quad \Rightarrow \quad Z_{eq}^{-1}(s) = \left(\frac{1}{s \cdot m}\right)^{-1} + \left(\frac{s}{k_1} + \frac{1}{b_1}\right)^{-1} + \left(\frac{s}{k_2}\right)^{-1}$$

$$Z_{eq}^{-1}(s) = s \cdot m + \frac{k_1 b_1}{s b_1 + k_1} + \frac{k_2}{s} = \frac{s^2 m\left(s b_1 + k_1\right) + s k_1 b_1 + k_2\left(s b_1 + k_1\right)}{s\left(s b_1 + k_1\right)}$$

$$Z_{eq}(s) = \frac{s\left(s b_1 + k_1\right)}{s^2 m\left(s b_1 + k_1\right) + s b_1\left(k_1 + k_2\right) + k_1 k_2}$$

Putting everything together, and using $R_{eq} = b_2^{-1} + b_3^{-1}$, we have

$$v(s) = \frac{Z_{eq} \cdot \dfrac{R_{eq} + Z_{eq}}{s \cdot m_B\left(R_{eq} + Z_{eq}\right) + 1}}{R_{eq} + Z_{eq}} \cdot F_{ext}(s) = \frac{Z_{eq}(s)}{s \cdot m_B\left[Z_{eq}(s) + b_2^{-1} + b_3^{-1}\right] + 1} \cdot F_{ext}(s)$$

To obtain an expression for $d(s)$, we take the Laplace transform of both sides of Equation (7.23). Thus,

$$d(s) = \mathcal{L}\{d(t)\} = \mathcal{L}\left\{d_0 + \int_0^t v(t)\,dt\right\} = d_0 \cdot \mathcal{L}\{1\} + \mathcal{L}\left\{\int_0^t v(t)\,dt\right\} = \frac{d_0}{s} + \frac{v(s)}{s}$$

where we used the identities $\mathcal{L}\{1\} = 1/s$ and $\mathcal{L}\left\{\int_0^t v(\tau)\,d\tau\right\} = v(s)/s$, which can be found in standard Laplace transform tables. Finally, we obtain the transfer function of the MEMS sensor as follows:

$$d(s) = \frac{d_0}{s} + \frac{v(s)}{s} \quad \Rightarrow \quad v(s) = s \cdot d(s) - d_0 = \frac{Z_{eq}(s)}{s \cdot m_B\left[Z_{eq}(s) + b_2^{-1} + b_3^{-1}\right] + 1} \cdot F_{ext}(s)$$

$$F_{ext}(s) = \frac{\left[s \cdot d(s) - d_0\right] \cdot \left(s \cdot m_B\left[Z_{eq}(s) + b_2^{-1} + b_3^{-1}\right] + 1\right)}{Z_{eq}(s)} \tag{7.24A}$$

$$\text{where} \quad Z_{eq}(s) = \frac{s(sb_1 + k_1)}{s^2 m(sb_1 + k_1) + sb_1(k_1 + k_2) + k_1 k_2} \quad \text{and} \quad \begin{cases} d(s) = \mathcal{L}\{d(t)\} \\ F_{ext}(s) = \mathcal{L}\{F_{ext}(t)\} \end{cases} \quad \text{(7.24B)}$$

To obtain $F_{ext}(t)$ from $C_{electrodes}(t)$, we have to first compute $d(t)$ using Equation (7.23):

$$d(t) = \epsilon_m \frac{A_{effective}}{C_{electrodes}(t)}$$

By applying the Laplace transform to get $d(s) = \mathcal{L}\{d(t)\}$ and using the transfer function of the MEMS sensor given in Equation (7.24), we can obtain $F_{ext}(s)$ from $d(s)$. Finally, we can apply the inverse Laplace transform to get $F_{ext}(t) = \mathcal{L}^{-1}\{F_{ext}(s)\}$.

(B) Modeling a Microfluidic System

In this example, we use a microfluidic system to illustrate the use of equivalent circuits for modeling incompressible fluidic microsystems. Unlike the MEMS sensor from Section 7.1.3(A), this microfluidic system is operated at DC (direct current) steady state. While electrical and mechanical systems can exhibit oscillatory behavior, this is rarely the case with microfluidic systems. In addition, microfluidic devices are typically operated at steady state because transient behavior is usually undesirable. DC steady state implies that

$$\text{frequency} = f = 0 \quad (\text{DC}) \quad \text{and} \quad \frac{\partial[\text{Potential}(t)]}{\partial t} = \frac{\partial[\text{Flow}(t)]}{\partial t} = 0 \quad (\text{steady state}) \quad (7.25)$$

Therefore, we have $\omega = 2\pi f = 0$. From Equation (7.16), we have

$$\text{Potential}(t) = P_0 \exp(\sigma t)\cos(\omega t + \theta) = P_0 \exp(\sigma t)\cos(\theta)$$

$$\frac{\partial[\text{Potential}(t)]}{\partial t} = \sigma P_0 \exp(\sigma t)\cos(\theta) = \sigma \cdot \text{Potential}(t) = 0 \quad \Rightarrow \quad \sigma = 0$$

since in general Potential $(t) \neq 0$. We can also reach the same result (i.e., $\sigma = 0$) using Equation (7.17). Furthermore, we use Equation (7.14) to obtain

$$s = \sigma + j\omega = 0 \quad \text{since} \quad \begin{cases} \omega = 2\pi f = 0 \quad (\text{DC}) \\ \sigma = 0 \quad (\text{steady state}) \end{cases} \quad (7.26A)$$

$$s = 0 \quad \Rightarrow \quad \begin{cases} Z_{capacitor}(s) = 1/(s \cdot C) \to \infty \quad (\text{open circuit}) \\ Z_{inductor}(s) = s \cdot L = 0 \quad (\text{short circuit}) \\ Z_{resistor}(s) = R \quad (\text{unaffected}) \end{cases} \quad (7.26B)$$

Thus, at DC steady state, capacitors become open circuits while inductors become short circuits. Resistors are unaffected because the impedance of a resistor is independent of s.

Before delving into the modeling of the microfluidic system, we need to derive expressions for the resistances, capacitances, and inductances in incompressible fluidic systems. We can use the volumetric flow rate Q_{PDF} due to pressure-driven flow as given in Section 2.5

to find an expression for the fluid resistance R_f in a cylindrical vessel (e.g., a channel, pipe, or tube) with radius r_0. From Equation (2.33), we have

$$Q_f = Q_{\text{PDF}} = \frac{\pi r_0^4 \Delta P}{8L\eta} \quad \Rightarrow \quad R_f = \frac{\Delta P}{Q_f} = \frac{8L\eta}{\pi r_0^4}$$

where L is the length of the cylindrical vessel, η is the dynamic viscosity of the fluid, and ΔP is the pressure drop across the vessel.

In addition, we can use Equation (7.4) to find an expression for the fluid vessel inertance L_f. Letting A be the cross-sectional area of the vessel, v_{fluid} be the fluid velocity, a_{fluid} be the fluid acceleration, and m_{fluid} be the fluid mass, we have

$$\Delta P = L_f \cdot \frac{dQ_f}{dt} \quad \Rightarrow \quad \frac{F}{A} = L_f \cdot \frac{d\left(v_{\text{fluid}}A\right)}{dt} \quad \Rightarrow \quad \frac{m_{\text{fluid}}a_{\text{fluid}}}{A} = L_f \cdot A \cdot a_{\text{fluid}} \quad \Rightarrow \quad L_f = \frac{m_{\text{fluid}}}{A^2}$$

For a cylindrical vessel with radius r_0, we have $A = \pi r_0^2$. Additionally, $m_{\text{fluid}} = \rho_{m(\text{fluid})} LA$, where L is the length of the cylindrical vessel and $\rho_{m(\text{fluid})}$ is the fluid density. Hence,

$$L_f = \frac{\rho_{m(\text{fluid})}LA}{A^2} = \frac{\rho_{m(\text{fluid})}L}{A} = \frac{\rho_{m(\text{fluid})}L}{\pi r_0^2}$$

From Equation (7.3) as provided below, we see that the fluid vessel compliance C_f is proportional to the change in fluid vessel volume ΔV_f corresponding to a change in pressure ΔP.

$$C_f = \frac{dV_{f(\text{vessel})}}{dP_{(\text{fluid})}} = \lim_{\Delta P_{(\text{fluid})} \to 0} \frac{\Delta V_{f(\text{vessel})}}{\Delta P_{(\text{fluid})}}$$

Therefore, the fluid vessel compliance C_f is a measure of the elasticity of the fluid vessel. If the fluid vessel is extremely stiff, we have $C_f \cong 0$. If the fluid vessel is highly elastic, C_f would be much larger.

In summary, we can express R_f, L_f, and C_f as shown below:

$$R_f = \frac{\Delta P}{Q_f} = \frac{8L\eta}{\pi r_0^4} \propto \frac{1}{r_0^4} \qquad L_f = \frac{\rho_{m(\text{fluid})}L}{A} = \frac{\rho_{m(\text{fluid})}L}{\pi r_0^2} \propto \frac{1}{r_0^2} \qquad C_f = \frac{dV_{f(\text{vessel})}}{dP_{(\text{fluid})}} \tag{7.27}$$

where the "$\propto$" symbol represents proportionality. Hence, relatively large vessels will have negligible (i.e., close to zero) R_f and L_f.

Now, we move on to discuss how to model a microfluidic system. As shown in Figure 7-5, we have a microfluidic system similar to those found in microfluidic and lab-on-a-chip devices. Depending on the exact configuration, this microfluidic system can be used for cell sorting and filtering via dielectrophoresis (DEP), for continuous perfusion to keep tissues alive in organ-on-a-chip devices, or as an automated fluid transport system in lab-on-a-chip biosensors.

This microfluidic system consists of a pump generating a volumetric flow rate of $Q_{f(\text{pump})}$, which pushes fluid through two cylindrical microchannels. Because the two microchannels have small radii r_0 relative to the rest of the system, microchannel 1 has a vessel fluid resistance of R_{f1} and a fluid vessel inertance of L_{f1}, while microchannel 2 has a vessel fluid resistance of R_{f2} and a fluid vessel inertance of L_{f2}. All conduits (including both microchannels) are highly stiff, and therefore have negligible (i.e., almost zero) compliance. The well connected to the right end of microchannel 1 is designed to collect the output of microchannel 1, which can then be extracted either manually or with another pump. This well is comprised

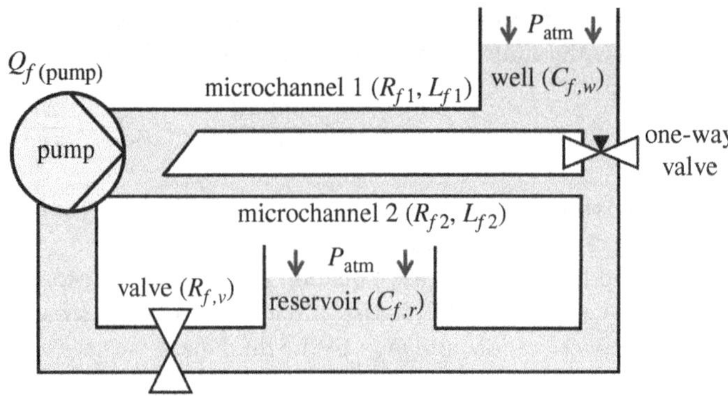

Figure 7-5 A typical microfluidic system similar to those found in microfluidic and lab-on-a-chip devices.

of an elastomer polymer, and has a fluid vessel compliance of $C_{f,w}$. Similarly, we have a reservoir filled with buffer solution to continuously feed the microfluidic system with fresh solution. The reservoir is comprised of a polymer with a fluid vessel compliance of $C_{f,r}$. Liquid in the well and reservoir is exposed to air, which exerts an atmospheric pressure of P_{atm}. Due to their relatively large dimensions, the well and reservoir have negligible R_f and L_f. There is a valve at the inlet side of the pump that can be used to start or shut off fluid circulation in the microsystem. The valve is non-ideal and has a vessel fluid resistance of $R_{f,v}$ and negligible L_f. Finally, there is a one-way valve designed to prevent the backflow of liquid from microchannel 2 into microchannel 1. The one-way valve is considered ideal and has negligible R_f and L_f. In addition, there is no pressure drop across the valve or the one-way valve.

The equivalent circuit of the microfluidic system is shown in Figure 7-6 (left) (please refer to Table 7-3 for a list of equivalent circuit elements for incompressible fluid flow). All vessel fluid resistances are represented by resistors, fluid vessel compliances represented by capacitors, and fluid vessel inertances represented by inductors. As with an electrical circuit, the ground is the point at which the (relative) potential is zero. For fluidic systems, the potential is the (relative) pressure. In Figure 7-6 (left), the ground pressure is defined to be zero pressure as found in vacuum chambers and outer space. If we were to instead define the ground pressure as atmospheric pressure P_{atm}, the two voltage sources would be removed and the two compliances $C_{f,w}$ and $C_{f,r}$ would be connected directly to ground. The ideal one-way valve is represented by an ideal diode, since diodes are circuit elements that allow current to flow in one direction only. The non-ideal valve is represented as a switch in series with a vessel fluid resistance of $R_{f,v}$, as switches can pass or block electrical current. There is no pressure drop across either valve.

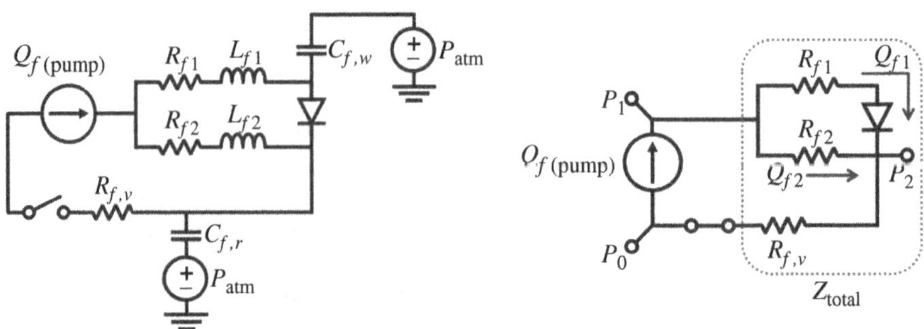

Figure 7-6 Two entirely equivalent circuit models of the microfluidic system. Since the microfluidic system is operated at steady state, the circuit on the right can be obtained from the circuit on the left.

Because the microfluidic system is operated at DC steady state, all capacitors become open circuits, and all inductors become short circuits, while the resistors are unaffected. Please refer to Equation (7.26) for more details. Therefore, we can redraw the equivalent circuit for the microfluidic system shown in Figure 7-6 (left), and obtain the simpler equivalent circuit shown in Figure 7-6 (right).

Choosing a suitable pump requires knowledge of the pressure drop across the pump given by $\Delta P_{\text{pump}} = P_1 - P_0$. Moreover, we want to know the fluid flow rates Q_{f1} and Q_{f2} in microchannels 1 and 2, respectively. To begin, we first compute ΔP_{pump} as

$$\Delta P_{\text{pump}} = Q_{f(\text{pump})} \cdot Z_{\text{total}} = Q_{f(\text{pump})} \cdot \left(R_{f,v} + R_{f1} \| R_{f2} \right) = Q_{f(\text{pump})} \cdot \left(R_{f,v} + \frac{R_{f1}R_{f2}}{R_{f1} + R_{f2}} \right)$$

$$\Delta P_{\text{pump}} = \left(R_{f,v} + \frac{R_{f1}R_{f2}}{R_{f1} + R_{f2}} \right) Q_{f(\text{pump})} \quad \text{where} \quad R_f = \frac{8L\eta}{\pi r_0^4} \tag{7.28}$$

where we used Equation (7.22) to compute $R_{f1} \| R_{f2}$. To obtain Q_{f1} and Q_{f2}, we first use Kirchhoff's generalized voltage law given in Equation (7.18) as follows:

$$\Delta P_{\text{pump}} = \left(P_1 - P_2 \right) + \left(P_2 - P_0 \right) \quad \Rightarrow \quad P_1 - P_2 = \Delta P_{\text{pump}} - \left(P_2 - P_0 \right) = \Delta P_{\text{pump}} - Q_{f(\text{pump})} R_{f,v}$$

since the full "current" of $Q_{f(\text{pump})}$ flows through $R_{f,v}$. We have

$$P_1 - P_2 = \Delta P_{\text{pump}} - \left(P_2 - P_0 \right) = Q_{f(\text{pump})} \left(R_{f,v} + \frac{R_{f1}R_{f2}}{R_{f1} + R_{f2}} \right) - Q_{f(\text{pump})} R_{f,v}$$

$$P_1 - P_2 = \frac{R_{f1}R_{f2}}{R_{f1} + R_{f2}} Q_{f(\text{pump})} \qquad Q_{f1} = \frac{P_1 - P_2}{R_{f1}} \qquad Q_{f2} = \frac{P_1 - P_2}{R_{f2}}$$

$$Q_{f1} = \frac{R_{f2}}{R_{f1} + R_{f2}} Q_{f(\text{pump})} \quad \text{and} \quad Q_{f2} = \frac{R_{f1}}{R_{f1} + R_{f2}} Q_{f(\text{pump})} \quad \text{where} \quad R_f = \frac{8L\eta}{\pi r_0^4} \tag{7.29}$$

Note that we could have obtained Q_{f1} and Q_{f2} in fewer steps using "current" division. Because we are operating the microfluidic system at DC steady state, we have $s = \sigma + j\omega = 0$. Hence, *none* of the equivalent circuit parameters depend on s. Using the above results, we can choose a suitable pump based on the expected ΔP_{pump}, and predict the volumetric flow rates Q_{f1} and Q_{f2} through each microchannel.

(C) Modeling a Thermal Microsystem

Thermal microsystems are heated microsystems such as heated microfluidic/MEMS devices and microreactors. Before delving into modeling a thermal microsystem, we first derive expressions for the resistances and capacitances in thermal systems. As mentioned in Section 7.1.1, thermal inductances can theoretically exist, but are uncommon enough to be typically excluded from thermal equivalent circuit models.

In thermal systems, there are two different kinds of thermal resistances R_t. The first kind of thermal resistance applies to immobile objects (e.g., immobile fluids and solids), while the second kind applies to moving fluids (e.g., flowing gases and liquids). Analogous to an electrical resistance $R_{\text{electrical}}$, the thermal resistance R_t of an immobile object is

$$R_t \equiv R_{\text{thermal}} = \left(\frac{1}{\kappa} \cdot \frac{\ell}{A} \right)_{\text{object}} \qquad \left[\text{analogous to } R_{\text{electrical}} = \left(\rho_r \frac{\ell}{A} \right)_{\text{resistor}} \right] \tag{7.30}$$

where ℓ is the length of the object, A is the cross-sectional area of the object, and κ is the thermal conductivity [W/(m · K)] of the material comprising the object.

To derive an expression for the thermal resistances of moving fluids, we start with the definition of the specific heat capacity c_h as follows:

$$c_h = \frac{Q_t}{m_{\text{fluid}}\Delta T} \quad \Rightarrow \quad Q_t = \Delta T \cdot m_{\text{fluid}} c_h \quad \Rightarrow \quad \frac{dQ_t}{dt} = \frac{d}{dt}\left(\Delta T \cdot m_{\text{fluid}} c_h\right)$$

where m_{fluid} is the mass of the fluid, Q_t is the thermal energy, and T is the temperature. Letting the mass flow rate of the fluid be $\dot{m}_{\text{fluid}}$, we have

$$q_t = \Delta T \cdot c_h \frac{dm_{\text{fluid}}}{dt} = c_h \dot{m}_{\text{fluid}} \Delta T \quad \text{where} \quad \dot{m}_{\text{fluid}} = \frac{dm_{\text{fluid}}}{dt}$$

Finally, we can derive the thermal resistance R_t of moving fluids using Equation (7.2) as

$$R_t = \frac{\Delta T}{q_t} = \left(\frac{1}{c_h \dot{m}}\right)_{\text{fluid}} = \left(\frac{1}{c_h \rho_m \dot{V}}\right)_{\text{fluid}} \quad \text{with} \quad \left\{ \begin{array}{l} \dot{m}_{\text{fluid}} = dm_{\text{fluid}}/dt = \rho_m \dot{V}_{\text{fluid}} \\[2mm] \dot{V}_{\text{fluid}} = dV_{\text{fluid}}/dt \end{array} \right. \tag{7.31}$$

where $\dot{V}_{\text{fluid}}$ is the volumetric flow rate of the fluid and ρ_m is the mass density of the fluid.

Let us consider the movement of fluid from the inlet of a vessel to the outlet. If the fluid at the inlet is stationary (i.e., not moving), there is no fluid heat flow (i.e., no "current") from the inlet to the outlet, and we expect the thermal resistance to be infinite representing an open circuit that allows no "current" flow. This is indeed the case with $\dot{m}_{\text{fluid}} = 0$ for stationary fluids; based on Equation (7.31), we have $R_t \to \infty$. On the other hand, let us consider the case where a large volume of fluid moves quickly from the inlet to the outlet of the vessel. With $\dot{m}_{\text{fluid}}$ being very large, we have $R_t \cong 0$ from Equation (7.31). In this case, heat from the moving fluid is transferred from the inlet to the outlet with virtually no thermal resistance.

The thermal "capacitance" C_t of an object is its heat capacity as defined by Equation (7.11). We have

$$C_t = \text{heat capacity} = m_{\text{object}} \cdot c_h = \rho_m V_{\text{object}} \cdot c_h = \rho_m c_h (\ell A)_{\text{object}} \tag{7.32}$$

where m_{object} is the mass of the object, c_h is the specific heat capacity [J/(kg · K)] of the material comprising the object, and ρ_m is the mass density [kg/m^3] of the object.

Now, we model a thermal microsystem using an equivalent circuit. As illustrated in Figure 7-7, we have a thermal microsystem similar to heated microfluidic devices, heated MEMS devices, and microreactors. Such thermal microsystems can be used to purify or separate biomolecules such as proteins and DNA, study the effect of temperature on live tissues, or perform important enzyme-catalyzed reactions.

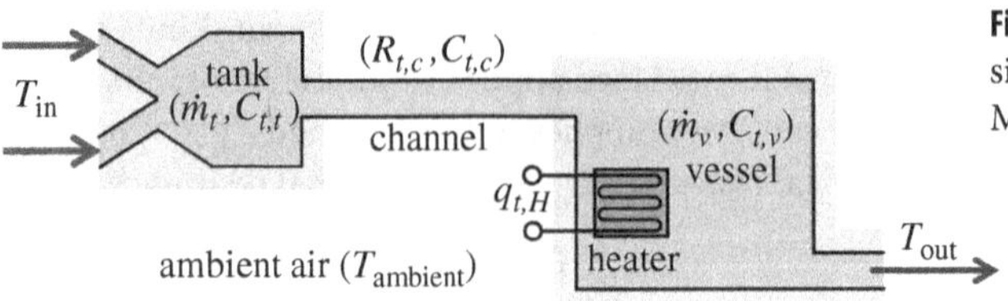

Figure 7-7   A thermal microsystem similar to heated microfluidic/MEMS devices and microreactors.

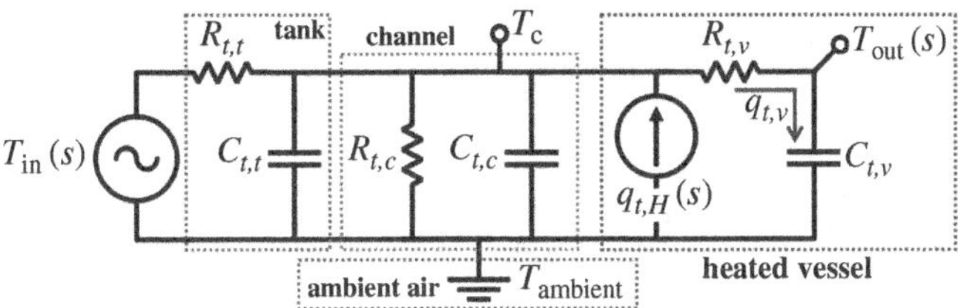

Figure 7-8 An equivalent circuit model of the thermal microsystem comprised of the tank, channel, heated vessel, and ambient air.

In this thermal microsystem, reactants all having temperatures of T_{in} relative to the ambient air temperature are mixed in an insulated tank. The mass flow rate of fluid through the tank is $\dot{m}_t$, and the heat capacity of fluid in the tank is $C_{t,t}$ (the heat capacity of the tank itself is negligible in comparison). After the reactants are mixed in the tank, the resulting solution is passed through a channel into an insulated vessel. The channel is both long and poorly insulated, and thus allows a significant amount of heat from the solution to be transferred into the surrounding air as represented by a thermal resistance of $R_{t,c}$. The fluid-filled channel also has a heat capacity of $C_{t,c}$. Upon being transferring into the insulated vessel, the solution is heated by a heater in order to facilitate further reactions. The heater generates a heat flow rate of $q_{t,H}$ [W]. The mass flow rate of fluid through the vessel is $\dot{m}_v$, and the heat capacity of fluid in the tank is $C_{t,t}$ (the heat capacity of the vessel by itself is negligible in comparison). Throughout the tank, channel, and vessel, the density ρ_m and specific heat capacity c_h of the solution fluid are approximately constant. Since T_{in} and $q_{t,H}$ are controlled by real-time temperature feedback systems, this thermal microsystem *does not* operate at DC steady state. Hence, $s \neq 0$ in the Laplace domain.

The equivalent circuit of this thermal microsystem is depicted in Figure 7-8. In thermal systems, the potential is represented by temperature. Here, the thermal ground is defined to be the ambient air temperature surrounding the tank, channel, and vessel. The temperature T_{in} of the input reactants at the inlet side of the tank is represented by a voltage source. For simplicity, we define the following parameters:

$$
\left\{
\begin{aligned}
R_{t,t} &\equiv R_{t,\text{tank}} = \left(\frac{1}{c_h \dot{m}_t}\right)_{\text{fluid}} \\
R_{t,c} &\equiv R_{t,\text{channel}} = \left(\frac{1}{\kappa} \cdot \frac{\ell}{A}\right)_{\text{channel}} \\
R_{t,v} &\equiv R_{t,\text{vessel}} = \left(\frac{1}{c_h \dot{m}_v}\right)_{\text{fluid}}
\end{aligned}
\right.
\qquad
\left\{
\begin{aligned}
C_{t,t} &\equiv C_{t,\text{tank}} = (\rho_m c_h V)_{\text{fluid}} \cdot V_{\text{tank}} \\
C_{t,c} &\equiv C_{t,\text{channel}} = (\rho_m c_h V)_{\text{fluid-filled channel}} \\
C_{t,v} &\equiv C_{t,\text{vessel}} = (\rho_m c_h)_{\text{fluid}} \cdot V_{\text{vessel}}
\end{aligned}
\right.
\qquad (7.33)
$$

The insulated mixing tank is represented by thermal resistance $R_{t,t}$ and thermal capacitance $C_{t,t}$. The thermal resistance $R_{t,t}$ is connected from the tank inlet to the tank outlet, since $R_{t,t}$ represents the transfer (i.e., loss) of heat as the fluid moves from the inlet to the outlet of the tank. Because the insulated tank is surrounded by ambient air (i.e., thermal ground), one end of the thermal capacitance $C_{t,t}$ must be grounded. The reaction vessel is represented in a similar fashion by a thermal resistance $R_{t,v}$ and thermal capacitance $C_{t,v}$. The heater within the vessel is represented as a current source with heat flow rate $q_{t,H}$ [W]. The heat capacity $C_{t,c}$ of the channel is represented in the same way. Finally, the continuous

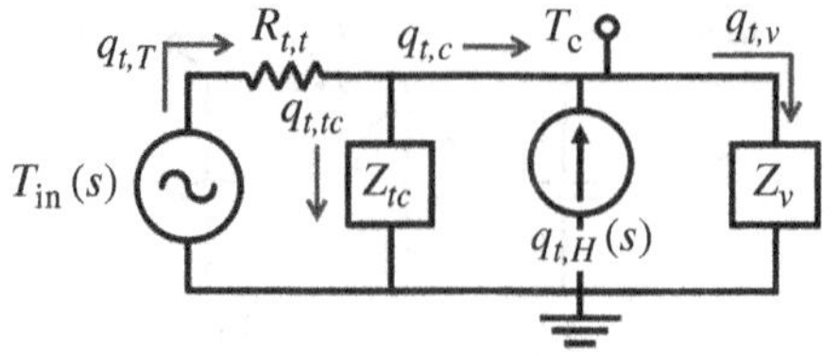

$$Z_{tc} = C_{t,t} \parallel R_{t,c} \parallel C_{t,c}$$

$$Z_{tc}(s) = \frac{1}{sC_{t,t}} \parallel R_{t,c} \parallel \frac{1}{sC_{t,c}}$$

$$Z_v(s) = R_{t,v} + \frac{1}{sC_{t,v}}$$

Figure 7-9   A simplified equivalent circuit model of the thermal microsystem.

heat loss to ambient air from the long and poorly insulated channel is represented by a shunt thermal resistance $R_{t,c}$ connected to ground (i.e., the ambient air).

The fluid output from this thermal microsystem is fed into another heated system. As such, we want to control the real-time temperature $T_{out}(t)$ of fluid leaving this thermal microsystem by adjusting $T_{in}(t)$ and $q_{t,H}(t)$ via temperature feedback control. To allow for the real-time control of $T_{out}(t)$, we need to derive a transfer function relating $T_{out}(s)$ to $T_{in}(s)$ and $q_{t,H}(s)$ in the Laplace domain. First, we simplify the thermal equivalent circuit shown in Figure 7-8 to obtain the equivalent circuit shown in Figure 7-9.

As can be obtained from Figure 7-8, $T_{out}(s)$ is given by

$$T_{out}(s) = q_{t,v}(s) \cdot \frac{1}{sC_{t,v}}$$

Using Figure 7-9 and Kirchhoff's generalized current law given in Equation (7.19), we have

$$q_{t,v} = q_{t,c} + q_{t,H} \quad \text{and} \quad q_{t,c} = q_{t,T} - q_{t,tc} \quad \Rightarrow \quad q_{t,v} = \left(q_{t,T} - q_{t,tc}\right) + q_{t,H}$$

Using Kirchhoff's generalized voltage law given in Equation (7.18), we obtain

$$T_{in} = T_c + R_{t,t}q_{t,T} \quad \Rightarrow \quad T_c = T_{in} - R_{t,t}q_{t,T} \quad \Rightarrow \quad q_{t,T} = \frac{T_{in} - T_c}{R_{t,t}}$$

Furthermore, we have

$$T_c = q_{t,v}Z_v = q_{t,tc}Z_{tc} \quad \Rightarrow \quad q_{t,tc} = q_{t,v}\frac{Z_v}{Z_{tc}} \quad \text{and} \quad q_{t,T} = \frac{T_{in} - T_c}{R_{t,t}} = \frac{T_{in} - q_{t,v}Z_v}{R_{t,t}}$$

$$q_{t,v} = q_{t,T} - q_{t,tc} + q_{t,H} = \frac{T_{in} - q_{t,v}Z_v}{R_{t,t}} - q_{t,v}\frac{Z_v}{Z_{tc}} + q_{t,H}$$

$$q_{t,v}\left(1 + \frac{Z_v}{R_{t,t}} + \frac{Z_v}{Z_{tc}}\right) = \frac{T_{in}}{R_{t,t}} + q_{t,H} \quad \Rightarrow \quad q_{t,v} = \frac{T_{in}/R_{t,t} + q_{t,H}}{1 + Z_v\left(1/R_{t,t} + 1/Z_{tc}\right)}$$

Our next task is to obtain expressions for Z_{tc} and Z_v. Using Equation (7.21) to combine the three parallel impedances of $Z_{tc}(s)$, we get

$$Z_{tc}(s) = \frac{1}{sC_{t,t}} \parallel R_{t,c} \parallel \frac{1}{sC_{t,c}} \quad \Rightarrow \quad Z_{tc}^{-1} = \left(\frac{1}{sC_{t,t}}\right)^{-1} + R_{t,c}^{-1} + \left(\frac{1}{sC_{t,c}}\right)^{-1} = sC_{t,t} + \frac{1}{R_{t,c}} + sC_{t,c}$$

$$\frac{1}{Z_{tc}} = s\left(C_{t,t} + C_{t,c}\right) + \frac{1}{R_{t,c}} \quad \text{and} \quad Z_v(s) = R_{t,v} + \frac{1}{sC_{t,v}} = \frac{sR_{t,v}C_{t,v} + 1}{sC_{t,v}}$$

Putting everything together, the transfer function of the thermal microsystem is obtained as follows:

$$T_{\text{out}}(s) = q_{t,v}(s) \cdot \frac{1}{sC_{t,v}} = \frac{T_{\text{in}}(s)/R_{t,t} + q_{t,H}(s)}{1 + \dfrac{sR_{t,v}C_{t,v} + 1}{sC_{t,v}}\left[\dfrac{1}{R_{t,t}} + s\left(C_{t,t} + C_{t,c}\right) + \dfrac{1}{R_{t,c}}\right]} \cdot \frac{1}{sC_{t,v}}$$

$$T_{\text{out}}(s) = \frac{T_{\text{in}}(s)/R_{t,t} + q_{t,H}(s)}{sC_{t,v} + \left(sR_{t,v}C_{t,v} + 1\right)\left[s\left(C_{t,t} + C_{t,c}\right) + 1/R_{t,t} + 1/R_{t,c}\right]} \tag{7.34A}$$

where the thermal resistances and capacitances are given in Equation (7.33).

The above transfer function for $T_{\text{out}}(s)$ in terms of $T_{\text{in}}(s)$ and $q_{t,H}(s)$ allows us to control $T_{\text{out}}(t)$ of fluid leaving this thermal microsystem in real time. Because the thermal ground of our equivalent circuit is the ambient air temperature, both T_{in} and T_{out} are defined relative to the ambient air temperature T_{ambient}. Therefore, the actual temperatures are

$$\left\{ \begin{array}{l} T_{\text{in(actual)}}(t) = T_{\text{in}}(t) + T_{\text{ambient}} \\ T_{\text{out(actual)}}(t) = T_{\text{out}}(t) + T_{\text{ambient}} \end{array} \right. \quad \text{where} \quad \left\{ \begin{array}{l} T_{\text{in}}(t) = \mathcal{L}^{-1}\left\{T_{\text{in}}(s)\right\} \\ T_{\text{out}}(t) = \mathcal{L}^{-1}\left\{T_{\text{out}}(s)\right\} \end{array} \right. \tag{7.34B}$$

7.2 POLYMERASE CHAIN REACTION MICROREACTORS

Microreactors are small and highly portable reactors that can carry out biochemical reactions significantly quicker and more efficiently than macroscale reactors. As an example of microreactors and for illustrating the application of equivalent circuit models, we will focus on polymerase chain reaction (PCR) microreactors. In particular, we will model PCR microreactors using thermal equivalent circuits.

PCR is a highly important technique used in both medical science and biology for the amplification of DNA (or cDNA), which enables DNA (or RNA) sequencing and quantification. For a more detailed description of PCR and its applications, please refer to Section 5.2. In the PCR process, the temperature of the system has to ramp up or down to the desired values in the denaturing, annealing, and elongation/extension steps. Unfortunately, temperature ramping is time-consuming. However, once the desired temperature is reached, the DNA denaturing and annealing steps in a standard PCR process are completed in as fast as a few seconds. The DNA extension time is dependent on the DNA polymerase used and the length of the DNA segment to be amplified. The temperature cycles of a typical commercial macroscale PCR thermal cycler are shown in Figure 7-10, which shows that most of the total cycle time for a macroscale PCR system is spent on temperature ramping.

A miniaturized PCR setup (i.e., a microfabricated implementation of PCR) can dramatically reduce the temperature ramping time and the time required for the whole PCR cycle due to decreased thermal mass and response time. A reduction in the PCR cycle time translates directly into increased instrument throughput. Also, the reagents used in the PCR process are expensive. The application of miniaturized PCR setups can significantly reduce the amounts of reagents required and therefore reduce the overall cost of the PCR process.[5]

EXAMPLE 7-3 The temperature cycle for a commercial macroscale PCR system (i.e., thermal cycler) with heating and cooling rates of 1°C/s is shown in Figure 7-10. What is the total PCR cycle time if we exclude the time to warm up from room temperature? Excluding temperature ramp times, how long does

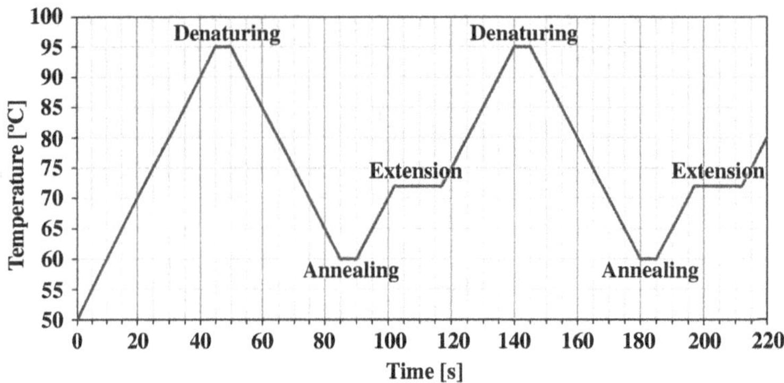

Figure 7-10   The temperature cycles for a commercial macroscale PCR system.

the denaturing, annealing, and extension steps take altogether? A type of DNA polymerase with an extension rate of 40 nucleotides per second (nts/s) is used, and the dsDNA segment to be amplified is 600 base pairs (bps) long.

Solution   From Figure 7-10, and excluding time to warm up from room temperature, the total PCR cycle time is 95 s since

$$t_{\text{total cycle}} = 140\ \text{s} - 45\ \text{s} = 95\ \text{s}$$

Excluding temperature ramp times, the time required for denaturing is 5 s, the time required for annealing is also 5 s, while the time required for extension is

$$t_{\text{extension}} = \frac{600\ \text{bps}}{40\ \text{bps/sec}} = 15\ \text{s} \quad \Rightarrow \quad t_{\text{denaturing}} + t_{\text{annealing}} + t_{\text{extension}} = 5\ \text{s} + 5\ \text{s} + 15\ \text{s} = 25\ \text{s}$$

Therefore, the denaturing, annealing, and extension steps require 25 s altogether. Also, the temperature ramping steps together require 70 s per PCR cycle because

$$t_{\text{temperature ramping}} = 95\ \text{s} - 25\ \text{s} = 70\ \text{s}$$

This implies that for a 95 s PCR cycle, 74% of the time (70 s) is used for temperature ramping while only 26% of the time (25 s) is used for the denaturing, annealing, and extension steps. Thus, utilizing miniaturized PCR setups can greatly reduce the PCR cycle time and increase throughput.   ▲

In the following sections, we will discuss two major types of PCR microreactor techniques used with miniaturized PCR setups: a batch PCR process and a continuous-flow PCR process. The two types of miniaturized PCR systems have unique advantages, disadvantages, and design challenges.

7.2.1 Batch PCR Microreactors

(A) Batch PCR Microreactor Overview

A batch PCR microreactor consists of one or more PCR microchambers that amplify desired strands of DNA batch by batch. The batch PCR microreactor was first reported by Northrup et al. in 1993. A single batch PCR microchamber is illustrated in Figure 7-11. Batch PCR microchambers are etched from a single silicon wafer using alkaline anisotropic wet etching. The top of the chamber is a glass cover sealed with silicone rubber. Two pieces of polyethylene microtubing which are embedded into the silicone rubber seal are used for sample input and output. The bottom of the chamber consists of a low-stress silicon nitride

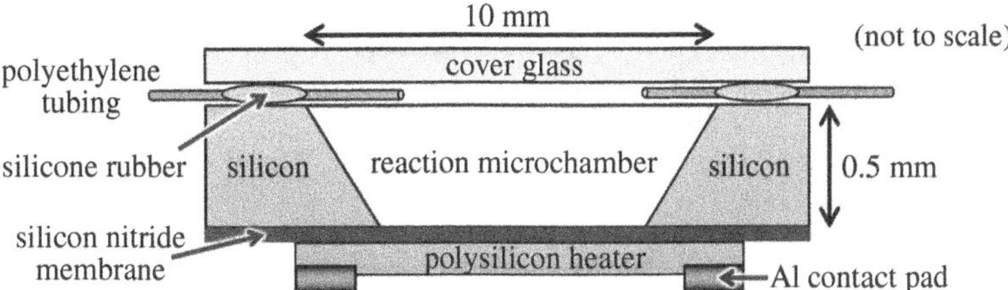

Figure 7-11   A side view of the batch PCR microreactor developed by Northrup et al. containing a single reaction microchamber. (*The schematic is redrawn with permission from M. A. Northrup et al.*[6])

membrane (2 to 3 μm thick) above a resistive polysilicon thin film heater (0.25 μm thick). At the bottom of the silicon wafer, there are two aluminum (Al) contact pads which act as electrodes for the resistive polysilicon heater. The volume of each microchamber is between 25 μL and 50 μL.[6]

The reaction temperature in the chamber is controlled by a resistance-based control circuit consisting of a Wheatstone Bridge combined with an amplifier and a driving transistor (Figure 7-12). R_{heater} is the resistance of the resistive polysilicon heater, while R_{fixed} is a fixed resistance. The resistors $R_{1,DAC}$ and $R_{2,DAC}$ are driven by the DC voltage (+15V) applied at the top of the bridge, and are voltage dividers made from a digital-to-analog converter (DAC). As the ratio of $R_{1,DAC}$ to $R_{2,DAC}$ is changed, the balance point of the bridge is modified. When the bridge is balanced, there must be just enough current passing through the R_{fixed}–R_{heater} arm of the bridge to raise the microchamber temperature via Joule heating of R_{heater}. Passive cooling of the microchamber is accomplished with ambient air. The miniature sizes of the batch PCR microchambers allow for high heating and cooling rates of 15 to 35 °C/s. Hence, the batch PCR microreactor amplifies DNA at least four times faster while drawing many times less power than commercial macroscale PCR systems.[6]

In 1998, Daniel et al. reported a modified batch PCR microchamber based on the design reported by Northrup et al. in 1993 (Figure 7-13). With a chamber volume of 2 μL, the modified microchamber is considerably smaller than the earlier version reported by Northrup et al. (which is 25 to 50 μL). The modified chamber is heated using the Joule heating of platinum (Pt) thin film resistors, and the temperature within the modified chamber is controlled with a fast feedback electronic circuit.[7]

To achieve superior thermal insulation, the modified microchamber has the following major features shown in Figure 7-13: (1) the four sides of the chamber are surrounded by air-filled cavities for better thermal isolation, since air with $\kappa = 0.03\,W/(m \cdot K)$ has a far lower thermal conductivity than silicon with $\kappa = 150\,W/(m \cdot K)$ for structural support, the microchamber is suspended on four silicon beams connected to the horizontal sides of

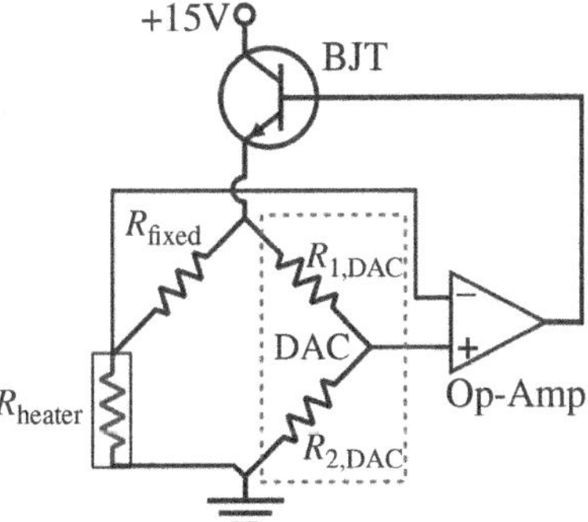

Figure 7-12   Temperature control circuit for the batch PCR microchamber developed by Northrup et al. The circuit is composed of a Wheatstone Bridge, an amplifier, and a driving transistor. (*The circuit diagram is redrawn with permission from M. A. Northrup et al.*[6])

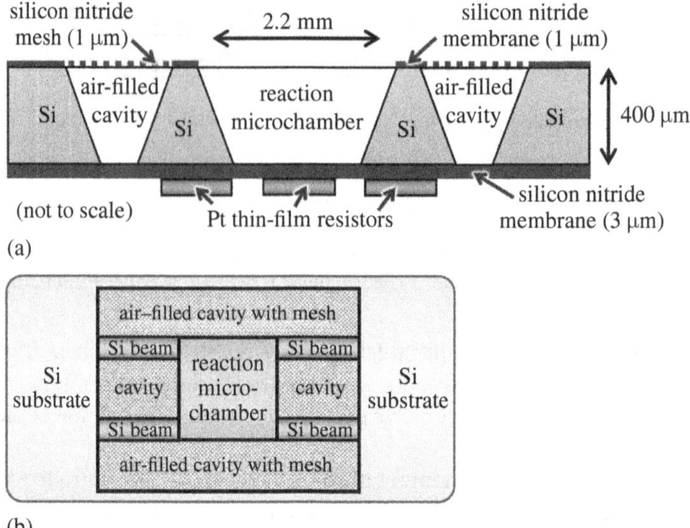

Figure 7-13   (a) Side view and (b) top view of the modified batch PCR microreactor. (*The illustrations are redrawn with permission from J. H. Daniel et al.*[7])

the chamber; (2) the top openings of the air-filled cavities are covered with silicon nitride mesh (1 μm thick) for support and additional thermal insulation; (3) the silicon substrate containing the chamber is coated with a low-stress transparent silicon nitride layer on the bottom (3 μm thick) for support and further thermal insulation.[7]

There are additional differences between the batch PCR microchamber used by Northrup et al. and the modified microchamber by Daniel et al. The modified microchamber surfaces are coated with silicon dioxide (200 nm thick) followed by bovine serum albumin (BSA) to prevent the adsorption of PCR reactants onto the surfaces. Instead of using a cover glass and silicone rubber to seal the microchamber, the modified chamber is sealed with a silicone oil droplet (~1 μL) to prevent evaporation of the PCR solution (~1.5 μL). The transparent bottom silicon nitride layer allows for optical readout of the modified microchamber, which is required since the oil droplet prevents optical readout from the top. Owing to the significantly smaller chamber size of 2 μL as well as improved thermal isolation, the modified batch PCR microchambers can achieve higher heating and cooling rates of 60 to 90°C/s.[7]

(B) Thermal Model of the Batch PCR Microreactor

To model the modified batch PCR microchamber reported by Daniel et al., we use a simplified thermal model (Figure 7-14) with the following assumptions:

(1)   The microchamber has a rectangular cross-section (ignore the sidewall slopes).

(2)   There is no heat conduction through the four horizontal sides of the microchamber, meaning that the four sides of the chamber are completely thermally insulated.

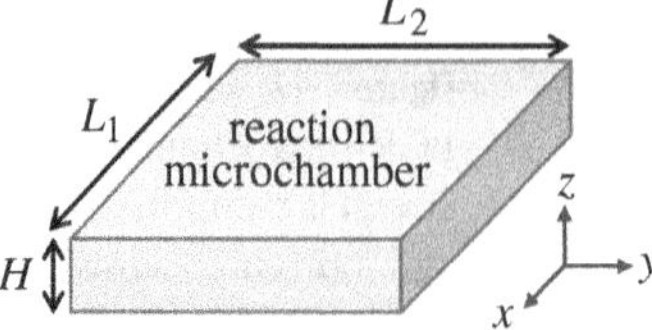

Figure 7-14   A simplified thermal model of the batch PCR reaction microchamber.

(3) The temperature within the chamber does not vary vertically (i.e., in the z-direction), and heat conduction through the top and bottom of the chamber is negligible.

Using these assumptions, we can model the fluid temperature $T(x, y, t)$ inside the batch PCR microchamber as a function of time t using two-dimensional heat flow.

First, we use the heat equation from Section 2.3.2 to model the modified batch PCR microchamber. In particular, we want to obtain the thermal resistance $R_{t,\text{chamber}}$ and heat capacity $C_{t,\text{chamber}}$ of fluid in the modified batch PCR microchamber. To do this, we start with the 2D heat equation with $T(x, y, t)$ representing the fluid temperature in the microchamber.

$$c_h \rho_m \frac{\partial T}{\partial t} = \kappa \nabla^2 T + S = \kappa \left(\frac{\partial^2 T}{\partial x^2} + \frac{\partial^2 T}{\partial y^2} \right) + S$$

where c_h is the specific heat capacity, κ is the thermal conductivity, S is the heat generation per unit volume, and ρ_m is the mass density of fluid in the microchamber. Note that for water and most water-based solutions such as PCR solutions, we have $c_h = 4180 \, \text{J}/(\text{kg} \cdot \text{K})$, $\kappa = 0.6 \, \text{W}/(\text{m} \cdot \text{K})$, and $\rho_m = 1000 \, \text{kg/m}^3$.

Since we are only interested in passive properties (i.e., $R_{t,\text{chamber}}$ and $C_{t,\text{chamber}}$) of fluid in the chamber, we can set the heat generation term S to zero. We have

$$\frac{c_h \rho_m}{\kappa} \frac{\partial T}{\partial t} = \frac{\partial^2 T}{\partial x^2} + \frac{\partial^2 T}{\partial y^2} \tag{7.35}$$

Due to its rectangular cross-section, we assume that the microchamber has lateral dimensions of $L_1 \times L_2$ and height H (Figure 7-14). Therefore, the boundaries of the microchamber are

$$\left\{ 0 \leq x \leq L_1 \quad 0 \leq y \leq L_2 \quad 0 \leq z \leq H \right\} \tag{7.36}$$

We need to solve Equation (7.35) for $t \geq 0$. Since there is no heat conduction through the four insulated horizontal sides of the chamber, the spatial temperature gradient must be zero at the four horizontal sides. Therefore, the boundary conditions are

$$\frac{\partial}{\partial x} T(0, y, t) = \frac{\partial}{\partial x} T(L_1, y, t) = 0 \qquad \frac{\partial}{\partial y} T(x, 0, t) = \frac{\partial}{\partial y} T(x, L_2, t) = 0 \tag{7.37}$$

To solve the partial differential Equation (7.35), we use separation of variables and let

$$T(x, y, t) \equiv X(x) Y(y) U(t) \tag{7.38}$$

Substituting Equation (7.38) into Equation (7.35), we get

$$\frac{c_h \rho_m}{\kappa} \frac{\partial}{\partial t} \left[X(x) Y(y) U(t) \right] = \frac{\partial^2}{\partial x^2} \left[X(x) Y(y) U(t) \right] + \frac{\partial^2}{\partial y^2} \left[X(x) Y(y) U(t) \right]$$

$$\frac{c_h \rho_m}{\kappa} X(x) Y(y) U'(t) = X''(x) Y(y) U(t) + X(x) Y''(y) U(t)$$

Dividing both sides by $X(x) Y(y) U(t)$, we have

$$\frac{c_h \rho_m}{\kappa} \frac{U'(t)}{U(t)} = \frac{X''(x)}{X(x)} + \frac{Y''(y)}{Y(y)} \tag{7.39}$$

For Equation (7.39), the left-hand side depends only on t, while the right-hand side depends only on x and y. Hence, Equation (7.39) is satisfied if and only if both sides are constant. Letting this constant be $-\lambda_+$ (as we will see later, this constant must be negative), we have

$$\frac{c_h \rho_m}{\kappa} \frac{U'(t)}{U(t)} = -\lambda_+ = \frac{X''(x)}{X(x)} + \frac{Y''(y)}{Y(y)}$$

Using a similar logic, the two terms on the right side of Equation (7.39) must also be constants:

$$\frac{X''(x)}{X(x)} = -k_x^2 \qquad \frac{Y''(y)}{Y(y)} = -k_y^2 \qquad \frac{c_h \rho_m}{\kappa} \frac{U'(t)}{U(t)} = -\lambda_+ = -\left(k_x^2 + k_y^2\right) \quad (7.40)$$

We start by solving the equation for $U(t)$. Since the first derivative $U'(t)$ is proportional to $U(t)$, $U(t)$ must be an exponential function. Letting $A_{m,n}$ be an arbitrary constant, we have

$$U'(t) = -\frac{\lambda_+ \kappa}{c_h \rho_m} U(t) \quad \Rightarrow \quad U(t) = A_{m,n} \exp\left(-\frac{\lambda_+ \kappa}{c_h \rho_m} t\right) \quad (7.41)$$

Because κ, c_h, and ρ_m are all positive physical constants, λ_+ must be a positive constant or else $U(t \to \infty)$ will diverge to infinity (note that $t \geq 0$). Thus, our assumption that the constant $-\lambda_+$ is negative must be correct. To solve the equation for $X(x)$, we have

$$X''(x) = -k_x^2\, X(x) \quad \Rightarrow \quad X(x) = A\sin(k_x x) + B\cos(k_x x)$$

Using the boundary condition in Equation (7.37), we get

$$\frac{\partial}{\partial x} T(0,y,t) = \frac{\partial}{\partial x} T(L_1,y,t) = 0 \quad \Rightarrow \quad X'(0)Y(y)U(t) = X'(L_1)Y(y)U(t) = 0$$

$$\text{Therefore, } X'(0) = X'(L_1) = 0$$

With $X'(x) = A\,k_x\cos(k_x x) - B\,k_x\sin(k_x x)$, we obtain

$$X'(0) = A\,k_x\cos(0) - B\,k_x\sin(0) = A\,k_x = 0 \quad \Rightarrow \quad A = 0$$

Note that we cannot have $k_x = 0$, or else we would end up with the incorrect solution $X(x) = B$. Furthermore, we have

$$X'(L_1) = A\,k_x\cos(k_x L_1) - B\,k_x\sin(k_x L_1) = -B\,k_x\sin(k_x L_1) = 0 \quad \Rightarrow \quad \sin(k_x L_1) = 0$$

To avoid the trivial solution $X(x) = 0$, we cannot have $B = 0$. Therefore,

$$k_x L_1 = m\pi \quad \Rightarrow \quad k_x = \frac{m\pi}{L_1} \quad \text{where} \quad m = 0,1,2,3,\ldots$$

Since $A = 0$, we have $X(x) = B\cos(k_x x)$ and

$$X(x) = B_m \cos\left(\frac{m\pi}{L_1} x\right) \quad \text{where} \quad m = 0,1,2,3,\ldots \quad (7.42)$$

Using the same procedure, we can obtain $Y(y)$:

$$k_y = \frac{n\pi}{L_2} \quad \Rightarrow \quad Y(y) = B_n \cos\left(\frac{n\pi}{L_2} y\right) \quad \text{where} \quad n = 0,1,2,3,\ldots \quad (7.43)$$

Putting everything together, we have

$$T_{m,n}(x,y,t) = X(x)Y(y)U(t) = \left[B_m \cos\left(\frac{m\pi}{L_1}x\right)\right]\left[B_n \cos\left(\frac{n\pi}{L_2}y\right)\right]\left[A_{m,n}\exp\left(-\frac{\lambda_+\kappa}{c_h\rho_m}t\right)\right]$$

$$T_{m,n}(x,y,t) = C_{m,n}\cos\left(\frac{m\pi}{L_1}x\right)\cos\left(\frac{n\pi}{L_2}y\right)\exp\left(-\frac{\lambda_+\kappa}{c_h\rho_m}t\right) \qquad \begin{cases} m = 0,1,2,3,\ldots \\ n = 0,1,2,3,\ldots \end{cases}$$

where $C_{m,n} = B_m B_n A_{m,n}$ is an arbitrary constant that depends on both m and n.

The full solution for the temperature $T(x,y,t)$ is obtained by a double sum of all eigenmodes of $T_{m,n}(x,y,t)$ which together contain all possible combinations of m and n:

$$T(x,y,t) = \sum_{m=0}^{\infty}\sum_{n=0}^{\infty}T_{m,n}(x,y,t) \quad \text{and if we let} \quad \tau_{m,n} = \frac{c_h\rho_m}{\lambda_+\kappa} = \frac{c_h\rho_m}{\left(k_x^2 + k_y^2\right)\kappa}$$

we have $\quad \tau_{m,n} = \dfrac{c_h\rho_m}{\left[\left(m\pi/L_1\right)^2 + \left(n\pi/L_2\right)^2\right]\kappa} = \dfrac{c_h\rho_m}{\left[\left(m/L_1\right)^2 + \left(n/L_2\right)^2\right]\kappa\pi^2}$

Therefore, the full solution $T(x,y,t)$ to the 2D heat equation is

$$T(x,y,t) = \sum_{m=0}^{\infty}\sum_{n=0}^{\infty}C_{m,n}\cos\left(\frac{m\pi}{L_1}x\right)\cos\left(\frac{n\pi}{L_2}y\right)\exp\left(-\frac{t}{\tau_{m,n}}\right) \tag{7.44A}$$

$$\text{where} \quad \begin{cases} m = 0,1,2,3,\ldots \\ n = 0,1,2,3,\ldots \end{cases} \quad \text{and} \quad \tau_{m,n} = \frac{c_h\rho_m}{\left[\left(m/L_1\right)^2 + \left(n/L_2\right)^2\right]\kappa\pi^2} \tag{7.44B}$$

When $m = 0$ and $n = 0$, we have $\tau_{0,0} \to \infty$ and

$$T_{0,0}(x,y,t) = C_{0,0}\cos(0)\cos(0)\exp(0) = C_{0,0} = \text{a constant}$$

The first eigenmode corresponds to $m = 1$ and $n = 1$. It is given by

$$T_{1,1}(x,y,t) = C_{1,1}\cos\left(\frac{\pi}{L_1}x\right)\cos\left(\frac{\pi}{L_2}y\right)\exp\left(-\frac{t}{\tau_{1,1}}\right) \quad \text{where} \quad \tau_{1,1} = \frac{c_h\rho_m}{\left(L_1^{-2} + L_2^{-2}\right)\kappa\pi^2} \tag{7.45}$$

For the temperature function $T(x,y,t)$, an important term is the exponential decay term $\exp(-t/\tau_{m,n})$ which describes the dissipation of heat through the fluid within the microchamber during the reaction. The time constant $\tau_{m,n} = R_t C_t$ can be considered as the product of thermal resistance R_t (i.e., generalized resistance) and heat capacity C_t (i.e., generalized capacitance). This is similar to the RC time constant of an electrical circuit which is the product of electrical resistance and capacitance. To find an approximate value for the thermal resistance $R_{t,\text{chamber}}$ and heat capacity $C_{t,\text{chamber}}$ of fluid in the microchamber, we consider only the first eigenmode corresponding to $m = 1$ and $n = 1$:

$$\tau_{1,1} = \frac{c_h\rho_m}{\left(L_1^{-2} + L_2^{-2}\right)\kappa\pi^2} \cong R_{t,\text{chamber}}C_{t,\text{chamber}} \tag{7.46}$$

Our next task is to find expressions for both $R_{t,\text{chamber}}$ and $C_{t,\text{chamber}}$. The heat capacity $C_{t,\text{chamber}}$ of fluid in the microchamber is defined as follows:

$$C_{t,\text{chamber}} = mc_h \cong \rho_m V_{\text{mode}(1,1)}c_h \tag{7.47}$$

where m is the mass, c_h is the specific heat capacity, ρ_m is the mass density, and $V_{\text{mode}(m,n)}$ represents the mode volume of the spatial temperature distribution of fluid in the microchamber. The mode volume $V_{\text{mode}(m,n)}$ is given by the following volume integral which is integrated over the entire volume of the microchamber. The absolute value sign ensures that the mode volume is always positive.

$$V_{\text{mode}(m,n)} = \iiint_{\text{Volume}} \left| \cos\left(\frac{m\pi}{L_1}x\right) \cos\left(\frac{n\pi}{L_2}y\right) \right| dV \tag{7.48}$$

It can be shown that

$$V_{\text{mode}(1,1)} = \frac{4}{\pi^2}L_1 L_2 H \quad \Rightarrow \quad C_{t,\text{chamber}} \cong \rho_m c_h V_{\text{mode}(1,1)} = \frac{4}{\pi^2}\rho_m c_h L_1 L_2 H \tag{7.49}$$

Combining Equations (7.46) and (7.49), we can obtain approximate expressions for the thermal resistance $R_{t,\text{chamber}}$ and heat capacity $C_{t,\text{chamber}}$ of fluid in the modified batch PCR microchamber. They are

$$R_{t,\text{chamber}} \cong \frac{\tau_{1,1}}{C_{t,\text{chamber}}} = \frac{\dfrac{c_h \rho_m}{\left(L_1^{-2} + L_2^{-2}\right)\kappa\pi^2}}{\dfrac{4}{\pi^2}\rho_m c_h L_1 L_2 H} = \frac{1}{4\left(L_1^{-2} + L_2^{-2}\right)\kappa L_1 L_2 H} = \frac{L_1 L_2}{4\kappa\left(L_1^2 + L_2^2\right)H}$$

$$R_{t,\text{chamber}} \cong \frac{1}{4\kappa_{\text{fluid}}}\left|\frac{L_1 L_2}{\left(L_1^2 + L_2^2\right)H}\right|_{\text{chamber}} \quad \text{and} \quad C_{t,\text{chamber}} \cong \frac{4\left(\rho_m c_h\right)_{\text{fluid}}}{\pi^2}\left(L_1 L_2 H\right)_{\text{chamber}} \tag{7.50}$$

EXAMPLE 7-4 Recall that we used the 2D heat equation as given below (left) to model the fluid temperature inside the modified batch PCR microchamber. In addition, we used the boundary conditions given below (right).

$$c_h \rho_m \frac{\partial T}{\partial t} = \kappa\nabla^2 T + S \quad \text{where} \quad \frac{\partial}{\partial x}T(0,y,t) = \frac{\partial}{\partial x}T(L_1,y,t) = \frac{\partial}{\partial y}T(x,0,t) = \frac{\partial}{\partial y}T(x,L_2,t) = 0$$

(a) Show that the solution we derived as given in Equation (7.44) satisfies both the 2D heat equation with no heat generation (i.e., $S = 0$) as well as the two boundary conditions.

(b) Use Equation (7.48) to prove that the mode volume of the first eigenmode is given by

$$V_{\text{mode}(1,1)} = \frac{4}{\pi^2}L_1 L_2 H$$

Solution

(a) We want to show that the full solution $T(x,y,t)$ as given by the double sum in Equation (7.44) satisfies the 2D heat equation and the two boundary conditions. To do this, we need to show that all eigenmodes $T_{m,n}(x,y,t)$ within the double sum satisfy the heat equation and the boundary conditions.

$$T(x,y,t) = \sum_{m=0}^{\infty}\sum_{n=0}^{\infty}T_{m,n}(x,y,t) \quad \text{where} \quad T_{m,n}(x,y,t) = C_{m,n}\cos\left(\frac{m\pi}{L_1}x\right)\cos\left(\frac{n\pi}{L_2}y\right)\exp\left(-\frac{t}{\tau_{m,n}}\right)$$

$$\frac{\partial T_{m,n}}{\partial t} = -\frac{1}{\tau_{m,n}}T_{m,n} \qquad \frac{\partial^2 T_{m,n}}{\partial x^2} = -\left(\frac{m\pi}{L_1}\right)^2 T_{m,n} \qquad \frac{\partial^2 T_{m,n}}{\partial y^2} = -\left(\frac{n\pi}{L_2}\right)^2 T_{m,n}$$

Using $S = 0$ and substituting $T = T_{m,n}$ into the 2D heat equation, we have

$$\frac{c_h \rho_m}{\kappa}\frac{\partial T_{m,n}}{\partial t} = \nabla^2 T = \frac{\partial^2 T_{m,n}}{\partial x^2} + \frac{\partial^2 T_{m,n}}{\partial y^2} \quad\Rightarrow\quad \frac{c_h \rho_m}{\kappa}\left(-\frac{1}{\tau_{m,n}}\right)T_{m,n} = -\left(\frac{m\pi}{L_1}\right)^2 T_{m,n} - \left(\frac{n\pi}{L_2}\right)^2 T_{m,n}$$

$$\frac{c_h \rho_m}{\kappa \tau_{m,n}} = \left[\left(\frac{m}{L_1}\right)^2 + \left(\frac{n}{L_2}\right)^2\right]\pi^2 \quad\Rightarrow\quad \tau_{m,n} = \frac{c_h \rho_m}{\left[\left(m/L_1\right)^2 + \left(n/L_2\right)^2\right]\kappa\pi^2}$$

Since the above equation (on the right) for $\tau_{m,n}$ matches the definition of $\tau_{m,n}$ in Equation (7.44B), all eigenmodes $T_{m,n}(x,y,t)$ and by extension the double sum given by $T(x,y,t)$ must satisfy the 2D heat equation with no heat generation. Next, we demonstrate that all eigenmodes $T_{m,n}(x,y,t)$ satisfy the two boundary conditions. Letting the "$\propto$" symbol represent proportionality, we have

$$\frac{\partial T_{m,n}}{\partial x} = -C_{m,n}\left(\frac{m\pi}{L_1}\right)\sin\left(\frac{m\pi}{L_1}x\right)\cos\left(\frac{n\pi}{L_2}y\right)\exp\left(-\frac{t}{\tau_{m,n}}\right) \quad\Rightarrow\quad \frac{\partial T_{m,n}}{\partial x} \propto \sin\left(\frac{m\pi}{L_1}x\right)$$

$$\frac{\partial}{\partial x}T_{m,n}(0,y,t) \propto \sin(0) = 0 \qquad\qquad \frac{\partial}{\partial x}T_{m,n}(L_1,y,t) \propto \sin(m\pi) = 0 \quad\text{since } m = 0,1,2,3,\ldots$$

$$\text{Thus,} \quad \frac{\partial}{\partial x}T_{m,n}(x=0,y,t) = \frac{\partial}{\partial x}T_{m,n}(x=L_1,y,t) = 0$$

We can use the same argument to show that

$$\frac{\partial}{\partial y}T_{m,n}(x,0,t) = \frac{\partial}{\partial y}T_{m,n}(x,L_2,t) = 0$$

(b) Starting with Equation (7.48) and letting $m = n = 1$, we have

$$V_{\text{mode}(1,1)} = \iiint_{\text{Volume}} \left|\cos\left(\frac{\pi}{L_1}x\right)\cos\left(\frac{\pi}{L_2}y\right)\right| dV = \int_0^H \int_0^{L_2} \int_0^{L_1} \left|\cos\left(\frac{\pi}{L_1}x\right)\right|\left|\cos\left(\frac{\pi}{L_2}y\right)\right| dx\, dy\, dz$$

$$\left\{0 \le x \le L_1 \quad 0 \le y \le L_2 \quad 0 \le z \le H\right\} \quad\text{(chamber boundaries)}$$

where we used the boundaries of the microchamber given in Equation (7.36). We can split the volume integral into three separate integrals as follows.

$$V_{\text{mode}(1,1)} = \left[\int_{x=0}^{x=L_1}\left|\cos\left(\frac{\pi}{L_1}x\right)\right| dx\right]\left[\int_{y=0}^{y=L_2}\left|\cos\left(\frac{\pi}{L_2}y\right)\right| dy\right]\left[\int_{z=0}^{z=H} dz\right]$$

Let $\theta_x = \frac{\pi}{L_1}x$ and $\theta_y = \frac{\pi}{L_2}y$ so that $dx = \frac{L_1}{\pi}d\theta_x$ and $dy = \frac{L_2}{\pi}d\theta_y$

$$V_{\text{mode}(1,1)} = \left[\int_{\theta_x=0}^{\theta_x=\pi}\left|\cos(\theta_x)\right|\frac{L_1}{\pi}d\theta_x\right]\left[\int_{\theta_y=0}^{\theta_y=\pi}\left|\cos(\theta_y)\right|\frac{L_2}{\pi}d\theta_y\right](H) = \frac{L_1 L_2 H}{\pi^2}\left[\int_0^\pi\left|\cos(\theta)\right| d\theta\right]^2$$

$$\text{Since } \begin{cases}\cos(\theta) \ge 0 \quad\text{for } 0 \le \theta \le \pi/2 \\ \cos(\theta) \le 0 \quad\text{for } \pi/2 \le \theta \le \pi\end{cases}, \text{ we can split the integral for } \left|\cos(\theta)\right| \text{ as follows:}$$

$$\int_0^\pi\left|\cos(\theta)\right| d\theta = \int_0^{\pi/2}\left|\cos(\theta)\right| d\theta + \int_{\pi/2}^\pi\left|\cos(\theta)\right| d\theta = \left|\sin(\theta)\right|_0^{\pi/2} + \left|\sin(\theta)\right|_{\pi/2}^\pi = |1-0| + |0-1| = 2$$

$$\text{Therefore,} \quad V_{\text{mode}(1,1)} = \frac{L_1 L_2 H}{\pi^2}(2)^2 = \frac{4}{\pi^2}L_1 L_2 H \quad\blacktriangle$$

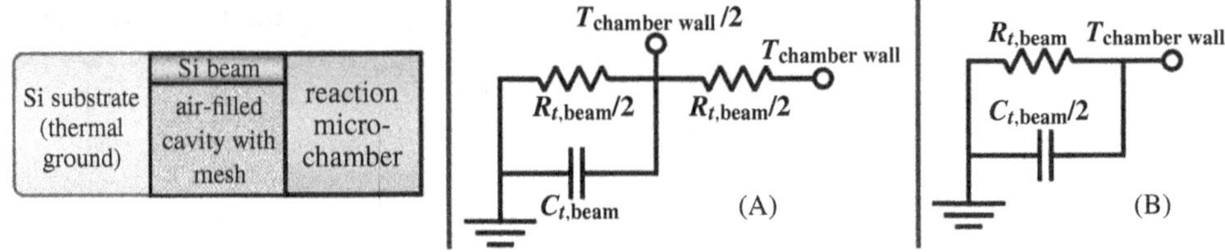

Figure 7-15   Modeling the silicon beam of the modified batch PCR microreactor developed by Daniel et al. (Left) Illustration of *a single silicon beam* connecting the silicon substrate (thermal ground) to the wall of the reaction microchamber. (A and B) Two lumped thermal equivalent circuit models representing *a single silicon beam* of the PCR microreactor.

(C) Thermal Equivalent Circuit of the Batch PCR Microreactor

We have shown in Example 7-3 that due to slow heating and cooling rates, the majority of PCR cycle time for macroscale PCR systems is spent on temperature ramping. If the temperature ramping is made faster and is controlled more precisely, the PCR system throughput will be improved. Northrup et al. accomplished this by utilizing PCR microreactors, while Daniel et al. used a combination of PCR microreactors and improved thermal isolation of each microreactor.[6,7]

The temperature response of the batch PCR microreactor can be understood using a lumped equivalent circuit comprised of various lumped circuit elements (i.e., discrete circuit components). As stated before, the modified PCR microchamber designed by Daniel et al. is supported by four silicon beams. We can use the lumped thermal equivalent circuit models shown in Figure 7-15 to model the thermal resistance $R_{t,\text{beam}}$ and heat capacity $C_{t,\text{beam}}$ of *one* beam. Since the potential variable in a thermal system is the temperature (analogous to voltage in electrical circuits), we can also include the microchamber wall temperature $T_{\text{chamber wall}}$ in our equivalent circuit. For simplicity, we will assume that all heat conduction between the silicon substrate and the microchamber is through the four silicon beams connected to the four horizontal sides of the chamber. Therefore, we ignore all heat conduction through the air-filled cavities that surround the four sides of the chamber, as well as through the top and bottom of the chamber. This assumption is reasonable since air with $\kappa = 0.03$ W/(m · K) has a far lower thermal conductivity than silicon with $\kappa = 150$ W/(m · K).

Beam Equivalent Circuit A[8]   This equivalent circuit of *one* silicon beam is shown in Figure 7-15A. In this circuit, the full heat capacity $C_{t,\text{beam}}$ of *one* beam in between two thermal resistors with resistances $R_{t,\text{beam}}/2$ is used. This circuit correctly models the full thermal resistance $R_{t,\text{beam}}$ between the substrate and the microchamber wall. Analogous to the ground reference point in electrical circuits, the silicon substrate is considered to be at thermal ground. At steady state, the temperature of the point where the capacitor is attached will be $T_{\text{chamber wall}}/2$. Using Equation (7.12), the steady-state thermal energy stored by the "capacitor" representing the beam with a temperature differential of $\Delta T_A = T_{\text{chamber wall}}/2$ is

$$\text{Energy Stored}_{(\text{Circuit A})} = C_{t,\text{beam}} \cdot \Delta T_A = \left(C_{t,\text{beam}}\right)\left(T_{\text{chamber wall}}/2\right) \qquad (7.51\text{A})$$

Beam Equivalent Circuit B[8]   This alternative equivalent circuit of *a single* silicon beam is shown in Figure 7-15B. Again, there is a thermal resistance of $R_{t,\text{beam}}$ between the microchamber wall and the substrate. However, the temperature differential across the "capacitor" is now $\Delta T_B = T_{\text{chamber wall}}$. To ensure that the thermal "capacitor" in circuit B stores the

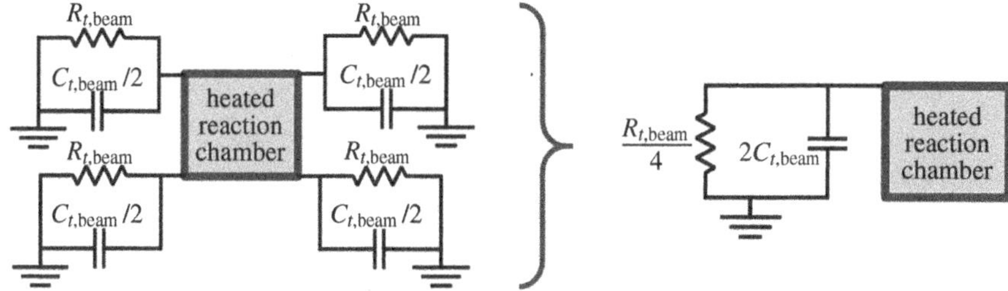

Figure 7-16   Modeling *all four silicon beams* of the modified batch PCR microreactor developed by Daniel et al. (Left) A thermal equivalent circuit of the PCR microreactor including all four beams. (Right) A simplified thermal equivalent circuit of the PCR microreactor *with all four beams* where we assume that the temperatures of the walls surrounding the four horizontal sides of the microchamber are the same.

same amount of thermal energy at steady state as the one in circuit A, the beam heat capacity is now given by $C_t/2$ such that

$$\text{Energy Stored}_{(\text{Circuit B})} = C_{t,\text{beam}} \cdot \Delta T_B = \left(C_{t,\text{beam}}/2\right)\left(T_{\text{chamber wall}}\right) \tag{7.51B}$$

Combined Equivalent Circuit   To model all four silicon beams together with fluid contained in the batch PCR microchamber, we will use **Circuit B** to represent each of the four beams, as shown in Figure 7-16 (left). For simplicity, we assume that the temperatures of the walls surrounding the four horizontal sides of the microchamber are the same, and let this chamber wall temperature be $T_{\text{chamber wall}}$. Analogous to electrical resistance, the thermal resistance $R_{t,\text{beam}}$ of the silicon beam can be expressed as

$$R_{t,\text{beam}} = \frac{1}{\kappa_{\text{Si}}}\left(\frac{\ell}{A}\right)_{\text{beam}} \qquad \left[\text{ analogous to } R_{\text{electrical}} = \rho_r\left(\frac{\ell}{A}\right)_{\text{resistor}}\right] \tag{7.52}$$

where κ_{Si} is the thermal conductivity of silicon, ℓ is the length of the beam, and A is the cross-sectional area of the beam. As shown in Figure 7-16, the parallel thermal resistances of the four silicon beams can be combined as

$$R_{t,\text{beam}}\| R_{t,\text{beam}}\| R_{t,\text{beam}}\| R_{t,\text{beam}} = R_{t,\text{beam}}/4 \tag{7.53}$$

The heat capacity $C_{t,\text{beam}}$ of the silicon beam (representing the thermal "capacitance" of the beam) is

$$C_{t,\text{beam}} = \left(m_{\text{beam}}\right)\left(c_{h,\text{Si}}\right) = \left(\rho_{m,\text{Si}}\right)\left(V_{\text{beam}}\right)\left(c_{h,\text{Si}}\right) = \left(\rho_{m,\text{Si}}\right)\left(c_{h,\text{Si}}\right)\left(\ell A\right)_{\text{beam}} \tag{7.54}$$

where $\rho_{m,\text{Si}}$ is the mass density of silicon, $c_{h,\text{Si}}$ is the specific heat capacity of silicon, and $(\ell A)_{\text{beam}}$ is the volume of *one* silicon beam.

Similar to the parallel thermal resistances, the parallel thermal "capacitances" (i.e., heat capacities) of the four beams can be combined as (Figure 7-16, right)

$$\frac{C_{t,\text{beam}}}{2}\left\|\frac{C_{t,\text{beam}}}{2}\right\|\frac{C_{t,\text{beam}}}{2}\left\|\frac{C_{t,\text{beam}}}{2}\right. = 2C_{t,\text{beam}} \tag{7.55}$$

Now, we model the fluid contained in the microchamber using the thermal resistance $R_{t,\text{chamber}}$ connected in series with the heat capacity $C_{t,\text{chamber}}$ attached between the chamber wall and thermal ground (i.e., the substrate). Recall that the microchamber design reported by Daniel et al. is heated using Joule heating of platinum thin film resistors. The thermal

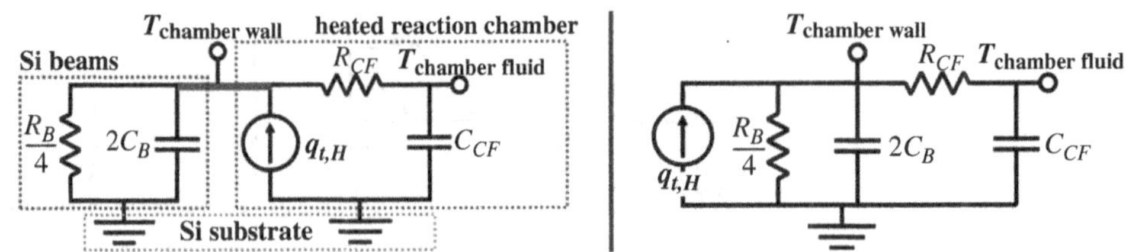

Figure 7-17   Two complete lumped-element thermal models of the modified batch PCR microreactor developed by Daniel et al. The left and right thermal circuit models are entirely equivalent.

power [i.e., heat flow rate (W)] $q_{t,H} = dQ_{t,H}/dt$ generated by Joule heating (H) of the resistors is modeled as a thermal current source.

Combining the thermal models of the microchamber and of the four silicon beams, a complete lumped-element model for the batch PCR microreactor developed by Daniel et al. can be generated, which is illustrated as a combined thermal equivalent circuit in Figure 7-17.

The four passive elements of the equivalent circuit are given as follows:

$$\begin{cases} \{R_B \equiv R_{t,\text{beam}} = \dfrac{1}{\kappa_{\text{Si}}}\left(\dfrac{\ell}{A}\right)_{\text{beam}} \\ C_B \equiv C_{t,\text{beam}} = (\rho_{m,\text{Si}})(c_{h,\text{Si}})(\ell A)_{\text{beam}} \end{cases} \quad \begin{cases} R_{CF} \equiv R_{t,\text{chamber}} \simeq \dfrac{1}{4\kappa_{\text{fluid}}}\left|\dfrac{L_1 L_2}{(L_1^2 + L_2^2)H}\right|_{\text{chamber}} \\ C_{CF} \equiv C_{t,\text{chamber}} \simeq \dfrac{4(\rho_m c_h)_{\text{fluid}}}{\pi^2}(L_1 L_2 H)_{\text{chamber}} \end{cases} \quad (7.56)$$

where B stands for beam and CF stands for chamber fluid. Using the equivalent circuit in Figure 7-17 along with standard circuit analysis techniques, it can be shown that the thermal transfer functions in the Laplace domain are given by

$$T_{\text{chamber wall}}(s) = \frac{\dfrac{1}{4}R_B\left(1 + sR_{CF}C_{CF}\right)}{\left(\dfrac{1}{2}R_B C_B R_{CF}C_{CF}\right)s^2 + \left[\dfrac{1}{2}R_B C_B + \left(R_{CF} + \dfrac{1}{4}R_B\right)C_{CF}\right]s + 1}\, q_{t,H}(s) \quad (7.57)$$

$$T_{\text{chamber fluid}}(s) = \frac{1}{1 + \left(R_{CF}C_{CF}\right)s}\, T_{\text{chamber wall}}(s) \quad (7.58)$$

where $T_{\text{chamber wall}}$ is the temperature of the microchamber walls, $T_{\text{chamber fluid}}$ is the temperature of fluid inside the microchamber, and $q_{t,H}$ is the thermal power generated by Joule heating of the Pt resistors. From Equation (7.58), the relationship between the chamber fluid temperature $T_{\text{chamber fluid}}(s)$ and the chamber wall temperature $T_{\text{chamber wall}}(s)$ corresponds to a single-pole response.

To carry out the denaturing, annealing, and extension steps of PCR cycles, the temperature of the PCR solution (i.e., fluid) within the microchamber needs to be accurately controlled. Control of the PCR fluid temperature can be accomplished with a temperature feedback loop in two different ways.

The first method is to use the microchamber wall temperature for feedback (Figure 7-18a). Because the silicon microchamber walls are thin and thermally isolated, the chamber walls respond quickly to temperature changes. However, the temperature of the PCR fluid within the microchamber lags far behind the wall temperature, indicating a great delay of the PCR fluid temperature response. As in an RC circuit, the time delay of the PCR fluid temperature response is about $3\,\tau_{\text{CF(batch)}} = 3\,R_{CF}C_{CF}$. This is the time required for the fluid to reach ~95% of the wall temperature. From (Figure 7-18a), it can be estimated that

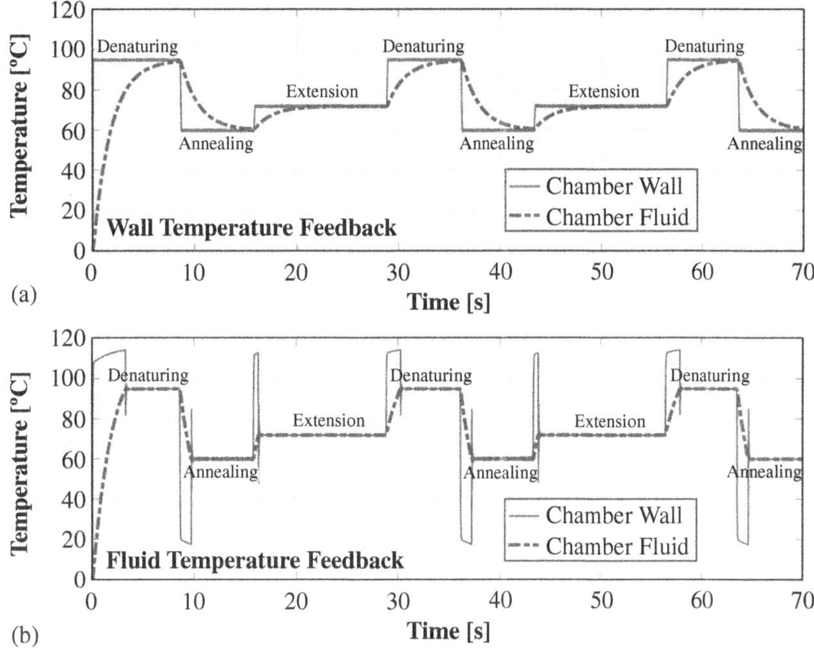

Figure 7-18   Microchamber wall temperature and PCR fluid temperature versus time with feedback temperature control.[7,8] (a) The microchamber wall temperature is used for feedback. (b) The PCR fluid temperature is used for feedback. (*The two plots were drawn using Simulink® in MATLAB® based on ideas from S. D. Senturia.*[8])

$3\,\tau_{CF(batch)} \cong 5$ s. This time delay is enough to slow down (i.e., increase) the time required for every PCR cycle. To fix this problem, other methods have been attempted to control the fluid temperature. The slow temperature response of the PCR fluid is due to the significantly lower thermal conductivity and higher specific heat capacity of water and water-based solutions compared to silicon, as shown below.[7,8]

$$\text{Water and water-based solutions:} \begin{cases} \kappa = 0.6 \text{ W}/(\text{m} \cdot \text{K}) \\ c_h = 4180 \text{ J}/(\text{kg} \cdot \text{K}) \end{cases} \text{Silicon:} \begin{cases} \kappa = 150 \text{ W}/(\text{m} \cdot \text{K}) \\ c_h = 700 \text{ J}/(\text{kg} \cdot \text{K}) \end{cases} \quad (7.59)$$

A second method is to use the temperature of the PCR fluid within the microchamber for feedback (Figure 7-18b). Compared with the first method, the main advantage of the second method is that the PCR fluid responds significantly faster to temperature changes, greatly reducing the time delays required to achieve the temperature set points. However, this feedback method is at the cost of wall temperature overshooting and undershooting. The wall temperature overshoots and undershoots to ensure that the PCR fluid temperature reaches the target temperature over a much shorter time span. Overshooting may adversely affect PCR reagents and can even cause boiling if the overshoot temperature exceeds the boiling point of water. Boiling of the PCR solution results in bubble formation, which causes large temperature differences in the PCR fluid as well as fluid loss.[5,8]

If the batch PCR microreactor system is to be used, there are a few options. First, one can use the first method (i.e., use wall temperature for feedback) and accept the time delay of the wall-to-fluid temperature response and lower throughput. Alternatively, one can use a more sophisticated temperature controller that uses both the wall temperature and the fluid temperature for feedback in order to reduce wall temperature overshoots while maintaining the faster temperature response of the second method. In addition, adding resistive heaters below the microchamber and/or reducing the microchamber volume would also speed up the temperature response of the PCR fluid inside the chamber.[8]

EXAMPLE 7-5 Characteristics of the modified batch PCR microreactor by Daniel et al.

(a) Use the equivalent circuits shown in Figure 7-17 to derive the thermal transfer function in the Laplace domain for $T_{\text{chamber wall}}(s)$ as shown in Equation (7.57).

(b) Derive the expression for $T_{\text{chamber fluid}}(s)$ as shown in Equation (7.58).

(c) Calculate the thermal time constant $\tau_{\text{CF(batch)}} = R_{CF}C_{CF}$ of PCR fluid within the heated reaction microchamber. Show that it takes $3\,\tau_{\text{CF(batch)}}$ for the fluid to reach ~95% of the microchamber wall temperature. Assume that the microchamber has dimensions of 2.2 mm × 2.2 mm × 400 μm.

Solution

(a) To derive the transfer function for $T_{\text{chamber wall}}(s)$ in the Laplace domain, we start by bundling all four passive circuit elements $R_B/4$, $2\,C_B$, R_{CF}, and C_{CF} together into a single equivalent impedance. As depicted in Figure 7-19, this equivalent impedance Z_{eq} is given by

$$Z_{\text{eq}} = \left(\frac{R_B}{4}\right) \| 2C_B \| (R_{CF} + C_{CF}) \quad \Rightarrow \quad Z_{\text{eq}}(s) = \left(\frac{R_B}{4}\right) \| \frac{1}{s(2C_B)} \| \left(R_{CF} + \frac{1}{sC_{CF}}\right)$$

Note that in the Laplace domain, the impedance of a resistor R is R (i.e., the same), while the impedance of a capacitor C is $1/(sC)$. From Figure 7-19 (right), we can deduce that

$$T_{\text{chamber wall}}(s) = Z_{\text{eq}}(s) \cdot q_{t,H}(s)$$

Our next task is to derive an expression for $Z_{\text{eq}}(s)$. We have

$$Z_{\text{eq}}^{-1}(s) = \left(\frac{R_B}{4}\right)^{-1} + \left[\frac{1}{s(2C_B)}\right]^{-1} + \left(R_{CF} + \frac{1}{sC_{CF}}\right)^{-1} = \frac{4}{R_B} + 2sC_B + \frac{sC_{CF}}{sR_{CF}C_{CF} + 1}$$

$$Z_{\text{eq}}^{-1}(s) = \frac{1}{R_B}\left(4 + 2sR_BC_B + \frac{sR_BC_{CF}}{sR_{CF}C_{CF} + 1}\right) = \frac{4}{R_B}\left[\frac{\left(1 + \frac{1}{2}sR_BC_B\right)(sR_{CF}C_{CF} + 1) + \frac{1}{4}sR_BC_{CF}}{sR_{CF}C_{CF} + 1}\right]$$

$$Z_{\text{eq}}(s) = \frac{\frac{1}{4}R_B(sR_{CF}C_{CF} + 1)}{\left(\frac{1}{2}R_BC_BR_{CF}C_{CF}\right)s^2 + \left[\frac{1}{2}R_BC_B + \left(R_{CF} + \frac{1}{4}R_B\right)C_{CF}\right]s + 1}$$

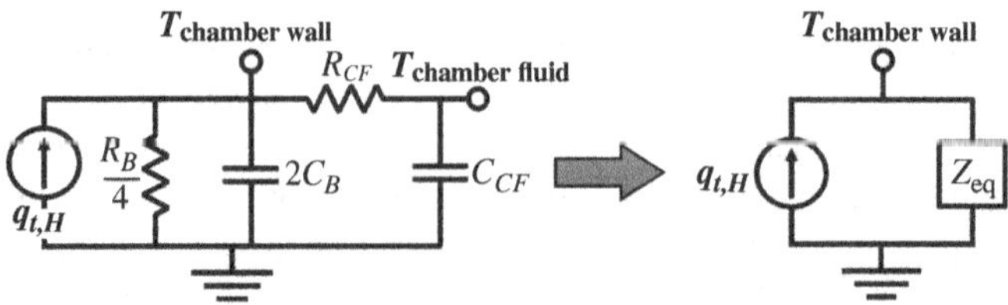

Figure 7-19 To simplify the lumped-element thermal model of the modified batch PCR microreactor developed by Daniel et al. (left), we combine all four passive elements $R_B/4$, $2\,C_B$, R_{CF}, and C_{CF} into a single equivalent impedance Z_{eq} (right).

Using $T_{\text{chamber wall}}(s) = Z_{eq}(s) \cdot q_{t,H}(s)$, we can finally prove Equation (7.57):

$$T_{\text{chamber wall}}(s) = \frac{\frac{1}{4}R_B\left(1 + sR_{CF}C_{CF}\right)}{\left(\frac{1}{2}R_BC_BR_{CF}C_{CF}\right)s^2 + \left[\frac{1}{2}R_BC_B + \left(R_{CF} + \frac{1}{4}R_B\right)C_{CF}\right]s + 1}\,q_{t,H}(s)$$

(b) To obtain $T_{\text{chamber fluid}}(s)$ and prove Equation (7.58), we can use a "voltage" divider as shown on the right. Noting that the impedance of R_{CF} is R_{CF} and that the impedance of C_{CF} is $1/sC_{CF}$, we have

$$T_{\text{chamber fluid}}(s) = \frac{\left(\dfrac{1}{sC_{CF}}\right)}{R_{CF} + \left(\dfrac{1}{sC_{CF}}\right)}\,T_{\text{chamber wall}}(s)$$

$$T_{\text{chamber fluid}}(s) = \frac{1}{1 + \left(R_{CF}C_{CF}\right)s}\,T_{\text{chamber wall}}(s)$$

(c) To calculate the thermal time constant $\tau_{CF(\text{batch})} = R_{CF}C_{CF}$, we will use Equation (7.46):

$$\tau_{CF(\text{batch})} = R_{CF}C_{CF} \cong \tau_{1,1} = \frac{c_h\rho_m}{\left(L_1^{-2} + L_2^{-2}\right)\kappa\pi^2} = \frac{1}{\pi^2}\left(\frac{\rho_m c_h}{\kappa}\right)_{\text{fluid}}\left(\frac{1}{L_1^{-2} + L_2^{-2}}\right)_{\text{chamber}}$$

Since the PCR fluid is a water-based solution, we have

$$\kappa \cong \kappa_{\text{water}} = 0.6\ \text{W}/(\text{m}\cdot\text{K}) \qquad c_h \cong c_{h(\text{water})} = 4180\ \text{J}/(\text{kg}\cdot\text{K})$$

Furthermore, we have $L_1 = L_2 = 2.2$ mm. Hence,

$$\tau_{CF(\text{batch})} \cong \frac{1}{\pi^2}\cdot\frac{\left(1000\ \text{kg}/\text{m}^3\right)\left[4180\ \text{J}/(\text{kg}\cdot\text{K})\right]}{\left[0.6\ \text{W}/(\text{m}\cdot\text{K})\right]}\cdot\frac{1}{2\cdot\left(2.2\times10^{-3}\ \text{m}\right)^{-2}} = 1.71\ \text{s}$$

Similar to an RC circuit, the time taken by the fluid to reach ~95% of the microchamber wall temperature is $n\cdot\tau_{CF}$, where n is given by

$$95\% = 0.95 = 1 - \frac{1}{e^n} \quad\Rightarrow\quad 0.05 = \frac{1}{e^n} \quad\Rightarrow\quad n = \ln\left(\frac{1}{0.05}\right) = 2.996 \cong 3$$

Thus, it takes about $3\tau_{CF(\text{batch})} \cong 5.13$ s for the fluid to reach ~95% of the wall temperature, which agrees with the estimate of $3\tau_{CF(\text{batch})} \cong 5$ s that we obtained from (Figure 7-18a). ▲

7.2.2 Continuous-Flow PCR Microreactors

(A) Continuous-Flow PCR Microreactor Overview

In the batch PCR microreactor, the denaturing, annealing and extension steps of a PCR cycle are carried out in a fixed volume chamber whose temperature is cycled. In 1998, Kopp et al. developed a continuous-flow PCR microreactor (Figure 7-20). In the continuous-flow microreactor, the denaturing (95°C), annealing (60°C) and extension (77°C) steps are completed in three well-defined zones while the PCR sample fluid flows in a single microchannel repetitively through the individual temperature zones. The microchannels etched into the glass chip substrate all have dimensions of 40 μm (depth) by 90 μm (width). The PCR fluid is introduced by syringe pumps into the microchannel through fused-silica capillaries

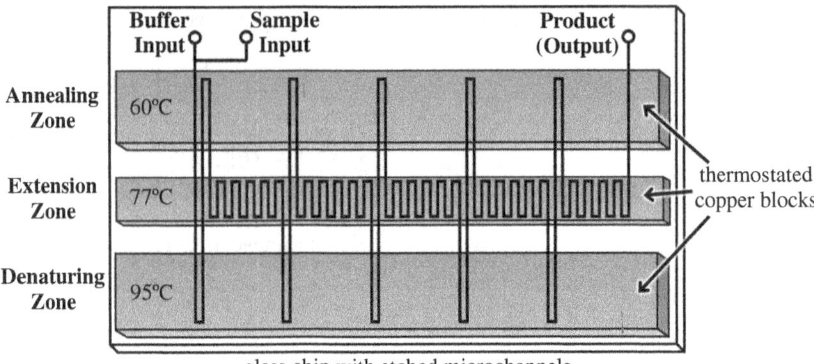

Figure 7-20   Layout of the continuous-flow PCR microreactor. (*The schematic is redrawn and reprinted with permission from M. U. Kopp et al.*[9])

glued to the holes in the cover plate. The glass chip substrate is clamped to a support containing three thermostated copper blocks for the three temperatures zones on the chip. That is, the temperatures of the copper blocks are controlled by thermostats. Heating cartridges are used to heat the copper blocks, while passive cooling fins are used to cool the blocks. The time spent on heating and cooling during every PCR cycle is less than 100 ms each.[9]

In the continuous-flow PCR microreactor, the path lengths in the three temperature zones are different. In the denaturing step of the first PCR cycle, extra length is given to allow sufficient time for the initial denaturing of the input room temperature PCR fluid. Similarly, the extension zone has longer path lengths because the extension step takes more time to complete than the denaturing or annealing steps. To reduce adsorption of PCR reactants onto the glass surfaces of microchannel walls, the microchannel wall surfaces are modified statically and dynamically. The static surface modification is achieved by silanization of the glass surface with dichlorodimethylsilane. For the dynamic surface modification, a nonionic surfactant mixed with a zwitterionic buffer is used as the PCR buffer. This buffer introduces a dynamic coating on the microchannel walls.[9]

The continuous-flow PCR microreactor can amplify DNA within tiny volumes of PCR solution. When 10 μL of PCR solution is run at 5.8 to 72.9 nL/s, the total flow-through time is 18.7 min to 1.5 min for 20 PCR cycles. In contrast, a fast commercial thermal cycler (Thermo Hybaid PCR Express) took a total of 50 min to complete 20 PCR cycles starting with 10 μL of PCR solution.[9]

(B) Modeling the Continuous-Flow PCR Microreactor

The continuous-flow PCR microreactor can be modeled in the same fashion as the batch PCR microreactor, but with L_1 = microchannel depth = 40 μm and L_2 = microchannel width = 90 μm. Similar to the reaction microchamber of the batch PCR microreactor, the thermal time constant τ_{CF} of fluid within the microchannels of the continuous-flow PCR microreactor is given by Equation (7.46). Letting CF represent channel fluid within the continuous-flow microreactor, we have

$$\tau_{CF(\text{continuous flow})} = R_{CF}C_{CF} \cong \tau_{1,1} = \frac{1}{\pi^2}\left(\frac{\rho_m c_h}{\kappa}\right)_{\text{fluid}}\left(\frac{1}{L_1^{-2}+L_2^{-2}}\right)_{\text{microchannel}} \tag{7.60}$$

$$\tau_{CF(\text{continuous flow})} \cong \frac{1}{\pi^2}\cdot\frac{\left(1000\ \text{kg/m}^3\right)\left[4180\ \text{J/(kg}\cdot\text{K)}\right]}{\left[0.6\ \text{W/(m}\cdot\text{K)}\right]}\cdot\frac{1}{\left(40\ \mu\text{m}\right)^{-2}+\left(90\ \mu\text{m}\right)^{-2}} = 0.943\ \text{ms}$$

Recall that fluid within the microchamber of the batch PCR microreactor had a thermal time constant of $\tau_{CF(batch)} \cong 1.71\,\text{s}$. As calculated below, the thermal response of the continuous-flow PCR microreactor is ~1800 times faster than the batch PCR microreactor.

$$\frac{\tau_{CF(batch)}}{\tau_{CF(continuous\ flow)}} = \frac{1.71\ \text{s}}{0.943\ \text{ms}} \cong 1800 \tag{7.61}$$

For the continuous-flow PCR microreactor, it takes about $3\,\tau_{CF}$ for the fluid to reach ~95% of the copper block temperature, since $1 - 1/e^3 \cong 95\%$. We can define a length $L_{\text{thermal equilibrium}}$ which corresponds to the length traveled by the PCR fluid through the microchannel during the time required for the fluid to reach ~95% of the copper block temperature. Therefore, we have

$$L_{\text{thermal equilibrium}} \cong 3\tau_{CF}v_{\text{fluid}} = 3\tau_{CF}\frac{Q_{\text{fluid flow}}}{A_{\text{channel}}} = 3\tau_{CF(continuous\ flow)}\frac{Q_{\text{fluid flow}}}{L_1 L_2} \tag{7.62}$$

where v_{fluid} is the velocity and $Q_{\text{fluid flow}}$ is the volumetric flow rate of PCR fluid in the microchannels. $A_{\text{channel}} = L_1 L_2$ is the cross-sectional area of the microchannels. Because the volumetric flow rate $Q_{\text{fluid flow}}$ is between 5.8 nL/s and 72.9 nL/s for the continuous-flow device, we have

$$L_{\text{thermal equilibrium (min)}} \cong 3(0.943\ \text{ms})\frac{5.8\times10^{-12}\,\text{m}^3/\text{s}}{(40\ \mu\text{m})(90\ \mu\text{m})} = 4.56\ \mu\text{m}$$

$$L_{\text{thermal equilibrium (max)}} \cong 3(0.943\ \text{ms})\frac{72.9\times10^{-12}\,\text{m}^3/\text{s}}{(40\ \mu\text{m})(90\ \mu\text{m})} = 57.3\ \mu\text{m}$$

$$L_{\text{thermal equilibrium}} \ll \text{microchannel length} \cong 5\ \text{to}\ 10\ \text{mm} \tag{7.63}$$

$L_{\text{thermal equilibrium}}$ is far smaller than the lengths of the microchannels within each temperature zone, which is on the order of 5 to 10 mm. Hence, the PCR fluid can reach the desired temperature for denaturing, annealing, or extension almost instantly after reaching the associated zone. This is a major advantage compared to the batch PCR microreactor. Using the approximation that the characteristic length $L \cong L_2 = 90\ \mu\text{m}$, we can compute the Reynolds number of fluid flow within the microchannels of the continuous-flow microreactor as follows.

$$\text{Re} = \frac{\rho_m L}{\eta}v_{\text{fluid}} \cong \frac{\rho_m L_2}{\eta}\left(\frac{Q_{\text{fluid flow}}}{L_1 L_2}\right) = \frac{\rho_m Q_{\text{fluid flow}}}{\eta L_1} \tag{7.64}$$

$$\text{Re}_{(min)} = \frac{(1000\ \text{kg/m}^3)(5.8\times10^{-12}\,\text{m}^3/\text{s})}{(0.89\times10^{-3}\ \text{Pa}\cdot\text{s})(40\ \mu\text{m})} = 0.163$$

$$\text{Re}_{(max)} = \frac{(1000\ \text{kg/m}^3)(72.9\times10^{-12}\,\text{m}^3/\text{s})}{(0.89\times10^{-3}\ \text{Pa}\cdot\text{s})(40\ \mu\text{m})} = 2.05$$

$$0.163 \le \text{Re} \le 2.05 \quad \Rightarrow \quad \text{Re} \ll 2100\ \ (\text{highly laminar}) \tag{7.65}$$

Since the Reynolds number is far below 2100, fluid flow within the microchannels is highly laminar. Thus, fluid motion of the PCR solution through the microchannels is constant and smooth with no significant turbulence or flow instabilities. For the continuous-flow PCR microreactor, laminar flow is highly desirable as it allows for precise temperature and flow velocity control for the PCR fluid moving through the microchannels.

7.2.3 **Comparison of Batch and Continuous-Flow PCR Microreactors**

The batch PCR microreactor and continuous-flow PCR microreactor each have advantages and drawbacks, as listed in Table 7-5. (1) The continuous-flow PCR microreactor offers far faster thermal response and better temperature control than the batch PCR microreactor. (2) The sample volume is flexible in the continuous-flow system, but is fixed in the batch system. Therefore, the continuous-flow PCR microreactor enables the applications of samples with varying volumes with the throughput controlled by the fluid flow rate. (3) The batch microreactor can suffer from temperature overshooting if the temperature controller is not well-designed. The continuous-flow microreactor can control temperature precisely without overshooting, only requiring a relatively simple control system because the three temperature zones are controlled separately. (4) For the continuous-flow PCR microreactor, the relative times that the PCR fluid spend in each temperature zone is fixed by the microchannel lengths in each zone; changing the relative times would require redesigning the continuous-flow PCR chip. In this sense, the protocol for the batch system is more flexible than that of the continuous-flow system. (5) Using the continuous-flow PCR microreactor, the sample can be analyzed dynamically, which is not possible with the batch PCR microreactor. (6) Cross-contamination is much less prevalent in the continuous-flow system than in the batch system as it is easier to clean the continuous-flow system. By injecting cleaning buffer between sample injections, the continuous-flow PCR chip can be reused many times before major cleaning is required. The batch PCR microreactor, however, needs to be manually cleaned before every use. For both systems, cleaning is required to remove sample residue buildup on the walls that can contaminate the next sample.[5,10]

It is also meaningful to compare the throughput of the two types of PCR microreactors. For the batch PCR microreactor, the throughput is mainly limited by the relatively slow thermal response as well as the time required to fill, empty, and clean the PCR reaction microchamber. For the continuous-flow PCR microreactor, the throughput is primarily limited by the volumetric flow rate of PCR solution through the microchannels. Overall, the maximum throughput of the continuous-flow PCR microreactor designed by Kopp et al. is 72.9 nL/s. If the time required for filling, emptying, and cleaning the PCR reaction microchamber is omitted, the throughput of the batch PCR microreactor designed by Daniel et al. is about 58 nL/s. If we consider the time saved from not having to fill or empty the

TABLE 7-5   Comparison of the Batch and Continuous-Flow PCR Microreactors

Batch PCR Microreactor		Continuous-Flow PCR Microreactor	
☒	Lower throughput	Greater (maximum) throughput	☑
☒	Poorer temperature control and far slower thermal response.	Better temperature control and far faster thermal response	☑
☒	Fixed sample volume and throughput	Flexible sample volume and throughput	☑
☑	More flexible protocol	Less flexible protocol; relative times spent in each temperature zone are fixed	☒
☒	Temperature overshooting issues	No temperature overshooting; temperature control is simplified	☑
☒	Static sample analysis	Dynamic sample analysis	☑
☒	More cross-contamination and harder to clean	Less cross-contamination and easier to clean	☑

reaction microchambers, the maximum throughput of the continuous-flow microreactor will be significantly greater than the batch microreactor throughput.[5,10]

In terms of performance, the continuous-flow PCR microreactor has many more advantages than the batch PCR microreactor. However, future developments and economic factors will ultimately determine whether either type of PCR microreactor will end up replacing commercial macroscale PCR systems.

7.3 DIABETIC GLUCOSE MONITORING WITH BIONANOTECHNOLOGY

Bionanotechnology can be applied to monitor a wide variety of diseases such as diabetes, cancer, and viral infections. Here, we discuss diabetic blood glucose monitoring as an example to illustrate the use of bionanotechnology for disease monitoring. Diabetes mellitus (also known as diabetes) refers to a group of metabolic disorders that affect how the body processes glucose, resulting in prolonged elevated levels of blood glucose. Over time, diabetes can damage blood vessels, nerves, and organs such as the heart, kidneys, and eyes. Diabetes is among the top ten leading causes of death in the world. The World Health Organization estimated that the number of adults with diabetes worldwide has increased from 108 million (4.7% prevalence) in 1980 to 422 million (8.5% prevalence) in 2014.[11] In 2018, the U.S. Centers for Disease Control and Prevention (CDC) reported that 13.0% (34.1 million) of all U.S. adults had diabetes, and that diabetes is the seventh leading cause of death in the United States.[12]

Glucose, a simple sugar (i.e., a monosaccharide), is an essential energy source for the body. Glucose combines with amino acids from fats to fuel physical exertion, and is the brain's primary source of energy. When a healthy human ingests carbohydrates, the body will break down the carbohydrates into glucose, which is absorbed into the bloodstream through the intestine. In response, the pancreas releases a hormone called insulin, which helps move glucose from the bloodstream into cells for fuel and storage. This mechanism is vital for regulating blood glucose levels. Without insulin, glucose levels in the blood may become dangerously high, a condition known as hyperglycemia. Chronic hyperglycemia presents many long-term complications such as nerve and kidney damage, an increased risk of cardiovascular disease, and problems with vision, such as cataracts and retinal damage.[13]

Diabetes occurs when the insulin-driven blood glucose regulating mechanism no longer works due to problems such as insulin insensitivity or insufficient insulin production. There are two common types of diabetes: type 1 and type 2. Type 1 diabetes describes the condition where the pancreas cannot produce insulin, whereas type 2 diabetes describes the situation where the body does not respond to insulin or is unable to produce a sufficient amount of insulin.[13]

Currently (as of 2022), there is no cure for diabetes. However, diabetes treatments are available that involve monitoring blood glucose levels combined with insulin injections, oral hypoglycemic medication, and/or exercise and dietary changes. The goal of diabetes treatments is to prevent long-term hyperglycemia. Blood glucose levels can be detected by optical (e.g., fluorescence), electrochemical (e.g., reverse iontophoresis), thermal, and nanomaterial-based biosensor methods.[14,15] As discussed in Section 6.2.2(A), blood glucose monitoring is most commonly accomplished using electrochemical lateral flow LOC biosensors. People afflicted with diabetes can extract a droplet of blood using a finger-prick and measure the blood glucose concentration using the lateral flow LOC biosensor. Due to the portability of lateral flow LOC biosensors, such a blood glucose measurement does not require a medical professional to administer and is known as self-monitoring of blood glucose (SMBG). Unfortunately, SMBG has some disadvantages: it is invasive, it may pose a risk of localized infections, and it only offers measurements at discrete times. Consequently, recent research and development has focused on non-invasive or minimally invasive continuous glucose monitoring (CGM) methods.[13]

A number of minimally invasive and non-invasive CGM methods have been reported. Here we focus on the application of nanotechnology in combination with optical and electrochemical techniques for CGM. One minimally invasive CGM method is called fluorescence-based glucose monitoring.[16] As the name suggests, fluorescence-based glucose biosensors rely on fluorescence. Fluorescent molecules or particles called fluorophores absorb incident light within a particular band of wavelengths and re-emit the absorbed energy as light at longer wavelengths. It is possible to construct glucose-sensing fluorophores so that the overall fluorescent effect—which can be measured—will decrease or increase in response to changes in glucose concentration. The main advantages of the fluorescence-based glucose monitoring system over the finger-prick SMBG are that it is minimally invasive and has high sensitivity to the blood glucose concentration. Although the small monitoring device has to be implanted underneath the skin through an invasive procedure, the blood glucose monitoring process performed via fluorescent light is non-invasive.[17]

Non-invasive CGM methods determine blood glucose concentration by detecting glucose levels in saliva, sweat, tears or skin interstitial fluid using sensors attached to the patient's skin. A promising development for non-invasive CGM is the reverse iontophoresis-based graphene–nanoparticle glucose biosensor, in which interstitial fluid is extracted through the skin via electro-osmosis and its glucose levels are monitored. Since the correlation between blood glucose concentration and the glucose levels in skin interstitial fluid is well established, the reverse iontophoresis-based biosensor can accurately provide the blood glucose concentration. This method of blood glucose level measurement is more accurate than other non-invasive CGM methods that detect glucose levels in saliva, sweat, or tears because the correlation between blood glucose concentration and glucose levels in saliva, sweat, or tears is uncertain. As of 2018, this technology has just passed the proof-of-concept stage and further developments are ongoing.[18]

7.3.1 Fluorescence-Based Minimally Invasive Glucose Monitoring

Prior to introducing this monitoring method, let us briefly review fluorescence, which has been discussed in greater detail in Section 4.2. Fluorescence refers to the emission of longer wavelength light in response to excitation from the absorption of incident light. Particles that exhibit fluorescence are known as fluorophores. The emission of light by a fluorophore occurs when incoming energy in the form of a photon excites an electron, and the electron jumps into a higher orbital. Shortly after, the fluorophore returns to a lower energy level when the electron relaxes to a lower orbital. For the fluorophore, this process releases energy in the form of fluorescent photons. Because some energy is lost (mainly as heat) through the absorption and re-emission processes, the emitted fluorescent photons have lower energies and therefore longer wavelengths than the incident photons.

In addition to the release of energy via photoemission, excited fluorophores can also emit energy in the form of heat. This phenomenon is known as fluorescence resonance energy transfer (FRET). FRET describes the transfer of energy between neighboring fluorophores—referred to as a donor–acceptor fluorophore pair—in response to excitation from incoming light. Energy is transferred from the excited donor fluorophore to the acceptor fluorophore, the amount of which is related to the distance between the fluorophores. When FRET is present, the fluorescence intensity of the donor is reduced as energy is transferred to the acceptor instead of being emitted as light. In glucose monitoring, FRET is an effect that describes the suppression of one molecule's fluorescence by another molecule.[19]

Biosensors used for molecular detection typically require four components: an analyte, a recognition mechanism, a recognition signal, and an architecture for housing the components. In fluorescence-based glucose monitoring, the analyte is glucose, the recognition mechanism is photodetection, and the recognition signal consists of fluorescence photons. Because fluorescence-based biosensors for glucose monitoring are under active development, biosensor architectures can vary greatly. Next, we will discuss the recognition signal and architecture utilized by one fluorescence-based glucose biosensor design.

Many studies have acknowledged FRET as a highly suitable analytical technique for correlating fluorescence intensity with glucose concentration. As such, FRET is commonly used as a recognition signal. One such technique is called FRET quenching. The process of FRET quenching requires a donor fluorophore, an acceptor fluorophore, and a glucose receptor in close proximity. In the absence of glucose, the receptor is empty which induces FRET quenching, such that the fluorescence emission by the donor is low. When glucose is present, glucose reversibly binds to the empty receptor; upon binding to the receptor, electron sharing between the acceptor–donor pair decreases, resulting in less FRET and more intense fluorescence. Therefore, glucose concentration is positively correlated with the fluorescence emission intensity.[17] FRET quenching is illustrated in Figure 7-21.

The FRET quenching mechanism shown in Figure 7-21 is a general technique that can be used to correlate glucose concentration with fluorescence intensity. Research has been carried out to develop novel ways of implementing this technique. Some of the current research explores the use of [17]

- Quantum dot (QD) fluorophores due to their photostability and wide absorption spectra.
- Glucose-binding proteins to serve as receptors for reversible glucose binding.
- Single-walled carbon nanotube (SWCNT) fluorophores that emit (i.e., fluoresce) near-infrared (NIR) light, which easily penetrates soft tissues.

In June 2018, the U.S. FDA–approved Senseonics' Eversense® CGM system.[20] The Eversense® CGM system uses a small cylindrical (3.5 mm diameter by 18.3 mm length) subcutaneous sensor implanted within the skin of the upper arm. The cylindrical sensor

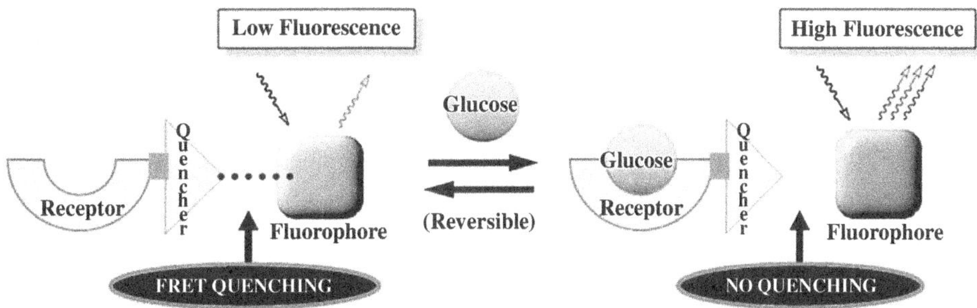

Figure 7-21   The fluorescence resonance energy transfer (FRET) quenching process. (Left) The glucose receptor is empty due to the absence of glucose, and FRET is induced leading to low fluorescence intensity. (Right) By reversibly binding to the receptor, glucose greatly reduces FRET quenching which results in high fluorescence intensity. (*The illustration is from D. C. Klonoff.*[19])

houses optoelectronics and a miniaturized spectrofluorometer. A fluorescent copolymer matrix which contains receptors for reversible glucose binding covers the outside of the sensor encasement. The implanted CGM sensor uses fluorescence (more specifically FRET) to measure the glucose concentration in skin interstitial fluid. A small battery-powered transmitter worn on the skin above the implanted sensor wirelessly powers the implanted sensor, calculates the blood glucose concentration, and reports it to the user via a mobile application at 5-minute intervals. Since the implanted sensor is wirelessly powered by the transmitter worn on the skin, the implanted sensor can function for up to 90 days, which is many times longer than previous CGM systems.[21]

During clinical trials, the Eversense® CGM system underwent a 90-day, unblinded and non-randomized study with adult participants who had a clinically confirmed diagnosis of either type 1 or type 2 diabetes. The study consisted of clinical visits to insert the sensor, accuracy assessments, and sensor removal. The accuracy of the sensor was evaluated by comparing glucose measurements from the CGM system with measurements taken by a bedside glucose monitor—a system that directly takes blood samples to obtain blood glucose concentration measurements. The study found that 85.7%, 93.3%, and 98.1% of the measurements from the CGM system were within ±15%, ±20%, and ±30%, respectively, of the values obtained by the reference bedside system over blood glucose concentrations of 40 to 400 mg/dL. Moreover, all of the implanted sensors were functional and provided reliable readings throughout the advertised lifetime of 90 days, and the study found that there was no impact from physical exercise on the sensor's recordings. The corresponding Clarke Error Grid Analysis—a technique established in 1987 for evaluating the accuracy of blood glucose monitoring relative to a reference method—found that 99.3% of the measurements from the Eversense® CGM system were within clinically acceptable error. This study and the subsequent success of the CGM system in the consumer marketplace demonstrate that the fluorescence-based technique is a viable option for minimally invasive CGM.[22]

7.3.2 Reverse Iontophoresis-Based Non-Invasive Glucose Monitoring

For a non-invasive CGM method, measurement of blood glucose levels must avoid the usual finger-prick procedure as well as the need for an implanted subcutaneous sensor, since implanted sensors carry the risk of potential pain, inflammation, and discomfort to the user.[14] Reverse iontophoresis is a non-invasive electrochemical technique for CGM which uses electro-osmosis with a small electric field applied across the skin. The applied electric field causes skin interstitial fluid to flow from the net negatively charged skin to a cathode placed on the skin surface. The glucose level in the skin interstitial fluid is detected by the cathode, and the blood glucose concentration is then obtained based on its correlation with the glucose concentration in the interstitial fluid.[23,24]

During the process of reverse iontophoresis, skin interstitial fluid can travel through multiple paths including intercellular, transcellular, and hair follicle pathways to the skin surface for detection (Figure 7-22, left). In comparison to the intercellular and transcellular pathways, the hair follicle pathway has a much lower resistance to fluid flow, so that most of the electro-osmotic flow of interstitial fluid is directed toward hair follicle pathways. Therefore, measuring glucose levels at hair follicle sites will provide the most accurate glucose concentration measurements. Hair follicles are semi-randomly distributed throughout a given area of skin. Assuming that each sensor "pixel" has an area of 2 to 5 mm², and that there are 27 hair follicles per cm², sensor "pixels" arranged in a 4×4 array and placed over the skin should cover at least one hair follicle. Larger arrays of sensor "pixels" will cover more hair follicles and improve the accuracy of glucose level detection.[18]

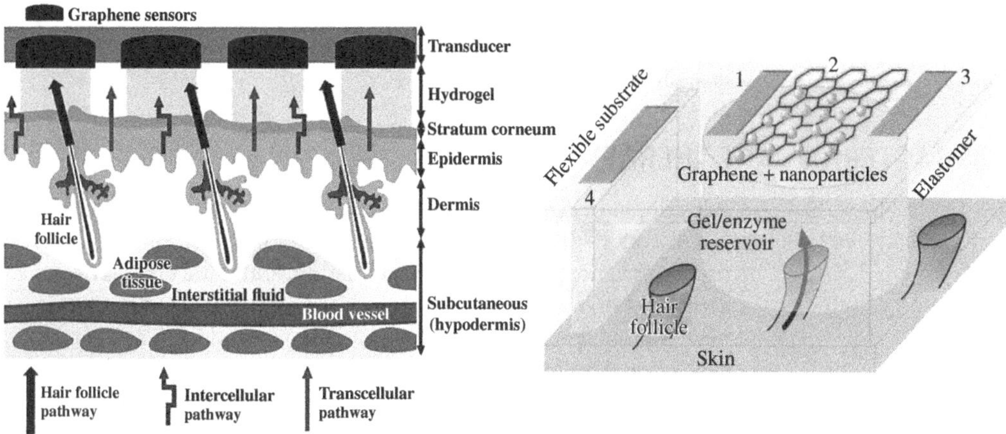

Figure 7-22 (Left) The three main pathways for skin interstitial fluid movement, with hair follicles being the primary pathway. (Right) A single graphene–nanoparticle glucose biosensor pixel, where 1 and 4 are electrodes that drive electro-osmosis of interstitial fluid, 2 is the working electrode made of the graphene–nanoparticle hybrid material, and 3 is the counter electrode. (*The figures are reprinted with permission from L. Lipani et al.*[18])

The biosensors used for reverse iontophoresis-based CGM can be formed by composite (i.e., hybrid) nanomaterials including (graphene)–(metal oxide nanoparticle), (graphene)–(platinum nanoparticle), or other (graphene)–(metal nanoparticle) nanomaterials. Graphene offers a number of desirable properties superior to traditional materials. Graphene as an inexpensive material has high electrical and thermal conductivity, superb mechanical properties, low capacitive background currents resulting in less noise, and is relatively easy to pattern into desired shapes and structures. In addition, graphene has a high surface-area-to-volume ratio, and can provide a desirable environment to pattern and integrate sensor devices which detect and monitor the levels of chemicals and molecules found within body fluids. With the addition of metal or metal oxide nanoparticles to form a (graphene)–(nanoparticle) composite material, the sensitivity of the biosensor to electro-chemical changes from reverse iontophoresis can be greatly enhanced.[25,26]

The glucose sensor "pixel" array described above could be formed by placing (graphene)–(platinum nanoparticle) biosensors in an array formation on top of a flexible substrate, with a hydrogel that contains glucose oxidase beneath the sensors. As the skin interstitial fluid is extracted via the process of electro-osmosis, the glucose oxidase enzyme present in the hydrogel converts the extracted glucose within the fluid into hydrogen peroxide. The concentration of hydrogen peroxide could then be measured by the biosensors to determine the glucose level within the interstitial fluid, which is then used to calculate the blood glucose concentration. The (graphene)–(platinum nanoparticle) biosensor arrays can be created with standard micro/nano fabrication techniques. Figure 7-22 (right) illustrates one sensor "pixel" of the (graphene)–(platinum nanoparticle) glucose sensor array.[18,27]

Over a large range of blood glucose levels from hypoglycemic to hyperglycemic levels, the non-invasive CGM (graphene)–(platinum nanoparticle) biosensor arrays worked as designed and produced clinically acceptable results when compared with benchmark test results from traditional finger-prick blood glucose tests. However, this technology is still in the early prototyping stage, and has only been demonstrated to provide 6 h of continuous monitoring. To be competitive with other CGM systems, the graphene–nanoparticle array CGM biosensor would need to work continuously for at least a few days. One possible way to increase the duration of CGM for this technology is to have multiple "sets" of arrays in a single device. By turning off one set of pixels once it has passed its period of reliable monitoring and immediately turning on a new set, the total duration of glucose monitoring can be easily extended.[18]

7.4 BACTERIOPHAGE THERAPY

Bacteriophage therapy is a type of targeted therapy that can treat antibiotic-resistant bacterial infections. The discovery of antibiotics has been one of the greatest achievements of modern science. Ever since its formulation, antibiotic use has become widespread due to its ability to kill multiple types of bacteria. People exploited antibiotics due to their effectiveness, leading to their overuse in both humans and farm animals, which caused bacteria to evolve and develop resistance against antibiotics. Over time, bacteria have gained resistance to many classes of antibiotics, while the rate of new antibiotics production is declining. Since 1962, only two new types of antibiotics have been discovered and approved for clinical use. Even if governments were to fund research for new types of antibiotics, it would not likely be sufficient to satisfy the required demand for new antibiotics. To combat this problem, a new solution that has gained popularity is the use of bacteriophages (also known as phages) for administering phage therapy to kill bacteria.[28]

Unlike antibiotics, which are chemical compounds, bacteriophages are viruses that specifically target bacteria. Bacteriophages are very specific in their targeting of bacteria. Because of this high specificity, more recent attention was given to bacteriophages. Bacteriophages are the most abundant organisms in nature, with their concentration estimated to be ~2.5×10^8 phages/mL in natural water.[29] Bacteriophage therapy uses viruses that adsorb onto the surface of a target host bacterium, inject their genome, and force the host bacterium to create about 10 to 100 phage virions (i.e., viruses) until it bursts to release these virions causing a chain reaction.[28] This will eventually lead to an exponential growth in the phage virus population until all of the target bacteria have been exterminated.

Phage–bacteria interactions are already abundant in both nature and the food industry. Bacteriophages are estimated to kill half of the Earth's bacteria population every day, and the food industry already uses some commercially available phage cocktails in the decontamination and storage of certain products.[30] Bacteriophages hold great potential in regards to individual therapy, and it is extremely important to consider this further as bacteria become more resistant to antibiotics and challenging to fight. Furthermore, there are different methods of engineering and administering phages, each with different benefits.

7.4.1 Bacteriophage Therapy Procedure

To administer phages, phages typically have to be created and mass-produced to have any viable impact against bacteria. One of the simplest ways of doing this is to collect samples from an environment and attempt to find and isolate naturally occurring phages.[28] This is simple and extremely effective given the large impact that phages already have on the environment. Taking advantage of the amount of computational storage we have today, it is easy to build up a library of phages, their characteristics, and the strains of bacteria they target. A phage is discovered through screening against potential bacterial strains. The bacteria strains against which a phage can be used are referred to as the "host range" of the bacteriophage.[28] Scientists can analyze the proteins that make up the surface of the virus and compare them with the proteins of potential bacteria hosts. When there is a match, the bacterial host will accept the phage and allows it to pass through, and the phage can begin to replicate within the bacterial host.

Next, the use of phages must be tested and mass-produced from the captured sample. To do this, accepted host bacteria are grown in a bioreactor. Typically, the bacteria are suspended in a medium and environment that will promote the growth and replication of the sample bacteria. From here, the phage(s) are administered into the sample so that they can begin to spread among the bacteria. This process continues until all the bacteria have been destroyed, and the only biological matter remaining are the phages and debris from phage-bacteria interactions. Centrifugation is then used to filter the bacterial cell debris from the phages, and the phages can then be refrigerated and put in storage for later use.

The administration of phages can be a powerful tool, but the effect can be minimal when the phage can only work on one type of bacteria. In general, there can be many forms of bacteria that a phage is trying to counteract, depending on the application. In the creation of phage cocktails, certain methods can be utilized to increase the host range which the cocktail affects. The simplest approach is to find a variety of phages and combine them to produce a phage cocktail. The many small host ranges of each phage combine to create a solution that can impact many varieties of bacteria. The second approach is to use genome engineering to mix and match the tail fibers of different phages so that they can work on more types of bacteria hosts. This is done by specifically altering a portion of one phage's DNA to match that of another, ideally creating phages with a combination of desirable characteristics from both.[32] The third approach is similar to the second, except it instead engineers random mutations in the genetic code of phages to produce strains that may or may not change the host range. Once the mutated varieties have been created, they can be recombined into one phage using homologous recombination (a type of genetic recombination).[32] This merges all of the DNA of the phage into a new phage that may have more beneficial properties than the first phage encountered. Figure 7-23 demonstrates the three types of phage cocktails for targeting a wider range of bacteria and what they look like.

7.4.2 Applications of Bacteriophage Therapy

Bacteriophage therapy spans a diverse set of applications for treating bacterial infections. The process begins with doing some preliminary tests on the patient to determine what kind or kinds of bacteria are predominantly responsible for the infection. Then, suitable phages are grown in a bioreactor and allowed to multiply in numbers, so that their concentration is potent enough to kill the desired bacteria. Depending on the infection, a phage cocktail or other combination meant to increase host bacteria range can be used to attack bacteria more efficiently. The uniqueness of phage therapy is the ability of the phages to multiply in the patient's body, given that the phages target the desired bacteria. As the phages multiply, the potency of the therapy increases proportionally without the need for repetitive dosage administration as the bacteria themselves provide the necessary processes for their own destruction by enabling phage replication. Bacteriophage therapy research has focused on the effects of bacterial infections on animals resulting from wounds, respiratory infections, or gastrointestinal illnesses.

A common disease for phage therapy research is bacterial respiratory infection due to cystic fibrosis. Cystic fibrosis is a genetic disease which causes high amounts of mucus in the lungs. Bacteria can enter the lungs and breed due to the excess mucus. The pulmonary pathogens responsible for infection can form biofilms, which make it difficult for antibiotics to kill the bacteria in the lung. Bacteriophage therapy is being studied to combat this issue. Another disease is ventilator-associated pneumonia that afflicts intensive care unit (ICU) patients. Many ICU patients suffer from bacterial infections. These bacteria can breed easily due to the weaker immune systems of ICU patients and can have high antibiotic resistance. Research with animal models is being carried out to combat ventilator-associated

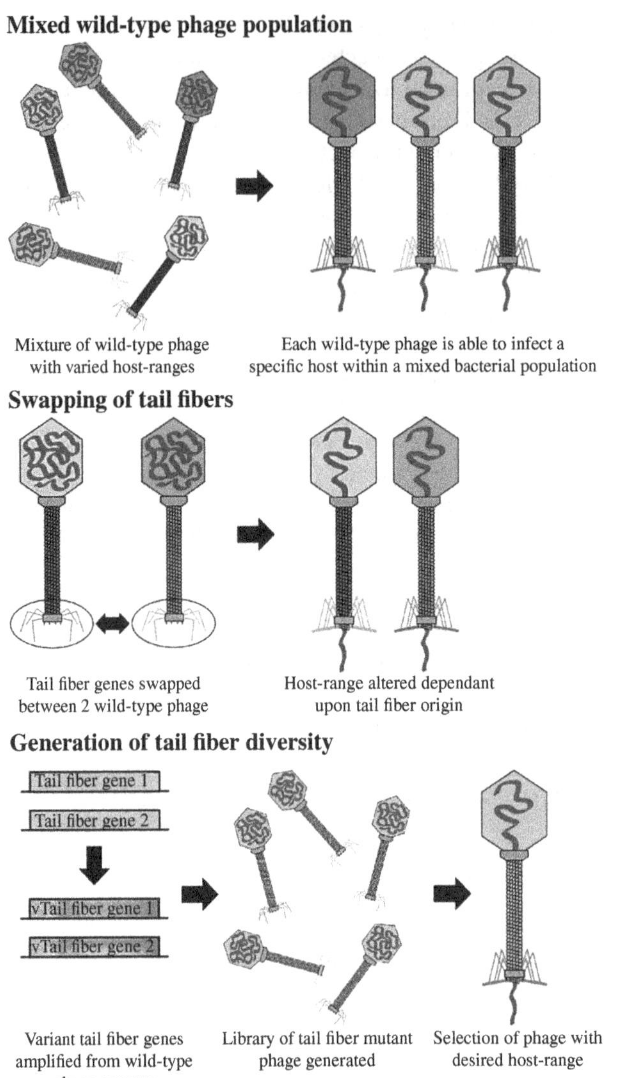

Figure 7-23 Creation of phage cocktails for targeting a wider range of bacteria. (*The illustration is reprinted with permission from R. Brown et al.*[31])

pneumonia using phage therapy because of their ability to target specific bacteria that have antibiotic immunity. Finally, a common condition among a third of the world's population—tuberculosis—is another disease that has been targeted as a suitable candidate for phage therapy. Tuberculosis-causing bacteria are multidrug-resistant, making them harder to treat. Data gathered by the World Health Organization shows that some strains have extensive drug resistance. Treatment for this kind of disease requires long-term antibiotic use (6 to 24 months) and has adverse side effects. Phage therapy can provide fast and efficient treatment without adverse side-effects because it only infects certain targeted strains of bacteria, leaving the patient's cells unharmed.

Most bacteria-infected wounds generate biofilms, which significantly reduces antibiotic efficacy and slows down tissue repair because antibiotics diffuse poorly through these biofilms. Bacteria in the biofilms are less metabolically active, which limits the efficacy of antibiotics that target metabolic pathways. To make matters worse, the use of antibiotics to treat bacterial infections can force bacteria to evolve antibiotic resistance, which could create new and highly resistant bacteria strains in the future. Phage therapy is being applied to treat these infections so that the therapy is completed in a timely manner without increasing antibiotic resistance.[28]

Bacterial gastrointestinal infections are very common in less developed countries due to the less hygienic food available. Most gastrointestinal infections are caused by infected food products that make their way through the gastrointestinal tract to the infection site. As with other types of bacterial infections, overuse of oral antibiotics has caused these bacteria to resist medication. These bacteria are not restricted to humans and affect other species like farm animals as well. The widespread use of antibiotics in feed for farm animals results in an increased rate of antibiotic resistance.

Although phages target bacterial and archaeal cells in nature, phages can be engineered to target other cells such as mammalian (e.g., human and mouse) cells. Other exciting applications of phages are drug delivery, gene therapy and targeted imaging. The idea is to use phages as vehicles for the delivery of drugs, genes, and tags/labels (such as radioactive tracers and fluorophores) targeting very specific cells. That way, the contents carried by the phages are protected while being transported and the phages with their contents are absorbed only by the targeted cells. Studies with cancerous cells have demonstrated the use of phages to deliver anti-cancer drugs, silence cancer genes, and image cancerous tumors in the battle against cancer. A study showed that the use of phages for gene therapy was extremely successful when targeting cancerous breast cells and conducting gene silencing.[30] Growth-halting drugs carried by phages were able to stop specific cells from growing. Moreover, phages have been used to transport imaging agents (such as labeled folic acid) into specific tissues, helping map cancerous cells and aiding in tissue visualization.

7.5 BIOMEDICAL APPLICATIONS OF NANOPARTICLES

Nanoparticles are currently applied to improve existing medical technologies, such as medical imaging enhancement. Nanoparticles are also used to create entirely new medical technologies. For example, nanoparticles are used in cancer treatments and personalized medicines. As shown in Figure 7-24, one of the most common biomedical applications of nanoparticles is for targeted drug or gene delivery.

Radiation therapy and chemotherapy are two commonly used cancer therapies. These therapies are not targeted, meaning that they kill cancer tumor cells as well as healthy cells. Researchers are now using nanoparticles to deliver radioactive elements to tumors, thus

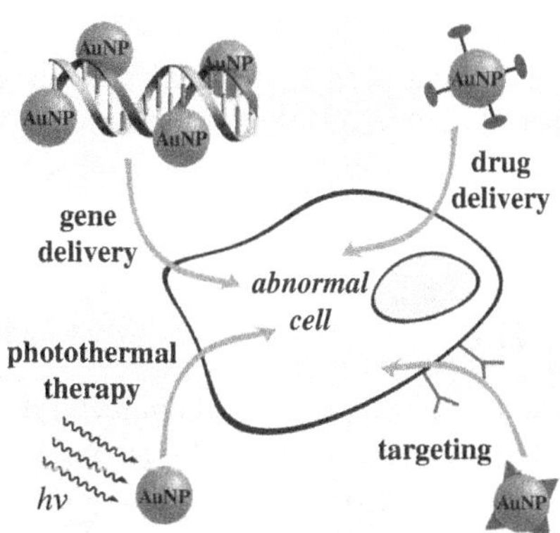

Figure 7-24 Using gold nanoparticles (AuNPs shown as spheres) as targeted nanocarriers for drug delivery, gene delivery, photothermal therapy, and other targeted purposes. (*The illustration is reprinted with permission from X. J. Loh et al.*[33])

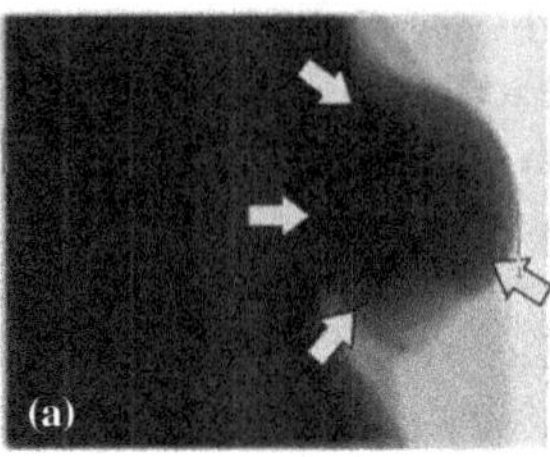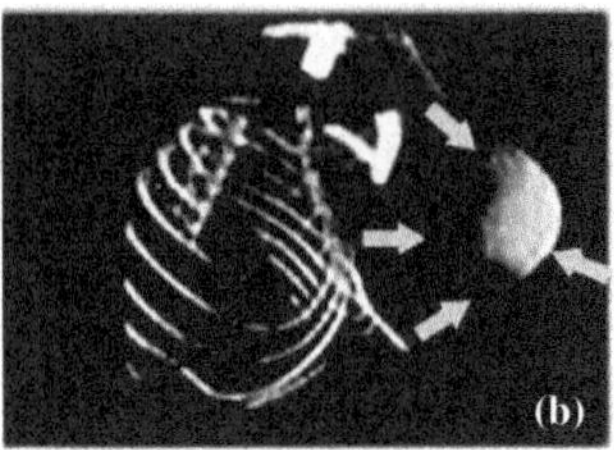

Figure 7-25 Breast CT images of an immune-suppressed mouse. (a) Original image; (b) Enhanced image after applying nanoparticles. (*The images are reprinted with permission from G. Feng et al.*[35])

TABLE 7-6 Current Gene Delivery Techniques[36]

Method	Advantages	Disadvantages	Status
Viral Delivery	Highly efficient	Potentially unsafe	Some therapies going through clinical trials
Microinjection	Highly reliable	Only one cell can be transfected at a time	Used when a few cells need to be transfected
Gene Gun	Works on large groups of cells	Kills many target cells; few animal tests	Used to transfect plant cells
Electroporation	Improved reliability	Does not help transfect the nuclear membrane	Some commercial products
Sonoporation	Improved reliability	Still unreliable	Some commercial products
Magnetofection	Improved reliability	Variable results	New method
Calcium Phosphate	Relatively inexpensive	Highly inefficient	Used for easier transfections
Liposomal Delivery	Varied efficiencies for individual products	Toxicity; low percentage recovery of cells; off-target activities	Some therapies going through clinical trials

sparing healthy tissues from radiation-induced damage. Since the metabolism of cancer cells is many times faster than that of healthy cells, glucose-labeled gold nanoparticles (GNPs) have been used to distinguish tumors from healthy cells. Experimental results show that tumor cells uptake glucose-coated GNPs at least ten times more than healthy cells do. Figure 7-25 shows the breast CT images of an immune-suppressed mouse before and after applying glucose-coated GNPs. By comparison, we can clearly identify the contour of the tumor from the image where nanoparticles were applied. When an external X-ray beam hits the GNPs, highly reactive radicals are generated locally (i.e., within the tumor) and targeted cancer therapy is achieved.[34]

Another example of nanoparticles in biomedical applications is gene delivery. The cell wall of plant cells or the cell membrane of mammalian cells blocks foreign substances from entering the cells. Various gene delivery methods have been proposed to increase delivery efficiency (Table 7-6).

7.6 TARGETED CANCER THERAPIES AND DRUG DELIVERY SYSTEMS

One of the most important applications of bionanotechnology is the targeted treatment of cancers. Cancer is a widespread illness, and is the second leading cause of death worldwide and in the United States. In 2018, 9.6 million deaths, or one in six deaths globally, were due to cancer.[37] In Canada, cancer is the leading cause of death and accounts for 30% of deaths nationwide. The Canadian Cancer Society estimates that 628 Canadians will be diagnosed with cancer and 232 Canadians will die from cancer every day in 2021.[38]

Cancer cells are cells with damaged cell division genes due to genetic mutations or DNA damage which causes them to multiply abnormally quickly and uncontrollably. While normal cells divide and multiply as needed at a healthy rate, cancer cells continue to grow out of control and form tumors (i.e., tissues formed by abnormal cells). Since tumors require large amounts of energy and nutrients for their survival, they create blood vessels through a process called angiogenesis to supply nutrients for themselves. This process starves the healthy cells around the tumors of nutrients, causing healthy tissues to stop functioning properly. Cancer cells can also pass through blood vessels and spread to other parts of the body in a process known as metastasis.[39] The new blood vessels created via angiogenesis are relatively far apart, and create a porous vasculature which increases permeability to other molecules. At the same time, tumors can impede lymphatic vessels (which help carry excess fluid out) by compressing against them. The two effects together result in the enhanced permeability and retention (EPR) effect.[40]

Traditionally, cancer is treated by surgery, chemotherapy, radiation therapy, or a combination of these methods. Chemotherapy and radiation therapy are non-targeted treatments which kill healthy cells just as easily as cancer cells. In addition to killing cancer cells, traditional treatments also damage healthy tissues, causing debilitating side effects such as nausea, vomiting, edema (swelling), pain, and increased risk for secondary infections. Therefore, it is important to develop targeted cancer therapies which are more effective and have less serious side effects than traditional treatments. Researchers have now developed novel targeted cancer therapies including immunotherapy, hormone therapy, and personalized therapy. Personalized therapy provides medical doctors with the ability to customize cancer medicine for their patients and allows them to tailor their methods to improve imaging capabilities and circulation half-life and to reduce toxicity.[41,42]

A promising approach for targeted cancer therapy is to use nanotechnology. This approach relies on nanoparticles which are used as drug carriers. The nanoparticles carry drugs to the cancer cells and the drugs are released there by environmental or physical stimuli such as changes in pH, hyperthermia, ultraviolet or near-infrared irradiation, ultrasound, and/or magnetic fields. The nanoparticles which are stimuli-responsive include DNA nanoparticles, liposomes, and biodegradable polymer-based micelles (i.e., nanoemulsions). The encapsulation of drugs within the nanoparticles allows drugs of low aqueous solubility to be effectively delivered to the target sites (i.e., within cancerous tumors), preventing drug degradation in body fluids and reducing side effects. In addition, imaging agents can be encapsulated along with therapeutic drugs within the nanoparticles to achieve therapeutic effects as well as enhanced imaging contrast for precise treatment assessment.[42]

7.6.1 Nanoparticle-Mediated Thermal Cancer Therapy

Cancer therapy is an evolving field of research influenced by many different areas in science and engineering. One type of cancer therapy called thermal cancer therapy utilizes cell hyperthermia to damage and kill cancer cells. For example, heating cancer cells to a temperature between 41°C and 47°C can cause irreversible damage to the cancerous cells by destroying cell membranes and denaturing cellular proteins. Based on studies with different heat sources, it was found that the use of light in thermal cancer therapy is most promising. To create heat within organic tissue that targets specific cells, we must increase the kinetic energy of targeted molecules within the desired cells while leaving the surrounding healthy cells unaffected.[43]

Photothermal therapy (PTT) is one of the most popular techniques for thermal cancer therapy. In PTT, photo-absorbing agents delivered into selectively targeted cells convert incident laser light into molecular vibrations known as phonons. Phonons are quasi-particles and thermal energy carriers, so energy from the incident laser photons are converted into heat. This conversion is achieved by using the laser light to excite electrons within the photo-absorbing agent to higher energy states, and then return to ground states upon the electrons relaxing. The change in potential energy of the electrons is released as phonons. The photo-absorbing agents used in PTT include natural chromophores and dye molecules such as indocyanine green. These compounds excel in converting light to heat, but they are unfortunately highly susceptible to photo-bleaching through which organic molecule photo-absorbing agents become progressively less efficient at converting light into heat over time.[43]

Advancements in nanotechnology in recent decades showcased a phenomenon known as surface plasmon resonance (SPR). Like the light-to-heat conversion obtained from using photo-absorbing agents, SPR induces the surface electrons of noble metals such as gold and silver to oscillate in accordance with the incident light. Noble metal nanoparticles—such as gold nanoparticles (GNPs) in the form of nanospheres, nanorods, nanostars, and nanocages—induce SPR oscillations and convert the incoming light into phonons. SPR overcomes the issue of photo-bleaching since it does not rely on the reaction between light and a photosensitive compound; instead, the incident light is directly converted into heat and no photo-absorbing agents are needed. Since GNPs are highly hydrophobic, GNPs need to be coated with a hydrophilic or amphiphilic compound to increase uptake within cancerous tumors. In addition to these coatings to assist nanoparticle uptake within the body, additional compounds can be used to disassemble the coatings to allow for easier renal filtering, enabling the nanoparticles to exit the body via urine after treatment. Nanoparticle buildup is an issue when the sizes of particulates exceed roughly 100 nm and can, in turn, cause acute inflammation or even cell apoptosis (i.e., programmed cell death). The delivery of GNPs to targeted cancer sites is also critical, which can be facilitated by attaching cancer cell-binding biomolecules to the GNPs. Since these biomolecules have a high affinity to both the GNPs and cancer cells, they can help bring an increased amount of nanoparticles into the cancerous area.[43,44]

Another advantage of GNPs is that they can be tuned to resonate at different frequencies to match the frequency of the light source. This property is especially useful for treating deep tissue tumors. Due to components of the human body such as water and hemoglobin, light within the visible spectrum (i.e., 400 to 700 nm wavelength light) has low transmissivity within the human body. In contrast, the skin is essentially optically transparent in the near-infrared (NIR) range. This "window" of transparency opens the door for *in vivo* cancer therapy since NIR light has the capability of penetrating up to 10 cm in soft tissue.[45] Therefore, resonating GNPs with light in the NIR range may be used for cancer treatment. It has been found that 20 minutes of NIR illumination on cancer cells can ablate 75% of the total cancerous cells within a 4-hour time frame. This finding shows great promise for using GNPs in the realm of thermal cancer therapy, and specifically in plasmonic photothermal therapy.[44]

The foundation of the plasmonic photothermal therapy (PPTT) method is surface plasmon resonance (SPR) caused by incident photons interacting with the conduction band electrons of noble metal nanoparticles. Although a variety of materials have been examined for cancer treatment with PPTT, only noble metal nanoparticles are commonly used in PPTT due to their low toxicity to the body. These noble metal nanoparticles are typically used in conjunction with NIR irradiation to achieve a penetration depth of as much as 10 cm in soft tissues. With the proper frequency of light incident upon the particles, electrons will oscillate at the given resonant frequency (Figure 7-26, left). The electrons are then

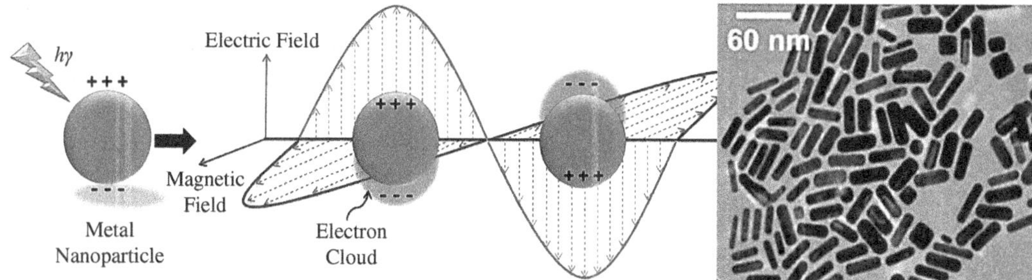

Figure 7-26   (Left) Light (i.e., electromagnetic waves) with frequency matching the surface plasmon resonance (SPR) frequency interacts with the surrounding electron clouds of gold nanoparticles (GNPs). This results in SPR oscillations of the polarized electron clouds at the same frequency as the incident light. The figure is reprinted with permission from S. Peiris et al.[46] (Right) Transmission electron microscope (TEM) image of gold nanorods. (*The image is reprinted with permission from M. A. Mackey et al.*[45])

raised to higher energy states, in which they release their excess energy as phonons (i.e., quantized crystal lattice vibrations). These oscillations and phonons, coupled with adjacent particles, work together to raise the kinetic energy and hence temperature of the surrounding environment. The resonant frequency of a particular GNP is highly dependent not only on its size, but also on its geometry. Therefore, the size and shape of GNPs used in PPTT can be optimized. The optimal NIR transmission window for human tissue is between 650 nm and 900 nm. By adjusting the shape and size of the nanoparticles, it can be assured that the nanoparticles absorb NIR light in this transmission window.[45,47]

For PPTT, the nanoparticles can be in the form of a variety of structures, including nanorods, nanocages, and nanoshells. Based on theoretical calculations, the absorption cross-sections of nanorods at NIR plasmon resonance are slightly greater than those of nanocages and over double those of nanoshells, making nanorods the optimal shape.[47] Thus, of all of the common shapes of GNPs, rod-shaped GNPs (Figure 7-26, right) have shown the most promising PPTT results for incident NIR light. Similarly, some important factors need to be considered when designing the size of the nanoparticle. As the nanoparticle size decreases, a greater fraction of the incident light is absorbed and a smaller fraction is scattered. However, the conversion efficiency of absorbed light energy into thermal energy is reduced for smaller nanoparticles. Larger nanoparticles absorb a smaller fraction of the incident light due to increased scattering, but the absorbed light energy is more efficiently converted into heat. Therefore, there is an optimal nanoparticle size where a fixed number of nanoparticles can generate the most heat using NIR.[45]

Mackey et al. (2014) studied the optimal size of GNP rods used in PPTT. In their studies, a gold nanorod of 38 nm (length) by 11 nm (diameter) was synthesized using the seed-mediated growth method, whereas two smaller gold nanorods were synthesized with a seedless growth method, one being 28 nm by 8 nm, and the other 17 nm by 5 nm. After synthesis, 10 nM of the nanorods were each placed in a solution, and then exposed to an 808 nm NIR laser. The temperature of the solutions was then measured. As a control, the laser was also exposed to a solution without any nanorods to account for the non-SPR heat generated by the laser itself. From the experiment, it was found that far more heat was generated by the gold nanorod solutions over time than the control when exposed to the NIR laser. In addition, the 28 nm by 8 nm nanorod solution generated significantly more heat than the other two nanorod solutions, proving that there is an optimal nanoparticle size for heat conversion at which the ratio of total incident light energy to the amount of thermal energy generated via SPR is maximized.[45]

One of the challenges for PPTT is to find a way to control and limit the damage to healthy cells in the body. To utilize this therapy for killing cancerous tumors, nanoparticles are planted in the tumors and then hit by laser radiation, generating hyperthermia at temperatures of 41°C to 47°C in the cancerous tissue. During this process, healthy tissues can be damaged by nanoparticles diffusing into the body from the tumor as well as unwanted absorption of laser light and thermal conductivity in healthy tissue. To prevent healthy tissue from being damaged, it is important to consider the optical and thermal properties of various tissues in the body.[48]

For this purpose, an experiment was conducted with artificial brain tissue as well as different porcine cerebral tissues. The tissue samples were exposed to an 806 nm NIR laser and their temperatures were recorded simultaneously. For the artificial brain tissue without nanoparticles, it was found that the steady-state temperature change was 1.7 K. For artificial brain tissue with added GNPs, a temperature change of 7.8 K was observed, which was more than enough to induce hyperthermia in cancerous cells. The laser power was then varied from 0.5 W to 2 W, and the heating rate (i.e., tissue temperature change per unit laser power) was measured. This procedure was applied for the artificial brain tissue as well as cerebellum, cerebrum, and brain stem tissues. It was found that the heating rate varied drastically (i.e., by as much as a factor of two) between the different types of brain tissue. This finding indicated that different types of brain tissue require different amounts of laser energy to induce hyperthermia, which could be attributed to differences in tissue properties such as density. For instance, dissimilar types of brain tissue contain different concentrations of white and gray matter which have different extinction coefficients as well as scattering coefficients. Overall, the experiment shows that the optical and thermal properties of different types of tissue have a major effect on PPTT.[48] As such, these properties must be taken into consideration when determining how to better attack tumors. A balance has to be maintained between destroying tumors and protecting healthy cells during PPTT.

PPTT is often used because cancerous cells are highly vulnerable to hyperthermia due to their far higher metabolic rates compared to healthy cells. Furthermore, only a relatively small amount of thermal energy is needed to cause significant destruction of cancer cells. The key advantages of PPTT compared with conventional cancer therapies such as chemotherapy and radiotherapy are that PPTT has vastly greater selectivity (i.e., kills cancer cells while preserving healthy cells) and far fewer side effects while offering comparable effectiveness.[47]

To demonstrate the effectiveness of PPTT, an experiment involving inoculating mice with cancerous tumor cells has been conducted. In the experiment (published in 2008), human squamous carcinoma cells were cultivated and injected into mice. The mice were then divided into three groups: the mice in the first group had GNPs injected directly into the tumor, the mice in the second group had intravenous injections of GNPs, and the mice in the third group were injected a saline solution as a control. All the mice were subjected to NIR at a wavelength of 808 nm after injection of GNPs. It was found that for the mice with injected GNPs, 10 to 15 min of irradiation using a laser power of 0.9 to 1.1 W/cm^2 (first group) and 1.7 to 1.9 W/cm^2 (second group) was required to destroy the tumor while minimizing damage to healthy tissues. The results also showed that average tumor growth by volume decreased by 96% and 74% for the mice in the first group and second group, respectively. Therefore, injecting GNPs directly into tumors reduces the laser energy required and is more effective than intravenously injecting GNPs.[47]

Although gold nanorods are most commonly used for PPTT, GNPs with different geometries can also be used. For instance, gold nanostars can be used to combine both photodynamic therapy (PDT) and plasmonic photothermal therapy (PPTT) in a single treatment. PDT is another type of light-induced cancer treatment that relies on photosensitizer

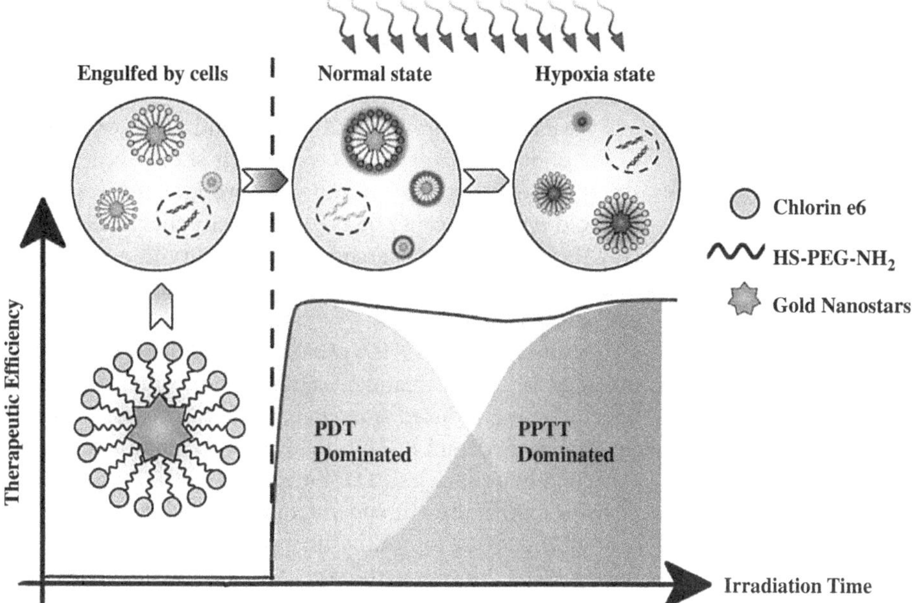

Figure 7-27 Combining photodynamic therapy (PDT) and plasmonic photothermal therapy (PPTT) in a single treatment using pegylated gold nanostars coated with Chlorin e6 photosensitizers. Upon exposure to a continuous wave NIR laser, the tumor-killing effect of the photosensitizer (via PDT) is powerful but short-lived, while the gold nanostars (via PPTT) continue to produce tumor-killing heat and become more effective over time. (*The illustration is reprinted with permission from S. Wang et al.*[50])

molecules delivered into cancerous cells. By irradiating photosensitizer molecules with a red or NIR laser, the photosensitizers convert the oxygen within the cells into highly reactive singlet oxygen that kills the targeted cells by reacting with essential organic compounds within the cell and depleting the oxygen required for cellular metabolism. Like PPTT, PDT also has superior selectivity and less side effects than chemotherapy or radiotherapy. However, the tumor-killing effect of photosensitizer molecules in PDT quickly wears off upon exposure to laser light as the photosensitizers self-destruct. The cancer cell-killing effect of noble metal nanoparticles in PPTT increases over time with exposure to laser light through the generation of more thermal energy over time. By combining PPTT with PDT (Figure 7-27), tumors can be killed with greater effectiveness and more control than either therapy alone. PDT delivers an initial blow to the tumor by reacting with essential cellular components and with oxygen depletion, while PPTT kills the remaining cancerous cells in the tumor with thermal energy.[49]

Gold nanostars can hold a high volume of photosensitizers owing to their surface roughness and high surface-area-to-volume ratio. These photosensitizers work in conjunction with the nanoparticles' inherent plasmonic (i.e., SPR) effect to combine PPTT with PDT for killing cancerous cells. One issue that arises is the mismatch between the operating light frequencies for the photosensitizer (i.e., PDT) and nanostar (i.e., PPTT). A simple solution is to use two separate lasers, but this would make the technique complex, cumbersome and expensive as it is challenging to focus two laser beams onto the same location. Another expensive solution is to use two-photon excitation with femtosecond laser pulses. However, it was observed *in vitro* that the rapid bursts of energy generated with femtosecond laser pulses could easily melt the nanostars into nanospheres, drastically changing their photothermal conversion capabilities.[50]

To match the resonance frequency of the gold nanostar with the activation frequency of the photosensitizer, Chlorin e6 photosensitizers were anchored onto the surface of a gold nanostar with resonant frequency tuned to fit that of the Chlorin e6. Thus, both the gold nanostar and Chlorin e6 photosensitizer could be activated by a single NIR continuous wave laser. When exposed to the continuous wave NIR laser, the tumor-killing effect of the photosensitizer was powerful but short-lived, while the gold nanostars remained structurally intact and continued to produce tumor-killing heat over time. In addition, the gold nanostar could be pegylated (i.e., chemically modified with polyethylene glycol (PEG)) to increase dispersivity and stability in a range of cellular and tissue mediums. Figure 7-27 depicts the entire process for combined PPTT/PDT treatment using Clorin e6–coated gold nanostars.[50]

In summary, PPTT is a promising alternative to conventional radiotherapy and chemotherapy for cancer treatment, offering comparable effectiveness combined with improved selectivity and reduced side effects. Since cancerous cells have very fast metabolism, the thermal energy from PPTT quickly destroys tumor cells. PPTT can also be combined with other methods such as PDT for greater tunability and effectiveness. However, the types of tissues afflicted with and surrounding the tumor must be taken into consideration to minimize damage to healthy tissues, since different tissue types heat up at different rates during PPTT. Moreover, the size and shape of the noble metal nanoparticles used for PPTT must be carefully considered to ensure that the nanoparticles effectively convert NIR light energy into tumor-killing heat. Additionally, coatings applied to the nanoparticles must be designed to increase uptake within cancer cells, improve biocompatibility, and allow for excretion in urine following treatment.

7.6.2 Targeted Cancer Treatment with Carbon Nanotubes

As outlined in Section 1.1, carbon nanotubes (CNTs) have many potential biomedical applications. Here, we focus on the application of CNTs in targeted cancer treatment. Due to their high surface area, high drug loading capacities, and the ability to easily penetrate cell membranes with a unique needle-like shape, CNTs have been studied as promising carriers for drug and gene delivery in targeted cancer therapy. CNTs interact with cancer cells through nano-penetration and endocytosis as shown in Figure 7-28. Nanotubes loaded with anticancer drugs or genes can either diffuse across the cellular membrane in an energy-independent passive nano-penetration process, or be engulfed by the cell in an energy-dependent active endocytosis process. As CNTs enter cancer cells, internal or external stimuli trigger the release of the loaded anticancer drugs or genes, which kills the cancer cells.[51]

To enhance the cellular uptake of CNTs by cancer cells, the surface of CNTs can be functionalized. Through functionalization, functional groups are covalently or non-covalently attached to the CNT surface to render the CNT soluble in water and allow the CNT to adapt to the internal environment of the human body. Many functionalization approaches have been reported. CNT PEGylation—the covalent attachment of polyethylene glycol (PEG) chains to the nanotubes—is a common method for surface modification. To carry out CNT PEGylation, the CNT surface is first oxidized to obtain carboxyl function groups. Next, PEG can be attached to the oxidized CNT surface either by esterifying the carboxyl groups with PEG having $-OH$ end groups or by amidating the carboxyl groups with PEG having $-NH_2$ end groups. Alternatively, non-covalent CNT PEGylation can be achieved by using van der Waals forces and/or hydrogen bonding to attach PEG to the oxidized surface of the CNTs.[52,53]

Razzazan et al. (2016) reported the application of PEGylated single-walled carbon nanotubes (SWCNTs) to successfully deliver an anticancer agent (gemcitabine) for treating

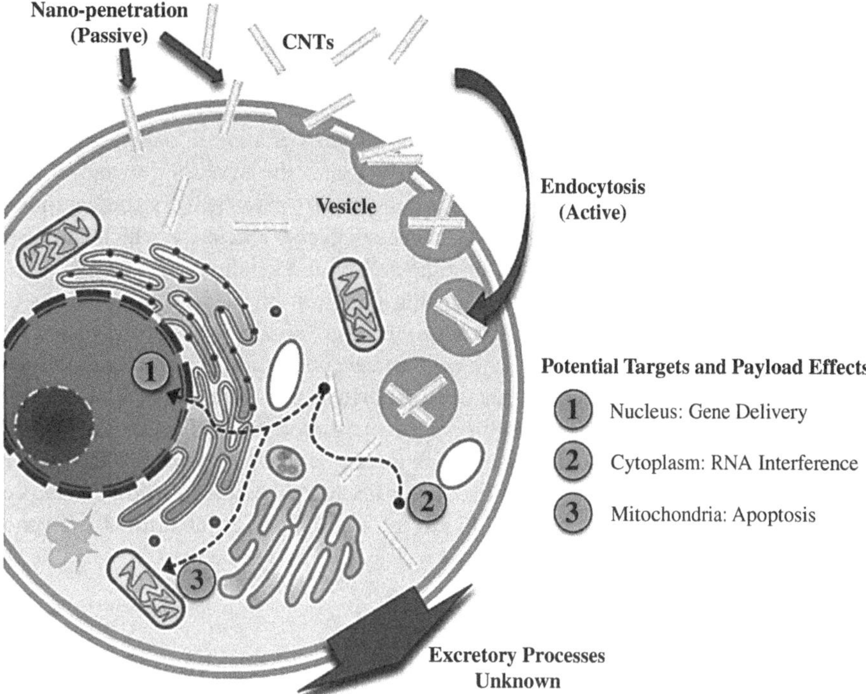

Figure 7-28 Carbon nanotubes (CNTs) can enter a cancer cell via nano-penetration (passive) or endocytosis (active). Next, CNTs release their payloads to kill the cancer cell. Currently, the mechanism by which CNTs are excreted by cancer cells is unknown. (*The illustration is reprinted with permission from C. P. Firme III and P. R. Bandaru.*[51])

lung and pancreatic cancers. As shown in Figure 7-29, gemcitabine was conjugated to both non-PEGylated SWCNTs (creating SWCNT-gemcitabine) and PEGylated SWCNTs (creating SWCNT-PEG-gemcitabine). It was found that the amount of gemcitabine by mass was 43.14% and 37.32% on the SWCNT-gemcitabine and SWCNT-PEG-gemcitabine, respectively. This finding indicated that PEGylated SWCNTs have a lower drug loading

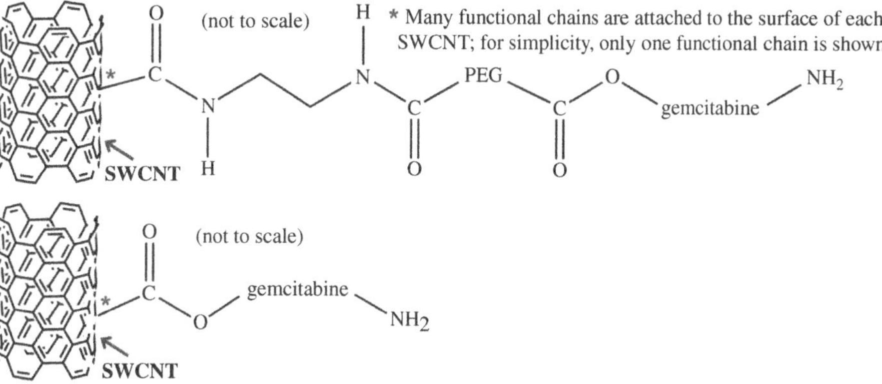

Figure 7-29 Gemcitabine-loaded single-walled carbon nanotubes (SWCNTs) for treating lung and pancreatic cancers. (Top) SWCNT-PEG-gemcitabine; (Bottom) SWCNT-gemcitabine. (*The figures are redrawn with permission from A. Razzazan et al.*[54])

capacity than non-PEGylated SWCNTs. Despite the lower drug loading capacity, the *in vivo* study demonstrated that SWCNT-PEG-gemcitabine was significantly more effective than SWCNT-gemcitabine in suppressing cancerous tumor growth in mice.[54]

CNT surface functionalization can also be achieved by grafting linear polyamidoamine (PAA) to the oxidized surfaces of a multi-walled carbon nanotube (MWCNT) to form amide linkages between PAA and the MWCNT surfaces. The resulting MWCNT-PAA is stable in aqueous solutions. *In vitro* gene delivery studies showed that MWCNT-PAA has a high transfection (i.e., gene delivery) efficiency, which can be ascribed to its low cytotoxicity, strong DNA binding ability, and small particle size.[55]

Although promising potential biomedical applications of CNTs have been demonstrated in many studies, there are concerns about the toxicity of CNTs—namely, their biocompatibility with cells and accumulation in tissues, as well as their biodegradability in the ecosystem. It has been reported that CNTs can be biodegradable in both cell cultures and mice, depending on how surfaces of the CNTs are functionalized. The *in vitro* biodegradation studies of CNTs in cell cultures showed that CNTs were degraded significantly by active enzymes (i.e., oxidases and peroxidases) within living cells. The *in vivo* biodegradation studies of CNTs in mice also demonstrated that CNTs underwent some degree of biodegradation. Further research is needed before CNTs can be safely applied to treat cancers and other diseases in humans.[56-58]

7.6.3 Ultrasound-Aided Phase-Shift Nanodroplets for Cancer Drug Delivery

Ultrasound was first used as an imaging tool for clinical purposes in the 1950s. The use of ultrasonic contrast agents such as microbubbles can significantly enhance the ultrasound reflectivity of structures in the human body, which consolidates ultrasound as a reliable medical diagnostic tool. After the technology of drug delivery by nanoparticles was discovered, ultrasound was also used as a tool to help release drugs from ultrasound-responsive nanoparticles within cancer cells and tumors. Both functions of ultrasound may be combined to achieve targeted drug delivery and improved imaging. In fact, nanoparticles (e.g., perfluorocarbon nanodroplets) can be used both as ultrasound contrast agents to enhance imaging and as ultrasound-activated drug delivery vehicles.[59]

In tumor-targeted drug delivery, ultrasound has been used to heat temperature-sensitive liposomes. In this case, a liposome is a spherical lipid bilayer encapsulating a drug-containing solution. Upon heating, the lipid membrane of a liposome undergoes a gel-to-fluid phase transition and thus the drugs encapsulated in the liposome are released at the target site. For example, ThermoDox®, a commercial product made from liposome nanoparticles with encapsulated doxorubicin (a common cancer drug), can be used to treat primary liver cancer, one of the deadliest and most common cancers. Heating the liposome nanoparticles to a temperature between 40°C and 45°C will allow doxorubicin in the liposomes to be released at the targeted tumor.[60]

In addition, the application of ultrasound generates acoustic oscillations. The absorption of high amplitude acoustic oscillations will generate acoustic streaming (i.e., steady fluid flow) in the fluid as well as acoustic radiation forces on particles in the fluid. Acoustic streaming together with acoustic radiation forces enhances the contact of drug-containing nanodroplets with tumor cells, promoting drug delivery into cell membranes.[59]

In the case of perfluorocarbon (PFC) nanodroplets used for drug delivery, ultrasound can be used to generate droplet-to-bubble phase transitions. The nanodroplets are made of PEG-PLLA copolymer, in which PEG (polyethylene glycol) serves as the hydrophilic shell while PLLA (poly-L-lactide) acts as the hydrophobic core. Both PFC and anti-cancer drugs (Genexol®-PM and paclitaxel) are encapsulated within the hydrophobic core. PFC has a

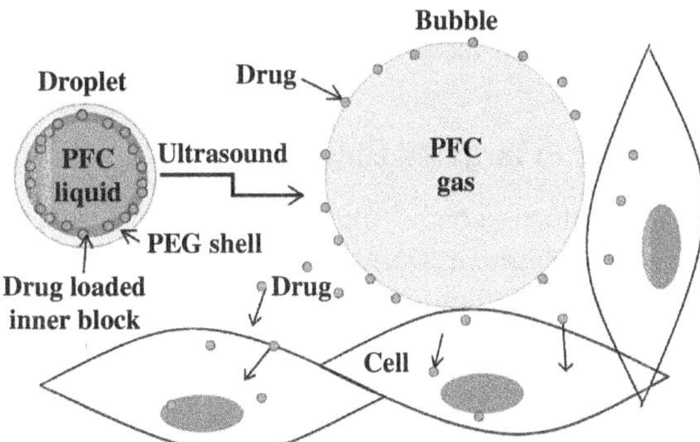

Figure 7-30 Illustration of drug release into cancer cells through ultrasound-aided droplet-to-bubble phase transition. (*The illustration is reprinted with permission from N. Y. Rapoport et al.[61]*)

boiling temperature of 29°C at atmospheric pressure. When nanodroplets arrive in the targeted region (i.e., within a tumor), ultrasound is used to trigger PFC droplet vaporization, by which the PFC nanodroplets transition from liquid to microbubbles (Figure 7-30). Due to the dramatic volume increase of PFC in the hydrophobic core, the thickness of the nanodroplet shell is reduced and the shell is partially broken, creating voids. As a result, the drug molecules contained in the nanodroplets migrate to the surface of the bubbles. Soon after, the drugs are released into tumor cells due to acoustic radiation forces and acoustic streaming.[62]

The efficacy of drug delivery by ultrasound-aided phase-shift nanodroplets was confirmed by an experiment with a mouse having bilateral ovarian carcinoma tumors. A photo of the mouse prior to treatment is shown in Figure 7-31a. Both tumors were treated for three weeks. The left tumor (control) was treated with nanodroplets without ultrasound application, while the right tumor was treated with nanodroplets plus ultrasound application. As can be seen from Figure 7-31b, the left tumor has grown significantly while the right tumor has shrunk following three weeks of treatment. The results indicate that ultrasound facilitated the release of drugs into the tumor, killing cancer cells. Without ultrasound application, the anti-cancer drugs encapsulated in the nanodroplets were less likely to be released into the tumor and hence the drug-tumor contact was limited, resulting in the uncontrolled growth of the left tumor.[61]

In general, ultrasound-aided nanodroplets for targeted drug delivery must have the following properties: (1) biocompatibility, so that the nanodroplets do not produce a toxic or immune response in the human body; (2) stability in circulation, such that nanodroplets remain stable before reaching the targeted areas; (3) drug retention, so that the nanodroplets safely retain the drugs inside them until the drugs are released; (4) responsiveness to

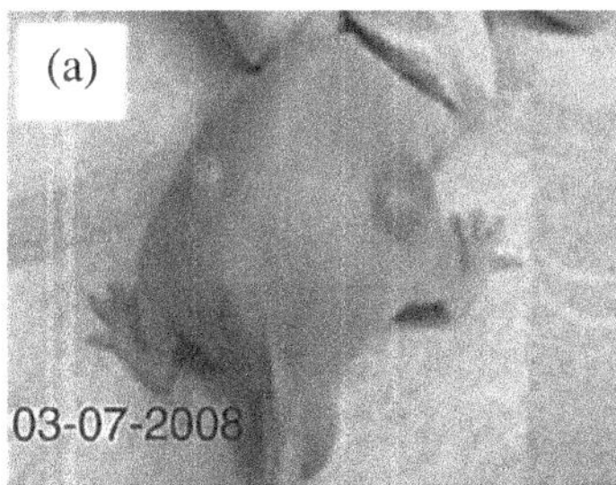

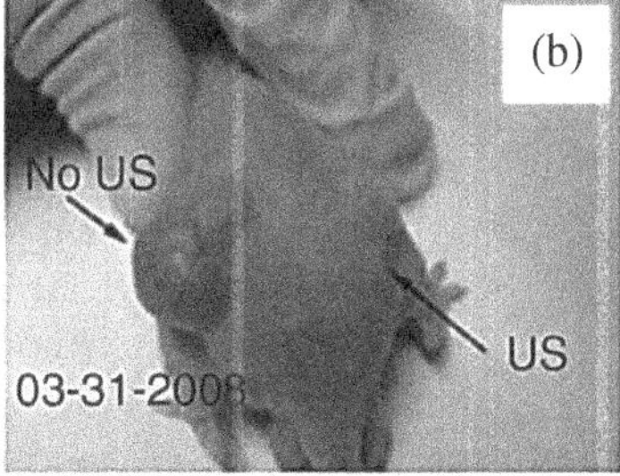

Figure 7-31 (a) A mouse with bilateral ovarian carcinoma tumors prior to treatment. (b) Mouse after three weeks of treatment with nanodroplets containing encapsulated anti-cancer drugs Genexol®-PM and paclitaxel; ultrasound irradiation was applied to the right tumor, but not to the left tumor (control). (*The images are reprinted with permission from N. Y. Rapoport et al.[61]*)

ultrasound; and (5) high penetration, allowing the nanodroplets to penetrate the target tissue (e.g., a tumor).[62]

7.6.4 Applications of DNA Nanotechnology in Targeted Cancer Treatment

In this section, we focus on the applications of DNA nanotechnology in targeted drug delivery for cancer treatment. DNA nanotechnology uses the unique chemical and physical properties of DNA for automated synthesis to create a variety of structures, including dendrimers, nanoshells, nanocages and other DNA nanostructures (please refer to Section 5.6 for more details). Promising DNA nanostructures developed for targeted drug delivery include tetrahedral nanostructures, honeycomb nanostructures, and nanotubes. DNA nanostructures are used as drug delivery vehicles to minimize toxicity, increase drug solubility, and add cell-targeting capabilities. For this purpose, DNA is constructed as boxes or other hollow geometries so that genes, drugs, or nanoparticles can be loaded into the DNA structures and are delivered to the targeted cancer cells via these vehicles. To effectively transport and reach the target cancer cells, the DNA nanostructures must survive the chemical and physical conditions in biological environments. Once the nanostructures reach the target cancer cells, they can either release drugs to kill cancer cells externally or break through the membranes of cancer cells and enter to release drugs within the cells and kill them internally. The second approach usually involves masquerading as a different common molecule that is frequently absorbed by cancer cells, adding surface features or creating geometries that increase the likelihood of the nanostructure being taken into cancer cells. In addition to these technical requirements, feasibility analysis must also be performed in terms of standard success indicators such as cost and ease of fabrication, as some technologies (e.g., the SELEX process for DNA nanostructure creation) can be effective but are complicated and expensive.[63,64]

Aside from nanostructures formed by DNA itself, DNA nanostructures can be combined with GNPs for targeted cancer therapy. A self-assembled gold-DNA nano-sunflower was reported for applications in gene interference therapy, which silences oncogenes within cancer cells to disrupt the functions of cancer cells and inhibit tumor growth. First, GNPs (each 2 nm in diameter) were attached to POY2T oligonucleotides via chemical modification to create gold-POY2T nanoparticles. The POY2T oligonucleotide is a 23 nucleotide-long strand of ssDNA which binds to the P2 promoter of the *c-myc* oncogene in cancer cells to form a triplex structure, silencing the *c-myc* oncogene. Next, the addition of strands of a different ssDNA (called CA) which complementarily binds to the tail part of the POY2T sequence results in the self-assembly (via cross-linking) of nano-sunflowers roughly 200 nm in size. In the nano-sunflower, most of the GNPs are distributed at the surface. The self-assembled nano-sunflower is easily disassembled by heat. Above the melting temperature (T_m) of DNA, the nano-sunflower will be destroyed and the gold-POY2T nanoparticles are released. The self-assembly (by cross-linking) and disassembly (by heat) of gold-DNA nano-sunflowers are illustrated in Figure 7-32 (top-left).[65]

Compared to the small size of the gold-POY2T nanoparticles, the much larger nano-sunflowers allow a greater number of gold-POY2T nanoparticles to be delivered to the tumor site. Once the nano-sunflowers accumulate at the tumor, near-infrared (NIR) light irradiation is applied, resulting in the release of gold-POY2T nanoparticles that bind to and silence the *c-myc* oncogenes of the cancer cells. This entire process is depicted in Figure 7-32 (bottom). It was found that the use of nano-sunflowers as delivery vehicles for gold-POY2T nanoparticles was far more effective than directly using the gold-POY2T nanoparticles. To demonstrate the efficacy of this experimental cancer therapy, nano-sunflowers were intravenously injected into tumor-bearing mice. After a 12-hour incubation

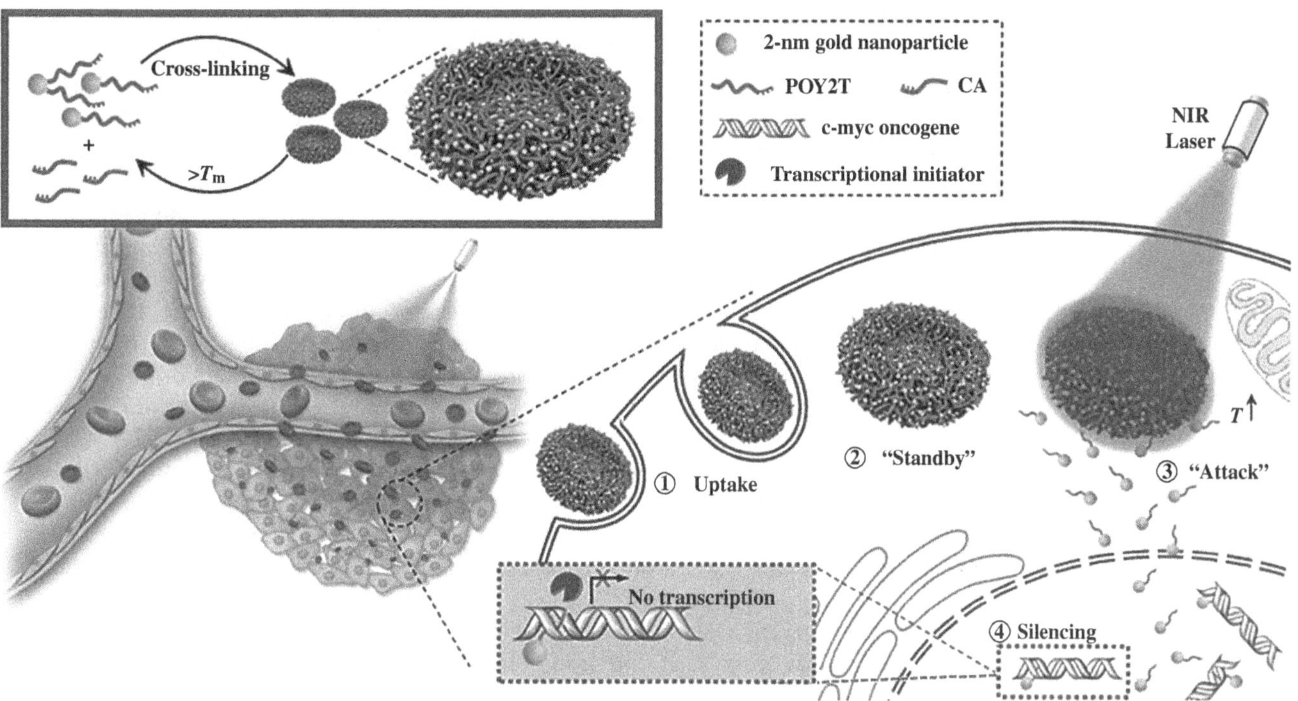

Figure 7-32   (Top-Left) Formation and disassembly of self-assembled gold-DNA nano-sunflowers. (Bottom) The uptake of nano-sunflowers into a cancer cell, followed by an incubation period ("standby"), and irradiation with NIR (near-infrared) light which liberates the gold-POY2T nanoparticles, silencing the *c-myc* oncogenes of the cancer cells. (*The figure is reprinted with permission from S. Huo et al.*[65])

period, NIR irradiation was applied for 3 min to breakdown the nano-sunflowers and release the gold-POY2T nanoparticles. 24 days later, the tumor volume in the mice treated with nano-sunflowers was reduced by 90% compared to the control. The results indicate that DNA-mediated self-assembled nanostructures provide a new and effective approach for targeted cancer treatment.[65]

Targeted cancer therapy is complex. In addition to the factors mentioned before, diagnosis and imaging capabilities, biocompatibility of drug delivery vehicles, the toxicity to non-targeted cells, and uptake and retention of the desired compounds in the targeted cells must all be considered. A successful targeted therapy would require high selectivity toward cancer cells, higher success rates than non-targeted therapies, minimal side effects, and an affordable cost. Currently, various types of nanostructures are being developed to contain and deliver cancer drugs directly to cancer cells without harming healthy cells. Emerging technologies are also combined to provide both therapeutic and diagnostic benefits. Aside from targeted cancer treatments, other applications such as vehicles to report the *in vivo* efficacy of therapeutic agents and detectors for molecular changes associated with diseases are under development.[66]

7.7 MITOCHONDRIA-TARGETED DELIVERY OF 2,4-DINITROPHENOL BY NANOPARTICLES

Traditional medication taken orally or intravenously requires the medicines to be highly soluble in water, so that they can diffuse through body fluids to the desired sites. However, many medicines have low solubility in water. To achieve therapeutic concentrations at target sites for effective treatment, it is easy to overdose the medicine, which may lead to poisoning or death. The application of targeted drug delivery through nanoparticles can avoid the overdose issue. Instead of relying on diffusion, nanoparticle delivery vehicles send medications directly to the target sites. Targeted drug delivery reduces the dose of medicine required for treatment as it drastically reduces the amount of medicine that reaches non-target sites. Thus, targeted drug delivery can improve the treatment success rate and reduce both the severity of side effects and cost of medications needed for treatment.[67]

For nanoparticle-based targeted drug delivery, medicines are loaded into nanoparticles which act as a therapeutic agent to repair or restore cell functionality. The therapeutic action of nanoparticles is dependent on the payload, namely the drugs they carry. Targeted drug delivery through nanoparticles is similar to the way through which viruses invade our bodies, but with benevolent rather than harmful purposes. Viruses are naturally occurring nanoparticles which carry payloads in the form of infectious strands of RNA or DNA. Once viruses attach to targeted cells, they deliver the payload to the cells in order to replicate, which overtakes and eventually destroys the cells.

Here we introduce the mitochondria-targeted delivery of 2,4-dinitrophenol (DNP) by nanoparticles. First of all, let us briefly review the history of DNP. In the early 1900s, DNP was initially used to produce dyes and explosives. From 1933 to 1938, DNP was used as a weight loss drug after it was reported that DNP could increase the metabolic rate substantially, which causes the body to rapidly lose fat. The increase in metabolic rate also causes human cells to produce significantly more heat, resulting in intracellular hyperthermia. It was observed that overdose of DNP led to a high death rate. This severe side effect resulted in the ban of DNP as a drug by the U.S. FDA in 1938.[68]

However, the mechanism of DNP function within cells was unknown until the 1960s when scientists elucidated the detailed functions of mitochondria. Mitochondria are organelles within cells which produce energy to support cellular functions through oxidative phosphorylation reactions, and the energy is stored in a small molecule called adenosine triphosphate (ATP). ATP synthesis is driven by the electrochemical gradient (i.e., potential) of protons across the mitochondrial inner membrane. Uncoupling mitochondrial membrane potential generation from ATP synthesis will inhibit ATP production. Now it is well-known that DNP is a mitochondrial uncoupler. Since DNP disrupts ATP generation and results in insufficient energy for cellular activities, the metabolic rate is increased in order to meet the energy demand.[68]

The toxicities caused by DNP are dose-dependent. Reducing the dose of DNP will decrease its detrimental effects. While DNP is still banned for use as a medicine for weight loss, scientists are trying to find its use in cancer treatment as well as safer ways to use it for weight control by taking advantage of its unique ability to cause mitochondrial uncoupling.[68] A report in 2008 showed that DNP was able to inhibit the growth of lung cancer cells.[69] Here we focus purely on the mitochondria-targeted delivery of DNP by nanoparticles for weight loss.

Figure 7-33 shows lipid (i.e., fat) accumulation in mouse adipocytes (i.e., fat cells) after 7 days in four distinct experimental groups: (1) control with no DNP applied, (2) free DNP is present, (3) DNP delivered by targeted nanoparticles (NPs), and (4) DNP delivered by non-targeted nanoparticles (NPs). Crucially, the concentrations of DNP used (0 to 100 μM) in this study are insufficient to exert cytotoxicity. In this study, mouse preadipocytes (i.e., precursors for fat cells) were differentiated into adipocytes, resulting in the accumulation of lipids. DNP in the three non-control experimental groups was used to hinder the accumulation of lipids to test its effectiveness for inducing weight loss. The non-targeted nanoparticle used is PLGA-*b*-PEG, while the targeted nanoparticle used is PLGA-*b*-PEG-TPP. PLGA is poly(lactic-co-glycolic acid), which is a biodegradable polymer approved by the U.S. FDA; PEG is polyethylene glycol; TPP (triphenylphosphonium) is a lipophilic cation

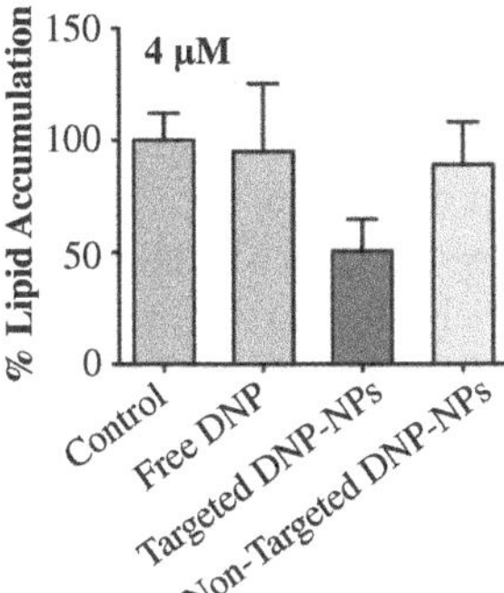
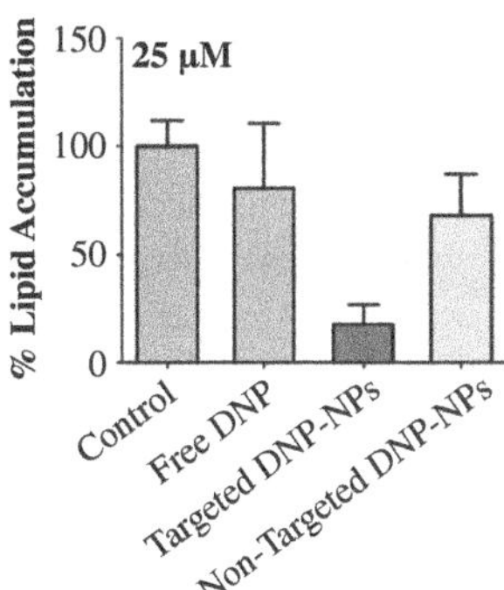

Figure 7-33 The effect of DNP on lipid (i.e., fat) accumulation within mouse adipocytes after 7 days with DNP or DNP-nanoparticle (DNP-NP) concentrations of 4 µM (left) and 25 µM (right). There are four distinct experimental groups. (*The plots are reprinted with permission from S. Marrache and S. Dhar.*[70])

which can cross into the mitochondrial matrix space and thus allows PLGA-*b*-PEG-TPP to target mitochondria. PLGA-*b*-PEG and PLGA-*b*-PEG-TPP each can form polymeric micelles having a hydrophobic core and a hydrophilic shell, with the hydrophobic core serving as a reservoir for DNP.[70]

The results in Figure 7-33 indicate that at low DNP concentrations, DNP delivered by targeted nanoparticles can inhibit lipid accumulation significantly more efficiently than free DNP or DNP delivered by non-targeted nanoparticles. For example, at 4 µM, DNP delivered by targeted nanoparticles reduced lipid accumulation by ~50%, whereas lipid reductions by free DNP or DNP delivered by non-targeted nanoparticles were not significant. Therefore, mitochondria-targeted delivery of DNP by nanoparticles makes it possible to achieve weight loss at safe doses.[70]

7.8 NEURAL IMPLANTS AND BRAIN–MACHINE INTERFACES

Another exciting application of bionanotechnology is the use of nanomaterials to improve biomedical devices such as neural implants and brain–machine interfaces. The brain remains the most physically untouched part of the human body, and a complete understanding of how it functions is still lacking. The brain controls the nervous system, which is the most complex system in the human body. The nervous system is composed of nerves and neurons which communicate signals between different parts of the body. Each neuron forms part of a neural network and produces an electric signal when triggered by internal or external stimuli. When there are abnormalities in communications between neurons, the human body can fall to severe illnesses such as movement disorders and changes of consciousness. To cure or control such illnesses, it is important to obtain and understand the electrical signals generated by neural activity in the targeted neurons and nerves. Such information can be obtained from neural implants. A neural implant is a surgically-implanted device containing micro- or nano-electrodes that can both record nerve signals in real time as well as stimulate nerves. Neural implants can provide either continuous nerve stimulation or only necessary nerve stimulation to restore lost body functions such as hearing or limb movement.

By interfacing neural implants with a computer, we can create a brain–machine interface (BMI). BMIs allow the human brain and by extension the nervous system to communicate with a computer. BMIs can interact with neural signals via microelectrodes so that we can obtain information about how the brain works. These neural signals occur when an action potential is triggered due to any stimulus from the internal or external environment. Each neuron forms part of a neural network and produces an electric signal when triggered (such as an action performed by a human). The signal can be measured by microelectrode threads placed extremely close to the neurons. Variations in the strength of neuronal electric signals are reflected in spikes, and the timing of these spikes provides useful quantitative information that needs to be analyzed. Once analyzed, the reverse can be achieved by synthesizing the signal and sending them back to specific parts of the brain.[71]

Cochlear implants are a well-known example of a BMI. To offset hearing loss, the implanted device produces electrical currents to relay audio signals past the inner ear to stimulate the cochlear nerve. Important issues to be considered are the biocompatibility of materials, and how the implant affects nearby tissue. High-intensity stimuli can cause permanent damage to the auditory nerve. Another example is the U.S. FDA–approved Utah array, which can record and stimulate a group of neurons. The Utah array is used to control a prosthesis. The problem is that the array can neither be inserted for too long nor be constantly reinserted because tissue scarring and neural damage can occur.[72]

Safety and long-term integration with the human brain are the main concerns when designing these micro-/nano-electrodes. Unfortunately, the typical instability of interfacing the brain with electrodes can render the electrodes useless due to cellular and vascular damage, inflammation, tissue response, neuronal degradation, and scar formation. If the electrodes are too large, they may cause glial scarring in the brain. However, if the electrodes are too small, they can easily break and be rendered useless. Figure 7-34 shows the effect of microelectrodes on the safety and long-term integration with brain or neural tissue. When a hard and noncompliant electrode is inserted into healthy tissue, inflammation is visible since many astrocytes and microglia are seen around the microelectrode (Figure 7-34b).[73]

To reduce the negative long-term impact of electrodes on neural tissue, nanomaterials including carbon nanotubes and various nanowires integrated with hydrogels are applied. Since the initial insertion of microelectrodes must be delicate and precise as local cells can be damaged during the insertion, soft conductive materials or ultra-thin and flexible electrodes can be used.[73] Figure 7-34c shows that porous and soft microelectrodes can achieve high biological integration with minimal inflammation.

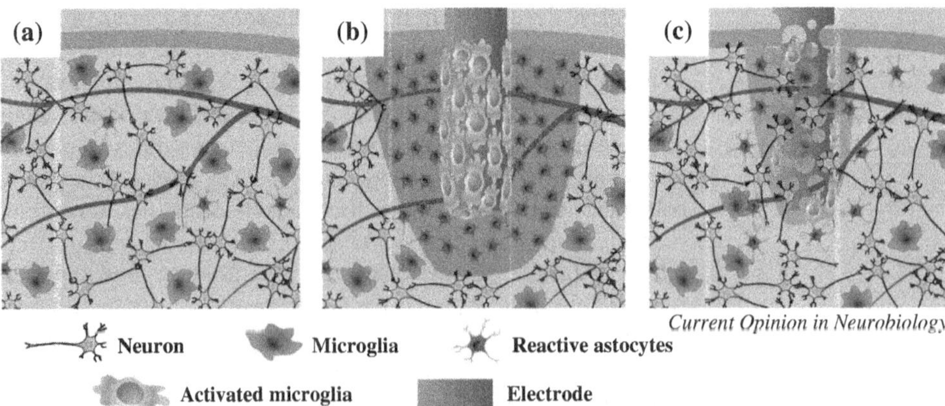

Figure 7-34 The effect of microelectrodes on the safety and long-term integration with brain or neural tissue. (a) healthy tissue; (b) inflamed tissue resulting from a noncompliant microelectrode; (c) noninflamed tissue integrated with a porous and soft microelectrode. (*The illustrations are reprinted with permission from D. Scaini and L. Ballerini.*[73])

Other important examples of BMIs are computer or microprocessor-controlled neural implants used for deep brain stimulation (DBS), vagus nerve stimulation, and mind-controlled prosthesis. DBS was first used in the 1990s. To implement DBS, a small and portable neurostimulator device is used with electrodes inserted into specific brain areas to deliver electrical pulses for suppressing abnormal nerve signals which cause symptoms. For instance, DBS can be effectively used to reduce uncontrollable movements with a neurostimulator device connected to electrodes inserted in the basal ganglia network of the brain (which controls motor behavior). Through insulated wires, the DBS electrodes are connected to a small battery-powered pulse generator controlled by a built-in microprocessor. The insulated wires and pulse generator are implanted under the skin near the collarbone or at other places in the body. DBS treatments have been used for patients with movement disorders such as Parkinson's disease, dystonia, essential tremor, and Tourette syndrome. The efficacy of DBS treatments depends on the appropriate target region of the brain as well as the stimulation settings which include intensity, pulse width, and frequency. The local field potentials (i.e., transient electrical signals) recorded by the electrodes are used to analyze the nervous system response to the stimulation, which can be used to determine optimal settings for individual patients. Even when DBS treatments are successful, the efficacy can be limited. A deeper understanding of the DBS mechanism of action in the brain is required to improve this therapy and avoid the side effects associated with DBS.[74]

Increasing the number of electrodes is being considered to improve DBS treatment. As electrodes are used to record the activity of neurons, the application of more electrodes will enable the collection of more signals from a greater number of neurons. Recently, Neuralink—a company focusing on BMIs—developed a device which has 3072 microelectrodes. These electrodes are distributed on 96 polymer threads, with each thread having 32 electrodes. The device is small, with 3072 channels (electrodes) in a space of 23 mm × 18.5 mm × 2 mm. The polymer threads are ultra-fine and flexible, offering greater biocompatibility compared to those made from metals or semiconductors. Since the microelectrodes are not stiff enough to penetrate the skull, a neurosurgical robot is used to implant the threads at a speed of 6 threads (i.e., 192 microelectrodes) per minute. The data collected is processed by an integrated circuit. At present, this device is mainly used as a research platform. Rodent studies using the device may pave the way for future applications in humans.[75]

In addition to DBS, BMIs can also be used for vagus nerve stimulation (VNS). The vagus nerve is located in the neck and regulates the functions of many internal organs as well as reflexes. VNS is a treatment for non-motor diseases such as epilepsy, pain, and neuropsychiatric disorders. It was first used for epilepsy treatment in 1988. In addition to vagus nerve electrodes inserted into the neck, the implantable VNS device includes a microprocessor-controlled pulse generator, lead wires, and a handheld magnetic controller accessory. Although the pulse generator is programmed by software, it also can be manually controlled by the user through the magnetic controller accessory. The magnetic accessory allows the user to increase or stop the vagus nerve stimulation. Increasing the stimulation level with the magnet right before the onset of seizures can shorten or stop the seizures. Unlike DBS neurostimulator devices, the battery-operated pulse generator of a VNS device is usually implanted in the upper chest or in the armpit. The vagus nerve is connected to the VNS pulse generator through lead wires. For the VNS device, the lead wires are positioned at the cervical portion of the trunk of the left vagus nerve above the clavicle. Due to its highly invasive nature and potentially serious side effects, VNS is usually used to treat drug-resistant epilepsy and treatment-resistant neuropsychiatric disorders.[76]

Finally, a mind-controlled prosthesis (e.g., an artificial limb, hand, or foot) can be used to restore extremity functions. In the 1900s, body-powered prostheses able to perform intended movements were developed. By the 1960s, myoelectric prostheses came into use. These prostheses could translate residual muscle electrical activity into movements. In myoelectric prostheses, surface electromyography electrodes are placed above residual muscles of the residual limb to record the muscle's electrical activity, which is used by the patient to control the prostheses. The accuracy of prostheses control can be improved using multi-channel surface electromyography electrodes or implanted electromyography electrodes.[77]

7.9 APPLICATIONS OF BIONANOTECHNOLOGY IN CROP AGRICULTURE

As the world population increases, demand for food increases as well. Unfortunately, the available land for agriculture worldwide is expected to decrease as a result of urban sprawl and climate change. To satisfy the increased demand for food, enhancing agricultural efficiency and improving soil health are required. Bionanotechnologies such as nanopesticides, nanofertilizers, nanobiosensors, and nanomaterials-based bioremediation of contaminated soils have been developed for these purposes. The main applications of bionanotechnology in crop agriculture are illustrated in Figure 7-35.[78]

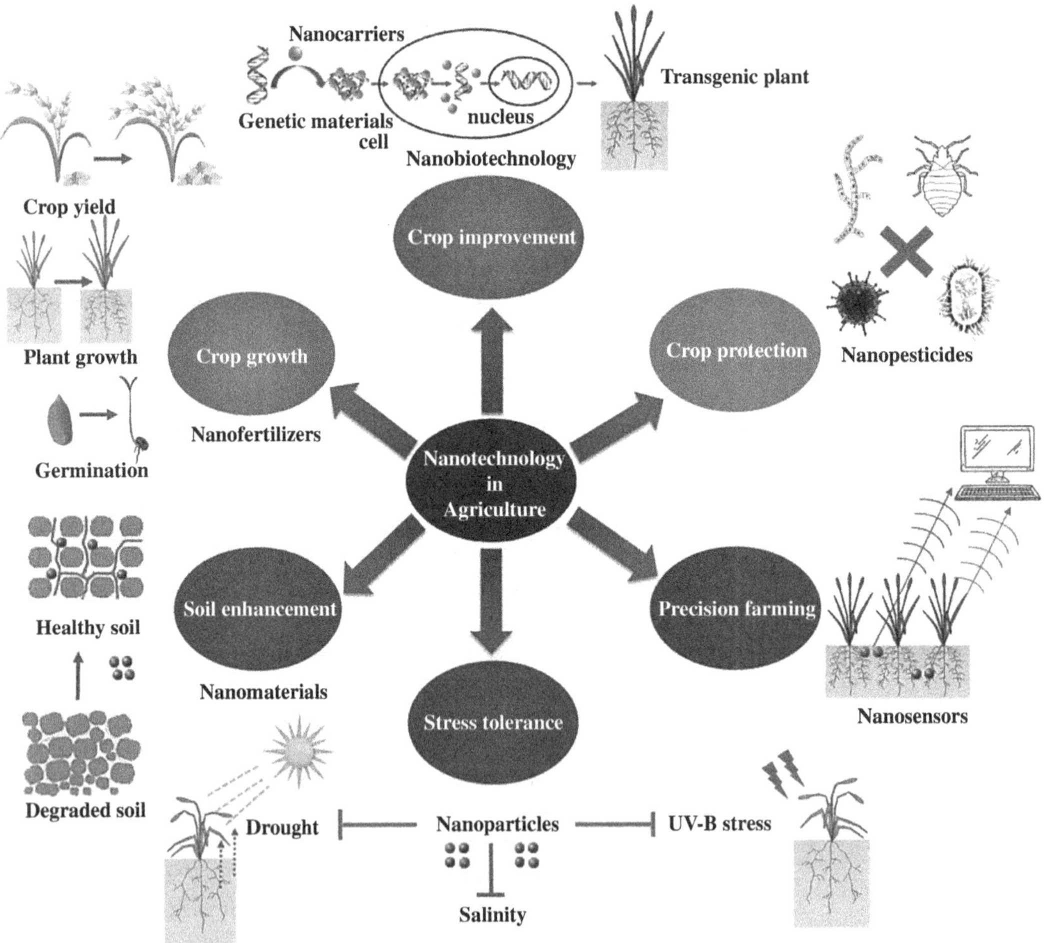

Figure 7-35 Applications of bionanotechnology in crop agriculture include crop improvement with genetic engineering, crop protection with nanopesticides, precision farming with nanobiosensors, improved crop stress tolerance with nanoparticles, soil enhancement with nanomaterials, and faster crop growth with nanofertilizers. (*The illustration is from Y. Shang et al.*[79])

Pesticides are routinely used in agriculture to kill or repel pests. Pesticides include herbicides for destroying pest plants such as weeds, and insecticides for controlling pest insects. In the application of pesticides, over 95% of herbicides and 98% of sprayed insecticides are lost to the environment instead of reaching target pest species.[80] Nanopesticides that provide effective pest control over long durations have been developed to minimize the use of pesticides, reducing their environmental impact. Nanopesticide technology can control the release of pesticides encapsulated in nanomaterials based on external stimuli such as light, temperature, pH, humidity, and the presence of enzymes. These nanopesticides are called intelligent pesticides.[81] In addition—due to their small size—nanopesticide droplets have better wettability and greater target adsorption on pest plants and pest insects. For instance, Pereira et al. encapsulated atrazine herbicide in poly(epsilon-caprolactone) nanoparticles to control weeds and reduce herbicide-associated environmental risks. The herbicide-containing nanoparticles were stable for 90 days because the polymer shell of each nanoparticle protected the herbicide inside from physio-chemical and microbiological degradation. It was found that the nanoparticles effectively controlled the growth of target weeds, while not affecting plant crops. It was proposed that the nanoparticles were absorbed by the roots of target weeds, after which atrazine herbicide was delivered to the weed plant tissues.[82]

As another example of nanopesticides, Stadler et al. successfully utilized nanostructured alumina (NSA) as a potent insecticide. While NSA is negatively charged, the bodies of insects are positively charged due to triboelectrification. When NSA comes into contact with insects, the NSA particles will adsorb strongly on insect bodies due to electrostatic attraction. The strong adsorption of NSA causes dehydration of the insects and their death. Due to their small particle size, NSA particles have relatively large surface area which grants them strong adsorption potential on insects and high insecticidal efficacy. However, the insecticidal efficacy of NSA particles decreases with increasing humidity.[83]

Nanofertilizers are another agricultural application of bionanotechnology. Fertilizers provide essential plant nutrients such as nitrogen, phosphorus, and potassium. Nanofertilizers are nanoscale fertilizer particles or fertilizers encapsulated in nanomaterials. Compared to conventional fertilizers, nanoscale fertilizer particles have much larger surface-area-to-volume ratio which significantly improves their application efficiency. Fertilizers encapsulated in nanomaterials can be released when triggered by internal stimuli from the plant such as the need for nutrients. The controlled and slow release of the nutrients effectively prevents the loss of fertilizers due to leaching, thereby increasing their efficiency and reducing environmental contamination.[84]

In order to protect environmental health, pesticides, fertilizers, and toxic metal ions in water and soil need to be monitored and controlled. Nanobiosensors can detect the quantity of residual pesticides, fertilizers, or toxic metal ions in both water and soil depending on the nanomaterials used in the nanobiosensors. Nanobiosensors can also detect soil moisture and soil nutrient status, providing useful information for farming.[78,85] For example, Yu et al. reported an atrazine herbicide biosensor which was used to detect trace atrazine in soil. The biosensor was fabricated by immobilizing tyrosinase enzymes on vertically grown TiO2 nanotubes, which have large available surface area for enzyme adsorption. The biosensor can detect atrazine concentrations of 0.2 parts per trillion to 2 parts per billion.[86]

To restore contaminated environments, water and soil must be decontaminated. Among many environmental remediation technologies, nanomaterials-based bioremediation of contaminants is the most remarkable technology. Integration of nanotechnology and biotechnology allows the contaminants to be remedied efficiently and in an environmentally friendly fashion. Nanomaterials can react with organic pollutants to change their properties or increase their bioavailability to bioagents. The nanomaterial-treated pollutants will subsequently be subjected to bioremediation. In phytoremediation, nanomaterials can improve the uptake of toxic heavy metals in contaminated soils by plants, while simultaneously reducing oxidative damage of heavy metals to the plants.[78,87]

7.10 REFERENCES

[1]   I. J. Busch-Vishniac, *Electromechanical Sensors and Actuators.* New York, NY, USA: Springer New York, 1999.

[2]   B. F. Romanowicz, *Methodology for the Modeling and Simulation of Microsystems.* Boston, MA, USA: Springer US, 1998.

[3]   A. C. Fairlie-Clarke, "Force as a flow variable," *Proceedings of the Institution of Mechanical Engineers, Part I: Journal of Systems and Control Engineering,* vol. 213, no. 1, pp. 77–81, 1999.

[4]   A. Schilling, X. Zhang, and O. Bossen, "Heat flowing from cold to hot without external intervention by using a 'thermal inductor,'" *Science Advances,* vol. 5, no. 4, article 9953, 2019.

[5]   C. Zhang and D. Xing, "Miniaturized PCR chips for nucleic acid amplification and analysis: latest advances and future trends," *Nucleic Acids Research,* vol. 35, no. 13, pp. 4223–4237, 2007.

[6]   M. A. Northrup, M. T. Ching, R. M. White, and R. T. Watson, "DNA amplification with a microfabricated reaction chamber," in *7th International Conference on Solid–State Sensors and Actuators (Transducers '93),* Yokohama, Japan, 1993, pp. 924–926.

[7]   J. H. Daniel, S. Iqbal, R. B. Millington, D. F. Moore, C. R. Lowe, D. L. Leslie, et al., "Silicon microchambers for DNA amplification," *Sensors and Actuators A: Physical,* vol. 71, no. 1–2, pp. 81–88, 1998.

[8]   S. D. Senturia, *Microsystem Design.* New York, NY, USA: Springer Science & Business Media, 2001.

[9]   M. U. Kopp, A. J. de Mello, and A. Manz, "Chemical amplification: continuous-flow PCR on a chip," *Science,* vol. 280, no. 5366, pp. 1046–1048, 1998.

[10]   J. Voldman. "BioMEMS case study: microdevices for PCR", MIT OpenCourseWare, Massachusetts Institute of Technology [Online]. Available: https://ocw.mit.edu/courses/electrical-engineering-and-computer-science/6-777j-design-and-fabrication-of-microelectromechanical-devices-spring-2007/lecture-notes/07lecture25.pdf, 2007.

[11]   "Health topics: diabetes," World Health Organization (WHO) [Online]. Available: http://www.who.int/topics/diabetes_mellitus/en, 2020.

[12]   "National Diabetes Statistics Report, 2020 Estimates of Diabetes and Its Burden in the United States," U.S. Centers for Disease Control and Prevention (CDC) [Online]. Available: https://www.cdc.gov/diabetes/pdfs/data/statistics/national-diabetes-statistics-report.pdf, 2020.

[13]   R. I. G. Holt, C. Cockram, A. Flyvbjerg, and B. J. Goldstein, Eds., *Textbook of Diabetes,* 4th ed. Chichester, West Sussex, UK: Wiley-Blackwell, 2010.

[14]   W. V. Gonzales, A. T. Mobashsher, and A. Abbosh, "The progress of glucose monitoring: a review of invasive to minimally and non-invasive techniques, devices and sensors," *Sensors,* vol. 19, no. 4, article 800, 2019.

[15]   M. Taguchi, A. Ptitsyn, E. S. McLamore, and J. C. Claussen, "Nanomaterial-mediated biosensors for monitoring glucose," *Journal of Diabetes Science and Technology,* vol. 8, no. 2, pp. 403–411, 2014.

[16]   J. C. Pickup, F. Hussain, N. D. Evans, O. J. Rolinski, and D. J. S. Birch, "Fluorescence-based glucose sensors," *Biosensors & Bioelectronics,* vol. 20, no. 12, pp. 2555–2565, 2005.

[17]   L. Chen, E. Hwang, and J. Zhang, "Fluorescent nanobiosensors for sensing glucose," *Sensors,* vol. 18, no. 5, 2018.

[18]   L. Lipani, B. G. R. Dupont, F. Doungmene, F. Marken, R. M. Tyrrell, R. H. Guy, et al., "Non-invasive, transdermal, path-selective and specific glucose monitoring via a graphene-based platform," *Nature Nanotechnology,* vol. 13, no. 6, pp. 504–511, 2018.

[19]   D. C. Klonoff, "Overview of fluorescence glucose sensing: a technology with a bright future," *Journal of Diabetes Science and Technology,* vol. 6, no. 6, pp. 1242–50, 2012.

[20]   "Eversense continuous glucose montioring system: P160048," U.S. FDA [Online]. Available: https://www.fda.gov/medical-devices/recently-approved-devices/eversense-continuous-glucose-monitoring-system-p160048, 2018.

[21]   "Eversense® XL continuous glucose monitoring system user guide," Eversense® by Senseonics Inc. [Online]. Available: https://global.eversensediabetes.com/sites/default/files/2019-09/LBL-1402-28-001_Rev_B_Eversense_User_Guide_mgdL_UAE_Web.pdf, 2018.

[22]   M. P. Christiansen, L. J. Klaff, R. Brazg, A. R. Chang, C. J. Levy, D. Lam, et al., "A prospective multicenter evaluation of the accuracy of a novel implanted continuous glucose sensor: PRECISE II," *Diabetes Technology & Therapeutics,* vol. 20, no. 3, pp. 197–206, 2018.

[23]   R. O. Potts, J. A. Tamada, and M. J. Tierney, "Glucose monitoring by reverse iontophoresis," *Diabetes/Metabolism Research and Reviews*, vol. 18, no. S1, pp. S49–53, 2002.

[24]   A. Sieg, R. H. Guy, and M. B. Delgado-Charro, "Electroosmosis in transdermal iontophoresis: implications for noninvasive and calibration-free glucose monitoring," *Biophysical Journal*, vol. 87, no. 5, pp. 3344–3350, 2004.

[25]   F. Wang, L. Liu, and W. J. Li, "Graphene-based glucose sensors: a brief review," *IEEE Transactions on Nanobioscience*, vol. 14, no. 8, pp. 818–834, 2015.

[26]   S. N. A. M. Yazid, I. M. Isa, S. Abu Bakar, N. Hashim, and S. Ab Ghani, "A review of glucose biosensors based on graphene/metal oxide nanomaterials," *Analytical Letters*, vol. 47, no. 11, pp. 1821–1834, 2014.

[27]   J. A. Tamada, S. Garg, L. Jovanovic, K. R. Pitzer, S. Fermi, R. O. Potts, et al., "Noninvasive glucose monitoring—Comprehensive clinical results," *Jama-Journal of the American Medical Association*, vol. 282, no. 19, pp. 1839-1844, 1999.

[28]   D. J. Malik, I. J. Sokolov, G. K. Vinner, F. Mancuso, S. Cinquerrui, G. T. Vladisavljevic, et al., "Formulation, stabilisation and encapsulation of bacteriophage for phage therapy," *Advances in Colloid and Interface Science*, vol. 249, pp. 100–133, 2017.

[29]   P. Tao, Y. Chen, H. Batra, J. Dong, C. Chen, and V. B. Rao, "Genetic engineering of bacteriophages against infectious diseases," *Frontiers in Microbiology*, vol. 10, p. 954, 2019.

[30]   R. Farr, D. S. Choi, and S.-W. Lee, "Phage-based nanomaterials for biomedical applications," *Acta Biomaterialia*, vol. 10, no. 4, pp. 1741–1750, 2014.

[31]   R. Brown, A. Lengeling, and B. Wang, "Phage engineering: how advances in molecular biology and synthetic biology are being utilized to enhance the therapeutic potential of bacteriophages," *Quantitative Biology*, vol. 5, no. 1, pp. 42–54, 2017.

[32]   S. Kilcher and M. J. Loessner, "Engineering bacteriophages as versatile biologics," *Trends in Microbiology*, vol. 27, no. 4, pp. 355–367, 2019.

[33]   X. J. Loh, T.-C. Lee, Q. Dou, and G. R. Deen, "Utilising inorganic nanocarriers for gene delivery," *Biomaterials Science*, vol. 4, no. 1, pp. 70–86, 2016.

[34]   F. Geng, K. Song, J. Z. Xing, C. Yuan, S. Yan, Q. Yang, et al., "Thio-glucose bound gold nanoparticles enhance radio-cytotoxic targeting of ovarian cancer," *Nanotechnology*, vol. 22, no. 28, p. 285101, 2011.

[35]   G. Feng, B. Kong, J. Xing, and J. Chen, "Enhancing multimodality functional and molecular imaging using glucose-coated gold nanoparticles," *Clinical Radiology*, vol. 69, no. 11, pp. 1105–1111, 2014.

[36]   A. Misra, *Challenges in Delivery of Therapeutic Genomics and Proteomics*. Burlington, MA, USA: Elsevier Inc., 2011.

[37]   "Cancer," World Health Organization (WHO) [Online]. Available: https://www.who.int/news-room/fact-sheets/detail/cancer, 2018.

[38]   "Cancer statistics at a glance," Canadian Cancer Society [Online]. Available: https://cancer.ca/en/research/cancer-statistics/cancer-statistics-at-a-glance, 2021.

[39]   D. Hanahan and R. A. Weinberg, "The hallmarks of cancer," *Cell*, vol. 100, no. 1, pp. 57–70, 2000.

[40]   H. Maeda, "The enhanced permeability and retention (EPR) effect in tumor vasculature: The key role of tumor-selective macromolecular drug targeting," *Advances in Enzyme Regulation*, vol. 41, no. 1, pp. 189–207, 2001.

[41]   P. Krzyszczyk, A. Acevedo, E. J. Davidoff, L. M. Timmins, I. Marrero-Berrios, M. Patel, et al., "The growing role of precision and personalized medicine for cancer treatment," *Technology*, vol. 6, no. 3–4, pp. 79–100, 2018.

[42]   S. Patricia Egusquiaguirre, M. Igartua, R. Maria Hernandez, and J. Luis Pedraz, "Nanoparticle delivery systems for cancer therapy: advances in clinical and preclinical research," *Clinical & Translational Oncology*, vol. 14, no. 2, pp. 83–93, 2012.

[43]   X. Huang, P. K. Jain, I. H. El-Sayed, and M. A. El-Sayed, "Plasmonic photothermal therapy (PPTT) using gold nanoparticles," *Lasers in Medical Science*, vol. 23, no. 3, p. 217, 2008.

[44]   S.-E. Kim, B.-R. Lee, H. Lee, S. D. Jo, H. Kim, Y.-Y. Won, et al., "Near-infrared plasmonic assemblies of gold nanoparticles with multimodal function for targeted cancer theragnosis," *Scientific Reports*, vol. 7, no. 1, pp. 1–10, 2017.

[45]   M. A. Mackey, M. R. Ali, L. A. Austin, R. D. Near, and M. A. El-Sayed, "The most effective gold nanorod size for plasmonic photothermal therapy: theory and in vitro experiments," *The Journal of Physical Chemistry B*, vol. 118, no. 5, pp. 1319–1326, 2014.

[46]   E. B. Dickerson, E. C. Dreaden, X. Huang, I. H. El-Sayed, H. Chu, S. Pushpanketh, et al., "Gold nanorod assisted near-infrared plasmonic photothermal therapy (PPTT) of squamous cell carcinoma in mice," *Cancer Letters*, vol. 269, no. 1, pp. 57–66, 2008.

[47]   S. Peiris, J. McMurtrie, and H.-Y. Zhu, "Metal nanoparticle photocatalysts: emerging processes for green organic synthesis," *Catalysis Science & Technology*, vol. 6, no. 2, pp. 320–338, 2016.

[48] Y. He, K. Laugesen, D. Kamp, S. A. Sultan, L. B. Oddershede, and L. Jauffred, "Effects and side effects of plasmonic photothermal therapy in brain tissue," *Cancer Nanotechnology*, vol. 10, no. 1, pp. 1–11, 2019.

[49] D. Yang, G. X. Yang, P. P. Yang, R. C. Lv, S. L. Gai, C. X. Li, et al., "Assembly of Au plasmonic photothermal agent and iron oxide nanoparticles on ultrathin black phosphorus for targeted photothermal and photodynamic cancer therapy," *Advanced Functional Materials*, vol. 27, no. 18, p. 14, 2017.

[50] S. Wang, P. Huang, L. Nie, R. Xing, D. Liu, Z. Wang, et al., "Single continuous wave laser induced photodynamic/plasmonic photothermal therapy using photosensitizer-functionalized gold nano-stars," *Advanced Materials*, vol. 25, no. 22, pp. 3055–3061, 2013.

[51] C. P. Firme III and P. R. Bandaru, "Toxicity issues in the application of carbon nanotubes to biological systems," *Nanomedicine: Nanotechnology, Biology and Medicine*, vol. 6, no. 2, pp. 245–256, 2010.

[52] K. A. S. Fernando, Y. Lin, and Y. P. Sun, "High aqueous solubility of functionalized single-walled carbon nanotubes," *Langmuir*, vol. 20, no. 11, pp. 4777–4778, 2004.

[53] D. Ravelli, D. Merli, E. Quartarone, A. Profumo, P. Mustarelli, and M. Fagnoni, "PEGylated carbon nanotubes: preparation, properties and applications," *RSC Advances*, vol. 3, no. 33, pp. 13569–13582, 2013.

[54] A. Razzazan, F. Atyabi, B. Kazemi, and R. Dinarvand, "In vivo drug delivery of gemcitabine with PEGylated single-walled carbon nanotubes," *Materials Science and Engineering C: Materials for Biological Applications*, vol. 62, pp. 614–625, 2016.

[55] M. Liu, B. Chen, Y. Xue, J. Huang, L. Zhang, S. Huang, et al., "Polyamidoamine-Grafted Multiwalled Carbon Nanotubes for Gene Delivery: Synthesis, Transfection and Intracellular Trafficking," *Bioconjugate Chemistry*, vol. 22, no. 11, pp. 2237–2243, 2011.

[56] H. Zare, S. Ahmadi, A. Ghasemi, M. Ghanbari, N. Rabiee, M. Bagherzadeh, et al., "Carbon Nanotubes: Smart Drug/GeneDelivery Carriers," *International Journal of Nanomedicine*, vol. 16, pp. 1681–1706, 2021.

[57] J. Russier, C. Menard-Moyon, E. Venturelli, E. Gravel, G. Marcolongo, M. Meneghetti, et al., "Oxidative biodegradation of single- and multi-walled carbon nanotubes," *Nanoscale*, vol. 3, no. 3, pp. 893–896, 2011.

[58] G. P. Kotchey, Y. Zhao, V. E. Kagan, and A. Star, "Peroxidase-mediated biodegradation of carbon nanotubes in vitro and in vivo," *Advanced Drug Delivery Reviews*, vol. 65, no. 15, pp. 1921–1932, 2013.

[59] P. A. Dayton, S. Zhao, S. H. Bloch, P. Schumann, K. Penrose, T. O. Matsunaga, et al., "Application of ultrasound to selectively localize nanodroplets for targeted imaging and therapy," *Molecular Imaging*, vol. 5, no. 3, pp. 160–174, 2006.

[60] "ThermoDox®: Enhancing the efficacy of doxorubicin with heat-activated liposome technology," Celsion Corporation [Online]. Available: https://celsion.com/thermodox/, 2020.

[61] N. Y. Rapoport, A. M. Kennedy, J. E. Shea, C. L. Scaife, and K.-H. Nam, "Controlled and targeted tumor chemotherapy by ultrasound-activated nanoemulsions/microbubbles," *Journal of Controlled Release*, vol. 138, no. 3, pp. 268–276, 2009.

[62] N. Rapoport, "Phase-shift, stimuli-responsive perfluorocarbon nanodroplets for drug delivery to cancer," *Wiley Interdisciplinary Reviews: Nanomedicine and Nanobiotechnology*, vol. 4, no. 5, pp. 492–510, 2012.

[63] V. Kumar, S. Palazzolo, S. Bayda, G. Corona, G. Toffoli, and F. Rizzolio, "DNA nanotechnology for cancer therapy," *Theranostics*, vol. 6, no. 5, p. 710, 2016.

[64] H.-M. Meng, H. Liu, H. Kuai, R. Peng, L. Mo, and X.-B. Zhang, "Aptamer-integrated DNA nanostructures for biosensing, bioimaging and cancer therapy," *Chemical Society Reviews*, vol. 45, no. 9, pp. 2583–2602, 2016.

[65] S. Huo, N. Gong, Y. Jiang, F. Chen, H. Guo, Y. Gan, et al., "Gold-DNA nanosunflowers for efficient gene silencing with controllable transformation," *Science Advances*, vol. 5, no. 10, article 6264, 2019.

[66] E. K.-H. Chow and D. Ho, "Cancer Nanomedicine: From Drug Delivery to Imaging," *Science Translational Medicine*, vol. 5, no. 216, p. 216rv4, 2013.

[67] J. K. Patra, G. Das, L. F. Fraceto, E. V. R. Campos, M. D. P. Rodriguez-Torres, L. S. Acosta-Torres, et al., "Nano based drug delivery systems: recent developments and future prospects," *Journal of Nanobiotechnology*, vol. 16, no. 71, 2018.

[68] J. G. Geisler, "2,4 Dinitrophenol as Medicine," *Cells*, vol. 8, no. 3, 2019.

[69] Y. H. Han, S. W. Kim, S. H. Kim, S. Z. Kim, and W. H. Park, "2,4-Dinitrophenol induces G1 phase arrest and apoptosis in human pulmonary adenocarcinoma Calu-6 cells," *Toxicology in Vitro*, vol. 22, no. 3, pp. 659–670, 2008.

[70] S. Marrache and S. Dhar, "Engineering of blended nanoparticle platform for delivery of mitochondria-acting therapeutics," *Proceedings of the National Academy of Sciences of the United States of America*, vol. 109, no. 40, pp. 16288–16293, 2012.

[71] S. Waldert, T. Pistohl, C. Braun, T. Ball, A. Aertsen, and C. Mehring, "A review on directional information in neural signals for brain-machine interfaces," *Journal of Physiology (Paris)*, vol. 103, no. 3–5, pp. 244–254, 2009.

[72]   E. M. Maynard, C. T. Nordhausen, and R. A. Normann, "The Utah intracortical electrode array: a recording structure for potential brain-computer interfaces," *Electroencephalography and Clinical Neurophysiology*, vol. 102, no. 3, pp. 228–239, 1997.

[73]   D. Scaini and L. Ballerini, "Nanomaterials at the neural interface," *Current Opinion in Neurobiology*, vol. 50, pp. 50–55, 2018.

[74]   M. Vissani, I. U. Isaias, and A. Mazzoni, "Deep brain stimulation: a review of the open neural engineering challenges," *Journal of Neural Engineering*, vol. 17, no. 5, article 051002, 2020.

[75]   E. Musk, "An integrated brain-machine interface platform with thousands of channels," *Journal of Medical Internet Research*, vol. 21, no. 10, article e16194, 2019.

[76]   D. H. Toffa, L. Touma, T. El Meskine, A. Bouthillier, and D. K. Nguyen, "Learnings from 30 years of reported efficacy and safety of vagus nerve stimulation (VNS) for epilepsy treatment: a critical review," *Seizure*, vol. 83, pp. 104–123, 2020.

[77]   M. Aman, C. Festin, M. E. Sporer, C. Gstoettner, C. Prahm, K. D. Bergmeister, et al., "Bionic reconstruction Restoration of extremity function with osseointegrated and mind-controlled prostheses," *Wiener Klinische Wochenschrift*, vol. 131, no. 23–24, pp. 599–607, 2019.

[78]   Y. Shang, M. K. Hasan, G. J. Ahammed, M. Li, H. Yin, and J. Zhou, "Applications of nanotechnology in plant growth and crop protection: a review," *Molecules*, vol. 24, no. 14, 2019.

[79]   M. Usman, M. Farooq, A. Wakeel, A. Nawaz, S. A. Cheema, H. U. Rehman, et al., "Nanotechnology in agriculture: current status, challenges and future opportunities," *Science of the Total Environment*, vol. 721, article 137778, 2020.

[80]   G. T. Miller and S. Spoolman, *Sustaining the Earth: An Integrated Approach*, 9th ed. Belmont, CA, USA: Brooks/Cole Publishing, 2009.

[81]   B. Huang, F. Chen, Y. Shen, K. Qian, Y. Wang, C. Sun, et al., "Advances in targeted pesticides with environmentally responsive controlled release by nanotechnology," *Nanomaterials*, vol. 8, no. 2, article 102, 2018.

[82]   A. E. S. Pereira, R. Grillo, N. F. S. Mello, A. H. Rosa, and L. F. Fraceto, "Application of poly(epsilon-caprolactone) nanoparticles containing atrazine herbicide as an alternative technique to control weeds and reduce damage to the environment," *Journal of Hazardous Materials*, vol. 268, pp. 207–215, 2014.

[83]   T. Stadler, "Particulate Nanoinsecticides: A new concept in insect pest management," in *Insecticides: Agriculture and Toxicology*, G. Begum, Ed., 1st ed. London, UK: IntechOpen, 2018.

[84]   M. C. DeRosa, C. Monreal, M. Schnitzer, R. Walsh, and Y. Sultan, "Nanotechnology in fertilizers," *Nature Nanotechnology*, vol. 5, no. 2, p. 91, 2010.

[85]   A. Antonacci, F. Arduini, D. Moscone, G. Palleschi, and V. Scognamiglio, "Nanostructured (Bio)sensors for smart agriculture," *TrAC Trends in Analytical Chemistry*, vol. 98, pp. 95–103, 2018.

[86]   Z. Yu, G. Zhao, M. Liu, Y. Lei, and M. Li, "Fabrication of a Novel atrazine biosensor and its subpart-per-trillion levels sensitive performance," *Environmental Science & Technology*, vol. 44, no. 20, pp. 7878–7883, 2010.

[87]   J. Singh and B.-K. Lee, "Influence of nano-TiO2 particles on the bioaccumulation of Cd in soybean plants (Glycine max): a possible mechanism for the removal of Cd from the contaminated soil," *Journal of Environmental Management*, vol. 170, pp. 88–96, 2016.

CHAPTER 8

Computer Simulations with COMSOL Multiphysics® Software

COMSOL Multiphysics® is a cross-platform software for modeling and simulating engineering and scientific problems governed by partial differential equations. Physical phenomena are typically described by systems of partial differential equations. With conventional graphical user interfaces, COMSOL Multiphysics® software numerically solves systems of non-linear partial differential equations using the finite element method. In addition, COMSOL Multiphysics® software provides a unified workflow and an integrated development environment for users to model and simulate systems involving electrical, mechanical, fluidic, thermal, chemical, and/or acoustic phenomena. The tutorials in this chapter were designed using COMSOL Multiphysics® 5.6 (Build 401). Depending on your COMSOL Multiphysics® version, the tutorial steps may differ slightly.

8.1 LAB #1: 2D SIMULATION OF INTERDIGITATED ELECTRODES

In this lab assignment, you will build and simulate a 2D model of interdigitated electrodes (IDEs) in COMSOL Multiphysics® simulation software. The overall steps are as follows.

(1) Define the geometry of the model to be used for the simulation.

(2) Select the materials used in the model and their boundaries.

(3) Select the appropriate "study" steps and associated settings to set up the simulation.

(4) Run the simulation and plot the results.

8.1.1 COMSOL Multiphysics® Software Tutorial #1

This tutorial introduces the process for building a 2D model, setting up the simulation, and plotting the results within COMSOL Multiphysics® simulation software.

Let us start with the IDE system shown in Figure 8-1. The tasks include the selection of materials (e.g., metal or liquid) and parameters (e.g., permittivity and conductivity). The setup of a "physics environment" for an IDE system will be shown in this lab. After setting up the model in COMSOL Multiphysics® software, compute and simulate different cases (e.g., varying the frequency and the supply voltage) to answer the lab assignments. An overview of the graphical user interface within COMSOL Multiphysics® simulation software is shown in Figure 8-2.

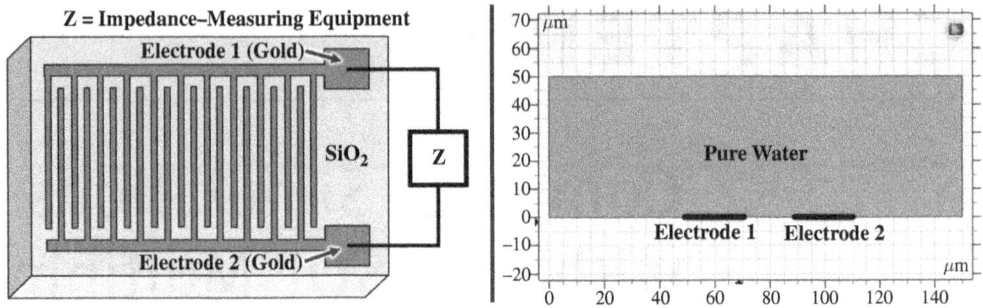

Figure 8-1   (Left) Simplified illustration of gold interdigitated electrodes (IDEs) on a SiO₂-coated silicon substrate. The IDEs are comprised of two interlocking comb-shaped microelectrode arrays (i.e., electrodes 1 and 2). (Right) 2D cross-sectional view of the IDE model in COMSOL Multiphysics® software.

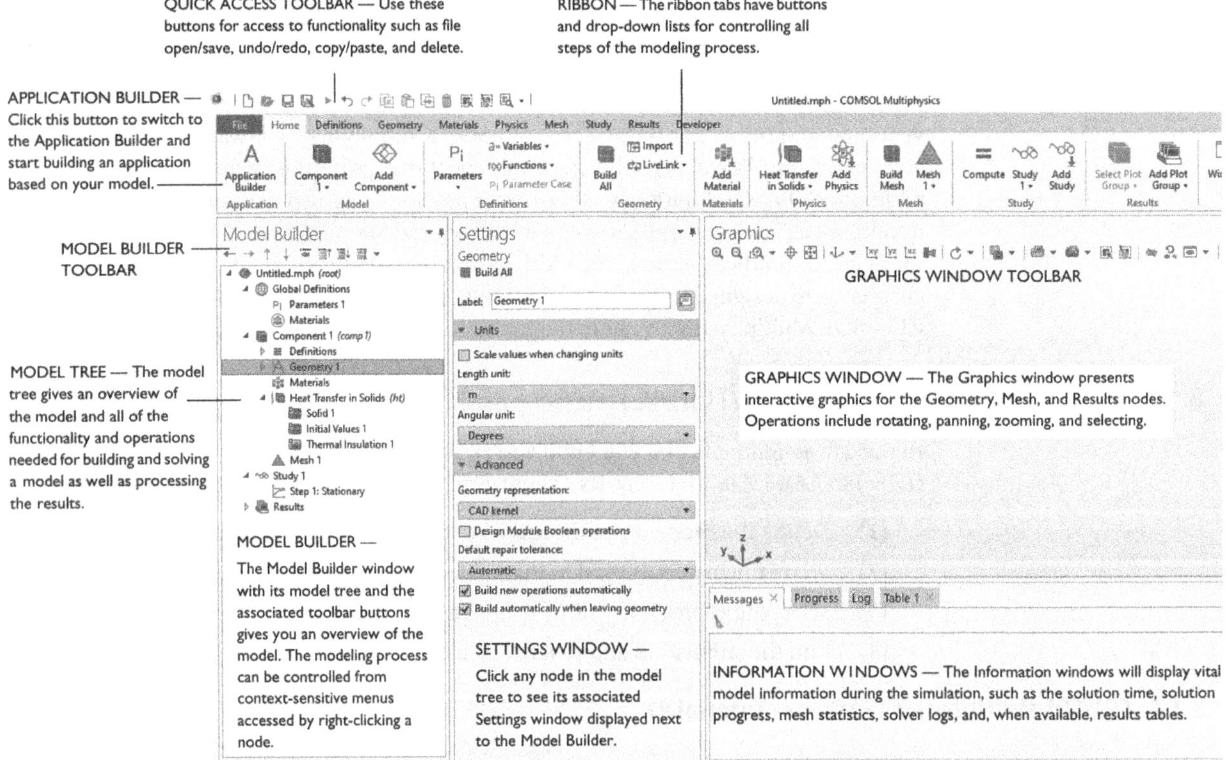

Figure 8-2   The graphical user interface of COMSOL Multiphysics® software reprinted with permission from https://cdn.comsol.com/doc/5.6/IntroductionToCOMSOLMultiphysics.pdf. (*This image was made using COMSOL Multiphysics® software and is provided courtesy of COMSOL®.*)

For all three labs in this chapter, we will use the "Electric Currents (ec)" physics interface, which can compute the electric field, potential, and current distributions. This interface can account for resistive and capacitive effects in the time and frequency domains, but excludes inductive effects.

(A) Building a 2D Model

The first step of creating a physical simulation in COMSOL Multiphysics® software is to build a geometric model. Here, we create a simple 2D model of an IDE.

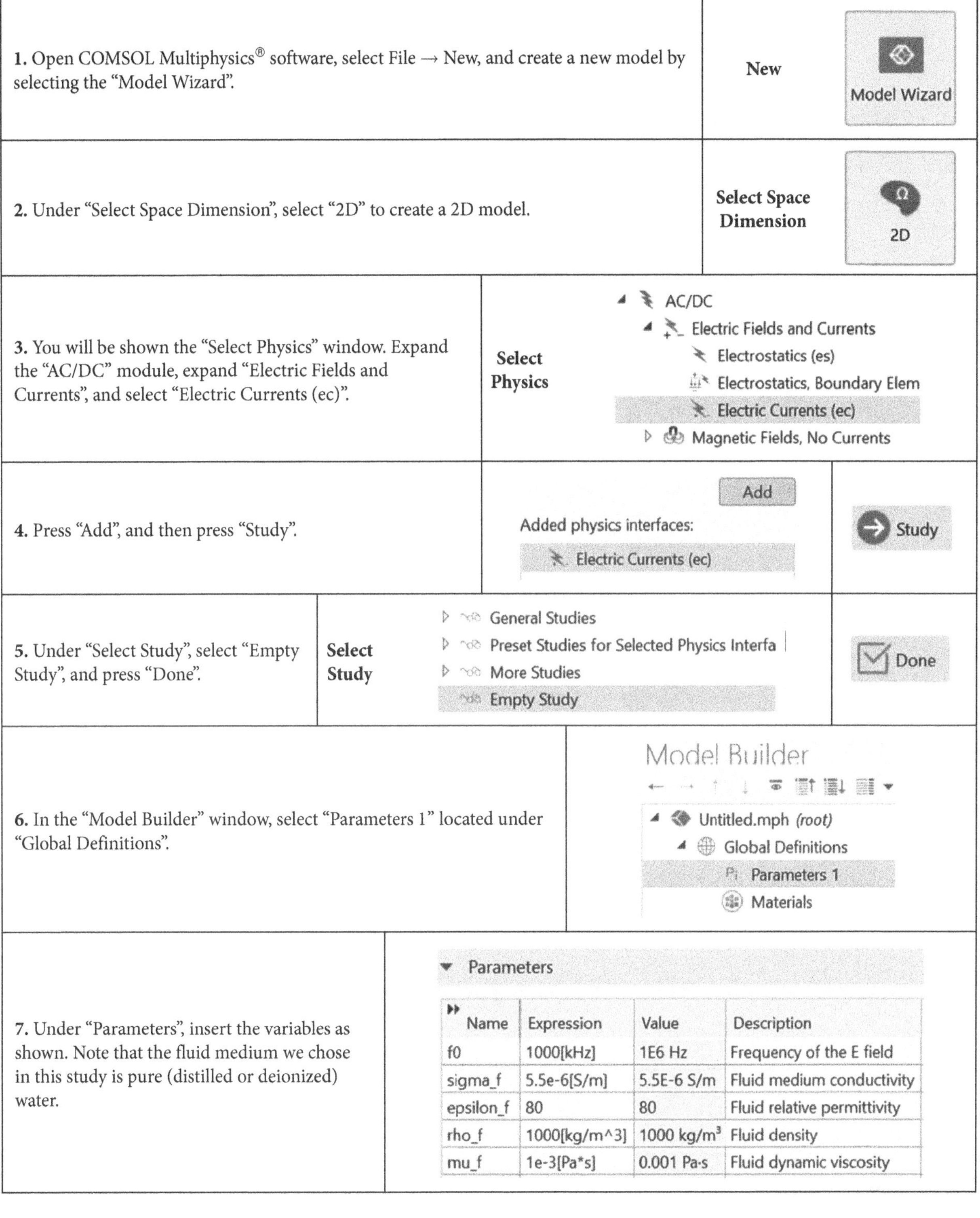

1. Open COMSOL Multiphysics® software, select File → New, and create a new model by selecting the "Model Wizard".	**New**
2. Under "Select Space Dimension", select "2D" to create a 2D model.	**Select Space Dimension**
3. You will be shown the "Select Physics" window. Expand the "AC/DC" module, expand "Electric Fields and Currents", and select "Electric Currents (ec)".	**Select Physics**
4. Press "Add", and then press "Study".	
5. Under "Select Study", select "Empty Study", and press "Done".	**Select Study**
6. In the "Model Builder" window, select "Parameters 1" located under "Global Definitions".	
7. Under "Parameters", insert the variables as shown. Note that the fluid medium we chose in this study is pure (distilled or deionized) water.	

Name	Expression	Value	Description
f0	1000[kHz]	1E6 Hz	Frequency of the E field
sigma_f	5.5e-6[S/m]	5.5E-6 S/m	Fluid medium conductivity
epsilon_f	80	80	Fluid relative permittivity
rho_f	1000[kg/m^3]	1000 kg/m³	Fluid density
mu_f	1e-3[Pa*s]	0.001 Pa·s	Fluid dynamic viscosity

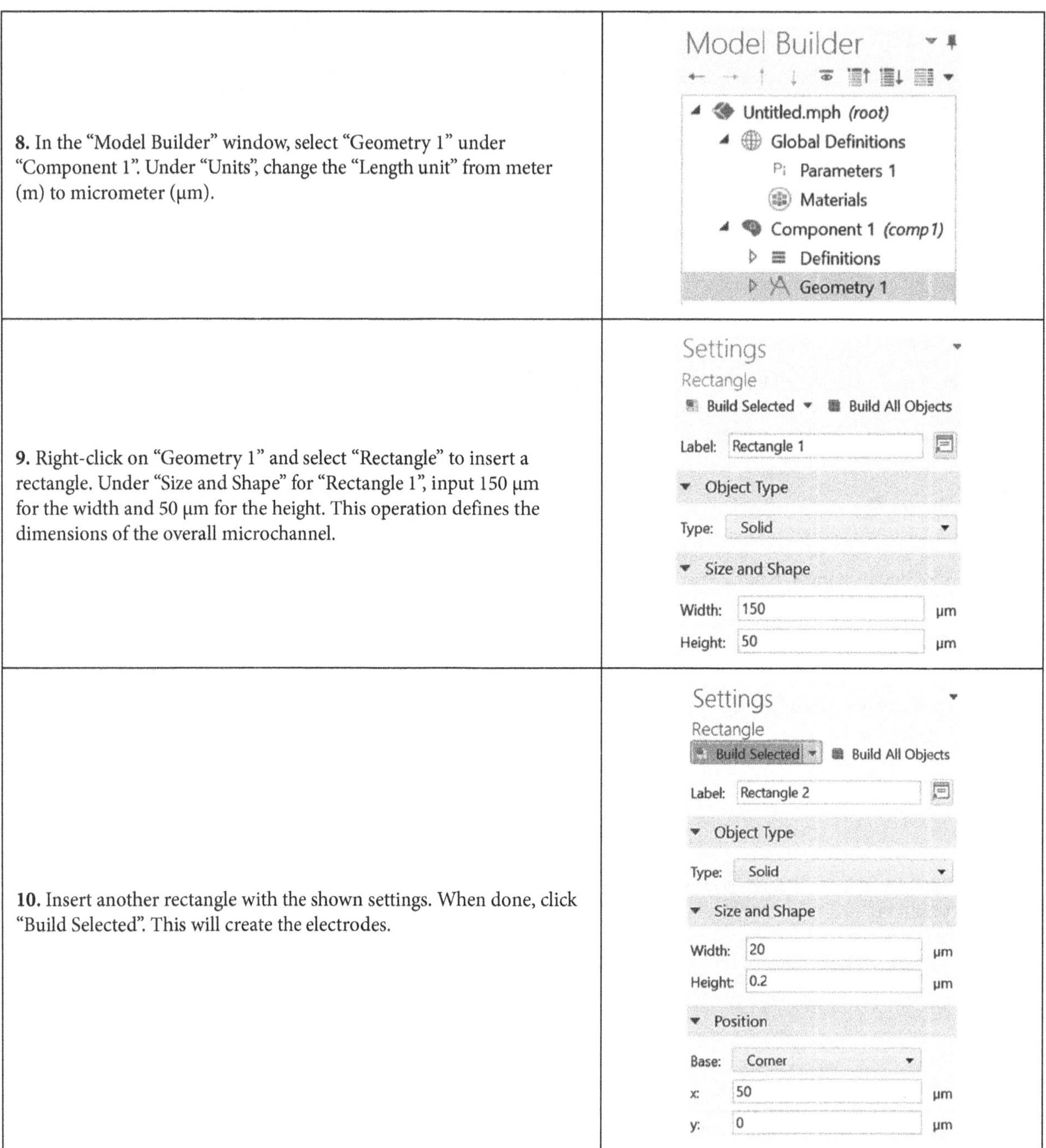

8. In the "Model Builder" window, select "Geometry 1" under "Component 1". Under "Units", change the "Length unit" from meter (m) to micrometer (μm).

9. Right-click on "Geometry 1" and select "Rectangle" to insert a rectangle. Under "Size and Shape" for "Rectangle 1", input 150 μm for the width and 50 μm for the height. This operation defines the dimensions of the overall microchannel.

10. Insert another rectangle with the shown settings. When done, click "Build Selected". This will create the electrodes.

11. Right click "Geometry 1" under "Component 1" in the "Model Builder" window. Select Transforms → Array. This will insert an array.

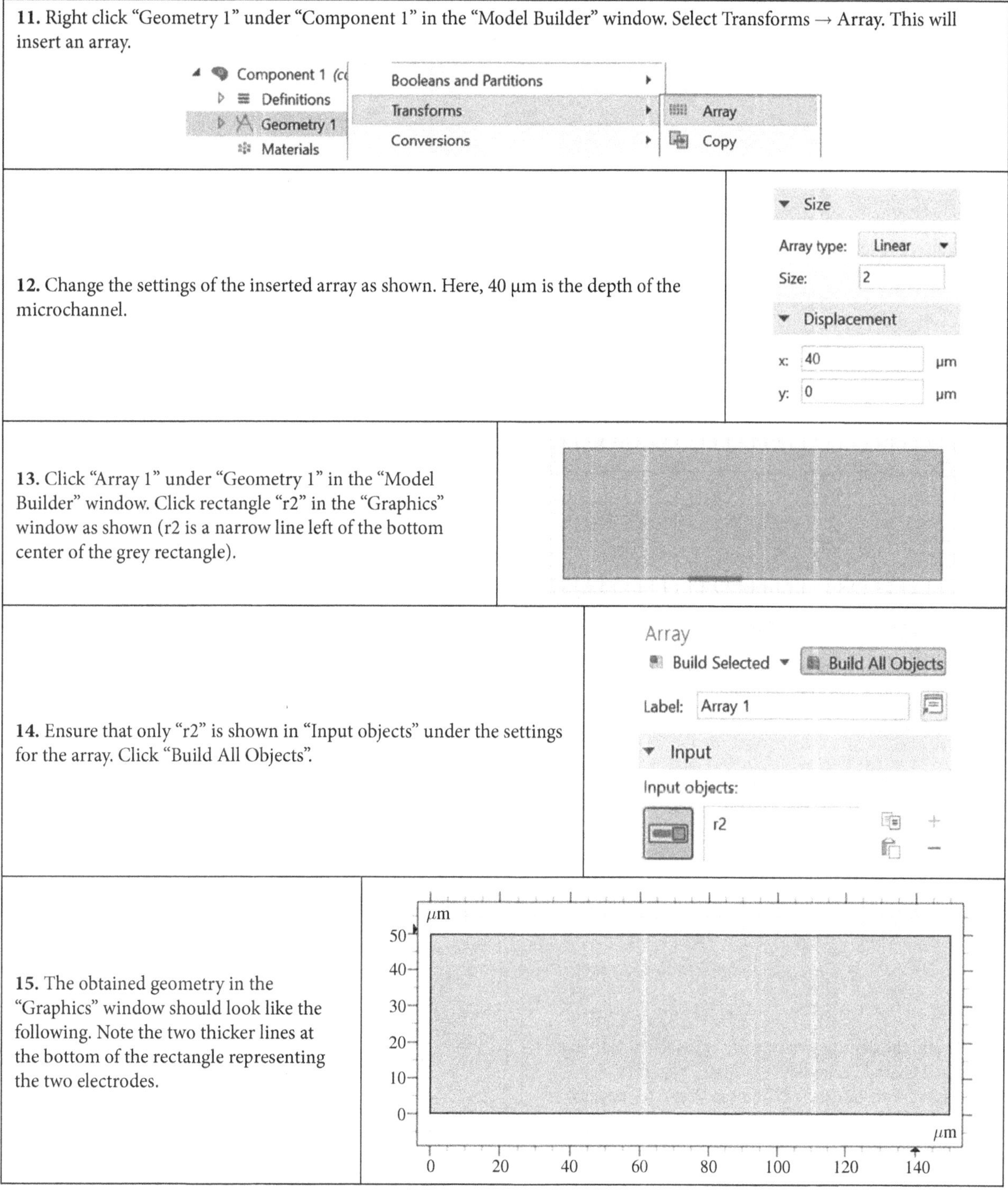

12. Change the settings of the inserted array as shown. Here, 40 μm is the depth of the microchannel.

13. Click "Array 1" under "Geometry 1" in the "Model Builder" window. Click rectangle "r2" in the "Graphics" window as shown (r2 is a narrow line left of the bottom center of the grey rectangle).

14. Ensure that only "r2" is shown in "Input objects" under the settings for the array. Click "Build All Objects".

15. The obtained geometry in the "Graphics" window should look like the following. Note the two thicker lines at the bottom of the rectangle representing the two electrodes.

(B) Simulation Setup

The second step is to set up the simulation within COMSOL Multiphysics® software.

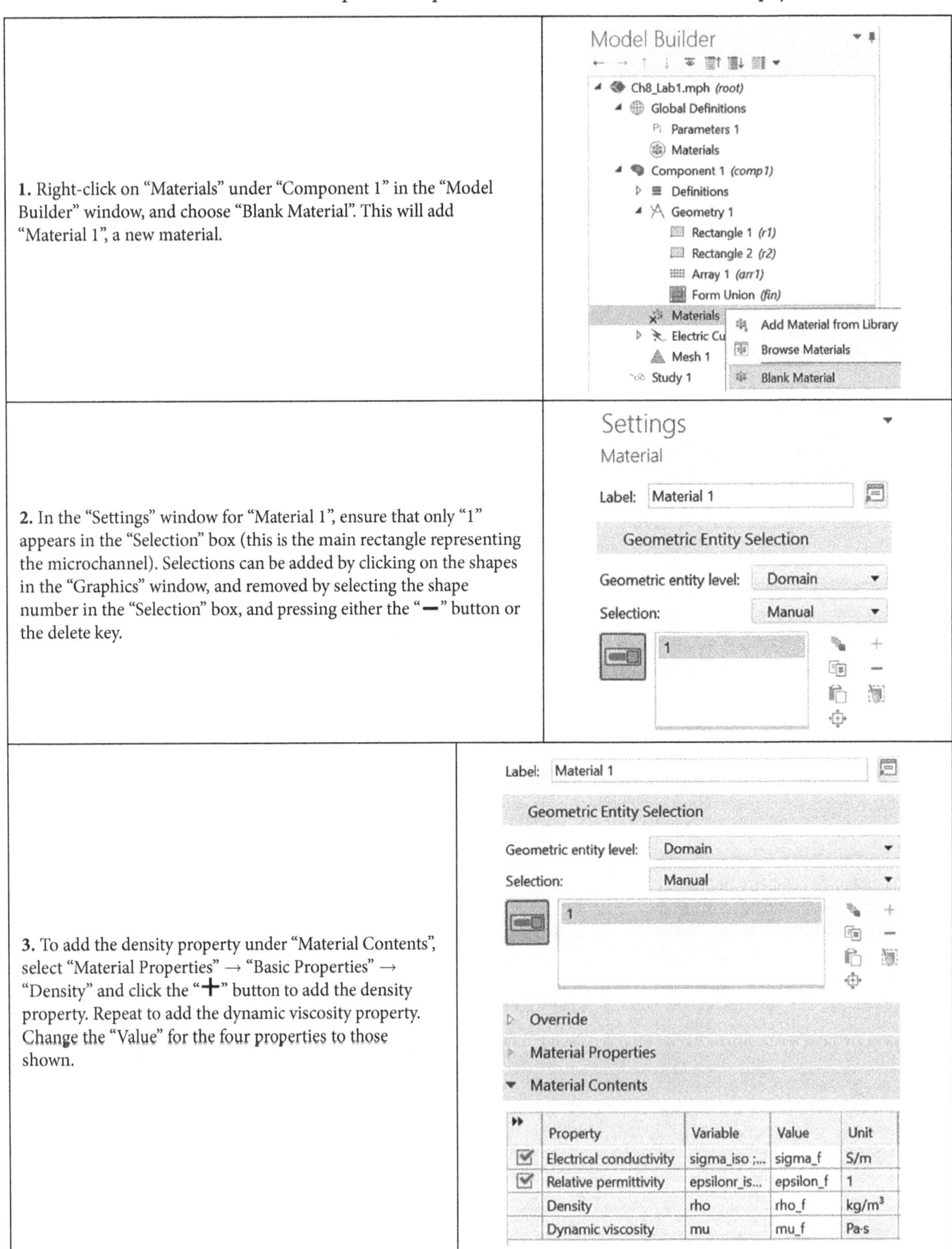

1. Right-click on "Materials" under "Component 1" in the "Model Builder" window, and choose "Blank Material". This will add "Material 1", a new material.

2. In the "Settings" window for "Material 1", ensure that only "1" appears in the "Selection" box (this is the main rectangle representing the microchannel). Selections can be added by clicking on the shapes in the "Graphics" window, and removed by selecting the shape number in the "Selection" box, and pressing either the "—" button or the delete key.

3. To add the density property under "Material Contents", select "Material Properties" → "Basic Properties" → "Density" and click the "+" button to add the density property. Repeat to add the dynamic viscosity property. Change the "Value" for the four properties to those shown.

4. Add another material from the material library by right clicking "Materials" under "Component 1". In the "Add Material" window, select "MEMS" → "Metals" → "Au - Gold". Press "Add to Component".

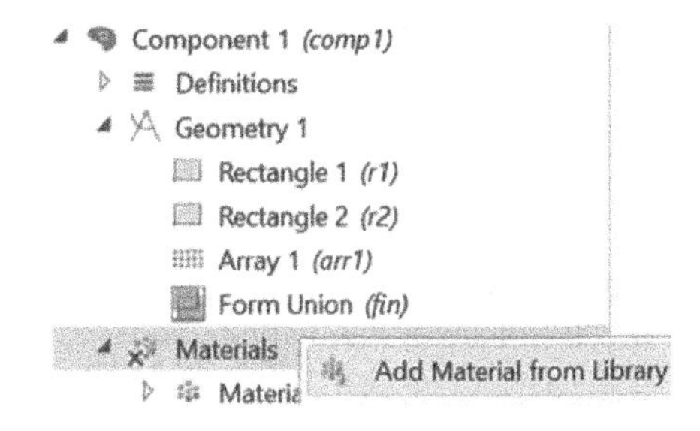
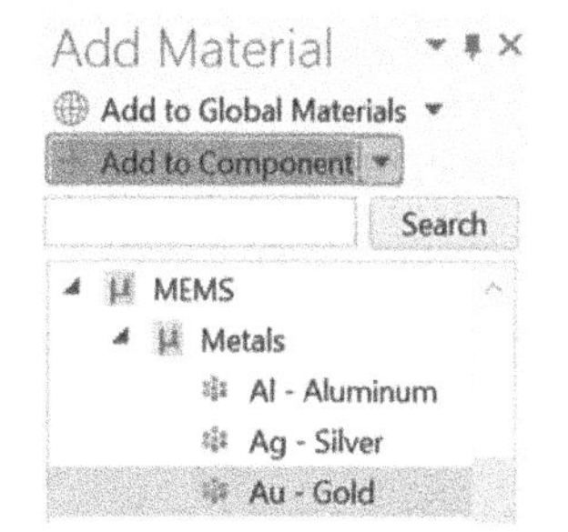

5. For the "Settings" window of the added gold material, choose both "2" and "3" (the two electrodes) in the "Selection" box by clicking on the two thicker lines at the bottom of the rectangle in the "Graphics" window. Fill out the value of "Relative permittivity" as 6.9.

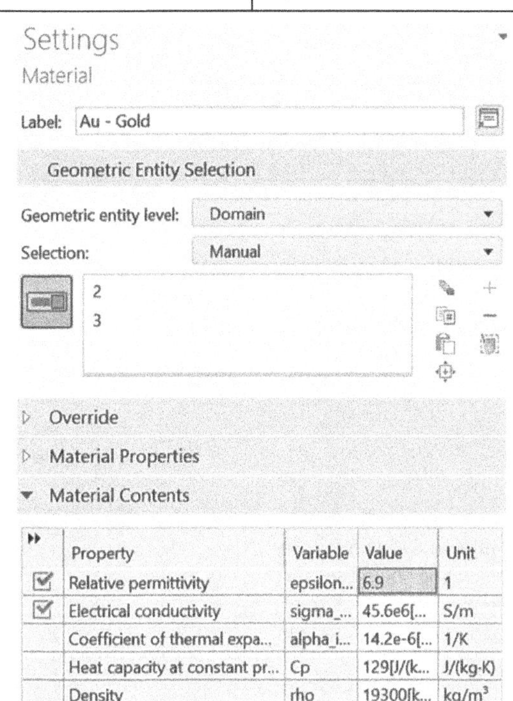

6. In the "Model Builder" window, right click "Electric Currents (ec)" and choose "Electric Potential". Set the "Electric Potential" V_0 to 1V, and click the line representing the left electrode in the "Graphics" window. Repeat for the right electrode, but change the electric potential to -1V.

Note: For AC voltages, the value of the "Electric Potential" V_0 represents the voltage amplitude (i.e., zero-to- peak value). If V_0 is negative, the polarity of the AC voltage will be reversed.

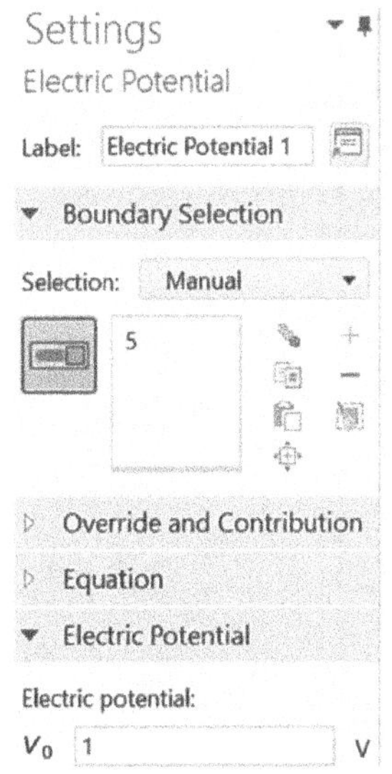
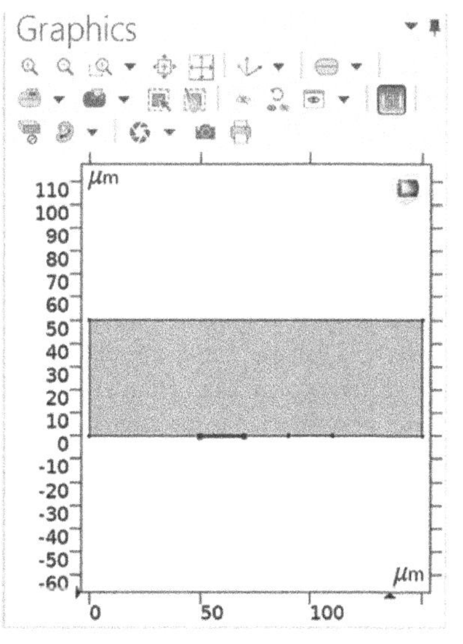

7. Right click "Study 1" in the "Model Builder" window. Select "Study Steps" → "Frequency Domain" → "Frequency Domain". In "Study Settings" of the "Settings" window, enter f0 to the right of "Frequencies".

(C) Plotting Results

The final step is to run the simulation and plot the results within COMSOL Multiphysics® software.

1. To simulate your model, select Home → Compute in the ribbon.

2. After the simulation is finished, you should see the following in the "Model Builder" window.

3. If your simulation has been successful, you should see the following surface plot of the electric potential amplitude in the "Graphics" window.

4. In the "Settings" window of "Surface 1" under "Electric Potential (ec)", you can change the plotted parameter from V (electric potential amplitude) to another parameter or expression by pressing either "Insert Expression" or "Replace Expression".

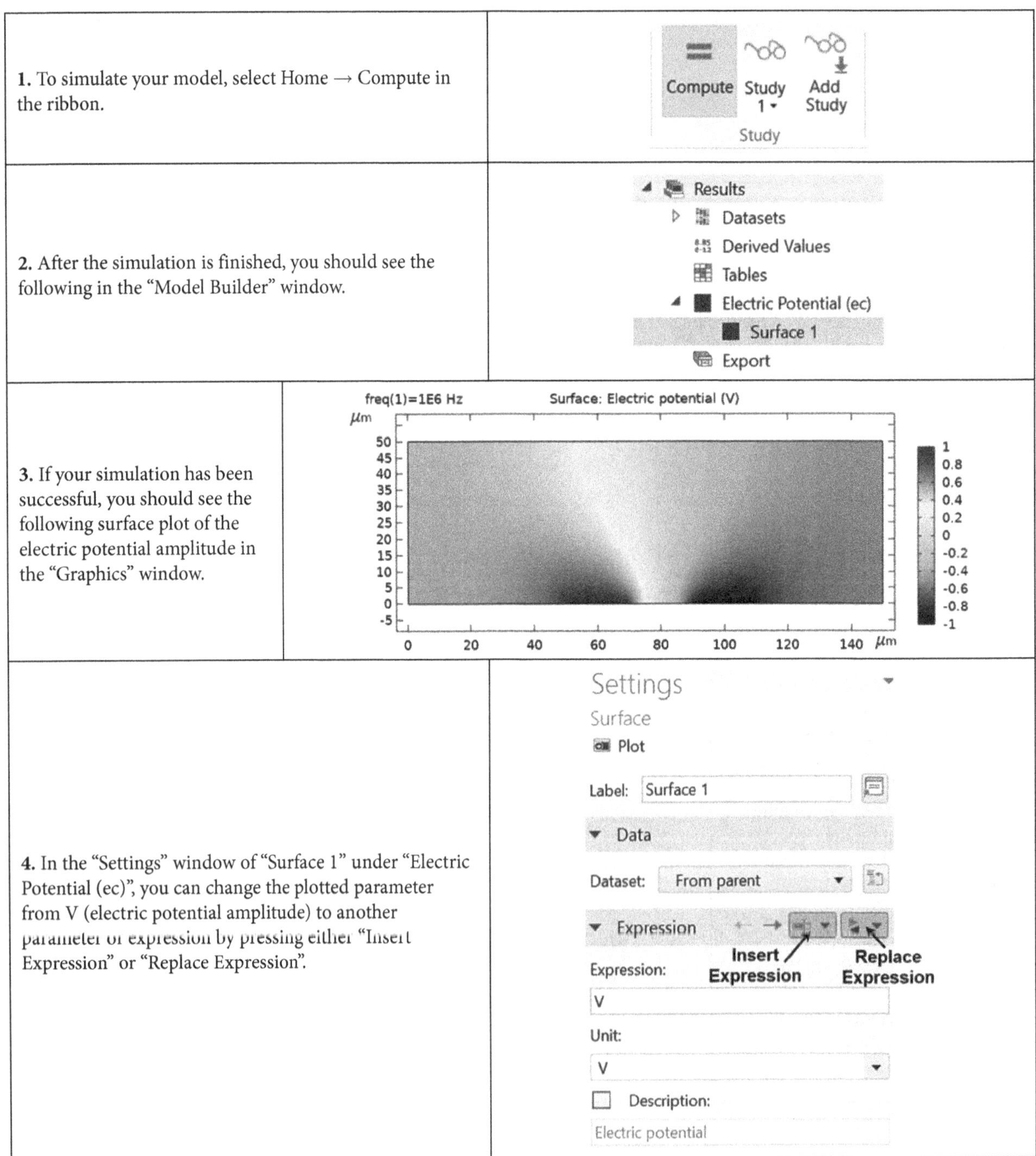

5. For instance, to plot the magnitude (norm) of the electric field instead of the electric potential amplitude (V), click "Replace Expression", type "electric field norm" (or select it from the list), and double click on "ec.normE - Electric field norm - V/m".

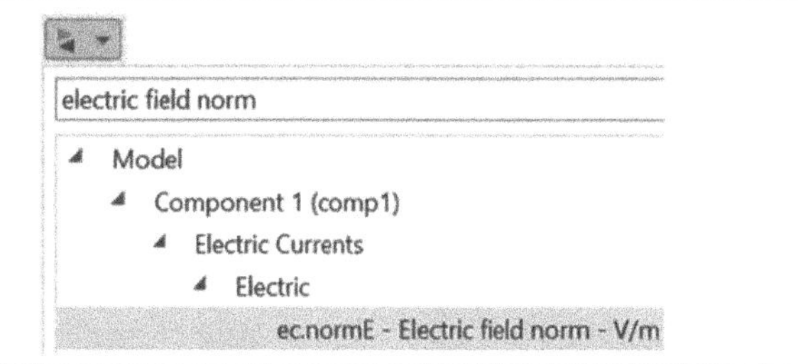

6. To add another plot (or overlay), select "Electric Potential (ec)" in the "Model Builder" window, select the "Electric Potential (ec)" tab in the ribbon, and click on the plot/overlay type you wish to add.

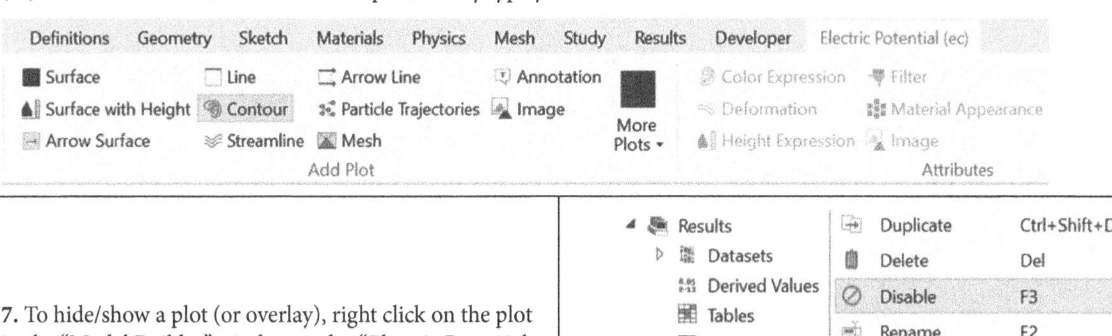

7. To hide/show a plot (or overlay), right click on the plot in the "Model Builder" window under "Electric Potential (ec)", and click "Disable" / "Enable".

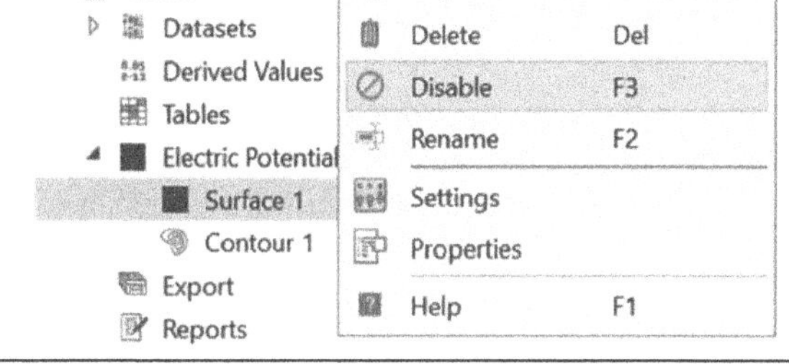

8. Save your model and simulation results by clicking File → Save.

Tip: In the "Settings" window of a selected plot, you can input a variety of operators and expressions to plot. For instance, the operator "d(variable, x)" represents the partial derivative $\partial(\text{variable})/\partial x$. As an example, the magnitude of the electric field gradient $|\nabla E(x,y)|$ is

$$\left|\nabla E(x,y)\right| = \sqrt{\left(\frac{\partial^2 V}{\partial x^2}\right)^2 + \left(\frac{\partial^2 V}{\partial x\,\partial y}\right)^2 + \left(\frac{\partial^2 V}{\partial y\,\partial x}\right)^2 + \left(\frac{\partial^2 V}{\partial y^2}\right)^2}$$

Enter the expression "sqrt(d(d(V,x),x)^2 + d(d(V,x),y)^2 + d(d(V,y),x)^2 + d(d(V,y),y)^2)" to plot $|\nabla E|$.

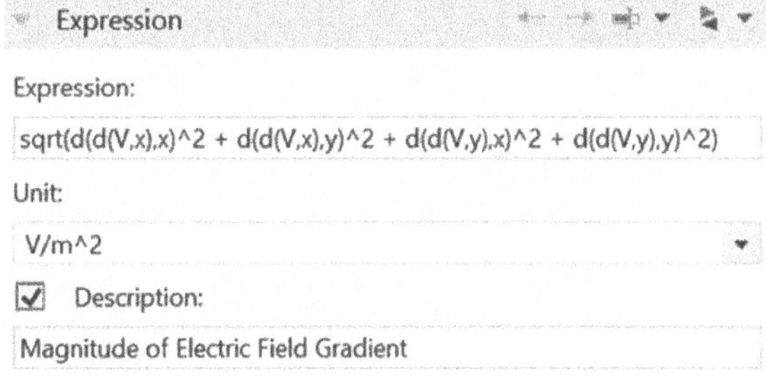

Note: Since the electric field $E(x,y)$ is a vector, the gradient of the electric field $\nabla E(x,y)$ is a 2×2 matrix. Using $E = -\nabla V$, we can obtain the magnitude of the electric field gradient $|\nabla E(x,y)|$ as follows:

$$E(x,y) = -\nabla V(x,y) = -\left(\frac{\partial V}{\partial x}\hat{x} + \frac{\partial V}{\partial y}\hat{y} \right) = E_x\hat{x} + E_y\hat{y} \;\Rightarrow\; E_x = -\frac{\partial V}{\partial x} \;\text{ and }\; E_y = -\frac{\partial V}{\partial y}$$

$$\nabla E(x,y) = \begin{bmatrix} \nabla E_x(x,y) \\ \nabla E_y(x,y) \end{bmatrix} = \begin{bmatrix} \partial E_x/\partial x & \partial E_x/\partial y \\ \partial E_y/\partial x & \partial E_y/\partial y \end{bmatrix}$$

$$|\nabla E(x,y)| = \sqrt{\left(\frac{\partial E_x}{\partial x}\right)^2 + \left(\frac{\partial E_x}{\partial y}\right)^2 + \left(\frac{\partial E_y}{\partial x}\right)^2 + \left(\frac{\partial E_y}{\partial y}\right)^2} = \sqrt{\left(\frac{\partial^2 V}{\partial x^2}\right)^2 + \left(\frac{\partial^2 V}{\partial x\,\partial y}\right)^2 + \left(\frac{\partial^2 V}{\partial y\,\partial x}\right)^2 + \left(\frac{\partial^2 V}{\partial y^2}\right)^2}$$

8.1.2 Lab Assignment #1

Part A (Building a 2D Model and Setting Up the Simulation)   A simplified 2D IDE model consists of a channel with dimensions of 150 μm (width) × 50 μm (height), plus two electrodes that are 20 μm (width) × 0.2 μm (height). There is a gap of 20 μm between the two electrodes. Build the 2D model in COMSOL Multiphysics® software by following Tutorial #1, and show a screenshot of your model in the "Graphics" window. Set the voltage amplitudes of the left/right electrodes to +1V/−1V, where negative voltage amplitudes represent reversed polarity. Set up the simulation using a frequency domain study set at f0 = 1000 kHz for your model.

Part B (Running the Simulation and Plotting Results)   Simulate your model at different frequencies (f0 = 0 Hz, 1 kHz, 1 MHz, and 1 GHz), as well as different electrode voltage amplitudes (+1V/−1V, +3V/−3V, and +5V/−5V). Does the frequency affect the simulation results? Show surface plots of the electric potential amplitude $V(x,y)$, arrow surface plots of the electric field $E(x,y)$ (i.e., the negative gradient of the electric potential, since $E = -\nabla V$), and contour plots of the magnitude of the electric field gradient $|\nabla E(x,y)|$.

Solution

Part A   Shown below is a screenshot of the 2D IDE model.

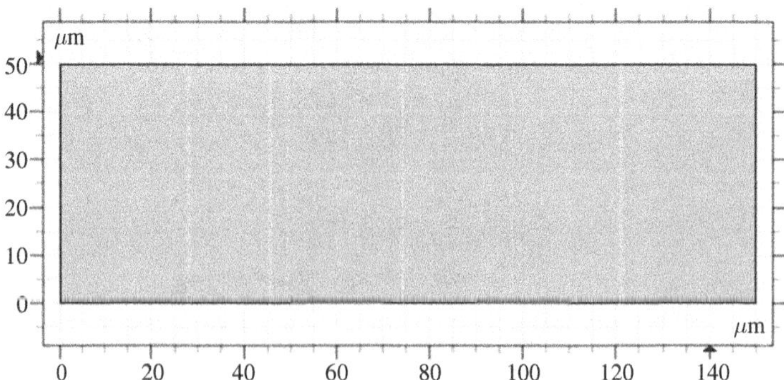

Part B   The frequency f0 does not make any difference at all in the simulation. Shown below are a surface plot of the electric potential amplitude *V*, arrow surface plot of the electric field ***E***, and two contour plots (one showing the entire channel, one zoomed-in at the corner of an electrode) of the magnitude of the electric field gradient $|\nabla E(x,y)|$. The plots are for electrode voltage amplitudes of +3V/−3V. Plots for other electrode voltage amplitudes will look similar. To obtain the plots shown, you will have to tweak some of the plot settings.

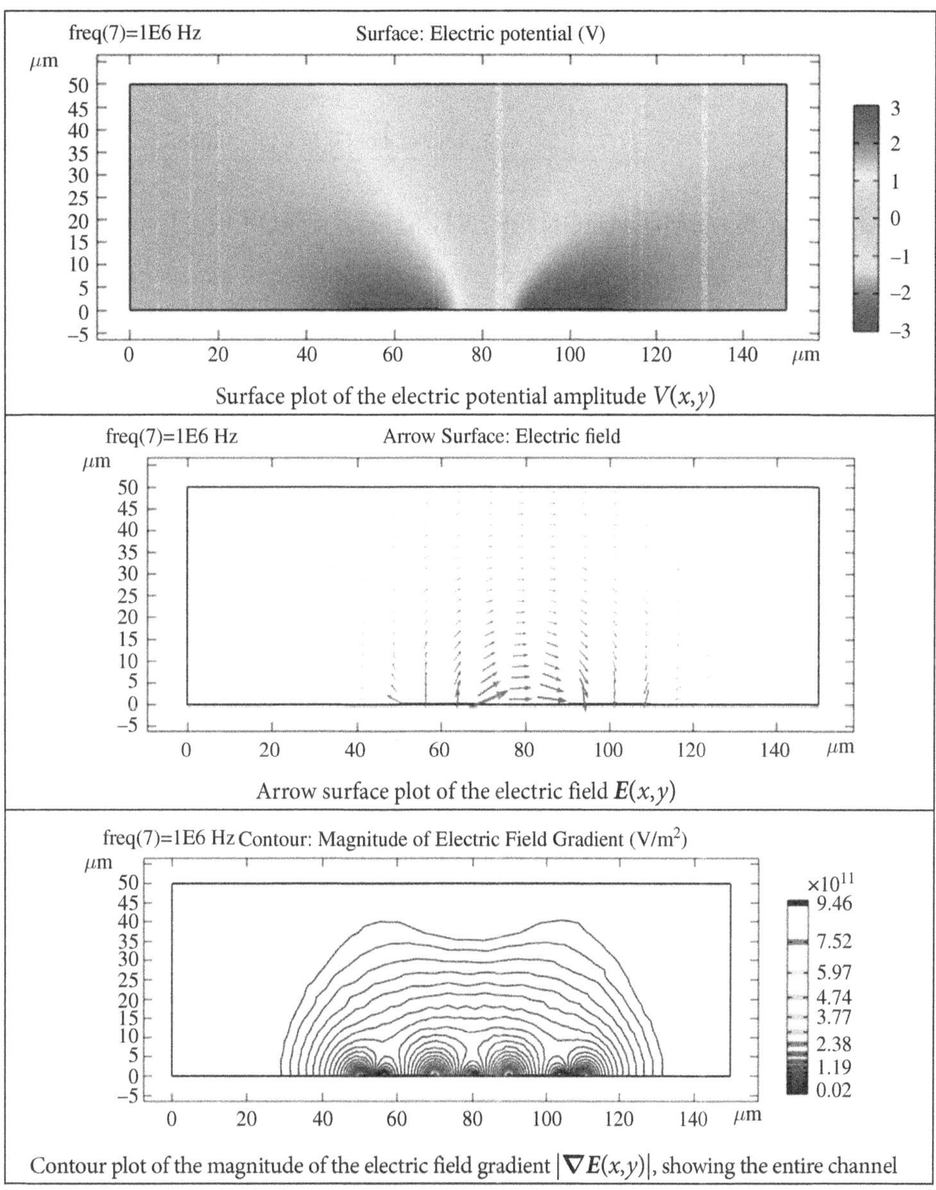

Surface plot of the electric potential amplitude $V(x,y)$

Arrow surface plot of the electric field $E(x,y)$

Contour plot of the magnitude of the electric field gradient $|\nabla E(x,y)|$, showing the entire channel

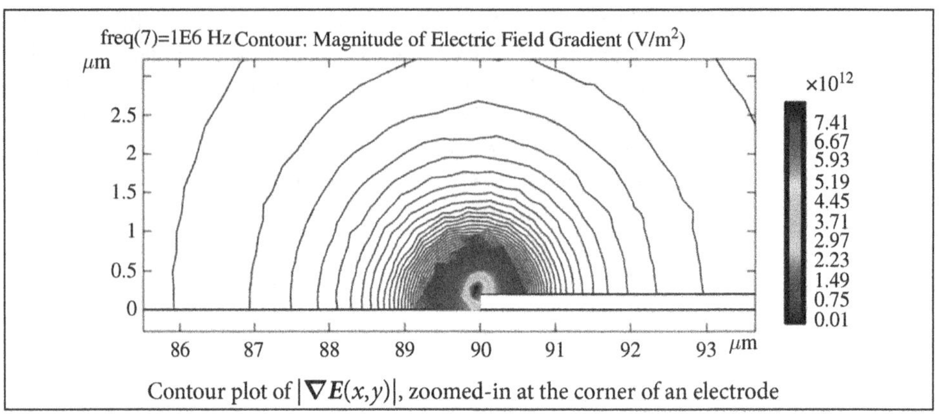

Contour plot of $|\nabla E(x,y)|$, zoomed-in at the corner of an electrode

8.2 LAB #2: 3D SIMULATION OF INTERDIGITATED ELECTRODES

In this lab assignment, you will build and simulate a 3D model of IDEs in COMSOL Multiphysics® simulation software. The 3D model of IDEs is shown in Figure 8-3. The steps for setting up the simulation and plotting the results will be similar to those shown in Lab #1.

8.2.1 COMSOL Multiphysics® Software Tutorial #2

This tutorial introduces the creation of a 3D IDE model in COMSOL Multiphysics® software, setting up the simulation, and plotting the results. Specifically, it involves building a 3D model representing the IDE system, selecting materials and model parameters, and

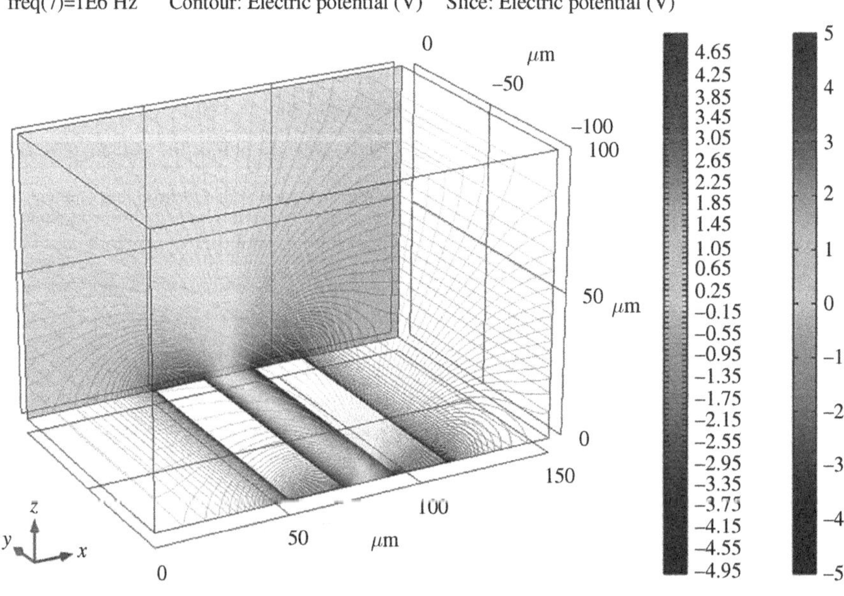

Figure 8-3   3D model of an IDE system in COMSOL Multiphysics® simulation software.

setting up a physics environment for the 3D model. Under the given physics environment, simulations will be conducted for different cases (e.g., varying the frequency and supply voltage) based on the 3D model.

---

1. Open COMSOL Multiphysics® software, select File → New, and create a new model by selecting the "Model Wizard". Under "Select Space Dimension", select "3D" to create a 3D model.

Select Space Dimension — 3D

---

2. You will be shown the "Select Physics" window. Expand the "AC/DC" module, expand "Electric Fields and Currents", and select "Electric Currents (ec)". Press "Add", and then press "Study". Under "Select Study", select "Empty Study", and press "Done".

---

3. In the "Model Builder" window, select "Parameters 1" located under "Global Definitions". Under "Parameters", insert the variables as shown. The fluid medium we chose in this study is pure (distilled or deionized) water.

Parameters

Name	Expression	Value	Description
f0	1000[kHz]	1E6 Hz	Frequency of electric field
sigma_f	5.5e-6[S/m]	5.5E-6 S/m	Fluid medium conductivity
epsilon_f	80	80	Fluid relative permittivity
rho_f	1000[kg/m^3]	1000 kg/m³	Fluid density
mu_f	1e-3[Pa*s]	0.001 Pa·s	Fluid dynamic viscosity

---

4. In the "Model Builder" window, select "Geometry 1" under "Component 1". Under "Units", change the "Length unit" from meter (m) to micrometer (μm). Right-click on "Geometry 1" and select "Work Plane" to insert a work plane.

---

5. Under the "Plane Definition" of the "Settings" window for "Work Plane 1", change the "Plane" to "xz-plane".

Label: Work Plane 1

Plane Definition

Plane type: Quick
Plane: xz-plane
Offset type: Distance
y-coordinate: 0   μm

6a. Right click "Plane Geometry" under "Work Plane 1" and click "Rectangle" to insert a rectangle within the work plane.

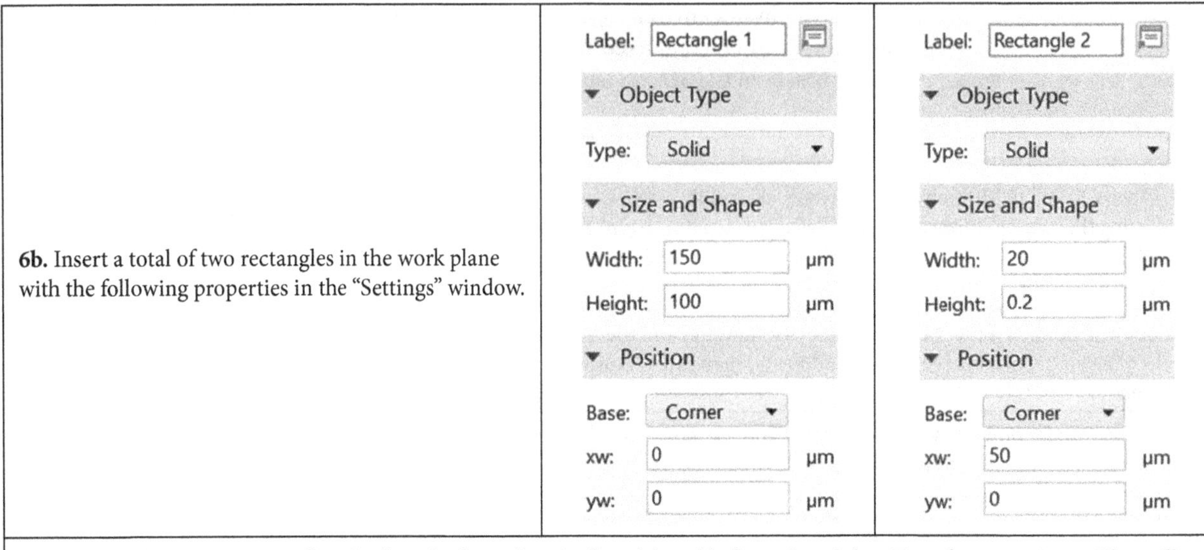

6b. Insert a total of two rectangles in the work plane with the following properties in the "Settings" window.

Rectangle 1:

Label:	Rectangle 1

Object Type

Type:	Solid

Size and Shape

Width:	150	µm
Height:	100	µm

Position

Base:	Corner
xw:	0	µm
yw:	0	µm

Rectangle 2:

Label:	Rectangle 2

Object Type

Type:	Solid

Size and Shape

Width:	20	µm
Height:	0.2	µm

Position

Base:	Corner
xw:	50	µm
yw:	0	µm

7. Right click "Plane Geometry" under "Work Plane 1" in the "Model Builder" window. Select Transforms → Array. This will insert an array in the work plane.

8. Change the settings of the inserted array as shown on the right. To add "r2" in "Input objects", click rectangle "r2" in the "Graphics" window as shown (r2 is a narrow line left of the bottom center of the grey rectangle).

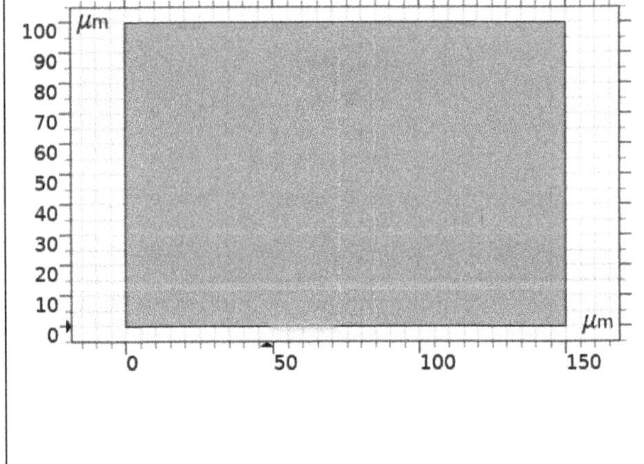

Label:	Array 1

Input

Input objects:

r2

Size

Array type:	Rectangular
xw size:	2
yw size:	1

Displacement

xw:	40	µm
yw:	0	µm

9. Right click "Geometry 1" in the "Model Builder" window and select "Extrude" to create 3D electrodes from the work plane. Under the "Settings" window for "Extrude 1", select "Work Plane 1 (wp1)" as the "Input objects" and change "Specify: Distances from plane" to 100 μm, the height of the 3D model.

Label: Extrude 1

General

Extrude from: Work plane

Work plane: Work Plane 1 (wp1)

Input objects:

wp1

Input object handling: Unite with

Distances

Specify: Distances from plane

Distances (μm)

100

10. In the "Settings" window for "Extrude 1", click "Build All Objects". This will create the 3D model.

Extrude

Build Selected ▼   Build All Objects

Label: Extrude 1

Graphics

11. In the "Graphics" window toolbar, click the "Transparency" button to enable transparency view of the 3D IDE model. The obtained geometry in the "Graphics" window should look like the following:

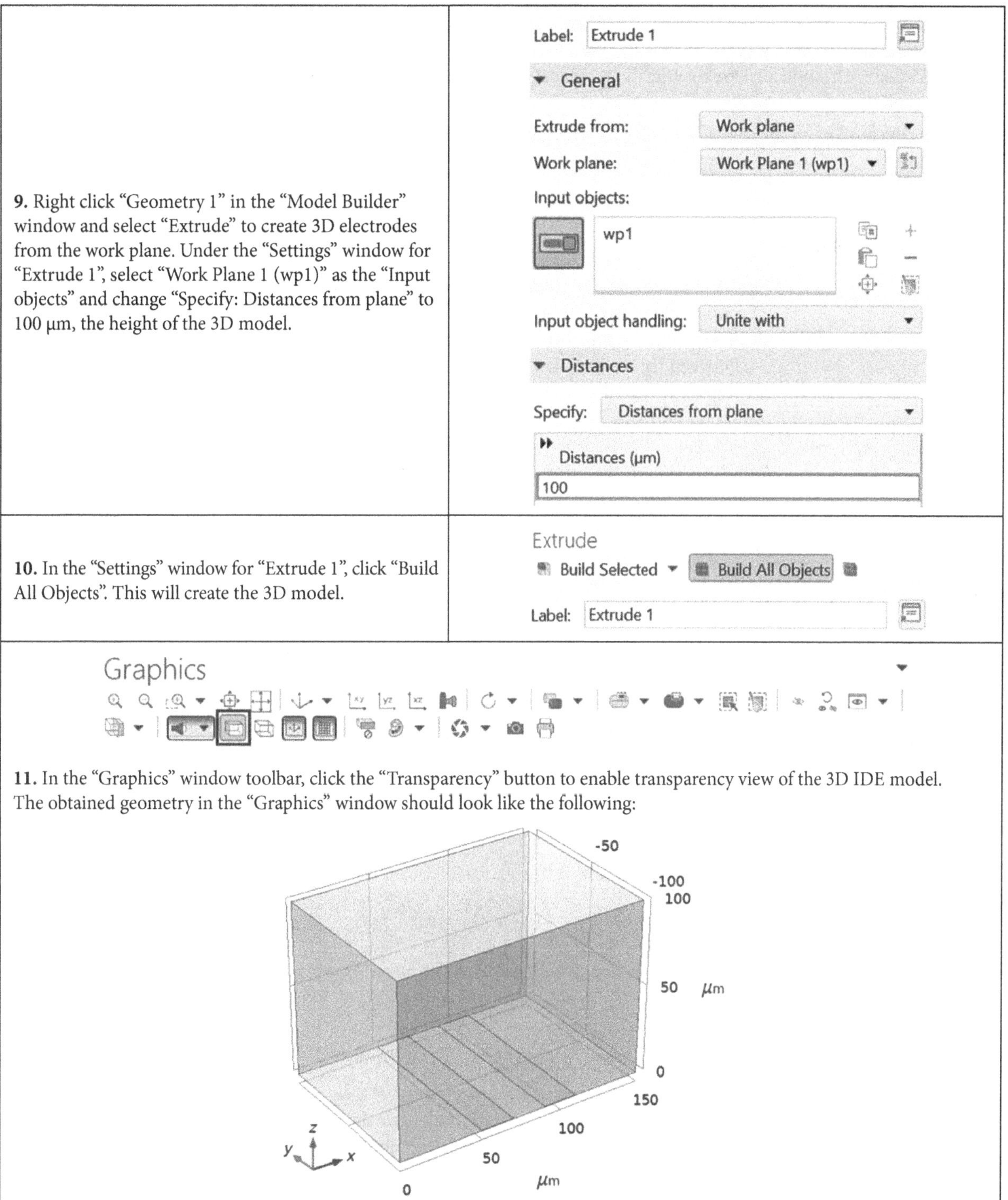

> **12.** Follow the procedure in Section 8.1.1(B) for Lab #1 to set up the simulation. The material for the entire volume is pure water, and the material for the electrodes is gold. If you have trouble selecting an electrode in the "Graphics" window to set the material or electric potential, try rotating the 3D model in the "Graphics" window. As with Lab #1, choose the "Frequency Domain" study.

> **13.** Follow the instructions in Section 8.1.1(C) for Lab #1 to run the simulation and plot the results. Compared to the 2D model, there are some additional plots for the 3D model, such as the "Multislice" plot and the "Volume" plot.

8.2.2 Lab Assignment #2

Part A (Building a 3D Model and Setting Up the Simulation)   A 3D IDE model is based on a work-plane consisting of one channel with 150 µm width and 100 µm height, and two electrodes with 20 µm width and 0.2 µm height. The two electrodes should have a gap of 20 µm between them. The 3D model should be extruded 100 µm from the work-plane. Follow the steps in Tutorial #2 to build the 3D model and set up the simulation in COMSOL Multiphysics® software. Show a screenshot of your model in the "Graphics" window.

Part B (Running the Simulation and Plotting Results)   Simulate your model at different frequencies (f0 = 0 Hz, 1 kHz, 1 MHz, and 1 GHz), as well as different electrode voltage amplitudes (+1V/−1V, +3V/−3V, and +5V/−5V). Does the frequency have an effect on the simulation results? Show multislice plots and contour plots of the electric potential amplitude $V(x,y,z)$, and contour plots of the electric field norm $|E(x,y,z)|$.

Solution

Part A   Shown below is a screenshot of the 3D IDE model.

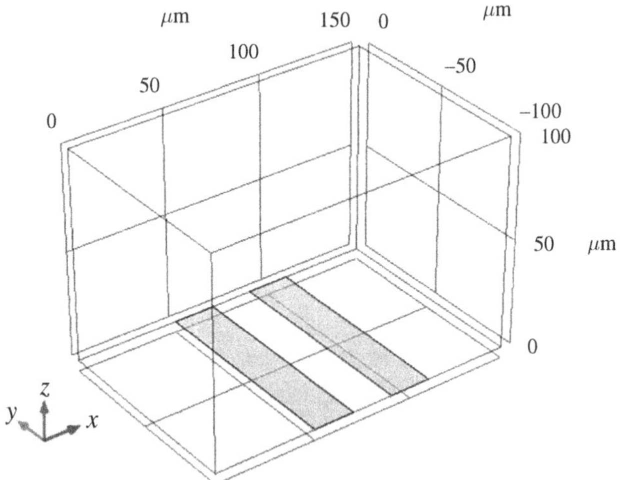

Part B   The frequency f0 does not make any difference at all in the simulation. The plots shown below are for electrode voltage amplitudes of +5V/−5V. Plots for other electrode voltage amplitudes will look similar. To obtain the plots shown, you will have to tweak some of the plot settings.

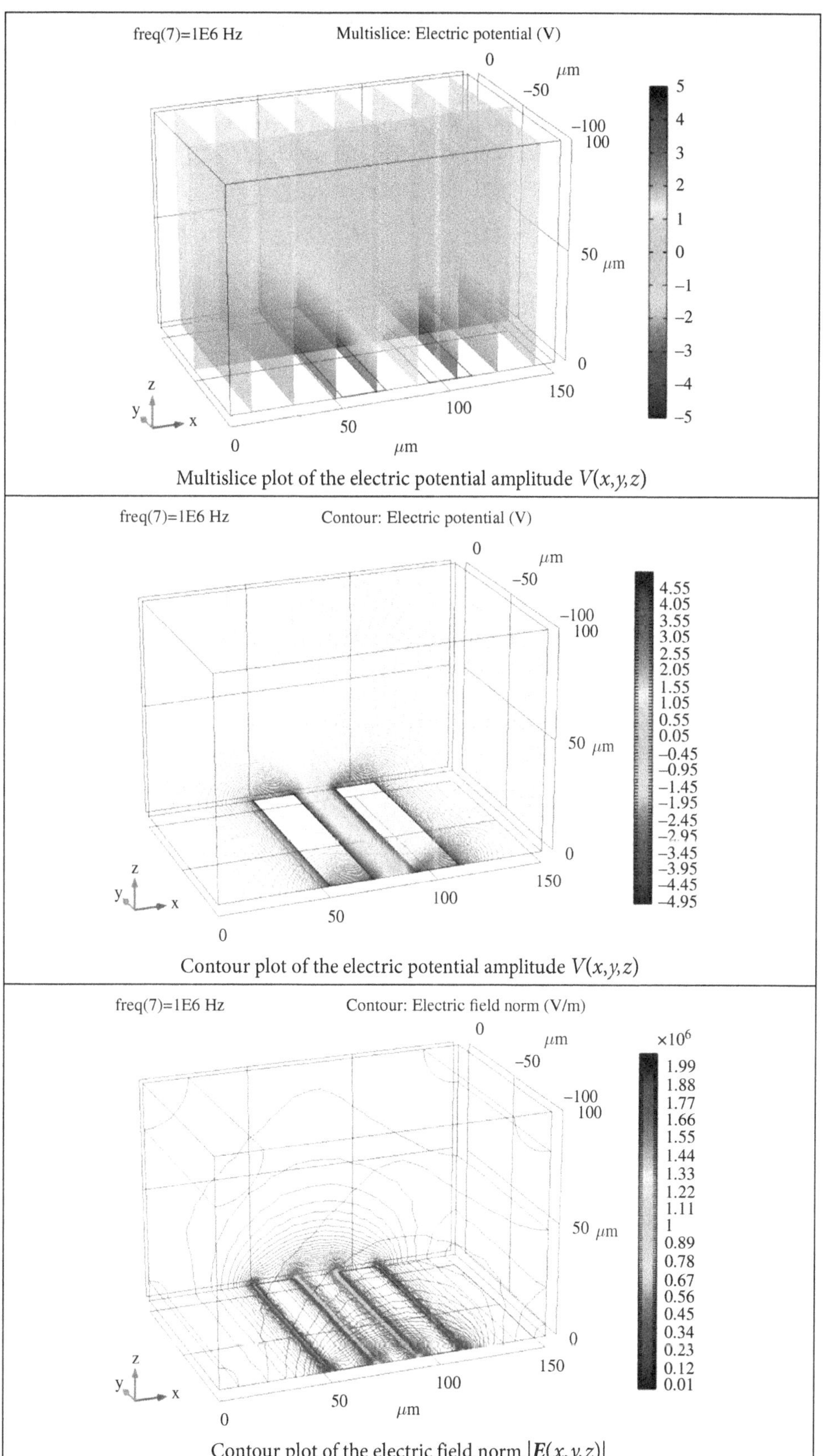

Multislice plot of the electric potential amplitude $V(x,y,z)$

Contour plot of the electric potential amplitude $V(x,y,z)$

Contour plot of the electric field norm $|E(x,y,z)|$

8.3 LAB #3: TRACING DIELECTROPHORETIC PARTICLE MOTION

In this lab assignment, you will use COMSOL Multiphysics® software to simulate particle motion in a microchannel. Recall from Section 3.5.2(B) that for spherical particles with radius R in a sinusoidal electric field given by $E(r,t) = E_0 \cos(\omega t)$, the time-averaged dielectrophoretic (DEP) force $\langle F_{\text{DEP}}(r) \rangle_{\text{Sphere}}$ in terms of the Clausius-Mossotti (CM) factor $\overline{K}_S(\omega)$ is

$$\langle F_{\text{DEP}}(r) \rangle_{\text{Sphere}} = \pi \epsilon_m R^3 \, \text{Re}\!\left[\overline{K}_S(\omega) \right] \nabla \left(\left| E_0(r) \right|^2 \right)$$

$$\text{where } \overline{K}_S(\omega) = \frac{\overline{\epsilon}_p - \overline{\epsilon}_m}{\overline{\epsilon}_p + 2\overline{\epsilon}_m} \text{ with } \overline{\epsilon}_p = \epsilon_p - j\frac{\sigma_p}{\omega} \text{ and } \overline{\epsilon}_m = \epsilon_m - j\frac{\sigma_m}{\omega}$$

Here, $\overline{\epsilon}_p$ and $\overline{\epsilon}_m$ are the complex permittivities of the particle and the medium, respectively. The real part of the CM factor $\text{Re}\!\left[\overline{K}_S(\omega) \right]$ results in either positive DEP (pDEP) when $\text{Re}\!\left[\overline{K}_S(\omega) \right] > 0$, or negative DEP (nDEP) when $\text{Re}\!\left[\overline{K}_S(\omega) \right] < 0$.

8.3.1 COMSOL Multiphysics® Software Tutorial #3

This tutorial introduces two other physics interface modules in COMSOL Multiphysics® simulation software. You can use the 2D simplified IDE model developed in Lab #1, or build your own 2D IDE model. In addition, you need to select the material and parameters for plastic bead particles which are supposed to be captured by the IDE system via microfluidic flow. The goal is to trace the motion of plastic beads moving through a microchannel within a 2D IDE system. Particle motion tracing simulations will be conducted for different cases (e.g., varying the frequency and supply voltage).

---

1. Open COMSOL Multiphysics® software, and load your 2D IDE model from Lab #1 by clicking File → Open, and selecting the .mph file from Lab #1.

2. In the "Model Builder" window, select "Parameters 1" located under "Global Definitions". Under "Parameters", insert the variables as shown. The fluid medium is pure (distilled or deionized) water, and the particle is a plastic bead.

▼ Parameters

Name	Expression	Value	Description
f0	1000[kHz]	1E6 Hz	Frequency of the E field
sigma_f	5.5e-6[S/m]	5.5E-6 S/m	Fluid medium conductivity
epsilon_f	80	80	Fluid relative permittivity
rho_f	1000[kg/m^3]	1000 kg/m³	Fluid density
mu_f	1e-3[Pa*s]	0.001 Pa·s	Fluid dynamic viscosity
rho_p	1175[kg/m^3]	1175 kg/m³	Particle density
dp1	2[um]	2E-6 m	Particle diameter
sigma_p1	0.25[S/m]	0.25 S/m	Particle conductivity
epsilon_p1	3	3	Particle relative permittivity

3. Click Home → Add Physics. "Electric Current (ec)" physics should already be under "Component 1" in the "Model Builder" window.

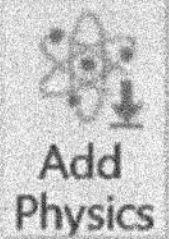

4. In the "Add Physics" window, add "Creepin Flow (spf)" and "Particle Tracing for Fluid Flow (fpt)" by clicking "Add to Component 1". This will add two more physics interfaces. You should see the following under "Component 1" in the "Model Builder" window.

5. Leave the "Electric Currents (ec)" physics interface unchanged since you have already set it up before. Click "Creeping Flow (spf)" in the "Model Builder" window. Under "Domain Selection" of the "Settings" window for "Creeping Flow", ensure that only the 2D channel is selected (deselect the two electrodes).

6. (a) Right click "Creeping Flow (spf)" in the "Model Builder" window and add one "Inlet" and one "Outlet". In the "Settings" window under "Boundary Selection" for the added "Inlet 1" and "Outlet 1", select the left-side wall of the channel as "Inlet 1" and the right-side wall of the channel as "Outlet 1".
(b) In the "Settings" window for "Inlet 1" under "Velocity", enter $U_0 = 10$ [um/s] as shown (right) to set an inflow velocity of 10 μm/s.

7. Click "Particle Properties 1" under "Particle Tracing for Fluid Flow (fpt)" in the "Model Builder" window. In the "Settings" window under "Particle Properties" and "Additional Material Properties", change the settings to those shown below.

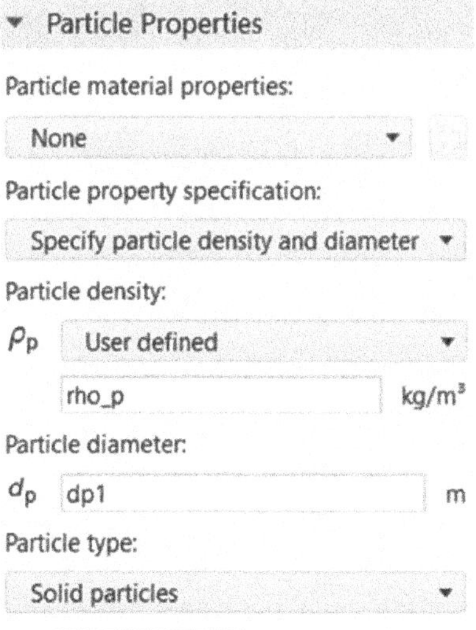

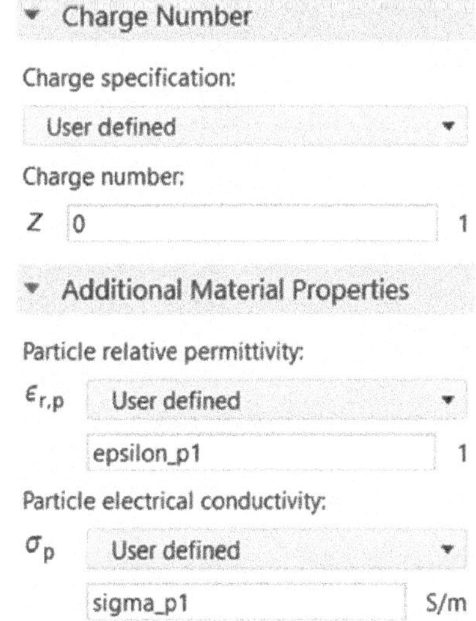

8. (a) By right clicking on "Particle Tracing for Fluid Flow (fpt)" in the "Model Builder" window, add an "Inlet", "Outlet", "Drag Force", and "Dielectrophoretic Force". *Note:* To add forces, select "Forces" in the right-click menu.
(b) For "Outlet 1", select the right boundary (right-side channel wall).

9. For "Drag Force 1", select the entire 2D channel, and change the "Velocity" setting from "User defined" to "Velocity field (spf)". This allows the "Creeping Flow" physics interface to control the particle velocity.

10. For "Dielectrophoretic Force 1", select the entire 2D channel, and change the "Electric field" setting from "User defined" to "Electric field (ec/cucn1)", so that the DEP force will be calculated based on the given "Electric Current (ec)" physics interface.

11. Select "Inlet 1" under "Particle Tracing for Fluid Flow (fpt)" in the "Model Builder" window. For "Inlet 1", select the left-side channel wall for the "Boundary Selection" and change the settings to those shown below. This will release a particle (a plastic bead) into the channel via the inlet every 0.5 s for 12 s.

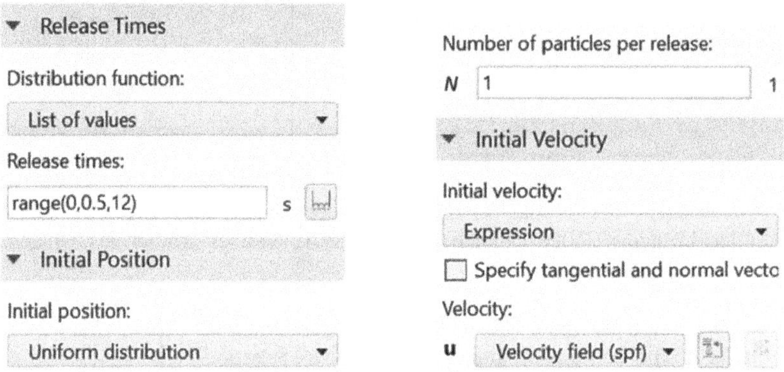

12. Study steps can be added by right-clicking "Study #" → "Study Steps", and choosing the desired step. "Study 1" should include two steps, which are "Step 1: Stationary" and "Step 2: Frequency Domain". Within a "Study #", study steps can be reordered by dragging them up or down in the "Model Builder" window.

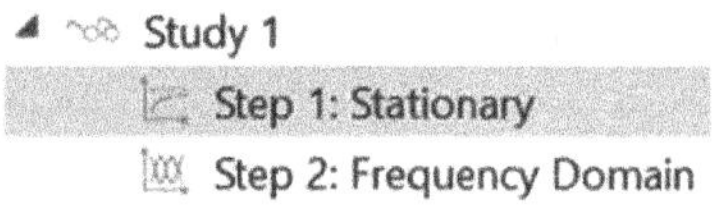

13. In the "Step 1: Stationary" study step, select only "Creeping Flow (spf)" as your "Physics Selection" and all "Dependent Variables" should be "Physics controlled".

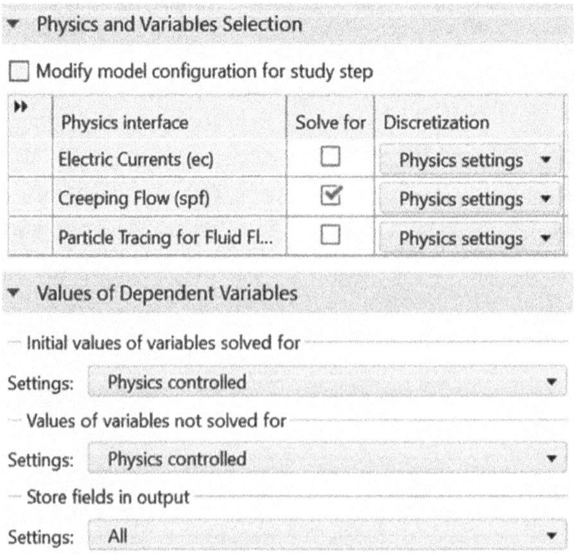

14. In the "Step 2: Frequency Domain" study step, enter f0 to the right of "Frequencies" under "Study Settings". Select only the "Electric Currents (ec)" as your "Physics Selection", and all "Dependent Variables" should be "Physics controlled".

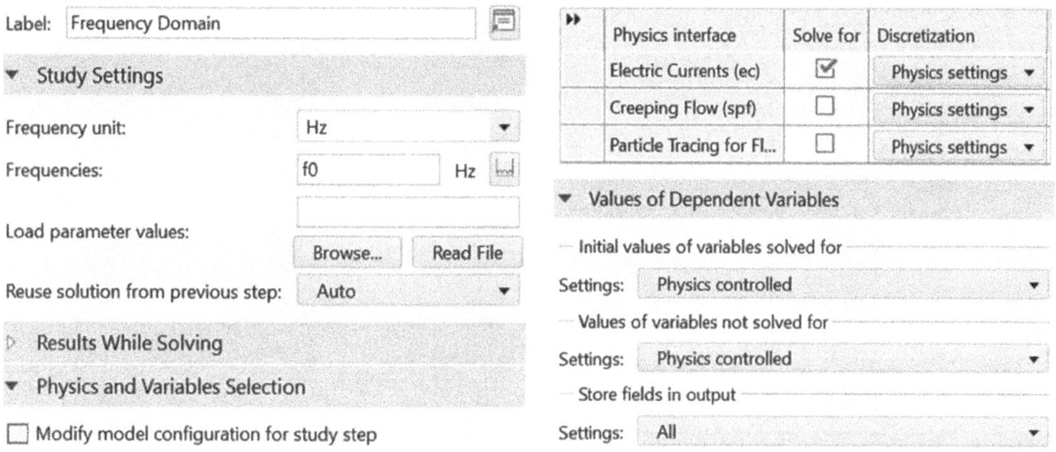

15. Add a second study by clicking Home → Add Study, and double clicking "Empty Study". Add a "Time Dependent" study step for "Study 2". In the "Step 1: Time Dependent" study step for "Study 2", adjust the settings as shown below.

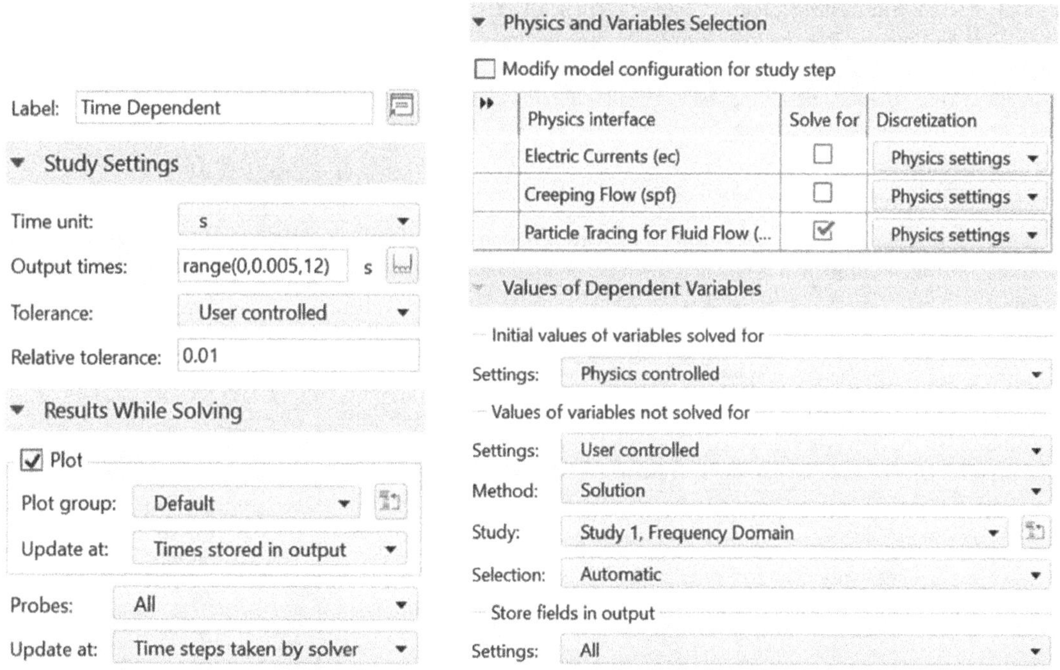

16. Right click "Study 2", and select "Statistics". Then select "Study 2" → "Solver Configurations" → "Solution 1 (sol1)" → "Time-Dependent Solver 1" → "Fully Coupled 1". In the "Settings" window for "Fully Coupled 1", change the "Termination technique" to "Iterations or tolerance".

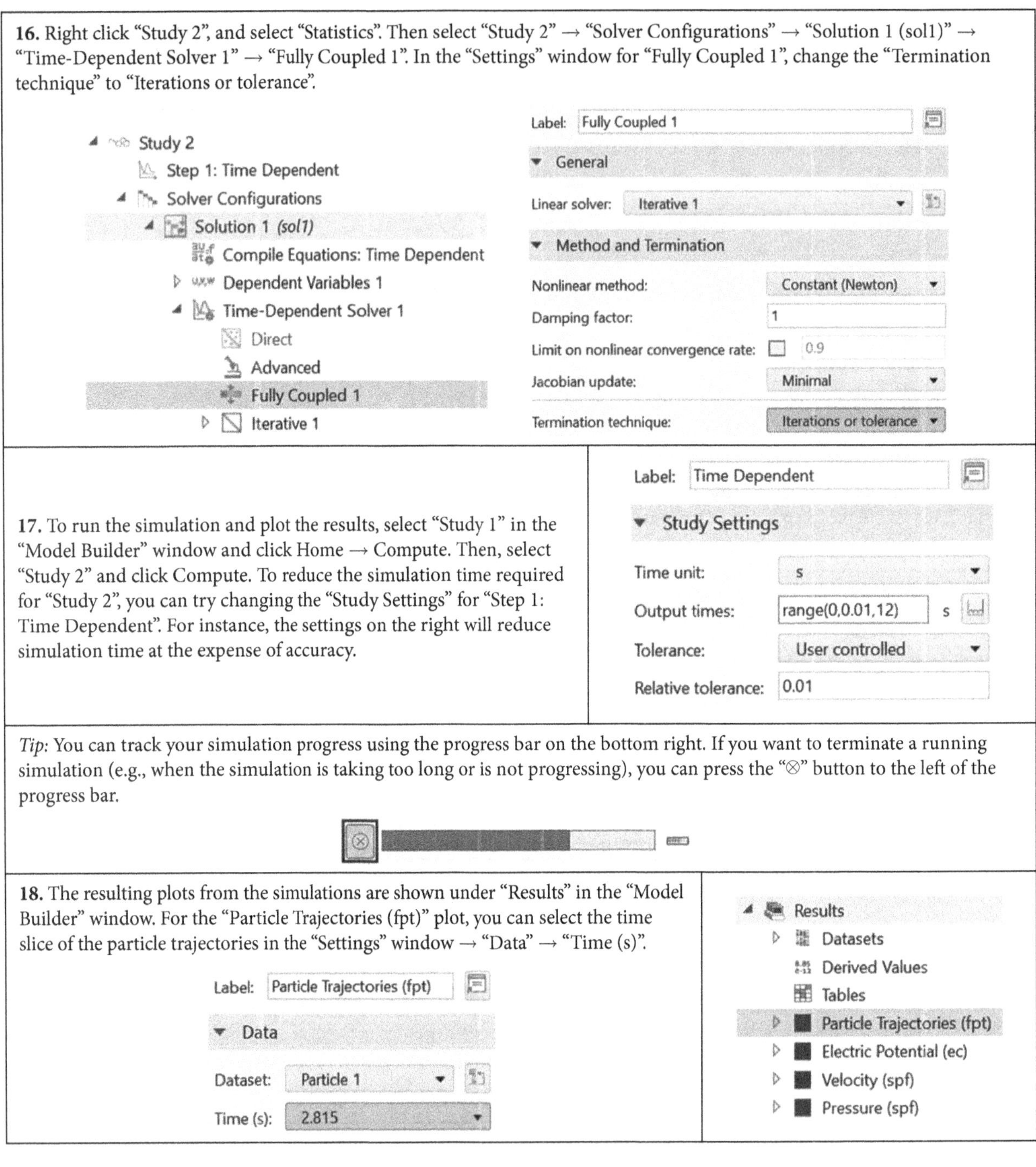

17. To run the simulation and plot the results, select "Study 1" in the "Model Builder" window and click Home → Compute. Then, select "Study 2" and click Compute. To reduce the simulation time required for "Study 2", you can try changing the "Study Settings" for "Step 1: Time Dependent". For instance, the settings on the right will reduce simulation time at the expense of accuracy.

Tip: You can track your simulation progress using the progress bar on the bottom right. If you want to terminate a running simulation (e.g., when the simulation is taking too long or is not progressing), you can press the "⊗" button to the left of the progress bar.

18. The resulting plots from the simulations are shown under "Results" in the "Model Builder" window. For the "Particle Trajectories (fpt)" plot, you can select the time slice of the particle trajectories in the "Settings" window → "Data" → "Time (s)".

8.3.2 Lab Assignment #3

Follow the steps in Tutorial #3 to set up the particle motion tracing simulation in COMSOL Multiphysics® simulation software. Simulate your model at different frequencies (f0 = 1 Hz, 1 kHz, 1 MHz, and 1 GHz), as well as different electrode voltage amplitudes (+0.5V/−0.5V, +1V/−1V, +2V/−2V, and +5V/−5V). Also try reversing the electrode voltage polarities. What are the effects of frequency and electrode voltage amplitude on the particle motion? Does reversing the electrode voltage polarities (e.g., from +2V/−2V to −2V/+2V) make any difference? *Briefly* justify your answers on a theoretical basis using the equation for the time-averaged DEP force $\langle F_{\mathrm{DEP}}(r)\rangle_{\mathrm{Sphere}}$. Show a single surface plot of the fluid velocity magnitude $\left|v_{\mathrm{fluid}}(x,y)\right|$ in the channel, and several plots of the particle trajectories.

Solution

Shown below is a plot of the fluid velocity magnitude $\left|v_{\mathrm{fluid}}(x,y)\right|$ in the channel. The fluid velocity does not depend on the electrode potential amplitudes or the frequency, and is entirely determined by the geometry of the channel and the setting for the inflow velocity $U_0 = 10\ \mu$m/s.

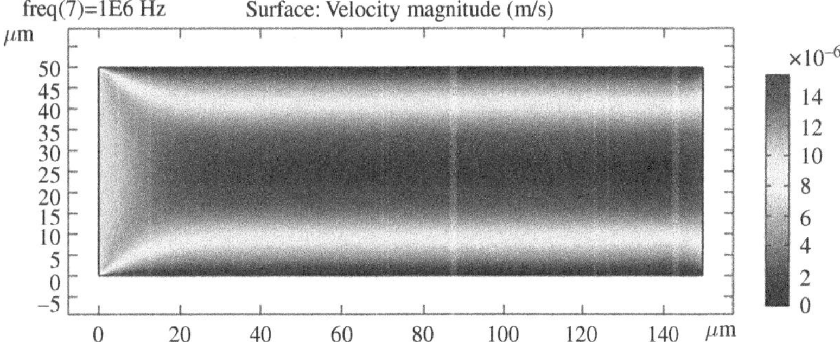

Reversing the electrode voltage polarities does not make any difference to the particle motion. This is because the time-averaged DEP force $\langle F_{\mathrm{DEP}}(r)\rangle_{\mathrm{Sphere}}$ depends on the gradient of the electric field magnitude, but not on the electric field direction. Reversing the electrode voltages will reverse the direction of the electric field, but does not affect the magnitude of the electric field.

$$\langle F_{DEP}(r)\rangle_{Sphere} = \pi\int_m R^3\ \mathrm{Re}\left[\bar{K}_S(\omega)\right]\nabla\left(\left|E_0(r)\right|^2\right)\ \mathit{with}\ \ E(r,t) = E_0\cos(\omega t)$$

Increased electrode voltage amplitudes will increase the gradient of the electric field magnitude, thereby increasing the DEP force $F_{\mathrm{DEP}}(r)$. Thus, the electrode voltage amplitudes affect the time and position at which the particles are captured by the IDEs. If the electrode voltage amplitudes are too low, the particles will pass through the channel without being captured. Higher electrode voltage amplitudes will cause the particles to be captured in less time and at a location closer to the left of the channel.

The AC frequency $f = \omega/2\pi$ affects the complex permittivities of the particle and the medium, which affects the real part of the CM factor. This in turn affects the DEP force $\langle F_{\mathrm{DEP}}(r)\rangle_{\mathrm{Sphere}} = \pi\epsilon_m R^3\ \mathrm{Re}\left[\bar{K}_S(\omega)\right]\nabla\left(\left|E_0(r)\right|^2\right)$.

$$\bar{K}_S(\omega) = \frac{\bar{\epsilon}_p - \bar{\epsilon}_m}{\bar{\epsilon}_p + 2\bar{\epsilon}_m}\ \ \mathrm{with}\ \ \bar{\epsilon}_p = \epsilon_p - j\frac{\sigma_p}{\omega}\ \ \mathrm{and}\ \ \bar{\epsilon}_m = \epsilon_m - j\frac{\sigma_m}{\omega}$$

If the frequency is at or below 1 MHz, the frequency makes little to no difference to the particle trajectory. However, when the frequency is at or above 1 GHz, the direction of the particle trajectory is reversed—the particles move up instead of down toward the electrodes. Very high frequencies can cause the sign of the DEP force to reverse by reversing the sign of the real part of the CM factor.

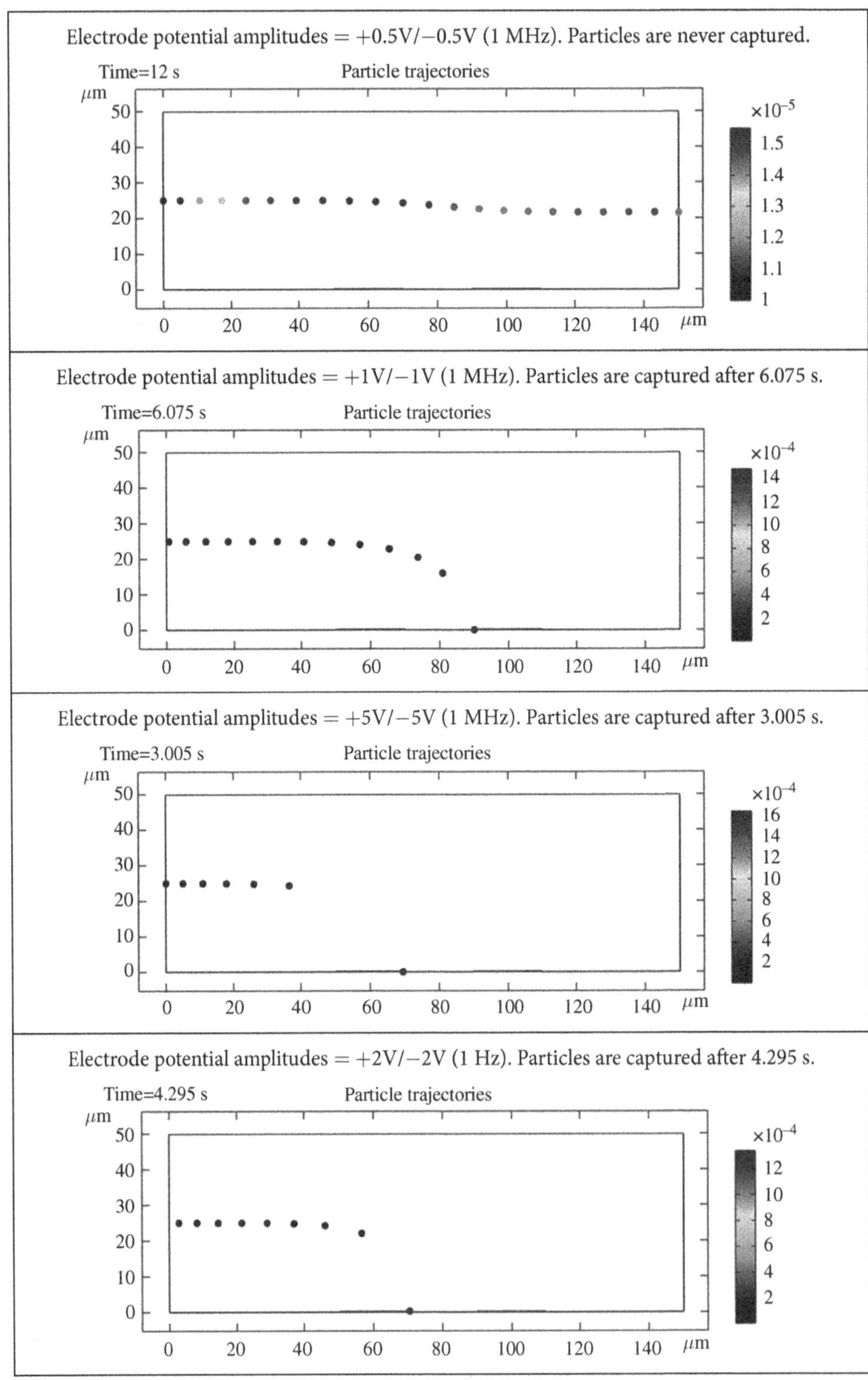

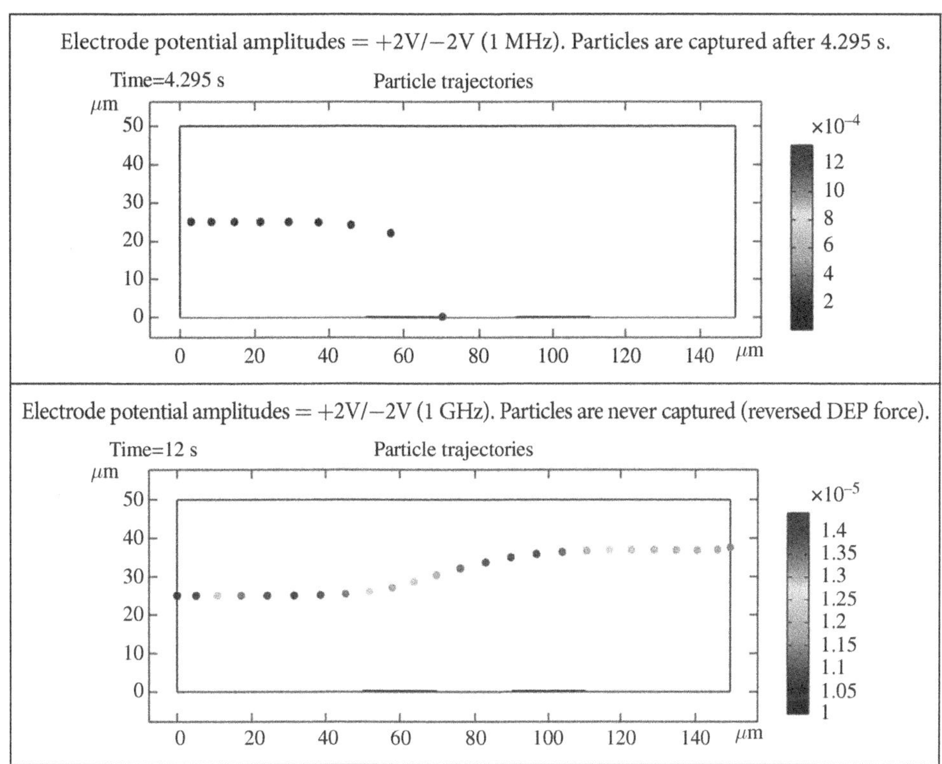

Electrode potential amplitudes = +2V/−2V (1 MHz). Particles are captured after 4.295 s.
Time=4.295 s
Particle trajectories
μm
×10⁻⁴
50
40
30
20
10
0
12
10
8
6
4
2
0
20
40
60
80
100
120
140
μm
Electrode potential amplitudes = +2V/−2V (1 GHz). Particles are never captured (reversed DEP force).
Time=12 s
Particle trajectories
μm
×10⁻⁵
50
40
30
20
10
0
1.4
1.35
1.3
1.25
1.2
1.15
1.1
1.05
1
0
20
40
60
80
100
120
140
μm

APPENDIX A

Abbreviations

µTAS	Micro total analysis system(s)
1D	One-dimensional
2D	Two-dimensional
3D	Three-dimensional
A	Adenosine (nucleotide)
AC	Alternating current
APCVD	Atmospheric-pressure chemical vapor deposition
ATP	Adenosine triphosphate
AuNP(s)	Gold (Au) nanoparticle(s)
BHF	Buffered HF (also known as BOE, wet etchant)
bioMEMS	Biomedical (or biological) micro-electro-mechanical system(s)
BJT(s)	Bipolar junction transistor(s)
BLAST	Basic local alignment search tool(s)
BMI	Brain–machine interface
BOE	Buffered oxide etchant (also known as BHF, wet etchant)
bp(s)	Base pair(s)
C	Cytosine (nucleotide)
CB	Conduction band
cDNA	Complementary DNA
CGM	Continuous glucose monitoring
CHO cells	Chinese hamster ovary cells
CM factor	Clausius-Mossotti factor
CMOS	Complementary metal-oxide-semiconductor
CMP	Chemical-mechanical polishing
CNT(s)	Carbon nanotube(s)
CRISPR	Clustered regularly interspaced short palindromic repeats
crRNA	CRISPR RNA
CT	Computerized tomography
CVD	Chemical vapor deposition
DBS	Deep brain stimulation
DC	Direct current
DCE	Downstream chemical etching
DEP	Dielectrophoresis (or dielectrophoretic)
didNTP	Di-deoxynucleotide triphosphate
DMSO	Dimethyl sulfoxide
DNA	Deoxyribonucleic acid

DNP	2,4-Dinitrophenol
dNTP	Deoxynucleotide triphosphate
DRIE	Deep reactive ion etching
dsDNA	Double-stranded DNA
e-beam	Electron beam
ECD	Electrochemical deposition
ECR-RIE	Electron cyclotron resonance–reactive ion etching
EDP	Ethylenediamine pyrocatechol (alkaline etchant)
EIS	Electrochemical impedance spectroscopy
ELISA	Enzyme-linked immunosorbent assay
EOF	Electro-osmotic flow
EPF	Electrophoretic flow
EtBr	Ethidium bromide
EUV	Extreme ultraviolet (light)
ex vivo	Within tissue in an external environment that mimics natural conditions
FET(s)	Field-effect transistor(s)
FRET	Fluorescence resonance energy transfer
FWHM	Full width at half maximum
G	Guanine (nucleotide)
GNP(s)	Gold nanoparticle(s)
gRNA	Guide RNA
HA	Heteroduplex analysis
HEK 293 cells	Human embryonic kidney 293 cells
HIV	Human immunodeficiency virus
HNA	Hydrofluoric-nitric-acetic acid mixture (wet etchant)
IC(s)	Integrated circuit(s)
ICP-RIE	Inductively coupled plasma–reactive ion etching
IDE(s)	Interdigitated electrode(s)
in vitro	Outside of a living organism (e.g., in a test tube or culture dish)
in vivo	Within a living organism
IPA	Isopropyl alcohol
IR	Infrared (light)
LCR	Inductance (L)–capacitance (C)–resistance (R)
LED(s)	Light-emitting diode(s)
LIGA	German acronym for lithography, electroplating, and molding
LOC(s)	Lab-on-a-Chip(s)
LOR	Lift-off resist
LPCVD	Low-pressure chemical vapor deposition
MEMS	Micro-electro-mechanical system(s)
MOSFET(s)	Metal-oxide-semiconductor field-effect transistor(s)
MRI	Magnetic resonance imaging
mRNA	Messenger RNA
MWCNT(s)	Multi-walled carbon nanotube(s)
nDEP	Negative dielectrophoresis
NIR	Near-infrared (light)
NSA	Nanostructured alumina
nt(s)	Nucleotide(s)
OOC(s)	Organ-on-a-chip(s) or organs-on-chip(s)

PAGE	Polyacrylamide gel electrophoresis
PCR	Polymerase chain reaction
pDEP	Positive dielectrophoresis
PDF	Pressure-driven flow
PDMS	Polydimethylsiloxane
PDT	Photodynamic therapy
PECVD	Plasma-enhanced chemical vapor deposition
PET	Positron emission tomography
pH	Potential (or power) of hydrogen
pI	Isoelectric point
poly-Si	Polycrystalline silicon (or polysilicon)
polysilicon	Polycrystalline silicon (or poly-Si)
PPTT	Plasmonic photothermal therapy
PR	Photoresist
PTFE	Polytetrafluoroethylene (also known as Teflon®)
PTT	Photothermal therapy
PVD	Physical vapor deposition
QD(s)	Quantum dot(s)
QE	Quantum efficiency
qPCR	Quantitative real-time polymerase chain reaction
QY	Quantum yield
RC	Resistance–capacitance (or resistor–capacitor)
RF	Radio frequency
RF AC	Radio frequency alternating current
RIE	Reactive ion etching
rms	Root-mean-square
RNA	Ribonucleic acid
RPM	Revolutions per minute
RT-PCR	Reverse transcription–PCR (polymerase chain reaction)
RT-qPCR	Quantitative real-time reverse transcription–PCR
SMBG	Self-monitoring of blood glucose
SNR	Signal-to-noise ratio
SPR	Surface plasmon resonance
SSCP	Single-strand conformation polymorphism
ssDNA	Single-stranded DNA
SU-8	An epoxy-based negative photoresist
SWCNT(s)	Single-walled carbon nanotube(s)
T	Thymine (nucleotide)
TMAH	Tetramethylammonium hydroxide (alkaline etchant)
tracrRNA	Trans-activating CRISPR RNA
U	Uracil (nucleotide)
UV	Ultraviolet (light)
VB	Valence band
via(s)	Vertical electrical interconnect(s)
VNS	Vagus nerve stimulation

APPENDIX B

Units in SI (International System of Units)

SI Unit Prefix	pico-	nano-	micro-	milli-	centi-	deci-	kilo-	mega-	giga-	tera-
Symbol	p	n	μ	m	c	d	k	M	G	T
Multiplication Factor	10^{-12}	10^{-9}	10^{-6}	10^{-3}	10^{-2}	10^{-1}	10^{3}	10^{6}	10^{9}	10^{12}

Unit Name	Symbol	Physical Quantity	SI Equivalents
mole	mol	amount of substance (base SI unit)	$1\ \text{mol} = N_A$ particles $1\ \text{mol} = 6.0221 \times 10^{23}$ particles
second	s	time	base SI unit
minute	min	time	$1\ \text{min} = 60\ \text{s}$
hour	hour	time	$1\ \text{hour} = 60\ \text{min} = 3600\ \text{s}$
hertz	Hz	frequency	s^{-1}
meter	m	length	base SI unit
angstrom	Å	length	$1\ \text{Å} = 10^{-10}\ \text{m} = 0.1\ \text{nm}$
liter	L	volume	$1\ \text{L} = 0.001\ \text{m}^3 = 1\ \text{dm}^3 = 1000\ \text{cm}^3$
molar	M	concentration	$1\ \text{M} = 1\ \text{mol} / \text{L} = 1000\ \text{mol} / \text{m}^3$
kilogram	kg	mass	base SI unit
ampere	A	electric current	base SI unit
kelvin	K	temperature	base SI unit
degree Celsius	°C	temperature	$T[^\circ\text{C}] = T[\text{K}] + 273.15$
radian (angle)	rad	angle	dimensionless
degree (angle)	°	angle	$1^\circ = \dfrac{\pi}{180}\ \text{rad}$
newton	N	force, weight	$\text{N} = \dfrac{\text{kg} \cdot \text{m}}{\text{s}^2}$

(Continued)

Unit Name	Symbol	Physical Quantity	SI Equivalents
pascal	Pa	pressure, stress	$Pa = \dfrac{N}{m^2} = \dfrac{kg}{m \cdot s^2}$
joule	J	energy, work, heat	$J = N \cdot m = \dfrac{kg \cdot m^2}{s^2}$
watt	W	power	$W = J / s = \dfrac{kg \cdot m^2}{s^3}$
coulomb	C	electric charge	$C = A \cdot s$
debye	debye or D	electric dipole moment	$1\ debye = 3.3356 \times 10^{-30}\ C \cdot m$
volt	V	electric potential (voltage)	$V = \dfrac{J}{C} = \dfrac{W}{A} = \dfrac{kg \cdot m^2}{s^3 \cdot A}$
farad	F	capacitance	$F = \dfrac{C}{V} = \dfrac{s^4 \cdot A^2}{kg \cdot m^2}$
ohm	Ω	(electrical) resistance, reactance, impedance	$\Omega = \dfrac{V}{A} = \dfrac{kg \cdot m^2}{s^3 \cdot A^2}$
siemens	S	(electrical) conductance, susceptance, admittance	$S = \Omega^{-1} = \dfrac{A}{V} = \dfrac{s^3 \cdot A^2}{kg \cdot m^2}$
weber	Wb	magnetic flux	$Wb = V \cdot s = \dfrac{kg \cdot m^2}{s^2 \cdot A}$
tesla	T	magnetic flux density	$T = \dfrac{Wb}{m^2} = \dfrac{kg}{s^2 \cdot A}$
henry	H	inductance	$H = \dfrac{Wb}{A} = \dfrac{kg \cdot m^2}{s^2 \cdot A^2}$

APPENDIX C

Fundamental Physical Constants

Fundamental Physical Constant	Symbol	Value (SI Units)
absolute zero	T_{0K}	$0\,K$ or $-273.15°C$
Avogadro's number	N_A	$6.0221 \times 10^{23}\,mol^{-1}$
Boltzmann constant	k_B	$1.3806 \times 10^{-23}\,J/K$
electron rest mass	m_e	$9.1094 \times 10^{-31}\,kg$
electron volt	eV	$1.6022 \times 10^{-19}\,J$
elementary charge	e	$1.6022 \times 10^{-19}\,C$
(Newtonian) gravitational constant	G	$6.6741 \times 10^{-11}\,N \cdot m^2/kg^2$
permeability of free space (magnetic constant)	μ_0	$4\pi \times 10^{-7}\,H/m$
permittivity of free space (electric constant)	ϵ_0	$8.8542 \times 10^{-12}\,F/m$
Planck constant	h	$6.6261 \times 10^{-31}\,J \cdot s$
reduced Planck constant	$\hbar = \dfrac{h}{2\pi}$	$1.0546 \times 10^{-34}\,J \cdot s$
speed of light in vacuum	c	$2.9979 \times 10^{8}\,m/s$
standard acceleration due to gravity	g	$9.81\,m/s^2$
(unified) atomic mass unit	Da or u	$1.6605 \times 10^{-27}\,kg$

APPENDIX D

Sign Convention for Fluid Flow

To distinguish the direction of fluid flow with a sign convention, let us consider fluid flow with velocity $\boldsymbol{v} = v\,\hat{\boldsymbol{x}}$ in a horizontal channel having a horizontal electric field $\boldsymbol{E} = E\,\hat{\boldsymbol{x}}$. If the fluid moves toward the right, the fluid velocity v is positive; if the fluid moves toward the left, v is negative. Similarly, if the electric field E points rightward (i.e., the left end of the channel has a higher electric potential V), E is positive; if E points leftward (i.e., the right end of the channel has higher potential V), E is negative.

Alternatively, we could have fluid flow with $\boldsymbol{v} = v\,\hat{\boldsymbol{z}}$ in a vertical channel having a vertical electric field $\boldsymbol{E} = E\,\hat{\boldsymbol{z}}$. If the fluid moves upward, v is positive; if the fluid moves downward, v is negative. Likewise, if E is directed upward (i.e., the bottom end of the channel has a higher potential V), E is positive; if E is directed downward (i.e., the top end of the channel has higher potential V), E is negative.

(1) *Pressure-Driven Flow (PDF):* For PDF (i.e., Hagen-Poiseuille flow), the fluid velocity is

$$v_{\text{PDF}}(r) = \frac{\Delta P\left(r_0^2 - r^2\right)}{4L\eta}$$

Because L and η are both positive physical quantities and $r \leq r_0$, the fluid velocity $v_{\text{PDF}}(r)$ due to PDF is in the direction of higher to lower pressure.

TABLE D-1 Sign Convention for Horizontal and Vertical Fluid Flow

Parameter [unit]	Horizontal Channel	Vertical Channel
Velocity v [m/s]	$(+)$ direction: rightward $(\rightarrow)$ $(-)$ direction: leftward $(\leftarrow)$	$(+)$ direction: upward $(\uparrow)$ $(-)$ direction: downward $(\downarrow)$
Electric Field E [V/m]	$(+)$ direction: rightward $(\rightarrow)$ $(-)$ direction: leftward $(\leftarrow)$	$(+)$ direction: upward $(\uparrow)$ $(-)$ direction: downward $(\downarrow)$
Constant Electric Field E from Electric Potential V	$E = \dfrac{V_{\text{left end}} - V_{\text{right end}}}{\text{channel length}}$	$E = \dfrac{V_{\text{bottom end}} - V_{\text{top end}}}{\text{channel length}}$
Pressure Differential ΔP [Pa]	$\Delta P = P_{\text{left end}} - P_{\text{right end}}$	$\Delta P = P_{\text{bottom end}} - P_{\text{top end}}$
Zeta Potential ζ [V]	reversing the sign of ζ will reverse v_{EOF}	
Electric Charge q [C]	reversing the sign of q will reverse v_{EPF}	

(2) *Electro-Osmotic Flow (EOF):* For EOF, the fluid velocity is given by

$$v_{EOF} = \frac{-\epsilon \zeta}{\eta} E$$

Noting that both ϵ and η are positive physical quantities, the negative sign in this equation indicates that if the zeta potential $\zeta > 0$, the direction of EOF fluid flow v_{EOF} will be opposite to the direction of the electric field E. Reversing the sign of the zeta potential will also reverse the sign of the fluid velocity v_{EOF} due to EOF.

(3) *Electrophoretic Flow (EPF):* The velocity of charged entities in a fluid due to EPF is given by

$$v_{EPF} = \frac{q}{6\pi\eta R_S} E$$

Here, η and R_S are both strictly positive physical quantities. If the electric charge of the entity is positive ($q > 0$), the EPF velocity v_{EPF} of the charged entities will be in the same direction as the electric field E. Reversing the electric charge q will reverse the flow direction of the charged entities.

In this book, we will follow this sign convention (as shown in Table D-1) for all electrokinetic forces (EOF, EPF, and dielectrophoresis) and for pressure-driven flow (PDF). For instance, if a voltage of V_0 is applied to the right side of a horizontal capillary with length L and the left side is grounded, the electric field E is given by

$$E = \frac{V_{left\ end} - V_{right\ end}}{channel\ length} = \frac{0 - V_0}{L} = \frac{-V_0}{L}$$

APPENDIX E

Coordinate Systems

Coordinate System	Identity
Cartesian Coordinates (x, y, z) $\boldsymbol{r} = x\,\hat{\boldsymbol{x}} + y\,\hat{\boldsymbol{y}} + z\,\hat{\boldsymbol{z}}$	$\boldsymbol{\nabla} f = \dfrac{\partial f}{\partial x}\hat{\boldsymbol{x}} + \dfrac{\partial f}{\partial y}\hat{\boldsymbol{y}} + \dfrac{\partial f}{\partial z}\hat{\boldsymbol{z}}$
	$\nabla^2 f = \dfrac{\partial^2 f}{\partial x^2} + \dfrac{\partial^2 f}{\partial y^2} + \dfrac{\partial^2 f}{\partial z^2}$
Cylindrical Coordinates (ρ, φ, z) $\boldsymbol{r} = \rho\,\hat{\boldsymbol{\rho}} + z\,\hat{\boldsymbol{z}}$	$\boldsymbol{\nabla} f = \dfrac{\partial f}{\partial \rho}\hat{\boldsymbol{\rho}} + \dfrac{1}{\rho}\dfrac{\partial f}{\partial \varphi}\hat{\boldsymbol{\varphi}} + \dfrac{\partial f}{\partial z}\hat{\boldsymbol{z}}$
	$\nabla^2 f = \dfrac{1}{\rho}\dfrac{\partial}{\partial \rho}\left(\rho\dfrac{\partial f}{\partial \rho}\right) + \dfrac{1}{\rho^2}\dfrac{\partial^2 f}{\partial \varphi^2} + \dfrac{\partial f^2}{\partial z^2}$
Spherical Coordinates (r, θ, φ) $\boldsymbol{r} = r\,\hat{\boldsymbol{r}}$	$\boldsymbol{\nabla} f = \dfrac{\partial f}{\partial r}\hat{\boldsymbol{r}} + \dfrac{1}{r}\dfrac{\partial f}{\partial \theta}\hat{\boldsymbol{\theta}} + \dfrac{1}{r\sin\theta}\dfrac{\partial f}{\partial \varphi}\hat{\boldsymbol{\varphi}}$
	$\nabla^2 f = \dfrac{1}{r^2}\dfrac{\partial}{\partial r}\left(r^2\dfrac{\partial f}{\partial r}\right) + \dfrac{1}{r^2\sin\theta}\dfrac{\partial}{\partial \theta}\left(\sin\theta\dfrac{\partial f}{\partial \theta}\right) + \dfrac{1}{r^2\sin^2\theta}\dfrac{\partial^2 f}{\partial \varphi^2}$

$\boldsymbol{r}$ = position vector $\qquad \boldsymbol{\nabla} f$ = gradient of $f \qquad \nabla^2 f = (\boldsymbol{\nabla}\cdot\boldsymbol{\nabla})f$ = Laplacian of f

Coordinate Transformation Identities

Cartesian (x, y, z) $\updownarrow$ Cylindrical (ρ, φ, z)		
	$x = \rho\cos\varphi$	$\hat{\boldsymbol{x}} = \cos\varphi\,\hat{\boldsymbol{\rho}} - \sin\varphi\,\hat{\boldsymbol{\varphi}}$
	$y = \rho\sin\varphi$	$\hat{\boldsymbol{y}} = \sin\varphi\,\hat{\boldsymbol{\rho}} + \cos\varphi\,\hat{\boldsymbol{\varphi}}$
	$z = z$	$\hat{\boldsymbol{z}} = \hat{\boldsymbol{z}}$
	$\rho = \sqrt{x^2 + y^2}$	$\hat{\boldsymbol{\rho}} = \cos\varphi\,\hat{\boldsymbol{x}} + \sin\varphi\,\hat{\boldsymbol{y}}$
	$\varphi = \arctan(y/x)$	$\hat{\boldsymbol{\varphi}} = -\sin\varphi\,\hat{\boldsymbol{x}} + \cos\varphi\,\hat{\boldsymbol{y}}$
	$z = z$	$\hat{\boldsymbol{z}} = \hat{\boldsymbol{z}}$

(Continued)

Coordinate Transformation Identities (*Continued*)

Cartesian (x, y, z) $\updownarrow$ Spherical (r, θ, φ)	$x = r\sin\theta\cos\varphi$	$\hat{x} = \sin\theta\cos\varphi\,\hat{r} + \cos\theta\cos\varphi\,\hat{\theta} - \sin\varphi\,\hat{\varphi}$
	$y = r\sin\theta\sin\varphi$	$\hat{y} = \sin\theta\sin\varphi\,\hat{r} + \cos\theta\sin\varphi\,\hat{\theta} + \cos\varphi\,\hat{\varphi}$
	$z = r\cos\theta$	$\hat{z} = \cos\theta\,\hat{r} - \sin\theta\,\hat{\theta}$
	$r = \sqrt{x^2 + y^2 + z^2}$	$\hat{r} = \sin\theta\cos\varphi\,\hat{x} + \sin\theta\sin\varphi\,\hat{y} + \cos\theta\,\hat{z}$
	$\theta = \arctan\left(\sqrt{x^2 + y^2}/z\right)$	$\hat{\theta} = \cos\theta\cos\varphi\,\hat{x} + \cos\theta\sin\varphi\,\hat{y} - \sin\theta\,\hat{z}$
	$\varphi = \arctan(y/x)$	$\hat{\varphi} = -\sin\varphi\,\hat{x} + \cos\varphi\,\hat{y}$

APPENDIX F

Complex Numbers

F.1 REVIEW OF COMPLEX NUMBERS

In general, a complex number z can be expressed in Cartesian form as

$$z = a + jb = \mathrm{Re}[z] + j\,\mathrm{Im}[z] \quad \text{where} \quad \begin{cases} \mathrm{Re}[z] = a \\ \mathrm{Im}[z] = b \end{cases}$$

where $j = \sqrt{-1}$ is the imaginary unit, $\mathrm{Re}[z]$ is the real part of z, and $\mathrm{Im}[z]$ is the imaginary part of z. Using Euler's formula given by

$$\exp(j\theta) = \cos\theta + j\sin\theta$$

we can express any complex number z in polar form as follows.

$$z = |z|\exp(j\theta) \quad \text{where} \quad \begin{cases} |z| = \sqrt{a^2 + b^2} \\ \theta = \arctan\left(\dfrac{b}{a}\right) \end{cases}$$

We can demonstrate that the Cartesian and polar forms of any complex number are equivalent as follows.

$$z = a + jb = |z|\exp(j\theta) = |z|(\cos\theta + j\sin\theta) = |z|\cos\theta + j|z|\sin\theta \;\Rightarrow\; \begin{cases} a = |z|\cos\theta \\ b = |z|\sin\theta \end{cases}$$

$$\frac{b}{a} = \frac{|z|\sin\theta}{|z|\cos\theta} = \tan\theta \quad \Rightarrow \quad \theta = \arctan\left(\frac{b}{a}\right)$$

$$a^2 + b^2 = \left(|z|\cos\theta\right)^2 + \left(|z|\sin\theta\right)^2 = |z|^2\left(\cos^2\theta + \sin^2\theta\right) = |z|^2 \quad \Rightarrow \quad |z| = \sqrt{a^2 + b^2}$$

F.2 (COMPLEX) PHASORS

For any time-dependent sinusoidal quantity $\mathbf{X}(t)$ which could be a vector or scalar function, we have

$$\mathbf{X}(t) = \mathbf{X}_0\cos(\omega t + \theta)$$

where $\omega = 2\pi f$ is the angular frequency, f is the frequency, and θ is the phase angle. Using Euler's formula, we have

$$\mathbf{X}_0\exp\left[j(\omega t + \theta)\right] = \mathbf{X}_0\cos(\omega t + \theta) + j\,\mathbf{X}_0\sin(\omega t + \theta)$$

Therefore,

$$\mathbf{X}(t) = \mathrm{Re}\left\{\mathbf{X}_0 \exp\left[\, j(\omega t + \theta)\right]\right\} = \mathrm{Re}\left\{\mathbf{X}_0 \exp(j\theta)\exp(j\omega t)\right\}$$

We can define a (complex) phasor $\bar{\mathbf{X}} = \mathbf{X}_0 \exp(j\theta)$ as follows.

$$\bar{\mathbf{X}} = \mathbf{X}_0 \exp(j\theta) \quad \Rightarrow \quad \mathbf{X}(t) = \mathrm{Re}\left\{\bar{\mathbf{X}} \exp(j\omega t)\right\}$$

One advantage of using (complex) phasors is that taking the time derivative is greatly simplified. That is,

$$\frac{\partial \mathbf{X}(t)}{\partial t} = \frac{\partial}{\partial t}\mathrm{Re}\left\{\bar{\mathbf{X}}\exp(j\omega t)\right\} = \mathrm{Re}\left\{\bar{\mathbf{X}}\frac{\partial \exp(j\omega t)}{\partial t}\right\} = \mathrm{Re}\left\{j\omega \cdot \bar{\mathbf{X}}\exp(j\omega t)\right\}$$

since $\bar{\mathbf{X}}$ does not depend on t. Therefore, the time derivative operator $\partial/\partial t$ is equivalent to multiplying by $j\omega$ when all variables have the same exponential time dependence $\exp(j\omega t)$. That is,

$$\frac{\partial}{\partial t} \rightarrow j\omega$$

Index

A

A-T base pair, 125
A-T bonding, 15–16
AC electric field, sphere with loss in, 61–63
Acid dissociation constant, 76
Acid strength, 76
Acidity constant, 76
Alkaline wet etchants, 206–207
Alkaline wet etching, 203, 206
Alzheimer's disease, 64
Amino acids:
  glycine, 77
  isoelectric point for, 76
  lysine, 77
Amorphous materials, 189
Anisotropic wet etching, 203–211
Annealing, 223
Antibiotics, 292, 295
Antibodies:
  as bioaffinity molecule, 106
  Cas9 response, 156
  coating of, 3
APCVD. *See* Atmospheric-pressure chemical vapor deposition
Array-type microchips, 164
Aspect ratio, 196
Atmospheric-pressure chemical vapor deposition, 188, 191
Autofluorescence, 95
Axons, microtubule arrangement in, 66

B

Bacon, Roger, 1
Bacteria, optical detection of, 97–100
Bacteriophages:
  definition of, 292
  description of, 121, 153
  therapeutic uses of, 292–294
Bandgap, of quantum dots, 101–103
Bandgap energy, 100, 103
Batch polymerase chain reaction microreactors:
  overview of, 270–272
  thermal equivalent circuit of, 278–283
  thermal model of, 272–278
Beer-Lambert law, 92–93
Bessel functions, 101–102
Bioaffinity molecules, 106
Bioconjugates, quantum dot, 106, 110
Bioelectrical signal detection, of organ-on-a-chip devices, 180, 185
Biofilms, 294

Biomarkers, 6–7
Bionanotechnology:
  applications of, 1–2, 251–252, 287–292, 309
  creation of, 1
  crop agriculture applications of, 312–314
  electromagnetic forces in, 14
  glucose monitoring applications of, 287–292
  gravity in, 14–15
  microfluidics in, 4
  neural implants, 309–312
Bioremediation, nanomaterials-based, 313–314
Biosensing. *See* Lab-on-a-chip biosensors
BLAST, 131–135
Blinking, 110
Blood glucose monitoring. *See* Glucose monitoring
Blood oxygen oximeter, 92–93
Body-on-a-chip systems, 182–183
BOE wet etching, 202–203, 230–231
Boltzmann constant, 33
Bosch process, 216–218
Brain-on-a-chip device, 179–180
Brain–machine interfaces, 309–312
BRCA1 gene, 118
Brus equation, 111
Bulk micromachining, of micro-electro-mechanical systems, 234

C

C-G bonding, 15–16
c-myc oncogene, 306
Cancer:
  chemotherapy for, 297
  deaths caused by, 296
  drug delivery in, ultrasound-aided phase-shift nanodroplets for, 304–306
  metastasis of, 297
  radiation therapy for, 297
  targeted therapies for:
    carbon nanotubes, 302–304
    description of, 296–297
    DNA nanotechnology applications in, 306–307
    gold nanoparticles, 298–302
    nanoparticle-mediated thermal therapy, 297–302
    nanoparticle therapies, 295–296, 298–302
    photothermal therapy, 298–302
    plasmonic photothermal therapy, 298–302
  tumor-on-a-chip devices for, 180–182
Cancer cells, 297

Capillaries:
    human, 18
    parabolic flow profile in, 28
    pressure-driven flow in, 27
Capillary action, 67
Capillary electrophoresis, 78–80
Capillary forces, 16–19
Capillary microfluidics, 11
Capillary pressure, 18
Carbon nanotubes:
    applications of, 3, 302
    description of, 2–3
    multi-walled, 3, 304
    PEGylated single-walled, 302–304
    semiconductor nanowires and, 4
    single-walled, 3, 289, 302–304
    surface functionalization of, 302, 304
    targeted cancer treatment using, 302–304
Carbon tetrafluoride, 213
Cartesian coordinates, 20
Cas proteins, 153
CB. *See* Conduction band
Cell capture and separation, dielectrophoresis
        for, 68–76
Centrifugal force, 12
Centrifugal microfluidics:
    description of, 11
    illustration of, 12
Cephedi, 11
"Chain-termination" sequencing, 138
Charged particles, electrophoretic flow of, 51
Chemical dry etching, 212–215
Chemical-mechanical polishing, 223
Chemical vapor deposition, 188, 190–192
Chemotherapy, 297
Chromosomes, 117, 119
Clarke Error Grid Analysis, 290
Clausius-Mossotti factor, 59, 62, 69–70, 72–73
CMOS lab-on-a-chip biosensors. *See* Complementary metal-
        oxide-semiconductor lab-on-a-chip biosensors
CMP. *See* Chemical-mechanical polishing
CNTs. *See* Carbon nanotubes
Cochlear implants, 310
Colloids, 32
Competition assays, 170–171
Complementary DNA, 135, 147
Complementary metal-oxide-semiconductor lab-on-a-chip
        biosensors:
    description of, 174, 226
    fabrication of, 241–246
Completely anisotropic etching, 196
COMSOL Multiphysics software, 319–343
Conduction band, 100–101, 103
Confocal laser-induced fluorescence, 95
Contact angle, 16

Contact photolithography, 199
Continuous-flow polymerase chain reaction microreactors:
    batch polymerase chain reaction microreactor versus, 286–287
    layout of, 284
    modeling of, 284–285
    overview of, 283–284
Continuous glucose monitoring. *See* Glucose monitoring
Copper, electrochemical deposition of, 192–193
Core quantum dots, 106
Core-shell quantum dots, 106
Coulomb force, 50
COVID-19 mRNA-based vaccines, 4
CRISPR-associated proteins, 153
CRISPR-Cas9, 153–155
CRISPR gene editing:
    applications of, 155
    challenges for, 155–156
    description of, 147, 153
    ethics of, 156
    limitations of, 155–156
CRISPR locus, 153
Crop agriculture, 312–314
Cry1Ab protein, 173–174
Cryogenic deep reactive ion etching, 216, 218–220
CVD. *See* Chemical vapor deposition
Cylindrical capillary, 23
Cylindrical coordinates, derivatives in, 20–21
Cystic fibrosis, 293

D
DBS. *See* Deep brain stimulation
Debye length, 29–34, 36
Deep brain stimulation, 311
Deep reactive ion etching:
    Bosch process, 216–218
    bulk micromachining using, 234
    for CMOS integrated circuits, 242
    cryogenic, 216, 218–220
    description of, 216
    inductively coupled plasma–reactive ion etching, 216
    passivation gases for, 216–217
Denaturants, 125
Deoxygenated hemoglobin, molar extinction coefficient of, 93
Deoxynucleotide triphosphates, 139
Deoxyribonucleic acid. *See* DNA
DEP. *See* Dielectrophoretic force
Derivatives in cylindrical coordinates, 20–21
Developer (for resists), 197, 200, 221
Di-deoxynucleotide triphosphates, 139
Diabetes mellitus:
    glucose monitoring for. *See* Glucose monitoring
    pathophysiology of, 287
    type 1, 287
    type 2, 287
DidNTPs. *See* Di-deoxynucleotide triphosphates

Dielectric constant, 29
Dielectric sphere, 57
Dielectrophoresis:
    cell capture and separation by, 68–76, 237–240
    force on infinitesimal dipole, 54–55
    induced dipole moment, 55–57
    insulating sphere in uniform electric field, 57–61
    principles of, 53
    schematic diagram of, 68
    sphere with loss in an AC electric field, 61–63
    theory of, 54–63
    torque on infinitesimal dipole, 55
Dielectrophoretic approximation, 55
Dielectrophoretic force:
    dielectrophoresis theory, 54–63
    microtubules, 64–66
    negative, 68
    non-uniform electric field for, 53
    overview of, 53–54
    positive, 68
    source of, 54
    for spherical particles, 73–76
    time-averaged, 63
Dielectrophoretic particle motion simulation, 336–343
Diffusion:
    characteristics of, 67
    description of, 47–49
    separation by, 67–68
Diffusion (doping), 222
Digital microfluidics, 233
Digital polymerase chain reaction, 11. *See also* Polymerase
        chain reaction
Dimethyl sulfoxide, 125
2,4-Dinitrophenol, mitochondria-targeted delivery using
        nanoparticles, 307–309
Dipole:
    definition of, 54
    induced dipole moment, 55–57
    infinitesimal:
        force on, 54–55
        torque on, 55
    net force on, 54
Dipole-dipole force, 15–16
Dipole moment:
    biological applications of, 64
    induced, 55–57
    of microtubules, 65
Direct-write lithography, 195, 199–201
DMSO. *See* Dimethyl sulfoxide
DNA:
    A-T base pair, 125
    backbone of, 122
    coating of, 3
    curved structures, 149
    denaturants, 125

DNA (*Cont.*):
    description of, 5
    dissociation, 124–127
    dissociation fraction of, 125–126
    dissolved ions, 125
    double-stranded, 117–118, 122, 124–127
    energy configuration diagrams of, 127
    experiments of, 119–121
    G-C base pair, 125
    hairpin, 146
    history of, 119–121
    long strands of, 124
    melting temperature for, 124–125
    mismatched bases, 125–126
    molecular structure of, 5, 117–118, 122–123
    nucleotides in, 5, 117, 122
    overview of, 119–123
    photoabsorption of, 94
    RNA and, comparison between, 123
    single-stranded, 124–126, 135
    strand length, 125
    technology involving, 5–6
    very short strands, 124
DNA bricks, 150
DNA gridirons, 150
DNA linkages, 15
DNA microarrays, 165
DNA mutations:
    heteroduplex analysis detection of, 137–138
    single-strand conformation polymorphism detection of, 138
DNA nanocages, 151
DNA nanostructures:
    description of, 148–151
    drug delivery uses of, 306
    gold nanoparticles and, 306
    targeted cancer treatment application of, 306–307
DNA origami, 148–149
DNA polymerase, 139, 147
DNA self-assembly, 148–151
DNA sequencing:
    applications of, 119
    definition of, 138
    description of, 5
    Maxam-Gilbert, 138, 142–145
    nanopore, 146
    next-generation, 145–146
    Sanger, 138–142
    second-generation, 145–146
    third-generation, 145–146
DNA silencing, 153–154
DNA tiles, 148
DNA tweezers, 151–152
DNase, 120
dNTPs. *See* Deoxynucleotide triphosphates
Doping, 222–223

Doping control method, for alkaline wet etching, 207–208
Double bonding, 15–16
Double-layer cellular model, 72–73
Double-stranded DNA:
    description of, 117–118, 122, 124–127
    in polymerase chain reaction, 131
Doxorubicin, 151
Drag force, 50
DRIE. *See* Deep reactive ion etching
Droplet microfluidics, 11
Drug delivery:
    2,4-dinitrophenol, mitochondria-targeted delivery using
        nanoparticles, 307–309
    DNA nanostructures for, 151, 306
    multifluidic systems in, 11
    nanoparticles for, 295–296
    nanoparticles in, 4
    ultrasound-aided phase-shift nanodroplets for, in
        cancer, 304–306
Dry etching:
    chemical, 212–215
    description of, 195–196, 211
    physical, 211–212
    physical-chemical, 212, 214
Dry oxidation, 194
Dynamic surface modification, 224

E
ECD. *See* Electrochemical deposition
EDP. *See* Ethylenediamine pyrocatechol
EIS. *See* Electrochemical impedance spectroscopy
Electric field:
    AC, sphere with loss in an, 61–63
    microtubule susceptibility to, 65
    sinusoidal, 73
Electric potential:
    on a charged surface. *See* Zeta potential
    description of, 31
    from finite electric dipole, 56
    total, 58
Electric potential energy, 103
Electrical screening, 33–34
Electrically screened point charge, 31
Electro-osmosis, 291
Electro-osmotic flow:
    characteristics of, 67
    Debye length, 29–34, 36
    description of, 28–29, 51
    electrical screening in, 33–34
    electrophoretic flow and, 66
    equation, 34–36
    microfluidic system application of, 34–35
    zeta potential, 33, 36–38
Electrochemical deposition, 192–193
Electrochemical impedance spectroscopy, 172
Electrochemical lab-on-a-chip biosensors, 167

Electromagnetic force, 13
Electromagnetic wave frequency of photons, 91
Electrons, 100, 103–104
Electrophoresis:
    capillary, 78–80
    gel, 49, 78–80
    microchip, 79–80
    in nanopore sequencing, 146
Electrophoretic flow:
    description of, 49–53, 66–67
    in gel electrophoresis, 78
Electrophoretic flow mobility, 51
Electroplating, 192
Electrostatic interactions, 32
Ellipsoidal particles, dielectrophoretic force for, 73–76
Emission spectrum, of quantum dots, 107–109
Emulsions, 31–32
ENIAC, 6
EOF. *See* Electro-osmotic flow
EPF. *See* Electrophoretic flow
Epitaxial chemical vapor deposition, 188, 191–192
Equivalent circuits:
    components, 256–259
    equations, 253
    formulas, 253
    micro-electrical-system sensor modeling uses of, 259–262
    microfluidic system modeling uses of, 262–265
    parameters of, 251–256
    thermal microsystem modeling uses of, 265–269
Equivalent impedances, 257
Etch masks, 194, 196–197, 213
Etch rate, 196
Etching:
    completely anisotropic, 196
    deep reactive ion:
        Bosch process, 216–218
        for CMOS integrated circuits, 242
        cryogenic, 216, 218–220
        description of, 216
        inductively coupled plasma–reactive ion etching, 216
        passivation gases for, 216–217
    definition of, 194
    dry:
        chemical, 212–215
        description of, 195–196, 211
        physical, 211–212
        physical-chemical, 212, 214
    isotropic, 196, 201–203
    partially anisotropic, 196
    reactive ion, 214–216
    sputter, 211
    wet:
        alkaline, 203, 206
        anisotropic, 203–211
        BOE, 202–203, 230–231
        description of, 195–196

Etching, wet (*Cont.*):
    HNA, 201–202
    isotropic, 201–203, 213
    of metals, 203
    of silicon nitride, 203
Ethylenediamine pyrocatechol, 207
Evaporative technique, of physical vapor deposition, 188–190
Eversense CGM system, 289–290

F
Fermi level, 105
Feynman, Richard, 1
Fick's second law, 47
"Fight or flight" response, 28
Flow:
    electrophoretic, 49–53
    Hagen-Poiseuille, 27
    pressure-driven, 4, 25–28
Fluid(s):
    in biomedical applications, 11–12
    motion of, 26
    separation by diffusion, 67–68
    viscosity of, 26
Fluid flow, 24
Fluid-handling microelectrodes, 233–234
Fluid transport:
    in biomedical applications, 11–12
    diffusion, 47–49
    electrophoretic flow, 49–53
    methods of, 66–67
    microfluidic system for, 12–13
Fluorescence, 94–100, 288
Fluorescence-based minimally invasive glucose monitoring, 288–290
Fluorescence resonance energy transfer, 288–289
Fluorescence resonance energy transfer quenching, 289
Fluorescent dyes:
    composition of, 100
    description of, 94–95
    optical absorption by, 107
    photostability of, 109
    quantum dots and, comparison between, 108–110
Fluorescent intercalators, 94
Fluorescent tags, 152
Fluorophores:
    definition of, 94
    organ-on-a-chip device, 185
    organic, 107–108
    quantum dots, 100. *See also* Quantum dot(s)
    for Sanger sequencing, 139
Force:
    capillary, 16–19
    centrifugal, 12
    dielectrophoretic. *See* Dielectrophoretic force
    dipole-dipole, 15–16

Force (*Cont.*):
    electromagnetic, 13
    fundamental types of, 13–14
    gravity, 13–14
    on infinitesimal dipole, 54–55
    intermolecular, 15–16
    mechanical, 24–25
    strong nuclear, 13
    van der Waals, 15
    weak nuclear, 13
Formamide, 125
Franklin, Rosalind, 121
FRET. *See* Fluorescence resonance energy transfer

G
G-C base pair, 125
Gauss's law, 58
Gel electrophoresis:
    description of, 49, 78–80
    four-lane, from Maxam-Gilbert DNA sequencing, 145
    in polymerase chain reaction, 127
Gemcitabine, 303
GenBank, 131–135
Gene, 117, 119, 147
Gene delivery, 295–296
Gene editing. *See* CRISPR gene editing
Genetics:
    definition of, 119
    history of, 119–121
GeneXpert, 11
Genomes, 5
Genomics, 117, 119
Glass:
    BOE wet etching of, 202–203, 230–231
    isotropic wet etching of, 230–233
Glucose, 287
Glucose-labeled gold nanoparticles, 296
Glucose meters, 7
Glucose monitoring:
    fluorescence-based minimally invasive, 288–290
    overview of, 287–288
    reverse iontophoresis-based non-invasive, 290–292
Glucose test strip, 168–169
Gluons, 13
Glycine, 77
Gold nanoparticles:
    cancer therapy uses of, 298–302
    description of, 295
    DNA nanostructures and, 306
    gold-POY2T nanoparticles, 306–307
Graphene, 2–3
Gravimetric lab-on-a-chip biosensors, 167
Gravity, 13–14
Griffith, Frederick, 119
Guide RNA, 154–155

H

H-filter, 67
HA. *See* Heteroduplex analysis
Hagen-Poiseuille flow, 27
Hairpin DNA molecule, 146
Hb. *See* Hemoglobin
Heart-on-a-chip device, 183
Heat equation, 22
HEK 293 cells, 69
HeLa cells, 151
Hemoglobin:
    definition of, 93
    molar extinction coefficient of, 93
α-Hemolysin nanopores, 146
Heteroduplex analysis, 127, 137–138
HIV. *See* Human immunodeficiency virus
HNA wet etching, 201–202
Holes (charge carriers), 100, 103–104
Holliday junctions, 148, 150
Home pregnancy test strip, 171
Human chorionic gonadotropin, 171
Human Genome Project, 138
Human immunodeficiency virus, 173
Hydrofluoric acid, 201
Hydrogen bonding, 15
Hydrophobic quantum dots, 106

I

ICP-RIE. *See* Inductively coupled plasma–reactive ion
        etching
ICs. *See* Integrated circuits
IDEs. *See* Interdigital electrodes
Impedimetric lab-on-a-chip biosensors, 171–174
In vitro RNA synthesis, 148
Induced dipole moment, 55–57
Inductively coupled plasma–reactive ion etching, 216
Infinitesimal dipole:
    force on, 54–55
    torque on, 55
Instantaneous conservation of charge, 61–62
Insulating sphere in uniform electric field, 57–61
Integrated circuits, 6
Integrated microchips:
    description of, 185
    fabrication of, 185
    of lab-on-a-chip biosensors, 175
    material biocompatibility for, 186
    micro/nano fabrication process for. *See* Micro/nano
        fabrication
    silicon for, 186
    substrate selection for, 185–187
    surface modification of, 187
Intelligent pesticides, 313
Interband transitions, 103, 105
Interdigital electrodes:
    description of, 171–172

Interdigital electrodes (*Cont.*):
    3D simulation of, 330–335
    2D simulation of, 319–330
Interdigitated electrode biosensor microchips:
    fabrication of, 226–229
    microelectrodes, 227–228
    sample loading wells for, 226–227
    surface modification, 228
Intermittent fluorescence, 110
Intermolecular forces, 15–16
Ion implantation, 222–223
Ion milling, 211
Isoelectric focusing, 77–78, 80
Isoelectric point, 76–78
Isopropyl alcohol, 200
Isotropic wet etching, 196, 201–203, 213

J

Joule heating in cylindrical capillary, 23

K

Kinetic energy, 101
Kirchhoff's current law, 257
Kirchhoff's voltage law, 257
"Knocking in," 153
"Knocking out," 153

L

Lab-on-a-chip biosensors:
    breakthroughs in, 174–176
    challenges for, 174–176
    complementary metal-oxide-semiconductor, 174
    components of, 165–166
    description of, 6–7
    design of, 165–168
    detection area of, 165–167
    detection methods for, 166–167
    electrochemical, 167
    electrochemical impedance spectroscopy, 172
    glucose test strip as, 168–169
    gravimetric, 167
    home pregnancy test strip as, 171
    impedimetric, 171–174
    integrated microchips of, 175
    interdigital electrodes in, 171–172
    lateral flow, 168–171, 174
    non-faradaic impedimetric, 171–174, 226
    optical detection, 167, 186
    optical lateral flow, 169–171
    purpose of, 165
    recognition molecules used by, 166
    sample preparation area of, 165
    signal processing platform of, 165–167
    signal-to-noise ratio of, 175
Lab-on-a-chip devices:
    advantages of, 164
    applications of, 163

Lab-on-a-chip devices (*Cont.*):
  biosensors. *See* Lab-on-a-chip biosensors
  description of, 4, 6–7
  examples of, 7
  fluid transport in, 12
  global market for, 165
  market for, 165
  microchips, 6, 163
  organ-on-a-chip, 4, 7
  overview of, 163–165
  reagent amounts for, 164
  types of, 164–165
Laminar flow, 13, 24
Laplace domain, 256
Laplacian operator, 21
Laser direct-write lithography, 200
Laser-induced fluorescence, 95
Lateral flow lab-on-a-chip biosensors, 168–171, 174
Leeuwenhoek, Antony van, 1
Legendre polynomials, 56–57, 70
Lennard-Jones potential diagram, 15
LIF. *See* Laser-induced fluorescence
Lift-off patterning, 194–195, 220–221
Lift-off resists, 220–221
LIGA, 235–237
Light:
  composition of, 91
  fundamentals of, 91
  photothermal therapy using, 298–302
  quantum dot absorption of, 104
  wavelength of, 92
Lithography:
  definition of, 194, 197
  direct-write, 195, 199–201
  photolithography, 195, 197–200
  soft, 231–233
Lithography, electroplating, and molding. *See* LIGA
LOC devices. *See* Lab-on-a-chip devices
Long DNA strands, 124
LOR. *See* Lift-off resists
Low-pressure chemical vapor deposition, 188, 191
LPCVD. *See* Low-pressure chemical vapor deposition
Lung-heart-bone-kidney-liver-gut organ-on-a-chip system, 182–183
Lung-on-a-chip device, 178–179
Lysine, 77

M
Machine learning algorithms, 174
Macrofluidic systems, 13
Magnetophoresis, 53
Magnetron sputtering, 190
Maxam-Gilbert DNA sequencing, 138, 142–145
Maxwell-Boltzmann distribution, 30
Mechanical forces, 24–25
Medical-device-on-a-chip, 165

Melting temperature, for DNA, 124–125
MEMS. *See* Micro-electro-mechanical systems
Mendel, Gregor, 119
Metabolomics, 119
Metal-oxide semiconductor field-effect transistor, 241
Metals, isotropic wet etching of, 203
Metastasis, 297
Methicillin-resistant *Staphylococcus aureus,* 155
Micro-electro-mechanical systems:
  bulk micromachining of, 234
  description of, 163, 178, 185
  fabrication of, 233–237
  sensor, equivalent circuits for modeling of, 259–262
  surface micromachining of, 234–235
  3D micromachining of, 234
  UV LIGA of, 235–237
Micro/nano fabrication:
  complementary metal-oxide-semiconductor lab-on-a-chip devices, 241–246
  interdigitated electrode biosensor microchips, 226–229
  microfluidic platforms, 229–240
  pattern transfer techniques for:
    aspect ratio of, 196
    description of, 187
    etching. *See* Etching
    lift-off patterning, 194–195, 220–221
    lithography. *See* Lithography
    purpose of, 194
    types of, 187
  process of, 186–187
  schematic diagram of, 187
  substrates for, 185–187
  surface modification, 224
  surface planarization, 223
  surface treatments:
    doping, 222–223
    ion implantation, 222–223
    piranha, 223–224
  thin film deposition/growth techniques for:
    chemical vapor deposition, 188, 190–192
    electrochemical deposition, 192–193
    overview of, 186–187
    physical vapor deposition, 188–190
    process substrate temperature, 188–189
    summary of, 188
    thermal oxidation, 188, 193–194
    thin film quality, 187–189
Micro total analysis system, 168
Microarrays, 4
Microchambers:
  isotropic wet etching fabrication of, 230–231
  soft lithography fabrication of, 231–233
Microchannels:
  isotropic wet etching fabrication of, 230–231
  soft lithography fabrication of, 231–233
  zeta potential of, 37

Microchips:
  design of, 5
  electrophoresis, 79–80
  integrated. *See* Integrated microchips
  interdigitated electrode biosensor, 226–229
  lab-on-a-chip, 6, 164
  organ-on-a-chip, 177
Microelectrodes:
  fabrication of, 227–228
  fluid-handling, 233–234
Microfluidic(s):
  capillary, 11
  centrifugal, 11
  definition of, 11
  description of, 4–5
  droplet, 11
  methods used in, 11
  pressure-driven, 11
Microfluidic microchips:
  description of, 165
  disposable, 12
Microfluidic platform:
  composition of, 11–12, 229
  fluid transport models used by, 166
  lab-on-a-chip biosensor, 166
  micro-electro-mechanical systems, 233–237
  micro/nano fabrication of, 229–240
  microchambers on, 230–233
  microchannels on, 230–233
  purpose of, 166
  for selective single-cell capture, 237–240
Microfluidic systems:
  applications of, 11
  components of, 263–264
  creation of, 12–13
  electro-osmotic flow in, 34–35
  equivalent circuits for modeling of, 262–265
  fluid movement in, 28
  function of, 12
  gravity in, 14
Microreactors:
  definition of, 269
  polymerase chain reaction. *See* Polymerase chain reaction
    microreactors
Microscopes, 1
Microtubules:
  in axons, 66
  definition of, 64
  dipole moment of, 65
  electric field susceptibility of, 65
  electrical properties of, 64–66
  polarity of, 64
  polymer structure of, 64
  tubulin protein of, 64
Miller indices, 204
Mind-controlled prosthesis, 311–312

Mismatched bases, 125–126
Mitochondria-targeted delivery of 2,4-dinitrophenol by
    nanoparticles, 307–309
Mitosis, 64
Mixing, 48
Mobility, electrophoretic flow, 51
Molar extinction coefficient value, 93
Moore's law, 6
MOSFET. *See* Metal-oxide semiconductor field-effect transistor
mRNA-based COVID-19 vaccines, 4
MRSA. *See* Methicillin-resistant *Staphylococcus aureus*
Multi-ink 3D printing, 183
Multi-layer cellular models, 69–73
Multi-organ organ-on-a-chip device, 182–183
Multi-walled carbon nanotubes, 3, 304
MWCNTs. *See* Multi-walled carbon nanotubes

N
Nanobiosensors, 313
Nanobiotechnology, 1. *See also* Bionanotechnology
Nanodroplets, ultrasound-aided phase-shift, 304–306
Nanofertilizers, 313
Nanomaterials:
  bioremediation using, 313–314
  description of, 2–4
Nanoparticles:
  biomedical applications of, 3, 295–296
  description of, 3–4, 297
  gold. *See* Gold nanoparticles
  mitochondria-targeted delivery of 2,4-dinitrophenol by, 307–309
  thermal cancer therapy uses of, 297–302
  types of, 297
Nanopesticides, 313
Nanopore DNA sequencing, 146
Nanopores, 146
Nanostructured alumina, 313
Nanostructures, DNA, 148–151
Nanotechnology:
  applications of, 1
  overview of, 1–2
Nanowires, semiconductor, 3–4
Native fluorescence, 95
Navier-Stokes equation, 26, 34
Nernst-Planck equation, 34
Neural implants, 309–312
Neuralink, 311
Neuron, 66
Neutrons, 13
Newtonian fluid, 25
Newton's law of viscosity, 25
Next-generation DNA sequencing, 145–146
Nickel, electrochemical deposition of, 193, 236
Nitric acid, 201–202
Non-faradaic impedimetric lab-on-a-chip biosensors,
    171–174, 226
Non-pyrogenic wet oxidation, 194

Non-uniform electric field:
   for dielectrophoretic force, 53
   dipole in presence of, 55
Nucleic acids, 94
Nucleotides, 5

O
Oligo(dT) primers, 135–136
OOC devices. *See* Organ-on-a-chip devices
Optical depth, 92
Optical detection:
   of bacteria, 97–100
   Beer-Lambert law for, 92
   confocal laser-induced fluorescence for, 95
   fluorophores used in, 94
   lab-on-a-chip biosensors, 167, 186
   organ-on-a-chip devices, 185
   photoabsorption for, 94
   purposes of, 92
Optical lateral flow lab-on-a-chip biosensors, 169–171
Optics, 91–94
Organ-on-a-chip devices:
   advantages of, 177
   applications of, 176–177, 180–182
   bioelectrical signal detection, 180, 185
   body-on-a-chip systems, 182–183
   brain-on-a-chip device, 179–180
   breakthroughs in, 182–185
   challenges for, 182–185
   description of, 4, 7, 164, 176–178
   design of, 176
   heart-on-a-chip, 183
   illustration of, 7
   lung-heart-bone-kidney-liver-gut, 182–183
   lung-on-a-chip device, 178–179
   macroscale cell cultures versus, 177
   market for, 165
   microchannels in, 177
   microchip of, 177
   multi-organ, 182–183
   optical detection, 177, 180, 185
   principles of, 178–180
   purpose of, 184
   real-time monitoring of tissues on, 180
   self-assembly of tissue structures, 184
   skin-intestine-liver-kidney, 182
   3D, 178, 182, 184
   tissue monitoring in, 185
   tumor-on-a-chip, 180–182
   validation protocols for, 184
Organic fluorophores, 107–108
Oxygenated hemoglobin, molar extinction coefficient of, 93

P
PAM. *See* Protospacer adjacent motif
Partially anisotropic etching, 196

Passivation gases, deep reactive ion etching with, 216–217
Pattern control method, for alkaline wet etching, 207
Pattern transfer techniques:
   aspect ratio of, 196
   description of, 187
   etching. *See* Etching
   lift-off patterning, 194–195, 220–221
   lithography. *See* Lithography
   purpose of, 194
   types of, 187
PCR. *See* Polymerase chain reaction
PDMS, 226
PDT. *See* Photodynamic therapy
PECVD. *See* Plasma-enhanced chemical vapor deposition
PEGylated single-walled carbon nanotubes, 302–304
Perfluorocarbon nanodroplets, 304
Pesticides, 313
Phages. *See* Bacteriophages
Phonons, 104–105, 298
Photoabsorption:
   description of, 94
   quantum dot, 107–108
Photodynamic therapy, 300–301
Photolithography, 195, 197–200
Photomask, 197, 199
Photons:
   definition of, 91
   electromagnetic wave frequency of, 91
   emission of, from fluorophores, 95
   fluorescent dyes for, 94
Photoresist, 197–199, 212
Photothermal therapy, for cancer, 298–302
Physical-chemical dry etching, 212, 214
Physical dry etching, 211–212
Physical vapor deposition, 188–190
pI. *See* Isoelectric point
Piranha surface treatment, 223–224
Planarization, of surface, 223
Plasma-enhanced chemical vapor deposition, 188, 191
Plasmid vector-based RNA synthesis, 147–148, 154
Plasmonic photothermal therapy, 298–302
Point charge, 29, 32
Poisson-Boltzmann method, 33
Poisson-Nernst-Planck method, 33
Poisson's equation, 32
Poly(A) tails, 135
Polycrystalline silicon, 186, 192
Polyethylene glycol. *See* PEGylated single-walled carbon nanotubes
Polymerase chain reaction:
   annealing step of, 128–130
   BLAST, 131–135
   cycle, 127–130
   definition of, 127, 269
   denaturing step of, 128–130
   description of, 11

Polymerase chain reaction (*Cont.*):
  double-stranded DNA in, 131
  extension/elongation step of, 128–130
  GenBank, 131–135
  modeling, 130–131
  primer selection for, 131–135
  procedure for, 128–130
  product, 127
  quantitative real-time, 127, 129
  reagents for, 128
  reverse transcription, 135–137
  steps involved in, 128–130
  time requirements for, 130
  virus, 133–134
Polymerase chain reaction microreactors:
  batch:
    continuous-flow polymerase chain reaction microreactor versus, 286–287
    overview of, 270–272
    thermal equivalent circuit of, 278–283
    thermal model of, 272–278
  continuous-flow:
    batch polymerase chain reaction microreactor versus, 286–287
    layout of, 284
    modeling of, 284–285
    overview of, 283–284
  overview of, 269–270
Polymers, Bosch process for etching of, 218
Potential energy, 103
POY2T oligonucleotides, 306
PPTT. *See* Plasmonic photothermal therapy
Pre-doped n-type silicon wafers, 222
Pre-doped p-type silicon wafers, 222
Pressure differential:
  description of, 14
  for pressure-driven flow, 28
Pressure-driven flow:
  characteristics of, 67
  description of, 4, 25–28
  electrophoretic flow versus, 49
  pressure differential for, 28
Pressure-driven microfluidics, 11
Primers:
  oligo(dT), 135–136
  polymerase chain reaction, 131–135
  reverse transcription–polymerase chain reaction, 135–136
  sequence-specific, 135
Projection photolithography, 199
Protein microarrays, 165
Proteomics, 119
Protons, 13
Protospacer adjacent motif, 154
Proximity photolithography, 199

Q
PTT. *See* Photothermal therapy
Pulse oximeter, 92–93
PVD. *See* Physical vapor deposition
Pyrogenic wet oxidation, 194

QDs. *See* Quantum dot(s)
QE. *See* Quantum efficiency
qPCR. *See* Quantitative real-time polymerase chain reaction
Quantitative real-time polymerase chain reaction:
  description of, 127, 129
  reverse-transcription, 136–137
Quantum confinement, 100–102
Quantum dot(s):
  advantages of, 109–110
  applications of, 109–110, 110–112
  band structure of, 100–102
  bandgap of, 101–103
  bioconjugates, 106, 110
  challenges associated with, 109–110
  composition of, 100
  conduction band for, 100–101, 103
  core, 106
  core-shell, 106
  description of, 4
  electrons of, 100–101, 103–104
  emission spectrum of, 107–109
  emission wavelength of, 100
  energy-level diagram of, 102
  holes of, 100–101, 103–104
  hydrophobic, 106
  intermittent fluorescence by, 110
  light absorption by, 104
  non-biodegradability of, 110
  optical absorption of, 107–108
  organic fluorescent dye and, comparison between, 108–110
  photoabsorption of, 107–108
  photostability of, 109
  polymer-coated, 110
  properties of, 107–109
  size distribution of, 108
  structure of, 106–107
  theory of, 100–105
  toxicity of, 110
  valence band for, 100–101, 103
  water-soluble, 106, 110
Quantum dot fluorescence:
  lifetime of, 109
  theory of, 100–105
Quantum efficiency, 94
Quantum yield, 94
Quarks, 13
Quartz, isotropic wet etching of, 230–233
QY. *See* Quantum yield

R

R-strain, 119–120
Radiation therapy, 297
Random primers, 136
Rastering, 200
Reactive ion etching:
    for CMOS integrated circuits, 242
    deep. *See* Deep reactive ion etching
    description of, 214–216
Rectangular capillary, 18
Resist removal, 200–201
Reverse iontophoresis, 290
Reverse iontophoresis-based non-invasive glucose monitoring,
        290–292
Reverse transcriptase enzymes, 135, 147
Reverse transcription, 135
Reverse transcription–polymerase chain reaction:
    description of, 135–137
    in RNA sequencing, 146–147
Reverse-transcription quantitative real-time polymerase chain
        reaction, 136–137
Reynolds number, 24–25
Ribonucleic acid. *See* RNA
RNA:
    DNA and, comparison between, 123
    in vitro synthesis, 155
    molecular structure of, 123
    nucleotides in, 117, 122
    photoabsorption of, 94
    plasmid vector-based synthesis, 147–148, 154
    technology involving, 5–6
RNA sequencing:
    applications of, 146
    description of, 6, 146–147
    nanopore, 146
    reverse transcription–polymerase chain reaction for, 135,
        146–147
RNase, 120
RT-PCR. *See* Reverse transcription–polymerase chain reaction

S

S-strain, 119–120
Salmonella Typhimurium, 117–118, 129
Sandwich assays, 170–171, 173
Sanger DNA sequencing, 138–142
Second-generation DNA sequencing, 145–146
Selective single-cell capture, microfluidic-platform-based
        microchip for, 237–240
Self-monitoring of blood glucose, 287
Semiconductor:
    doping of, 222
    nanowires, 3–4
    p-type, 222
Separation by diffusion, 67–68
Sequence-specific primers, 135

Silicon:
    BOE wet etching of, 202–203, 230–231
    Bosch process for etching of, 217–218
    chemical dry etching of, 212–213
    description of, 186
    dopants for, 222
    HNA wet etching of, 201–202
Silicon dioxide, 192
Silicon nitride, 192, 203
Silicon wafers, 194, 222
Single-cell capture, microfluidic platform for, 237–240
Single-crystal silicon, 186, 192, 205
Single-strand conformation polymorphism, 138
Single-stranded DNA:
    cleavage of, 142–143
    description of, 124–127, 135
Single-walled carbon nanotubes, 3, 289, 302–304
Sinusoidal electric field, 73
Skin-intestine-liver-kidney organ-on-a-chip systems, 182
SMBG. *See* Self-monitoring of blood glucose
Snyder, Michael, 119
Soft lithography, 231–233
Spectrophotometers, 93–94
Sphere:
    axes of, 74
    with loss in an AC electric field, 61–63
Spherical coordinates, 20
Spherical particle:
    dielectrophoretic force for, 73–76
    double-layer model of, 72–73
    multi-layer cellular models, 69–73
SPR. *See* Surface plasmon resonance
Sputter etching, 211
Sputtering technique, of physical vapor deposition, 188, 190
SSCP. *See* Single-strand conformation polymorphism
Staphylococcus aureus, 153, 155
Static surface modification, 224
Stationary point charge, 29
Steady-state temperature distribution, 22
Stokes' drag force, 50
Stokes radius, 51
Stokes shift, 107
Streptococcus pneumoniae, 119
Streptococcus pyogenes, 153, 155
Strong nuclear force, 13
Surface micromachining, of micro-electro-mechanical systems,
        234–235
Surface modification, 224
Surface planarization, 223
Surface plasmon resonance, 298
Surface tension, 16–18
Surface treatments:
    doping, 222–223
    ion implantation, 222–223
    piranha, 223–224

SWCNTs. *See* Single-walled carbon nanotubes

T
TALENs. *See* Transcription activator-like effector nucleases
Targeted cancer therapies:
   carbon nanotubes, 302–304
   description of, 295–296, 296–297
   DNA nanotechnology applications in, 306–307
   gold nanoparticles, 298–302
   nanoparticle-mediated thermal therapy, 297–302
   nanoparticle therapies, 295–296, 298–302
   photothermal therapy, 298–302
   plasmonic photothermal therapy, 298–302
Taylor series expansion, 56, 93
Tetramethylammonium hydroxide, 206
Thermal microsystems:
   definition of, 265
   equivalent circuit modeling of, 265–269
   thermal resistances in, 265
Thermal oxidation, 188, 193–194
Thermal oxide, 194
Thermodynamics:
   configuration of, 19
   derivatives in cylindrical coordinates, 20–21
   heat equation, 22
   joule heating in cylindrical capillary, 23
   Newton's law of viscosity, 25
   overview of, 19–20
Thermoplastic polyurethane, 182
Thin film deposition/growth:
   chemical vapor deposition, 188, 190–192
   electrochemical deposition, 192–193
   overview of, 186–187
   physical vapor deposition, 188–190
   process substrate temperature, 188–189
   summary of, 188
   thermal oxidation, 188, 193–194
   thin film quality, 187–189
Third-generation DNA sequencing, 145–146
3D diffusion, 47
3D DNA origami, 149
3D micromachining, of micro-electro-mechanical
     systems, 234
3D organ-on-a-chip devices, 178, 182, 184
Time-averaged dielectrophoretic force, 63
Time control method, for alkaline wet etching, 207
TMAH. *See* Tetramethylammonium hydroxide
Torque on infinitesimal dipole, 55
Total electric potential, 58
Trans-activating CRISPR RNA, 153
Transcription activator-like effector nucleases, 153
Transitional flow, 24
Triple bonding, 15–16
Triple-layer cellular model, 73

Tuberculosis, 294
Tubulin protein, 64
Tumor-on-a-chip, 180–182
Turbulent flow:
   description of, 13, 24
   diffusion, 48
2D diffusion, 47
2D DNA origami, 149
2D gel electrophoresis, 80

U
Undercutting, 201, 230
Uniform electric field, insulating sphere in, 57–61
UV LIGA, 235–237
UV light source, for photolithography, 197

V
Vagus nerve stimulation, 311
Valence band, 100–101, 103
van der Waals force, 15
VB. *See* Valence band
Very short DNA strands, 124
Viscosity, Newton's law of, 25
VNS. *See* Vagus nerve stimulation

W
Water-soluble quantum dots, 106, 110
Weak nuclear force, 13
Wet etching:
   alkaline, 203, 206
   anisotropic, 203–211
   BOE, 202–203, 230–231
   description of, 195–196
   of glass, 230–233
   HNA, 201–202
   isotropic, 201–203, 213, 230–233
   of metals, 203
   of quartz, 230–233
   of silicon nitride, 203

X
X-ray LIGA, 235–236
Xenon difluoride, 212, 214

Y
Yeast cells, 69
Young's equation, 16–17
Young's modulus, 2

Z
Zeta potential, 33, 36–38
ZFNs. *See* Zinc-finger nucleases
Zinc-finger nucleases, 153
Zwitterion, 76